Fundamental Skills and Concepts in Patient Care

Fundamental Skills and Concepts in Patient Care

Sixth Edition

Barbara Kuhn Timby, RN,C, BSN, MA

Nursing Professor
Glen Oaks Community College
Centreville, Michigan

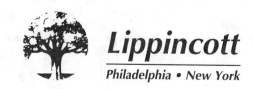

Lippincott
Philadelphia • New York

Sponsoring Editor: Mary P. Gyetvan, RN, MSN
Coordinating Editorial Assistant: Susan M. Keneally
Project Editor: Sandra Cherrey Scheinin
Indexer: Ellen Murray
Design Coordinator: Doug Smock
Interior Designer: Susan Hess Blaker
Cover Designer: Ilene Griff
Production Manager: Helen Ewan
Production Coordinator: Patricia McCloskey
Compositor: Circle Graphics
Printer/Binder: Courier Book Company/Kendallville
Cover Printer: Lehigh Press Lithographers

Edition 6th

Library of Congress Cataloging in Publications Data

Timby, Barbara Kuhn.
    Fundamental skills and concepts in patient care/Barbara Kuhn
Timby.—6th ed.
        p.   cm.
    ISBN 0-397-55168-1
    1. Nursing.   I. Title.
    [DNLM: 1. Nursing Care. WY 100 T583f 1996]
RT41.L67 1996
610.73—dc20
DNLM/DLC
for Library of Congress   95-25023
                                                                      CIP

The material contained in this volume was submitted as previously unpublished material, except in
the instances in which credit has been given to the source from which some of the illustrative material
was derived.

Any procedure or practice described in this book should be applied by the health-care practitioner
under appropriate supervision in accordance with professional standards of care used with regard to
the unique circumstances that apply in each practice situation. Care has been taken to confirm the accuracy of information presented and to describe generally accepted practices. However, the authors,
editors, and publisher cannot accept any responsibility for errors or omissions or for any consequences from application of the information in this book and make no warranty, express or implied,
with respect to the contents of the book.

The authors and publisher have exerted every effort to ensure that drug selection and dosage set
forth in this text are in accordance with current recommendations and practice at the time of publication. However, in view of ongoing research, changes in government regulations, and the constant
flow of information relating to drug therapy and drug reactions, the reader is urged to check the
package insert for each drug for any change in indications and dosage and for added warnings and
precautions. This is particularly important when the recommended agent is a new or infrequently
employed drug.

Materials appearing in this book prepared by individuals as part of their official duties as U.S. Government employees are not covered by the above-mentioned copyright.

9 8 7 6 5 4 3 2 1

Dedication
To LuVerne Wolff Lewis, who passed away in 1993 after contributing much to the education of countless nursing students.

CONTRIBUTORS

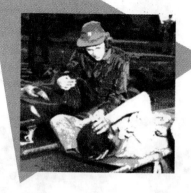

Roberta J. Renicker, RN, AAS
Instructor
Sanford-Brown College
Kansas City, Missouri

Marge Roark-Lofgreen, RN, BSN, Med
Clinical Instructor in Nursing
Spoon River College
Canton, Illinois

Adjunct Faculty
Western Illinois University
Macomb, Illinois

Dawn M. Specht, RN, MSN, CEN, CCRN
Clinical Nurse III
Thomas Jefferson University Hospital
Emergency Room
Philadelphia, Pennsylvania

Nursing Instructor
Episcopal Hospital School of Nursing
Philadelphia, Pennsylvania

REVIEWERS

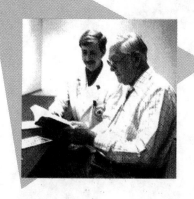

Penny Hood, RN, BSN
Instructor—Preclinical
Decatur School of Practical Nursing
Decatur, Illinois

Mary L. Micklus, RN, BSN
Nursing Instructor
Capital Area School of Practical Nursing
Springfield, Illinois

Roberta J. Renicker, RN, AAS
Instructor
Sanford-Brown College
Kansas City, Missouri

Judith D. Sawyer, RN, MS
Former Director
Isabella Graham Hart School of Practical Nursing
Rochester General Hospital
Rochester, New York

PREFACE

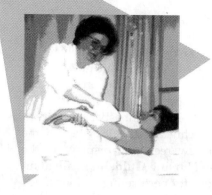

Fundamental Skills and Concepts in Patient Care is designed to assist beginning nursing students acquire a solid foundation of basic information. It is only when the student has demonstrated an understanding of the fundamentals of nursing practice, mastering both concepts and skills, that further depth and breath of knowledge can be added.

This holds true regardless of which entry level nursing program the student nurse selects—practical/vocational, associate degree, diploma, or baccalaureate—there is a core of content that is essential for the practice of nursing. This textbook has other potential applications. It can serve as a ready reference for updating the skills of practicing nurses, as well as reintroducing returning nurses to clinical practice after a period of inactivity.

There are several underlying philosophic concepts permeating the text that the reader should be aware of:

- The content supports the belief in holistic nursing to facilitate health and healing. This is founded on the belief that the human experience is a composite of physiologic, emotional, social, and spiritual aspects.
- Caring is the essence of nursing, and is extended to each and every patient. At the same time, the nurse recognizes the uniqueness of the individual and adapts care to best meet the individual needs of the patient. Although skills presented in the text are straightforward, the student needs to learn to adapt techniques when necessary, without compromising safety or effectiveness.
- A supportive environment promotes health and healing. Recognizing this, the text encourages nurses to include the patient's support network (family and friends), in teaching sessions, informal discussions, and provision of services.

- Ethical dilemmas and legal issues continue to increase, and they affect the practice of nursing. Nurses have an obligation to practice their profession safely and to protect their patients from harm. Therefore, this text attempts to reinforce the concept that nurses, including student nurses, are accountable for their actions and clinical decisions. An effort has been made to include recent legislation and recommendations affecting safe care.

The information contained in the sixth edition of **Fundamental Skills and Concepts in Patient Care** has been carefully planned. Overall, two broad goals directed the process. The first was to add new skills and concepts in order to provide an updated and comprehensive knowledge base for the beginning nursing student. The second was to increase the visual appeal and presentation so that students would learn more easily and effectively.

Several features of this text are designed to assist the reader in using the sixth edition with greater ease and with improved learning outcomes:

- To assist in locating information, there is a list of chapters in the Contents. A more detailed description is given in the expanded contents. A topical **Chapter Outline** is provided at the beginning of each chapter.
- Each chapter now also begins with a list of **Key Terms** important for the beginning student to learn. Each key term appears in bold face lettering and is defined when it is first used within the chapter. **Learning Objectives,** phrased in behavioral terms, alert the student to the expected outcomes, which can be achieved by mastering the chapter content.

- Each chapter concludes by adding two new features. **Key Concepts** summarizes information and helps reinforce learning of the most important content. It is designed to correlate with the Learning Objectives in the chapter opener. To prepare the students for analyzing and applying information rather then memorizing it, there are at least two **Critical Thinking Exercises** in each chapter. These exercises may be used in a variety of creative ways. They may become a focal point for group discussions, used as essay questions, or as an independent assignment.
- Each chapter includes **Suggested Readings**. These can be used to help supplement the text's information on a particular topic.
- A **Glossary** of terms now appears at the end of the text. It is limited to those key terms that appear in more than one chapter. The glossary provides a ready reference of technical terms.
- There are two **Appendices** which also serve as important reference tools. The first includes a list and explanation of commonly used symbols and abbreviations. The other contains the most current list of nursing diagnoses accepted by the North America Nursing Diagnosis Association.

The sixth edition of **Fundamental Skills and Concepts in Patient Care** has been substantially revised in other ways in an effort to provide the beginning student with a contemporary framework for developing strong initial skills and clinical thinking processes.

The Table of Contents has grown from 5 Units in the fifth edition to 12 Units in the sixth edition. This change now permits organization of clusters of chapters that relate to a common theme. Similarly, the previous 28 chapters now number 38. This resulted from dividing formerly long chapters into several shorter chapters to promote more focused learning. Additionally, most chapter titles have been changed to reflect more specifically the content they contain.

Two new chapters, one on *Homeostasis, Stress and Adaptation*, and another on *Culture and Ethnicity* have been added to define nursing's continuing concern with the individual's unique internal and external environment. Other new chapters were developed from content contained in previously longer chapters. This is an intentional effort to call attention to the importance of such topics as *Health and Illness, The Nurse-Patient Relationship*, and *Patient Teaching*.

A stronger focus on the nursing process is built into this edition. The chapter that introduces the concepts and paradigm for the nursing process now appears as the second chapter of the text. The premise is that early familiarity with its components will reinforce its use in the **Skills** and sample **Nursing Care Plans** that appear throughout the text. Each skill chapter also continues to display **Applicable Nursing Diagnoses** that correlate the types of problems recipients of the respective skills may have.

The **Skills**, formerly called Skill Procedures, continue to be a strength in the sixth edition. Screened in a second color, the Skills can now be immediately recognized and quickly accessed. The Skills are now formatted according to the steps of the nursing process; sample documentation is also provided.

Recognizing that other important aspects of patient care extend beyond technical skills has led to the development of two new recurring displays in the sixth edition. The first, **Nursing Guidelines**, are mini-procedures or directions for performing various kinds of nursing care, or suggestions for managing patient care problems. The second, **Patient Teaching**, recognizes that students need to prepare patients for self-care and health maintenance, especially since patients are being discharged from health care systems earlier and earlier.

Each skill and nursing guideline, along with accompanying illustrations, has been closely reviewed to make sure that it complies with *Standard Precautions*, new infection control guidelines proposed by the Centers for Disease Control and Prevention.

The sixth edition places a major emphasis on the geriatric population who comprise the fastest growing age group in America. Since they are most representative of the patients nursing students care for, a new recurrent display, **Focus on Older Adults**, has been included in this edition. This section addresses the unique characteristics and problems of aging adults as they pertain to the chapter contents.

Recognizing the growing importance of communication in all aspects of our lives, including the communication of safe, effective health care, a comprehensive chapter on Recording and Reporting is included. Additionally, the important information to document when performing each skill and a sample of that documentation is included throughout the text.

Numerous tables, displays and updated photographs are included in the sixth edition to provide supplemental information that adds breadth and depth to the text's discussion and to focus on the current health care scene.

The sixth edition of **Fundamental Skills and Concepts of Patient Care** is accompanied by a complete teaching/learning package. To augment teaching, The Instructor's Manual is three-hole punched and the pages are perforated to allow the development of individual lesson plans. A chapter conversion guide is included to assist the instructor who may be familiar with the fifth edition to relocate the rearranged material. To maximize learning, a Study Guide includes chapter summaries, behavioral objectives, and a variety of learning exercises. Performance checklists are included that correlate with the Skills in the text and assist with faculty evaluation or student/peer evaluation in the clinical laboratory. The Study Guide is also three-hole punched and perforated to allow the creation of individual learning packages and to permit easy reproduction of the Performance Checklists. Finally, a test bank is included that contains over 850 multiple-choice questions to assist faculty in developing and customizing their tests.

It is our sincere hope that this text and its ancillary package will facilitate learning and produce safe, effective practitioners, capable of providing quality care for a variety of patients in a variety of settings.

Barbara Kuhn Timby, RN,C, BSN, MA

ACKNOWLEDGMENTS

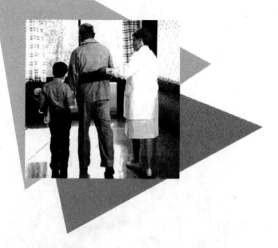

Thanks go to the following people and the agencies for which they work for their help in preparing this list:

- Donna Hilton, Vice President, Lippincott-Raven Publishers, for fresh ideas on reorganizing the content and creating pedagogical techniques in the sixth edition.

- Mary Gyetvan, Nursing Editor, Lippincott-Raven Publishers, for support and assistance during manuscript preparation.

- Susan Keneally, Editorial Assistant, for handling the details of manuscript compilation, tracking permissions, art, and photographs,

- Sandra Cherry Scheinin, Project Editor, for editing manuscript and preparing it for publication.

- Betsy Morgan, Director of the Learning Resources Center, Glen Oaks Community College, Centreville, Michigan, and her assistant, Judy Baumeister Fetch, for their assistance in literary searches of pertinent reference materials.

- Contributors Marjorie Roark-Lofgreen, Roberta Renicker, and Dawn Specht, who helped meet the deadlines and preserve my mental health by reorganizing and revising several chapters.

- Administrators and personnel from The Community Health Center of Branch County, Coldwater, Michigan; Three Rivers Area Hospital, Three Rivers, Michigan; and Riverview Manor, Three Rivers, Michigan; for extending the use of their facilities for the purposes of updating photographs within the new edition.

- Student nurses and their assigned patients, who agreed to be photographed during the course of nursing care.

- Ken Timby, whose skills as a photographer have proved to be an invaluable asset to the revision of this and previous editions.

- Jody, Brian, Erin, and Sheila Timby, who have managed to survive and flourish despite the lack of attention during the time of manuscript preparation.

CONTENTS

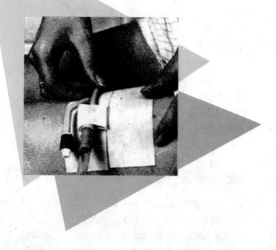

Fundamental Nursing Concepts

UNIT I

Exploring Contemporary Nursing

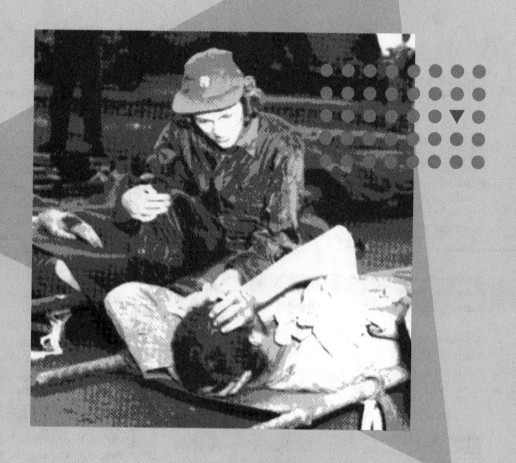

CHAPTER 1
Nursing Foundations
CHAPTER 2
Nursing Process

CHAPTER 1

Nursing Foundations

Key Terms

Active Listening	Empathy
Art	Nursing Skills
Assessment Skills	Science
Caring Skills	Sympathy
Comforting Skills	Theory
Counseling Skills	

Learning Objectives

An understanding of the content within this chapter will be evidenced by the student's ability to:

- Describe three factors that led to the demise of nursing in England before the time of Florence Nightingale
- Identify four reforms for which Florence Nightingale is responsible
- Describe at least five ways in which early U.S. training schools deviated from those established under the direction of Florence Nightingale
- List three ways that nurses used their skills in the early history of nursing in the United States
- Explain how art, science, and nursing theory have been incorporated into contemporary nursing practice
- Discuss the evolution that has occurred in definitions of nursing
- List four types of educational programs that prepare students for beginning levels of nursing practice
- Identify at least five factors that influence a person's choice of educational nursing program
- State three reasons that support the need for continuing education in nursing
- Describe four skills that all nurses use in clinical practice

Nursing is one of the youngest professions, yet oldest arts. It began in antiquity with family living and progressed as an extension of family nurturing. Surrogates were often called on to suckle healthy newborns and care for other family members as they became ill, aged, and helpless. Caring was needed more often than curing.

Eventually organized religious groups combined a commitment to care for the sick with saving souls. Some religious institutions engaged the penitent and disadvantaged to share the burden of care. However, the service of caring for the sick changed with the schism between King Henry VIII of England and the Catholic church when nuns and priests were extradited to continental Europe. Parochial hospitals in England and the patients within found themselves abandoned.

The administration of English hospitals became a duty of the state. Consequently, hospitals became poorhouses and eventually pesthouses. Attendants were recruited from the ranks of criminals, widows, and orphans who repaid the Crown for their meager food and

Timby BK: *Fundamental Skills and Concepts in Patient Care, Sixth Edition* © 1996 Lippincott-Raven Publishers

shelter by tending to the unfortunate sick. An example of the requirements for employment appears in Display 1-1.

For the most part, attendants were ignorant, uncouth, and apathetic to the needs of their charges. The quality of care reflected the caliber of its uncommitted labor force. Without supervision, nursing attendants rarely lived up to even the minimum of their job description. Infections, pressure sores, and malnutrition were a testimony of their neglect.

THE NIGHTINGALE REFORMATION

In the midst of these deplorable health care conditions, Florence Nightingale, an Englishwoman born of wealthy parents, announced that she had been called by God to become a nurse. Determined, despite her family's protests, she worked alongside nursing deaconesses, a Protestant order of women who cared for the sick, in Kaiserwerth, Germany.

After having become suitably prepared through her nursing apprenticeship, Nightingale embarked on the next phase of her career. She worked at reforming and managing the care of women who were retired from the service of their affluent employers.

The Crimean War (1854–1856)

At the same time Nightingale was proving her ability to improve the care and services provided to the residents at the Institution for the Care of Sick Gentlewomen in Distressed Circumstances, England found itself allied with Turkey, France, and Sardinia in defending the Crimea, a peninsula on the north shore of the Black Sea.

The British soldiers suffered terribly and their dire circumstances were made public by war correspondents at the front lines. The British public was outraged by the reports on the morbidity and mortality among its war casualties. As a result of the widespread pub-

licity, the government became the object of national criticism.

Meanwhile, Florence Nightingale proposed to Sidney Herbert, then Secretary of War and an old family friend, that the sick and injured British soldiers at Scutari (a military barracks in Turkey) would fare better if cared for by a team of women she would train with nursing skills (Fig. 1-1). With Herbert's approval, Nightingale selected women whose reputations would be beyond reproach. She intuitively realized that only individuals with devotion and idealism would be able to accept the discipline and hard work necessary for the task before them.

The medical staff at Scutari did not see this group of women as capable of providing adequate care. Jealousy and rivalry caused the British medical officers to refuse any help from Nightingale and her 38 volunteers. When it became clear that the daily death rate, which averaged about 60%, would not subside, Nightingale's nurses were allowed to work. Under her supervision, the band of women cleaned up the filth and vermin, and improved ventilation, nutrition, and sanitation; they staved off putrefaction—and lowered the death rate to 1%.

Servicemen and families alike were grateful; the country adored her. To show their appreciation, funds were donated to sustain the great work that Florence had begun. The funds were used to start the first Nightingale training school for nurses at St. Thomas Hospital in England. This school became the model for others in Europe and the United States.

ESTABLISHING NURSING IN THE UNITED STATES

The Civil War came on the heels of the Nightingale Reformation. Like England, the United States found itself involved in a war with no organized or substantial staff of trained nurses to care for its sick and wounded. The military had to rely on untrained corpsmen and

---

DISPLAY 1-1. *Rules of Employment for Nursing Attendants —1789*

- No dirt, rags, or bones may be thrown from the windows.
- Nurses are to punctually shift the bed and body linen of patients, viz., once in a fortnight (2 weeks), their shirts once in four days, their drawers and stockings once a week or oftener, if found necessary.
- All nurses who disobey orders, get drunk, neglect their patients, quarrel with men, shall be immediately discharged.

Goodnow M. Outlines of Nursing History. 5th ed. Philadelphia and London: WB Saunders, 1933, pp. 57–58.

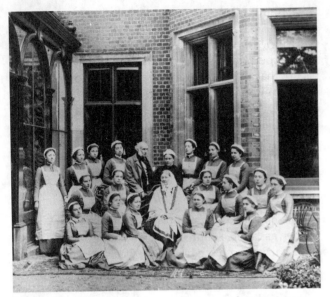

FIGURE 1-1
Florence Nightingale (*center*), her brother-in-law, Sir Harry Verney, and Miss Crossland, the nurse in charge of the Nightingale Training School at St. Thomas Hospital in 1886, with a class of student nurses. (Courtesy of The Florence Nightingale Museum Trust, London, England.)

civilian volunteers who often consisted of the mothers, wives, and sisters of inducted soldiers.

The Union government appointed Dorothea Lynde Dix, a social worker who had proved her worth earlier by reforming health conditions for the mentally ill, to select and organize women volunteers to care for the troops. In 1862 Dix followed Nightingale's advice and established the following selection criteria. Applicants were to be:

- between the ages of 35 and 50 years
- matronly and plain looking
- educated
- of serious disposition, neat, orderly, sober, and industrious, and were required to
- submit two letters of recommendation attesting to their moral character, integrity, and capacity to care for the sick.

Once selected, a volunteer nurse was to dress plainly in brown, gray, or black colors, and agree to serve for at least 6 months (Donahue, 1985).

U.S. Nursing Schools

After the Civil War, the country mended its wounds, and attention was turned to establishing training schools for nurses. Unfortunately, the United States deviated substantially from the Nightingale paradigm (Table 1-1). Whereas planned, consistent, formal education was the priority in Nightingale schools, the

training of American nurses was more an unsubsidized apprenticeship.

Eventually training schools became more organized and uniform in their curricula. The training period lengthened from 6 months to 3 full years. Graduate nurses received a diploma attesting to their successful completion of nurses' training.

Expanding Horizons of Practice

Diplomas in hand, American nurses entered the 20th century by distinguishing themselves in caring for the sick and disadvantaged outside the walls of hospitals (Fig. 1-2). Nurses moved into the communities and established "settlement houses" where they lived and worked among the immigrant poor. Others provided midwifery services, especially in the rural hills of Appalachia. The success of their public health efforts at prenatal and obstetric care, teaching child care, and immunizing children is well documented.

And, as other generations of nurses had done in the past, they continued to volunteer during wars. Nurses offered their services fighting yellow fever, typhoid, malaria, and dysentery during the Spanish–American War. They replenished the nursing staff in military hospitals during World Wars I and II (Fig. 1-3). They worked side-by-side with physicians in Mobile Army Service Hospitals (MASH) during the Korean War, acquiring knowledge about trauma care that would later help to reduce the mortality of American soldiers in Vietnam. And, most recently, nurses answered the call during Operation Desert Storm. Whenever and wherever there has been a need, nurses have put their own lives on the line.

CONTEMPORARY NURSING

Combining Nursing Art With Science

At first, the training of nurses consisted of learning the art of nursing. An **art** is the ability to perform an act skillfully. Nursing arts, the skills performed by nurses, were acquired under the guidance and direction of other experienced practitioners and passed on from mentor to student as a result of tradition. But contemporary nursing practice has added another dimension, that of science. The English word "science" comes from the Latin word *scio*, which means, "I know." A **science** is a body of knowledge unique to a particular subject. It develops from observing and studying the relation of one phenomenon to another. Through the development of a unique body of scientific knowledge, it is now possible to predict which nursing interventions are most appropriate for producing desired outcomes.

TABLE 1-1. *Differences in Nightingale Schools and U.S. Training Schools*

Nightingale Schools	U.S. Training Schools
Training schools were affiliated with a few selective hospitals.	Any hospital, rural or urban, could establish a training school.
Training hospitals relied on a staff of employees to provide patient care.	Students staffed the hospital.
Costs for education were borne by the student or endowed from the Nightingale Trust Fund.	Students worked without pay in return for training—which more often than not consisted of performing housekeeping chores.
Cooperating in the training of nurses provided no financial advantages to the hospital.	Hospitals profited by eliminating the need to pay employees.
Class schedules were planned separate from practical experience.	No formal classes were held; training was an outcome of work.
There was a uniform core of curricular content.	The curriculum was unplanned and the content varied according to current cases.
Formal instruction was provided by a previously trained nurse with a focus on nursing care.	Instruction was usually informal, at the bedside, from the physician's perspective.
The number of clinical hours during training was restricted.	Students were expected to work 12 hours a day and live in or adjacent to the hospital in case they were unexpectedly needed.
At the end of the training period, graduates became paid employees or were hired to train other students.	At the end of training, students were discharged from the training hospital and new students took their places; most graduates sought private-duty positions.

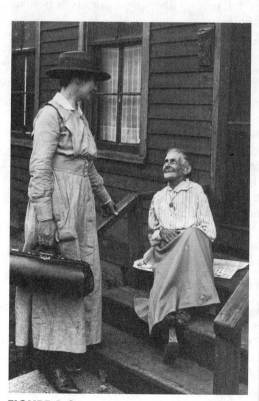

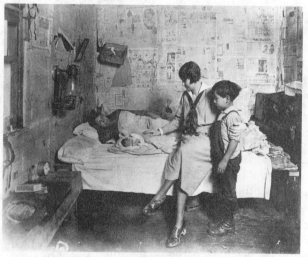

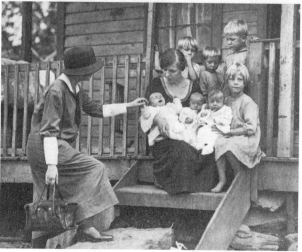

FIGURE 1-2
Community health nurses circa late 1800s to early 1900s. (Courtesy of Visiting Nurse Association, Inc. Detroit, MI.)

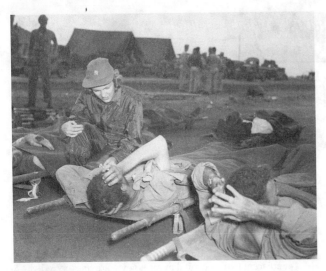

FIGURE 1-3
A military nurse comforts a soldier during World War II. (Courtesy of the National Archives, Washington, DC.)

Integrating Nursing Theory

The word theory comes from a Greek word that means "vision." A **theory** is an opinion, belief, or view that explains a process. For example, a scientist may study the relationship of sunlight and plants and arrive at a theory of photosynthesis, which explains the process of how plants grow. Others who believe the theorist's view to be true may then apply the theory for their own practical use.

Nursing has undergone a similar scientific review. Nursing theorists, like Florence Nightingale and others who are more contemporary, have examined the relationships between man, health, the environment, and nursing. The outcome of the analysis becomes the basis for a theory about nursing—in other words, a personal belief as to what the process called "nursing" is about. The theory may then be adopted by a nursing program to serve as the conceptual framework or model for the school's philosophy, curriculum, and, most important, nursing approaches with patients. A similar example can be seen in the manner in which psychologists have adopted Freud's psychoanalytic theory or Skinner's behavioral theory and used them as models to follow for diagnostic and therapeutic interventions with patients.

Table 1-2 summarizes some nursing theories and discusses how each theory has been applied to nursing practice. Those selected are only a representative sample of the accumulating theories of nursing. Additional information on this topic can be researched in more detail in current nursing literature.

Definitions of Nursing

In an effort to clarify for the public, and nurses themselves, just what nursing encompasses, various working definitions have been proposed. Florence Nightin-

gale, the person who restored dignity to caring for the sick, is credited with the earliest modern definition. She proposed that "nursing is putting individuals in the best possible condition for nature to restore and preserve health."

Other definitions have been offered by nurses who have come to be recognized as authorities and, therefore, qualified spokespeople on the practice of nursing. One such authority is Virginia Henderson. Her definition, which was eventually adopted by the International Council of Nurses (ICN), added a new dimension by broadening the description of nursing to include health promotion, not just illness care. She stated in 1966 that

> The unique function of the nurse is to assist the individual, sick or well, in the performance of those activities contributing to health or its recovery (or to a peaceful death) that he could perform unaided if he had the necessary strength, will or knowledge. And to do this in such a way as to help him gain independence as rapidly as possible.

In her writing and speaking, Henderson proposed that nursing is more than carrying out medical orders. It involves a special relationship and service between the nurse and those entrusted in his or her care. According to Henderson, the nurse acts as a temporary proxy, meeting health needs with knowledge and skills that neither the patient nor his or her family can provide.

The most recent definition of nursing comes from the American Nurses Association (ANA). In its published report, *Nursing: A Social Policy Statement* (1980), nursing is defined as "the diagnosis and treatment of human responses to actual or potential health problems." The position of the ANA is that in addition to nursing's traditional dependent and interdependent functions, there is an independent area of practice in which to use nursing skills. It may be expected that as the role of the nurse changes in the future, there will be further revisions to the definition of nursing so as to describe more succinctly the scope of nursing practice.

THE EDUCATIONAL LADDER

There are two basic educational options for those interested in pursuing a career in nursing: either practical (or vocational) nursing or one of several programs that prepare graduates for registered nursing. Each educational track provides the knowledge and skills for a particular entry level of practice. Some of the factors affecting the choice of a nursing program include:

- a person's career goals
- geographic location of schools
- costs involved

TABLE 1-2. *Nursing Theories and Applications*

Theorist	Theory	Explanation
Florence Nightingale 1820–1910	**Environmental Theory**	
	Man	Individuals whose natural defenses are influenced by a healthful or unhealthful environment
	Health	A state in which the environment is optimum for the natural body processes to achieve reparative outcomes
	Environment	All the external conditions that are capable of preventing, suppressing, or contributing to disease or death
	Nursing	Putting the patient in the best condition for nature to act
	Synopsis of Theory	External conditions such as ventilation, light, odor, and cleanliness are capable of preventing, suppressing, or contributing to disease or death.
	Application to Nursing Practice	Nurses modify unhealthy aspects of the environment to put the patient in the best condition for nature to act.
Virginia Henderson 1897–	**Basic Needs Theory**	
	Man	Individuals with human needs that have meaning and value unique to each person
	Health	The ability to independently satisfy human needs composed of 14 basic physical, psychological, and social elements
	Environment	The setting in which an individual learns unique patterns for living
	Nursing	Temporarily assisting an individual who lacks the necessary strength, will, and knowledge to satisfy 1 or more of 14 basic needs
	Synopsis of Theory	Individuals have basic needs that are components of health. Their significance and value are unique to each person.
	Application to Nursing Practice	Nurses assist in performing those activities the patient would perform if he or she had the strength, will, and knowledge.
Dorothea Orem 1914–	**Self-Care Theory**	
	Man	Individuals who use self-care to sustain life and health, recover from disease or injury, or cope with its effects
	Health	The result of practices that individuals have learned to carry out on their own behalf to maintain life and well-being
	Environment	External elements with which man interacts in his struggle to maintain self-care
	Nursing	A human service that assists individuals to progressively maximize their self-care potential
	Synopsis of Theory	Individuals learn behaviors that they perform on their own behalf to maintain life, health, and well-being.
	Application to Nursing Practice	Nurses assist patients with self-care to improve or maintain health.
Sister Callista Roy 1939–	**Adaptation Theory**	
	Man	Social, mental, spiritual, and physical beings who are affected by stimuli in the internal and external environment
	Health	The ability of an individual to adapt to changes in the environment
	Environment	Internal and external forces that are in a continuous state of change
	Nursing	A humanitarian art and expanding science that manipulates and modifies stimuli to promote and facilitate man's ability to adapt
	Synopsis of Theory	Man is a biopsychosocial being. A change in one component results in adaptive changes in the others.
	Application to Nursing Practice	Nurses assess biologic, psychological, and social factors interfering with health; alter the stimuli causing the maladaption; and evaluate the effectiveness of the action taken.

- length of programs
- reputation and success of past graduates
- flexibility in course scheduling
- opportunity for part-time versus full-time enrollment
- ease of matriculation into the next level of education

Practical or Vocational Nursing Education

During World War II, many registered nurses enlisted in the military. This left civilian hospitals, clinics, schools, and other health care agencies with an acute shortage of trained nurses. To fill the void as expeditiously as possible, abbreviated programs in practical nursing were developed across the country to teach essential nursing skills. The intent was that graduates of these programs would acquire the necessary skills to care for the health needs of well infants, children, and adults; and those mildly or chronically ill, or convalescing, so as to use registered nurses more effectively in areas where patients were acutely ill.

However, after the war, there continued to be a need for practical nurses because many registered nurses opted for part-time employment or resigned to become full-time housewives when American servicemen returned from the war. It became obvious that the role practical nurses were fulfilling in health care delivery would not be a temporary one. Consequently, leaders in practical nursing programs organized to form The National Association for Practical Nurse Education and Service (NAPNES), Inc. This group set about to standardize practical nurse education and facilitate licensure of their graduates. By 1945, eight states had approved practical nurse programs (Grippando, 1993). The need and quality of practical nursing education continues to be reaffirmed by the fact that currently there are 1098 LPN/LVN programs in the United States with a reported enrollment of 60,749 students—a figure that represents the highest growth rate in the previous 10 years (Fig. 1-4).

Career centers, vocational schools, hospitals, independent agencies, or community colleges usually offer practical nursing programs. Clinical experience is arranged at local community hospitals, clinics, and nursing homes. The average length of a practical nursing program is from 1 year to 18 months, after which graduates are qualified to take the national licensing examination (NCLEX-PN). And, because this is the shortest of all the nursing preparatory programs, it is considered by many to be the most economical. Licensed graduates provide direct health care for patients under the supervision of a registered nurse, physician, or dentist. To provide for career mobility, many schools for practical nursing have developed matriculation agreements facilitating the enrollment of their graduates into another school that offers a path to registered nursing.

Registered Nursing Education

There are three educational options available for becoming a registered nurse, all of which meet the requirements for taking the national licensing examination (NCLEX-RN). One may choose from a hospital-based diploma program, a program that awards an associate degree in nursing, or a baccalaureate nursing program. A person who is licensed as a registered nurse may work directly at the bedside or supervise others in managing the care of groups of patients.

HOSPITAL-BASED DIPLOMA PROGRAMS

Diploma programs were the traditional route for nurses up to and through the middle of this century. Their decline became obvious in the 1970s, and their

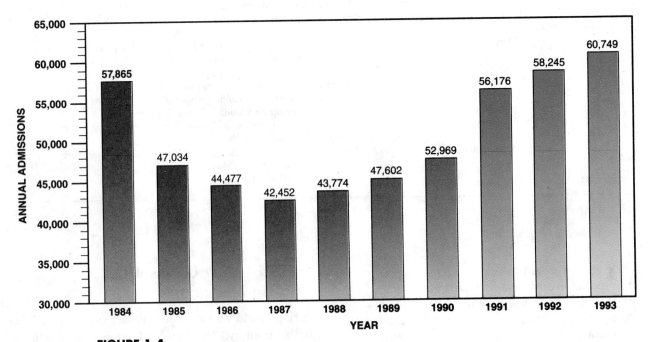

FIGURE 1-4
Trends in LPN/LVN enrollments 1984–1993. (National League for Nursing. Focus on Practical/Vocational Nursing, Vol. III, New York, 1994).

numbers continue to dwindle (Fig. 1-5). Their decline is partially the result of the drive to increase professionalism in nursing by encouraging education from degree-granting colleges and universities, and because hospitals are no longer financially able to subsidize schools of nursing.

Diploma nurses were, and are, well trained. Because of their vast clinical experience, compared to students from other types of programs, they are often characterized as more self-confident and more easily socialized into the role requirements of a graduate nurse.

A hospital-based diploma program usually is 3 years in length. Many hospital schools of nursing collaborate with nearby colleges to provide basic science and humanities courses that may transfer if a graduate chooses to pursue an associate or baccalaureate degree at a later time.

ASSOCIATE DEGREE PROGRAMS

During World War II, hospital-based schools accelerated the education of some registered nursing students through the Cadet Nurse Corps to accommodate the attrition of qualified nurses needed for the war effort. Afterward, Mildred Montag, a doctoral nursing student herself, began to question if it was actually necessary for students in a registered nursing program to spend 3 years acquiring a basic education. It was her hypothesis that nursing education could be shortened to 2 years and relocated to a vocational school or junior or community college. The graduate from this type of program would acquire an associate degree in nursing, be referred to as a technical nurse, and would not be expected to work in a management position.

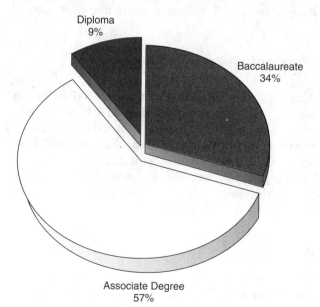

FIGURE 1-5
The distribution of basic RN programs. (National League for Nursing. Nursing Datasource, New York, 1993.)

This type of nursing preparation has proven extremely popular and now commands the highest enrollment among all registered nurse programs. Despite its condensed curriculum, graduates of associate degree programs have demonstrated a high level of competence in passing the national licensing examination for registered nurses (NCLEX-RN). However, employers have not seen fit to differentiate between the educational outcomes for which each program prepares its graduates. In other words, when hiring a new graduate, whether from a diploma, associate degree, or baccalaureate program, employers have demonstrated the attitude that "a nurse is a nurse." Table 1-3 describes how each level of education prepares its graduates to assume separate, yet coordinated, types of responsibilities.

BACCALAUREATE PROGRAMS

Although collegiate nursing programs were established at the beginning of the 20th century, they have not attracted large numbers of students. Their popularity is recently increasing, perhaps because of the proposals by the ANA and the National League for Nursing (NLN) to establish baccalaureate education as the entry level into nursing practice. The deadline for this goal, once set for 1985, has been temporarily postponed. The basis for the delay can be attributed to three factors: (1) the date for implementation coincided with a national shortage of nurses; (2) there was tremendous opposition from nondegreed nurses who felt threatened that their titles and positions might be jeopardized; and (3) employers of nurses feared that paying higher salaries to degreed personnel would escalate budgets beyond their financial limits. Consequently, the adoption of a unified entry level into practice is still in limbo.

But, although baccalaureate programs are the longest and most expensive preparatory programs, baccalaureate-prepared nurses have the greatest flexibility in qualifying for nursing positions, both staff and managerial. More often than not, a nurse with a baccalaureate degree is preferred in areas like public health in which there is a high degree of independent decision-making.

Currently, nondegreed nurses are returning to school to complete the requirements for a baccalaureate degree. Matriculation has been difficult for many because of the nontransferability of courses taken during their diploma or associate degree programs. To facilitate enrollment, some collegiate programs are offering nurses an opportunity to obtain credit by successfully passing challenge examinations. In addition, many colleges and universities are providing satellite or outreach programs beyond their main campuses to accommodate nurses who cannot go to school full-time or travel long distances.

TABLE 1-3. *Levels of Responsibilities for the Nursing Process**

	Practical/Vocational Nurse	Associate Degree Nurse	Baccalaureate Nurse
Assessing	Gathers data by interviewing, observing, and performing a basic physical examination of people with common health problems with predictable outcomes.	Collects data from people with complex health problems with unpredictable outcomes, their family, medical records, and other health team members.	Identifies the information needed from individuals or groups to provide an appropriate nursing data base.
Diagnosing	Contributes to the development of nursing diagnoses by reporting abnormal assessment data.	Uses a classification list to write a nursing diagnostic statement, including the problem, its etiology, and signs and symptoms. Identifies problems that require collaboration with the physician.	Conducts clinical testing of approved nursing diagnoses. Proposes new diagnostic categories for consideration and approval.
Planning	Assists in setting realistic and measurable goals. Suggests nursing actions that can prevent, reduce, or eliminate health problems with predictable outcomes. Assists in developing a written plan of care.	Sets realistic, measurable goals. Develops a written individualized plan of care with specific nursing orders that reflects the standards for nursing practice.	Develops written standards for nursing practice. Plans care for healthy or sick individuals or groups in structured health care agencies or the community.
Implementing	Performs basic nursing care under the direction of a registered nurse.	Identifies priorities. Directs others to carry out nursing orders.	Applies nursing theory to the approaches used for resolving actual and potential health problems of individuals or groups of patients.
Evaluating	Shares observations on the progress of the patient in reaching established goals. Contributes to the revision of the plan of care.	Evaluates the outcomes of nursing care on a routine basis. Makes revisions in the plan for care.	Conducts research on nursing activities that may be improved with further study.

*Note that each more advanced practitioner can perform the responsibilities of those identified previously.

Graduate Nursing Programs

Graduate nursing programs are available at both the master's and doctoral levels. Nurses with master's degrees fill the roles of clinical specialists, nurse practitioners, administrators, and educators. Doctoral degrees allow their recipients to conduct research, advise, administer, and instruct nurses pursuing undergraduate and graduate degrees. Although a graduate degree in nursing is preferred, some nurses pursue advanced education in non-nursing fields, such as business, leadership, and education, to enhance their nursing career.

CONTINUING EDUCATION

Continuing education is any planned learning experience that takes place beyond one's basic nursing program (ANA, 1974). Florence Nightingale is credited with having said, "to stand still is to move backwards." Although her remark was made over a century ago, the principle that learning is a life-long process still ap-

plies. Display 1-2 lists reasons why nurses, in particular, pursue opportunities for continuing education.

UNIQUE NURSING SKILLS

Although **nursing skills**, or those activities that are unique to the practice of nursing, may be used differently depending on a person's choice of educational program, all nurses share the same philosophical perspective. Keeping with the traditions of Florence Nightingale, contemporary nursing practice continues to include assessment skills, caring skills, counseling skills, and comforting skills.

Assessment Skills

Before the nurse can determine what nursing care a person requires, the patient's needs and problems must be determined. This requires the use of assessment skills. **Assessment skills** are those acts that involve collecting data. They involve interviewing, observing, and

---

DISPLAY 1-2. *Rationale for Acquiring Continuing Education*

- No basic program provides all the knowledge and skills needed for a lifetime career.
- Current advances in technology make previous practice obsolete.
- Assuming responsibility for self-learning demonstrates personal accountability.
- To ensure the public's confidence, nurses must demonstrate evidence of current competence.
- Practicing according to current nursing standards helps to ensure that care is legally safe.
- Renewal of state licensure is often contingent on evidence of continuing education.

---

examining the patient and, in some cases, the patient's family—a term used loosely to refer to those people with whom the patient lives and closely associates. Although the patient and the family are the primary resources for information, the nurse also uses the patient's medical record and other health workers as resources for facts. Assessment skills are discussed in more detail in Unit IV.

Caring Skills

Caring skills are those nursing interventions that restore or maintain a person's health. For some patients, this may involve something as minimal as assisting with activities of daily living (ADL). ADL is a term that refers to those acts that people do in the normal course of living, like bathing, grooming, dressing, toileting, and eating. More and more, however, the role of the nurse is being extended to include the safe care of patients who require invasive or highly technical equipment. This textbook introduces the beginning nurse to the concepts and skills needed to provide care for patients whose disorders have fairly predictable outcomes. Once this foundation has been established, students may add to their initial knowledge base.

Traditionally, nurses are—and always have been—providers of physical care for people unable independently to meet their own health needs. But caring also involves the concern and attachment that results from the close relationship of one human being with another. Despite the close relationship that caring involves, the nurse ultimately wants patients to become self-reliant. The nurse who assumes too much care for patients, like the mother who continues to tie a child's shoes, often delays his or her patients' independent status.

Counseling Skills

A counselor is one who listens to a patient's needs, responds with information based on their area of expertise, and facilitates the outcome that a patient desires. Nurses implement **counseling skills** by communicating with patients, actively listening to the exchange of information, offering pertinent health teaching, and demonstrating emotional support.

To get the patient's perspective on a situation, the nurse may use therapeutic communication techniques to facilitate a patient's verbal expression. Therapeutic and nontherapeutic communication techniques are discussed more fully in Chapter 7. The interaction is facilitated by the use of active listening. **Active listening** is demonstrating full attention to what is being said, hearing the content being communicated as well as the unspoken message. Giving patients the opportunity to be heard helps them to organize their thoughts and evaluate their situation more realistically.

Once the patient's perspective is clear, the nurse provides pertinent health information without offering specific advice. By reserving personal opinions, nurses promote the right of every person to make his or her own decisions and choices on matters affecting health and illness care. The role of the nurse is to share information on potential alternatives, allow patients the freedom to choose, and support the decision that is made.

While giving care, the nurse finds many opportunities to teach patients how to promote healing processes, stay well, prevent illness, and carry out ADL in the best possible way. People know much more about health and health care today than in the past, and they expect nurses to share accurate information with them.

Because patients do not always communicate their feelings to strangers, nurses may use empathy. **Empathy** is an intuitive awareness of what the patient is experiencing. The nurse uses empathy to perceive the patient's emotional state and need for support. This skill, which is different from sympathy, involves being able to remain compassionate yet detached. **Sympathy**, on the other hand, involves identifying so closely with the patient's feelings that the nurse becomes ineffectual in providing for the patient's needs.

Comforting Skills

Florence Nightingale's presence and the light from her lamp communicated comfort to the frightened British soldiers. As a result of that heritage, contemporary nurses understand that illness often causes feelings of insecurity that may threaten the patient's or the family's ability to cope. Either or both may feel very vulnerable. It is then that the nurse uses **comforting skills** (Fig. 1-6). Because previously supportive people may

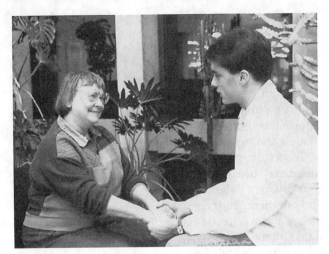

FIGURE 1-6
This nurse offers comfort and emotional support.

not be continuously available, the nurse becomes the stabilizing figure during a health-related crisis. The nurse becomes the guide, companion, and interpreter for those requiring nursing care. When provided, this supportive relationship generally evokes trust and reduces fear and worry.

Thus, as a result of one woman's efforts, modern nursing was born. It has continued to mature and flourish ever since. The skills performed by Florence Nightingale on a very grand scale are repeated today during each and every nurse–patient relationship.

KEY CONCEPTS

• The art of nursing declined in England with the exile of Catholic religious orders to Europe, which resulted in the government assuming responsibility for the care of the sick, aged, and infirm. Eventually, this care was delegated to untrained and, for the most part, uninterested people of questionable character.

• Florence Nightingale changed the image of nursing by (1) training people to care for the sick, (2) selecting only those with upstanding character as potential nurses, (3) improving the sanitary conditions within patients' environments, (4) significantly reducing the morbidity and mortality of British soldiers, (5) providing formal nursing classes separate from clinical experience, and (6) advocating that nursing education be a life-long process.

• Training schools in the United States deviated from the pattern established by Nightingale in the following ways: there were no criteria as to which hospitals were used for the training of nurses; students staffed the hospitals without being paid; there was no uniformity in what was taught; students learned more by experience than by formal instruction; what nursing students were taught was from a physician's per-

spective; students were required to work and live at the beck and call of the hospital's administrator; and after graduation, students were left to seek employment elsewhere.

• Besides being employed in hospitals, early graduates of nursing programs met the health needs of the immigrant poor by living in and among them in settlement houses located in the ghettos of large cities, by being midwives to rural women where medical care was unavailable, and caring for sick and wounded servicemen.

• What started initially as an art, passing on the skills of nursing from one practitioner to another, was soon joined by science, a unique body of knowledge making it possible to predict which nursing interventions would be most appropriate for producing desired outcomes. And, most recently, nursing has become theory-based, which means that nursing scholars are proposing what the process of nursing encompasses by explaining the relationship between four essential components: man, health, the environment, and nursing.

• One of the earliest definitions of nursing defined the scope of practice as caring for the sick; more recently, nursing has been redefined with the addition of the nurse's role in health promotion and as having an area of independent practice.

• Those who wish to pursue a career in nursing may choose from a practical/vocational nursing program or registered nursing program taught in a career center, hospital school, community or junior college, or university.

• The choice of a nursing educational program is often contingent on one's career goals, location of schools, costs involved, length of the program, reputation and success of graduates, flexibility in course scheduling, opportunities for part-time or full-time enrollment, and ease of matriculation to the next level of education.

• Continuing education is necessary for contemporary nurses because it demonstrates personal accountability, promotes the public's trust, ensures competence in current nursing practice, and keeps one abreast of how technology is affecting patient care.

• Regardless of from which educational program a nurse graduates, all nurses use assessment, caring, counseling, and comforting skills in clinical practice.

CRITICAL THINKING EXERCISES

• Describe the Nightingale reforms and explain which one you feel was most important.
• In what ways was the service of nurses during Operation Desert Storm similar to that provided by the Nightingale nurses during the Crimean War?
• How would you define nursing?

SUGGESTED READINGS

American Nurses Association. Nursing: A Social Policy Statement. Kansas City, MO: American Nurses Association, 1980.

American Nurses Association. Standards for Continuing Education in Nursing. Kansas City, MO: American Nurses Association, 1974.

Ashley J. Hospitals, Paternalism, and the Role of the Nurse. New York: Teachers College Press, 1976.

Donahue MP. Nursing: The Finest Art. St. Louis: CV Mosby, 1985.

Grippando G. Nursing Perspectives and Issues. 5th ed. Albany, NY: Delmar, 1993.

Henderson V. The Nature of Nursing. New York: Macmillan, 1966.

Marks G, Beatty W. Women in White. New York: Scribners, 1972.

Nightingale F. Notes on Nursing: What It Is, and What It Is Not. London: Harrisson, 1859. Commemorative edition: Philadelphia: JB Lippincott, 1992.

Stuart ME. Nursing: the endangered profession? Canadian Nurse April 1993;89:19–22.

CHAPTER 2
Nursing Process

Chapter Outline

 NURSING GUIDELINES

Nursing Guidelines for Using the Nursing Process

Key Terms

Actual Problem   Objective Data
Assessment   Planning
Diagnosis   Possible Problem
Evaluation   Potential Problem
Implementation   Short-term Goal
Long-term Goal   Signs
Nursing Diagnosis   Subjective Data
Nursing Process   Symptoms

Learning Objectives

An understanding of the content within this chapter will be evidenced by the student's ability to:

- Define nursing process
- List five steps in the nursing process
- Describe six characteristics of the nursing process
- Identify four sources for assessment data
- Differentiate between a data base and focus assessment
- Distinguish between a nursing diagnosis and a collaborative problem
- List three parts of a nursing diagnostic statement
- Describe the rationale for setting priorities
- Discuss the circumstances in which short-term and long-term goals are appropriate
- Identify four ways for documenting a plan of care
- Describe the information that is documented in reference to the plan of care
- Discuss three outcomes that result from evaluation

In the distant past, nursing practice involved actions that were based mostly on common sense and the examples set by older, more experienced nurses. The actual care of patients tended to be limited according to the medical orders given by a physician. Nurses today continue to work interdependently with other health practitioners. Now, however, nurses plan and implement patient care more independently. To put it in even stronger terms, nurses are being held responsible and accountable for providing appropriate patient care that reflects current accepted standards for nursing practice.

THE NURSING PROCESS

A **process** is a set of actions leading to a particular outcome. The nursing process is an organized sequence of steps, identified as assessment, diagnosis, planning, implementation, and evaluation, that nurses use to

Timby BK: *Fundamental Skills and Concepts in Patient Care, Sixth Edition* © 1996 Lippincott-Raven Publishers

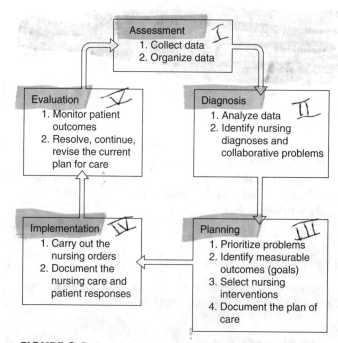

FIGURE 2-1

The steps in the nursing process.

solve the health problems of patients (Fig. 2-1). It is the accepted standard for clinical practice established by the American Nurses Association (ANA) (Display 2-1). When nursing practice models the nursing process, patients receive high-quality care within a minimum of time and at a maximum of efficiency.

Characteristics of the Nursing Process

The nursing process has seven distinct characteristics:

1. *It is within the legal scope of nursing.* The definitions of nursing in most state nurse practice acts describe nursing in terms of a more independent problem-solving role that involves the diagnosis and treatment of human responses to actual or potential health problems.
2. *It is based on knowledge.* The ability to solve patient problems requires the application of a unique knowledge base in nursing. By thinking critically, a process of carefully analyzing situations, nurses are able to determine what problems necessitate collaboration with the physician and which ones fall within the independent domain of nursing. Critical thinking further enables nurses to select appropriate nursing interventions for achieving predictable outcomes.
3. *It is planned.* The steps of the nursing process are organized and systematic. One step leads to the next in an orderly fashion.
4. *It is patient centered.* The nursing process facilitates a comprehensive plan of care for each patient as a unique individual. Patients are expected, whenever possible, to be active participants in their care.
5. *It is goal directed.* The nursing process facilitates a united effort between the patient and the nursing team in achieving desired outcomes.

Based on Laws of science

DISPLAY 2-1. *Standards of Clinical Nursing Practice*

Standard I. Assessment

The nurse collects client health data.

Standard II. Diagnosis

The nurse analyzes the assessment data in determining diagnoses.

Standard III. Outcome Identification

The nurse identifies expected outcomes individualized to the client.

Standard IV. Planning

The nurse develops a plan of care that prescribes interventions to attain expected outcomes.

Standard V. Implementation

The nurse implements the interventions identified in the plan of care.

Standard VI. Evaluation

The nurse evaluates the client's progress toward attainment of outcomes.

Reprinted with permission from Standards of Clinical Nursing Practice. © 1991, American Nurses Association, Washington, D.C.

DISPLAY 2-2. *Examples of Objective and Subjective Data*

Objective Data	Subjective Data
Weight	Pain
Temperature	Nausea
Skin color	Depression
Blood cell count	Fatigue
Vomiting	Anxiety
Bleeding	Loneliness

6. *It is prioritized.* When the nursing process is used, it provides a focused strategy for resolving those problems that represent the greatest threat to health.
7. *It is dynamic.* Because the health status of any patient is constantly changing, the nursing process acts like a continuous loop. Evaluation, the last step in the nursing process, involves data collection, and the process begins again.

ASSESSMENT

Assessment, the first step in the nursing process, is the systematic collection of information, or *data*, for the purpose of identifying current and potential health problems. Assessment begins with the nurse's first contact with a patient, and is ongoing.

Types of Data

Data are either objective or subjective. **Objective data** refer to information that is observable and measurable, such as the patient's blood pressure. Objective data are

often referred to as **signs** of a disorder. **Subjective data** comprise information that only the patient feels and can describe, such as pain. Subjective data may also be called **symptoms** (Display 2-2).

Sources for Data

The primary source for information is the patient. Secondary sources include the patient's family, reports, test results, information in current and past medical records, and discussions with other health care workers.

Types of Assessments

There are two types of assessments: a data base assessment and a focus assessment (Table 2-1).

DATA BASE ASSESSMENT

A **data base assessment** provides an extensive amount of information about the patient's physical, emotional, social, and spiritual health. The data are lengthy and comprehensive.

Data base information is obtained during the initial interview and physical examination (see Chap. 12). Hospitals usually provide a printed form (Fig. 2-2) to use as a guide while collecting information. Information obtained during a data base assessment serves as a reference for comparing all future data and provides the evidence from which the patient's initial problems are identified.

FOCUS ASSESSMENT

A **focus assessment** expands the data base by providing more details about specific problems. For instance, if during the initial interview the nurse is informed that constipation is more often the rule than the exception for a patient, more questions may be asked

TABLE 2-1. *Comparison of Data Base and Focus Assessments*

Data Base Assessment	Focus Assessment
• Obtained on admission	• Compiled throughout subsequent care
• Performed once	• Repeated each shift or more often
• Findings are documented on an admission assessment form	• Findings are documented on a checklist or in progress notes
• Time-consuming; may be as much as an hour or more	• Completed in a brief amount of time; 15 minutes, more or less
• Supplies a broad, comprehensive volume of amassed data	• Limited in the amount of data that is collected
• Provides breadth for future comparisons	• Adds depth to the initial data base
• Reflects the condition of the patient on entering the health care delivery system	• Provides comparative trends for evaluating the patient's response to treatment

Community Health Center of Branch County

ADMISSION ASSESSMENT RECORD

RESPIRATION

[ ] PROBLEM

HISTORY OF — [ ] CHEST PAIN   [ ] PNEUMONIA   [ ] BRONCHITIS   [ ] ASTHMA   [ ] EMPHYSEMA

SHORTNESS OF BREATH
[ ] YES   [ ] WITH EXERCISE   [ ] WITHOUT EXERCISE
[ ] NO

[ ] POTENTIAL FOR REFERRAL

COUGH
[ ] YES   [ ] PRODUCTIVE   [ ] NON-PRODUCTIVE   [ ] SPUTUM COLOR
[ ] NO

BREATH SOUNDS (DESCRIBE)

RATE	RHYTHM	QUALITY	SKIN COLOR
		[ ] LABORED [ ] SHALLOW	[ ] PINK [ ] PALE [ ] CYANOTIC

ACCESSORY MUSCLES

COMMENTS

CIRCULATION

[ ] PROBLEM

HISTORY OF — [ ] BLOOD CLOTS   [ ] EDEMA   [ ] ABNORMAL EKG   [ ] NUMBNESS   [ ] TINGLING   [ ] POOR CIRCULATION   [ ] FATIGUE   [ ] HYPERTENSION

[ ] POTENTIAL FOR REFERRAL

APICAL RATE	APICAL RATE [ ] REGULAR [ ] IRREGULAR	RHYTHM

NECK VEIN DISTENSION   [ ] PRESENT   [ ] ABSENT
NAIL BEDS   [ ] PINK   [ ] PALE   [ ] CYANOTIC

PEDAL EDEMA   [ ] PRESENT   [ ] ABSENT

PEDAL PULSES
LEFT   [ ] PRESENT   [ ] WEAK   [ ] ABSENT
RIGHT   [ ] PRESENT   [ ] WEAK   [ ] ABSENT

COMMENTS

NUTRITIONAL/METABOLIC

[ ] PROBLEM

HISTORY OF — [ ] DIABETES   [ ] HYPOGLYCEMIA   [ ] THYROID PROBLEMS

NUTRITIONAL STATUS   [ ] WELL NOURISHED   [ ] EMACIATED   [ ] OBESE

MEALS PER DAY	DIET AT HOME	DIET PREFERENCE	LAST MEAL [ ] A.M. [ ] P.M.	RECENT WEIGHT CHANGES

[ ] POTENTIAL FOR REFERRAL

NUTRITIONAL DISTURBANCES
[ ] VOMITING   [ ] NAUSEA   [ ] ANOREXIA   [ ] CHEWING PROBLEMS   [ ] OTHER (DESCRIBE)

JAUNDICE PRESENT [ ] YES [ ] NO	DENTAL HYGIENE (DESCRIBE)	TEETH [ ] OWN [ ] DENTURES	TONGUE CONDITION [ ] DRY [ ] COATED [ ] MOIST [ ] SWOLLEN	ORAL MUCOSA [ ] DRY [ ] MOIST COLOR

COMMENTS

ELIMINATION

[ ] PROBLEM

BOWEL HABITS
STOOLS PER DAY _____   COLOR   [ ] SOFT FORMED   [ ] DIARRHEA   [ ] CONSTIPATED   [ ] USE LAXATIVE
LAST BOWEL MOVEMENT

BLADDER   [ ] URGENCY   [ ] CALCULI   [ ] HEMATURIA
[ ] DYSURIA   [ ] NOCTURIA   [ ] FREQUENCY   [ ] PROSTATE PROBLEM

BOWEL SOUNDS   [ ] PRESENT   [ ] ABSENT
OSTOMIES OR TUBES (DESCRIBE)

[ ] POTENTIAL FOR REFERRAL

ABDOMEN
[ ] TENDER   [ ] SOFT   [ ] FIRM   [ ] DISTENDED   [ ] NOT DISTENDED

URINARY DEVICES (DESCRIBE)

COMMENTS

COGNITIVE/PERCEPTUAL

[ ] PROBLEM

HISTORY OF — [ ] SEIZURES [ ] FREQUENT [ ] INFREQUENT   [ ] HEADACHES [ ] FREQUENT [ ] INFREQUENT

LIMITATION OR RESTRICTION RELATED TO
[ ] HEARING - IMPAIRED   [ ] YES   [ ] NO
[ ] VISION - IMPAIRED   [ ] YES   [ ] NO

[ ] POTENTIAL FOR REFERRAL

LEVEL OF CONSCIOUSNESS
[ ] ALERT   [ ] LETHARGIC   [ ] CONFUSED   [ ] LISTLESS   [ ] RESPONDS TO PAIN   [ ] UNRESPONSIVE

ORIENTED TO
[ ] TIME   [ ] PLACE   [ ] PERSON
AFFECT   [ ] WITHDRAWN   [ ] CALM   [ ] APPREHENSIVE   [ ] OTHER (DESCRIBE)

BEHAVIOR
[ ] COOPERATIVE   [ ] UNCOOPERATIVE
PUPILS   [ ] EQUAL   [ ] REACTIVE   [ ] OTHER (DESCRIBE)

COMMUNICATION
[ ] SPEAKS ENGLISH   [ ] ABLE TO READ   [ ] ABLE TO WRITE   [ ] COMMUNICATES ADEQUATELY

AWARENESS
[ ] NO PROBLEM WITH MEMORY   [ ] PROBLEM WITH MEMORY

DISCOMFORT/PAIN
[ ] YES   WHERE   TYPE
[ ] NO
PAIN MANAGEMENT
POTENTIAL RISK OF FALLS   [ ] YES   [ ] NO

COMMENTS

FIGURE 2-2

One page of a multipage admission assessment form is shown. (Courtesy of the Community Health Center of Branch County, Coldwater, MI.)

DISPLAY 2-3. *Organization of Data*

Assessment Findings

Lassitude; distended abdomen; dry, hard stool passed with difficulty; fever; weak cough; thick sputum

Related Clusters

Lassitude, fever

Weak cough, thick sputum

Distended abdomen; dry, hard stool passed with difficulty

---

concerning elimination patterns or the characteristics of the stool. The nurse may ask the patient to save a stool specimen for subsequent inspection, and institute a record for monitoring bowel elimination.

Focus assessments may be repeated frequently or on a scheduled basis to determine trends in a patient's condition. For instance, it is customary to perform specific assessments on patients at the beginning and near the end of each shift, but not as comprehensively as during admission. Another example is the routine assessments that are repeated after surgery to determine if the patient's condition is stable or deteriorating (see Chap. 27).

Organizing Data

Interpreting the data is easier if the information is organized. Organization involves grouping related information. For example, consider the following list of words: apple, wheels, orchard, pedals, tree, and handlebars. At first glance, they appear to be a jumble of terms. However, if asked to cluster the terms that are related, most would correctly group "apple," "tree," and "orchard" together.

Nurses organize assessment data in much the same way (Display 2-3). Using knowledge and past experiences, nurses group clusters of related data. By organizing the data into small groups, the information is more easily analyzed and takes on more significance than when each fact is considered separately or the group is examined as a whole.

DIAGNOSIS

Diagnosis, the second step in the nursing process, involves identifying problems. This step is an outcome of having analyzed the collected data and interpreting whether the data suggest normal or abnormal findings.

Nursing Diagnoses

Nurses analyze data to identify one or more nursing diagnoses. A **nursing diagnosis** is a health problem that can be prevented, reduced, or resolved through independent nursing measures.

Nursing diagnoses can refer to existing problems or those that are very likely to develop. The terms "actual," "potential," and "possible" are used to describe the status of the identified problem. An **actual problem** refers to one that is currently present; a **potential problem** is one for which the patient is at risk for developing; and a **possible problem** is one that the nurse is unsure exists and believes more data must be gathered before making a final decision. Physicians use the same intellectual process for the purpose of identifying diseases that are treated using medical interventions (Table 2-2).

The NANDA List

The ANA has designated the North American Nursing Diagnosis Association (NANDA) as the authoritative organization for developing and approving nursing diagnoses. NANDA is the clearing house for proposals suggesting diagnoses that fall under the independent domain of nursing practice. The proposals are debated for their appropriateness. They are incorporated into a list that is published for clinical use. The most recent list, which usually is revised every 2 years, can be found in Appendix B.

Although entries in the NANDA list may change, most authorities believe that the language of approved diagnoses should be used whenever possible. When a patient's problem does not fit any of the categories approved by NANDA, the nurse can use his or her own terminology when stating a nursing diagnosis.

TABLE 2-2. *Analysis of Data*

Data	Analysis	Nursing Diagnosis	Medical Diagnosis
Distended abdomen, dry, hard stool passed with difficulty	Actual problem	Colonic Constipation	Diverticulosis
Weak cough, thick sputum	Potential problem	Risk for Ineffective Airway Clearance	Emphysema
Lassitude, fever	Possible problem	Possible Activity Intolerance	Infection

---

> **DISPLAY 2-4. *Parts of a Nursing Diagnostic Statement***
>
> 1. Sleep pattern disturbance = problem
> 2. Related to excessive intake of coffee = etiology
> 3. As manifested by difficulty in falling asleep, feeling tired during the day, and irritability with others = signs and symptoms

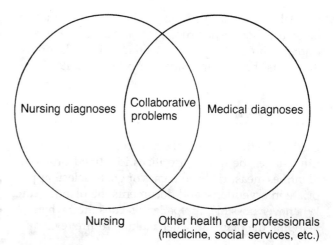

Nursing   Other health care professionals
(medicine, social services, etc.)

FIGURE 2-3

These two overlapping circles illustrate that the nurse independently treats nursing diagnoses. Doctors, other health professionals, and nurses work together on collaborative problems. (Carpenito LJ. Nursing Diagnosis: Application to Clinical Practice. 3rd ed, p 28. Philadelphia: JB Lippincott, 1989.)

The Nursing Diagnostic Statement

A diagnostic statement includes three parts: the problem portion, the etiology, and the signs and symptoms. They are collectively referred to as the **PES** (Display 2-4). One of the hallmarks of a nursing diagnosis is that the etiology is something that nurses can treat *independently.*

Potential problems are prefaced with the terms *Risk for . . .* , as in: Risk for Impaired Skin Integrity related to inactivity. The word *Possible* is used before the problem portion of a diagnostic statement to indicate uncertainty, as in, for example, Possible Sexual Dysfunction related to anxiety.

Potential and possible nursing diagnoses do not include the third part of the statement. In potential nursing diagnoses, the signs or symptoms have not yet been manifested; in possible nursing diagnoses, the data are still incomplete. However, those factors that place the patient at risk or make the nurse suspect that a diagnosis is possible are identified somewhere within nursing assessment documentation.

Collaborative Problems

Collaborative problems are physiologic complications that nurses monitor to detect (Carpenito, 1993). Because definitive treatment of a collaborative problem is beyond the independent scope of nursing practice, management requires the combined expertise of the nurse and the physician (Fig. 2-3). The nurse is specifically responsible and accountable for:

- Correlating medical diagnoses or medical treatment measures with the risk for unique complications
- Documenting the potential complications for which patients are at risk
- Making pertinent assessments to detect the complications
- Reporting trends that suggest a complication is being manifested
- Managing the emerging problem with nursing and physician-prescribed measures
- Evaluating the outcomes

Collaborative problems are often identified on a patient's plan for care with the abbreviation *PC*, which stands for "potential complication" (Table 2-3). Because

TABLE 2-3. *Correlation of Collaborative Problems*

Medical Diagnosis or Medical Treatment	Possible Consequence	Collaborative Problem
Myocardial infarction (heart attack)	Abnormal heart rhythm	PC: Dysrhythmias
Heart failure	Fluid in the lungs	PC: Pulmonary edema
Severe (3°) burns	Serum moves into tissue, depleting blood volume	PC: Hypovolemic shock
HIV positive (infected with AIDS virus)	Decreased blood cells that fight infection	PC: Immunodeficiency
Gastric decompression (suctioning stomach fluid)	Removes acid and electrolytes	PC: Alkalosis
		PC: Electrolyte imbalance
Cardiac catheterization (inserting a catheter into the heart)	Arterial bleeding	PC: Hemorrhage

AIDS, acquired immunodeficiency syndrome; HIV, human immunodeficiency virus; PC, potential complication.

a collaborative problem, in a sense, requires that the nurse use diagnostic processes, there are some nursing leaders who are proposing that the term "collaborative diagnosis" be used instead (Alfaro-LeFevre, 1994).

PLANNING

During the third step of the nursing process, the **planning** stage, the nurse prioritizes identified problems, identifies measurable outcomes or goals, selects appropriate interventions, and documents the plan for care. Whenever possible, the patient is consulted when developing the plan and when making future revisions.

Setting Priorities

Not all of the patient's problems may be resolved during a typically short hospitalization period. Therefore, it is important to determine which problems require the most attention. This is done by setting priorities. Prioritization involves ranking from most to least important.

There may be more than one way to determine priorities. One method, which is frequently used by nurses, is to rank nursing diagnoses according to Maslow's (1968) Hierarchy of Human Needs (see Chap. 4). Those problems that interfere with physio-

logic needs have priority over those that affect other levels of needs (Display 2-5). The rank can change as problems are resolved or new problems develop.

Establishing Goals

A **goal** is an expected or desired outcome. Although the terms "goal" and "outcome" are sometimes used interchangeably, outcomes are usually more specific (Display 2-6). Regardless of the term that is used, what is important is that the statement contain the criteria or objective evidence for verifying that a goal has been reached.

Goals help the nursing team know when, and if, the nursing care has been appropriate for resolving the patient's problem. Therefore, a goal accompanies each identified problem. Depending on the health agency, nurses may identify short-term goals, long-term goals, or both.

SHORT-TERM GOALS

Short-term goals are those that can be met in a few days to a week. Sometimes only short-term goals are identified in acute care settings, because most hospitalizations do not extend beyond a week's time.

DISPLAY 2-5. *Prioritizing Nursing Diagnoses*

Human Need*	Examples of Nursing Diagnoses
Physiologic	Altered Nutrition: Less than Body Requirements Ineffective Breathing Pattern Pain Impaired Swallowing Urinary Retention
Safety and Security	Risk for Injury Impaired Verbal Communication Altered Thought Processes Anxiety Fear
Love and Belonging	Social Isolation Impaired Social Interactions Altered Family Processes Parental Role Conflict
Esteem and Self-Esteem	Body Image Disturbance Powerlessness Caregiver Role Strain Ineffective Breastfeeding
Self-Actualization	Altered Growth and Development Spiritual Distress

Categories of human needs reflect those described by Abraham Maslow (1968).

DISPLAY 2-6. *Goals versus Outcomes*

Goal

The patient will be well hydrated by 8/23.

Outcome

The patient will have adequate hydration as evidenced by an oral intake between 2,000–3,000 mL/24 hours and a urine output ± 500 mL of the intake amount by 8/23. *labout*

Short-term goals have the following characteristics (Display 2-7):

- *They are developed from the problem portion of the diagnostic statement.*
- *They are patient centered*; that is, they reflect what will be accomplished from the patient's perspective, not the nurse's.
- *They are measurable* in that they identify specific criteria that provide evidence that the goal has been reached.
- *They are realistic* or logically accomplishable; setting unattainable goals is self-defeating and creates frustration.
- *They are accompanied by a target date* for accomplishment. The target date is the predicted time by which the goal will be met. The target date builds a time line for evaluation into the nursing process.

LONG-TERM GOALS

Long-term goals predict a desirable outcome that may take weeks or months to accomplish. They generally are identified for patients who have chronic health

Chronic dialysis diabetic

problems that require extended care in a nursing home or who receive community health services or home health care.

An example of a long-term goal for the patient with a cerebrovascular accident (CVA, or stroke) is the return of (full or partial) function to a paralyzed limb. This goal is not likely to be achieved at the time of discharge. However, by progressively accomplishing short-term goals while in the hospital, long-term goals are more likely to be achieved.

Selecting Nursing Interventions

Planning measures for accomplishing identified goals involves critical thinking. The nursing interventions are directed at eliminating the etiologies. The selection of strategies is based on the knowledge that certain nursing actions produce a desired effect. Whatever interventions are planned, they must be safe, within the legal scope of nursing practice, and compatible with medical orders.

The initial interventions usually are limited to selected measures that have the potential for achieving success. Some interventions are held in reserve in case the goal is not accomplished.

Documenting the Plan of Care

The plan for care can be handwritten (Fig. 2-4), standardized, computer generated, or based on an agency's *Standards for Care*. Whatever system is used, the Joint Commission on Accreditation of Health Organizations (JCAHO), requires that every patient's medical record provide evidence of the planned nursing interventions for meeting the patient's needs (Carpenito, 1991).

Nursing orders are the directions for a patient's care; they identify the what, when, where, and how for performing nursing measures. Nursing orders must be specific so that all health team members understand ex-

---

DISPLAY 2-7. *Components of Short-Term Goals*

Nursing Diagnostic Statement

Constipation related to decreased fluid intake, lack of dietary fiber, and lack of exercise as manifested by absence of a normal bowel movement for the past 3 days, abdominal cramping, and straining to pass stool.

Short-Term Goal

The patient will ————————— *patient centered*

have a bowel movement ————— identifies *measurable* criteria that reflect the *problem portion* of the diagnostic statement

in 2 days ————————————— identifies a *target date* for achievement

(specify date) within a *realistic* time frame

Name: Mrs. Rita Willard   Age: 68   Date of Admission: 11/10

Diagnosis on admission: CVA c̄ left-sided weakness

Nursing diagnosis: Impaired Physical Mobility, High Risk for Injury, Situational Low Self-esteem

Long-term goals: Independent mobility using walker or quad cane, record of personal safety, positive self-regard

DATE	PROBLEM	GOAL	TARGET DATE	NURSING ORDERS
11/10	#1 Impaired Physical Mobility related to left-sided weakness as manifested by decreased muscle strength in left leg and arm, slowed gait, dragging foot.	Will stand and pivot from bed to wheelchair or commode.	11/24	1) Passive ROM t.i.d. to left arm and leg 2) Physical therapy b.i.d. for practice at parallel bars 3) Apply left leg brace and sling to left arm when up 4) Assist to balance on right leg at bedside before and after physical therapy daily C. Meyer, RN
11/10	#2 High Risk for Injury related to Motor deficit	Will transfer from bed to wheelchair without injury	12/1	1) Keep side rails up and trapeze over bed 2) Use shoe c̄ nonskid sole on right foot (leg brace on left) before transfer 3) Dangle for 5 minutes before attempting to stand 4) Lock wheels on wheelchair before transfer 5) Obtain help of second assistant 6) Block left foot to avoid slipping during pivot 7) Place signal light on right side within reach at all times C. Meyer, RN
12/2	#3 Situational Low Self-Esteem related to dependence on others as manifested by statements "I need as much help as a baby; I feel so useless; how embarrassing to be so dependent."	Will identify one or more examples of improved mobility and self-care	12/18	1.) Allow to express feelings without disagreeing or interrupting. 2.) Reinforce concept that the right side of body is unaffected. 3.) Help to set and accomplish one realistic goal daily. S. Moore, RN

FIGURE 2-4
Sample nursing care plan. (Scherer JC, Timby BK. Introductory Medical–Surgical Nursing. 6th ed, p 13. Philadelphia: JB Lippincott, 1995.)

DISPLAY 2-8. *Nursing Orders*

Nursing Order	Weakness	Improvement
Encourage fluids.	Lacks specificity	Provide 100 mL of oral fluid every hour while awake.
	Likely to be interpreted differently	
	May result in inconsistent or less-than-adequate care	

[handwritten margin note: give specific hours]

actly what to do for the patient (Display 2-8). Nursing orders are also signed to indicate accountability.

Standardized care plans are preprinted. Both computer-generated and standardized plans provide general suggestions for managing the nursing care of patients with a particular problem. It is up to the nurse to transform the generalized interventions into specific nursing orders and eliminate whatever is inappropriate or unnecessary.

Agency-specific *Standards for Care* also relieve the nurse from having to write time-consuming plans. The printed standards identify the nursing interventions that will be implemented within that agency depending on the patient's identified problems. The standards provide for an efficient use of nursing time and ensure consistency in providing high-quality care.

Communicating the Plan

Goal achievement depends on consistency and continuity of care. Therefore, the nurse shares the plan for care with nursing team members, the patient, and the patient's family. In some clinical agencies, the patient co-signs the written care plan.

The plan for care is a permanent part of the patient's medical record. It may be placed within the patient's chart, kept separate at the patient's bedside, or kept in a temporary folder at the nurses' station for easier access. Wherever the plan of care is located, it is referred to daily by each nurse assigned to the patient's care, reviewed for its appropriateness, and revised according to the changes in the patient's condition.

IMPLEMENTATION

Implementation, the fourth step in the nursing process, involves carrying out the plan for care. This includes the medical orders as well as the nursing orders, which should complement each other.

Implementing the plan involves the patient and one or more members of the health care team. In essence,

there is a wide circle of care providers with assorted roles who may be called on to participate, either directly or indirectly, in carrying out one patient's plan for care.

Documentation

The medical record must show that the plan for care has been more than just a paper trail. There must be a correlation between the plan and the documented care; in other words, the nurse's charting (see Chap. 9) is a mirror image of the written plan. If nursing orders have not been carried out, the reason should be explained. Accountability for carrying out nursing orders should not be any less than that for doctor's orders.

In addition to identifying what care has been provided, the record also describes the quantity and quality of the patient's response. Quoting the patient helps identify what is occurring from the patient's point of view and safeguards against making incorrect assumptions.

Appropriate documentation maintains open lines of communication among members of the health care team, ensures the continuing progress of the patient, complies with accreditation standards, and facilitates reimbursement from government or private insurance companies.

EVALUATION

Evaluation is the process of determining if, or how well, a goal has been reached. By analyzing the patient's response, evaluation helps to determine the effectiveness of the plan for care (Display 2-9). Although it is considered the last step in the nursing process, it is actually one that is ongoing.

Before revising a plan of care, it is important to discuss the lag or lack of progress with the patient. In this way, both the nurse and the patient can speculate on what activities need to be discontinued, added, or

DISPLAY 2-9. *Outcomes From Evaluation*

Analysis	Reason	Action
Goals have been reached	Plan was effective and implemented consistently	Discontinue the nursing orders
Some progress has been made	Care has been inconsistent	Check that nursing orders are clear and specific
	Target date was too ambitious	Continue care as planned; readjust target date
	Patient's response has been less than expected	Revise the plan by adding additional nursing interventions or more frequent implementation
No progress has occurred	Inaccurate initial diagnosis	Revise problem list; write new goals and nursing orders
	New problems have occurred	Add new problems, goals, and nursing orders
	Unrealistic target date	Revise expected date for achievement
	Ineffective nursing interventions	Add new nursing orders; discontinue ineffective measures; readjust target date

changed. Other health team members who are familiar with a particular patient or problems similar to those of the patient's may offer their expertise as well. The evaluation of a patient's progress may be the subject of a nursing team conference. Some progressive units even invite the patient and his or her family to attend and participate.

USING THE NURSING PROCESS

Use of the nursing process is generally accepted as the standard for determining the quality of nursing care. More detailed discussions of the nursing process can be found in specialty texts and in some of the bibliographic entries at the end of this chapter. Guidelines follow that describe the essential steps for using the nursing process.

NURSING GUIDELINES FOR USING THE NURSING PROCESS

- Collect information about the patient.
  Rationale: Provides the basis for identifying problems
- Organize the data.
  Rationale: Simplifies the process of analysis
- Analyze the data for what is normal and abnormal.
  Rationale: Provides clues to the patient's problems

- Identify actual, potential, possible nursing diagnoses, and collaborative problems.
  Rationale: Directs the nurse to select methods for maintaining or restoring the patient's health
- Prioritize the problem list.
  Rationale: Targets those problems that require the most attention
- Set goals with specific criteria for evaluating whether the problems have been prevented, reduced, or resolved.
  Rationale: Predicts the expected outcomes from nursing care
- Select a limited number of appropriate nursing interventions.
  Rationale: Uses scientific knowledge to determine which measures will be most effective in accomplishing the goals of care
- Give specific directions for nursing care.
  Rationale: Promotes consistency and continuity among caregivers
- Document the plan for care using whatever written format is acceptable.
  Rationale: Provides a reference for the nursing team to follow
- Discuss the plan with nursing team members, the patient, and family.
  Rationale: Ensures that everyone is informed and goal-directed
- Put the plan into action.
  Rationale: Promotes goal achievement
- Observe the patient's responses.

Rationale: Forms the basis for determining the effectiveness of the plan for care
- Chart all nursing activities and the patient's responses.
  Rationale: Demonstrates that the planned care has been implemented and provides information as to the patient's progress
- Compare the patient's responses with the goal criteria.
  Rationale: Indicates progress toward accomplishing goals
- Discuss the progress, or lack of it, with the patient, family, and other nursing team members.
  Rationale: Provides a forum for better alternatives when revising the plan for care
- Change the plan in areas that are no longer appropriate.
  Rationale: Ensures the care plan is current
- Continue to implement and evaluate the revised plan for care.
  Rationale: Promotes a continuous sequence of actions that is repeated until the goals have been met

KEY CONCEPTS

- The nursing process is an organized sequence of steps used to solve health problems.
- The steps in the nursing process include assessment, diagnosis, planning, implementation, and evaluation.
- The nursing process is within the legal scope of nursing, based on unique knowledge, planned, patient centered, goal directed, prioritized, and dynamic.
- Resources for data include the patient, the patient's family, medical records, and other health care workers.
- A data base assessment provides a vast amount of information about a patient at the time of admission. Focus assessments, which are ongoing, expand the data base with additional information.
- A nursing diagnosis is a health problem that nurses can independently treat. A collaborative problem is a physiologic complication that requires the skills and interventions of both nurses and physicians.
- A nursing diagnostic statement consists of (1) the problem portion, (2) the etiology for the problem, and (3) the signs and symptoms, or evidence for the problem.
- Because hospitalizations are exceedingly short, setting priorities for care helps to maximize efficiency in a minimum amount of time.
- Short-term goals are those the nurse expects to accomplish in a few days to a week when caring for pa-

tients in an acute-care setting like a hospital. Long-term goals are those that may take weeks to months to accomplish. They are identified when caring for patients with chronic problems who are receiving nursing care in a long-term health facility, through community health agencies, or through home health care.
- The plan for care may be documented by writing all the problems, goals, and nursing orders by hand; referring to an agency's *Standards for Care;* or using a standardized or computer-generated care plan.
- Implementation of the plan of care is demonstrated by correlating the written plan with the nurse's documentation in the medical record.
- When evaluating the patient's progress, nursing orders may be discontinued if the goal has been met and the problem no longer exists; the care plan may be revised if there has been progress but the goal remains unmet, or if there has been no progress in reaching a desired outcome.

CRITICAL THINKING EXERCISES

- If an unconscious patient is brought to the nursing unit, explain how you would develop a data base.
- There are three nursing diagnoses on a patient's plan of care. They are Ineffective Breathing, Social Isolation, and Anxiety. Which one has the highest priority, and why?
- When a nurse reviews a patient's plan of care, it is noted that no progress has been made in accomplishing the goal by its projected target date. Discuss what actions would be appropriate at this time.

SUGGESTED READINGS

Alfaro-LeFevre R. Applying Nursing Process: A Step-by-Step Guide. 3rd ed. Philadelphia: JB Lippincott, 1994.

Booth B. Nursing diagnosis: one step forward . . . adopting a system of approved nursing diagnoses. Nursing Times February 12–18, 1992;88:32–33.

Carpenito LJ. Has JCAHO eliminated care plans? American Nurse June 1991;23:6.

Carpenito LJ. Nursing Diagnosis: Application to Clinical Practice. 5th ed. Philadelphia: JB Lippincott, 1993.

Maslow A. Toward a Psychology of Being. 2nd ed. New York: D Von Nostrand, 1968.

McKenna H, Deeney P. The heart of communication . . . primary nursing cannot exist without good care plans. Nursing Times July 8–14, 1992;88:54, 56–58.

Walker D. A-ND-I-O: linking nursing notes and care plans. Nursing Management August 1993;24:58–59.

Worthy MK, Siegrist-Mueller L. Integrating a "plan of care" into documentation systems. Nursing Management October 1992;23:68–70, 72.

UNIT II

Integrating Basic Concepts

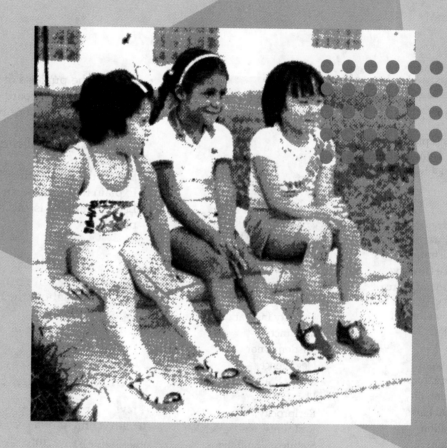

CHAPTER 3
Laws and Ethics

Key Terms

Administrative Laws
Advance Directive
Allocation of Scarce
Resources
Anecdotal Record
Assault
Battery
Civil Laws
Code of Ethics
Confidentiality
Criminal Laws
Defamation
Defendant
Ethics
False Imprisonment
Felony
Good Samaritan Laws

Incident Report
Intentional Torts
Invasion of Privacy
Law
Liability Insurance
Malpractice
Misdemeanor
Negligence
Nurse Practice Act
Plaintiff
Reciprocity
Restraints
Statute of Limitations
Tort
Truth Telling
Unintentional Torts
Whistle-blowing

Learning Objectives

An understanding of the content within this chapter will be evidenced by the student's ability to:

- Differentiate between administrative, criminal, and civil laws

- Discuss the purpose of nurse practice acts and the role of the state's board of nursing
- Explain the difference between intentional and unintentional torts
- Describe the difference between negligence and malpractice
- Define the term "ethics"
- Explain the purpose for a code of ethics
- List five ethical issues that are common in nursing practice

Laws, ethics, patient rights, and nursing duties affect nurses throughout their careers. This chapter introduces basic legal and ethical concepts as well as issues that affect the practice of nursing.

LAWS

A **law** is a rule of conduct established and enforced by the government of a society. Administrative, criminal, and civil laws are intended to protect both society as a whole and private individuals.

Administrative Laws

Administrative laws empower federal and state governments with legal authority to ensure the health and safety of citizens. For example, the Food and Drug Administration is authorized by the federal government to protect the public from the sale of impure or dangerous substances. State governments, on the other hand, uphold the duty to protect their respective residents by regulating the licensing and practice of people who provide health services within the state.

Timby BK: *Fundamental Skills and Concepts in Patient Care, Sixth Edition* © 1996 Lippincott-Raven Publishers

DISPLAY 3-1. *Sample Nurse Practice Act*

The term "the practice of practical nursing" means the performance for compensation of any of those services in observing and caring for the ill, injured or infirm, in applying counsel and procedures to safeguard the life and health in administering treatment and medication prescribed by a licensed physician or dentist which are commonly performed by licensed practical nurses and which require specialized knowledge and skill such as are taught or acquired. (Adopted by the Indiana General Assembly, 1974.)

NURSE PRACTICE ACTS

A **nurse practice act** is a form of state legislation that legally defines the unique role of the nurse and differentiates it from those of other health care practitioners, such as physicians, pharmacists, and physical therapists (Display 3-1). Although each state's nurse practice act is unique, all usually contain three elements: (1) they define the scope of nursing practice; (2) they establish the limits to that practice; and (3) they identify the titles that nurses may use, such as licensed practical nurse (LPN), licensed vocational nurse (LVN), or registered nurse (RN).

State Boards of Nursing

Each state's board of nursing is the regulatory agency for managing the provisions of its nurse practice act. The board of nursing develops rules and regulations for the education and licensing of individuals who wish to practice as nurses within the state.

The state board of nursing also has the responsibility for suspending and revoking licenses and reviewing applications requesting reciprocity. **Reciprocity** refers to obtaining a license to practice nursing based on evidence of having met similar criteria for licensure in another state.

Although the intent of reciprocity is primarily to facilitate employment for nurses who live in one state and work in another, or who move from one state to another, the practice has been subject to abuse. For example, it was not impossible for people relieved of their licenses as a punitive measure in one state, to move to another and obtain a license. Recently, however, legislation has been enacted to track incompetent practitioners. Since 1989, the names of licensed health care workers, such as nurses, who are disciplined by hospitals, courts, licensing boards, professional associations, insurers, and peer review committees are submitted to a National Practitioner Data Bank. This data bank is a computerized resource sponsored by the Office of Quality Assurance, a branch within the Department of Health and Human Services. The information that is compiled is made available to licensing boards and health care facilities who hire nurses throughout the nation.

Criminal Laws

Criminal laws protect the public's welfare. Violation of a criminal law is referred to as a crime. The state represents "the people" when prosecuting individuals accused of crimes. Crimes may be either misdemeanors or felonies.

MISDEMEANORS VERSUS FELONIES

A **misdemeanor** is a minor offense, like shoplifting. If convicted, a small fine, short-term incarceration of usually less than 1 year, or both, may be levied. The fine is paid to the state.

A **felony** is a serious offense, like murder, falsifying medical records, insurance fraud, and stealing narcotics. Conviction of a felony is punishable by imprisonment for longer than 1 year, or even execution. The state generally prohibits convicted felons from obtaining an occupational license, or revokes licenses after a conviction.

Civil Laws

Civil laws are statutes that protect the personal freedoms and rights of individuals. Some examples include the right to be left alone, freedom from threats of injury, freedom from offensive contact, and freedom from character attacks. Civil infractions are called torts. A **tort** is litigation in which one citizen asserts that an injury, which may be physical, emotional, or financial, occurred as a consequence of another citizen's actions or failure to act.

Torts may be considered intentional or unintentional. The accused person is the **defendant**; the individual claiming injury is called the **plaintiff**. Each person involved in a tort is personally responsible for legal fees. If found guilty of a tort, the defendant is required to pay the plaintiff restitution for damages.

INTENTIONAL TORTS

Intentional torts refer to lawsuits in which a plaintiff charges that the defendant committed a deliberately aggressive act. Examples of intentional torts include assault, battery, false imprisonment, invasion of privacy, and defamation.

Assault

Assault is an act in which there is a threat or attempt to do bodily harm. This may be in the form of physical intimidation, a verbal remark, or a gesture the plaintiff interprets to mean that force may be forthcoming. A nurse may be accused of assault if she or he makes a verbal threat to restrain a patient unnecessarily, for example to curtail the use of the signal light.

Battery

Battery occurs when there is unauthorized physical contact. The contact can include touching a person's body, clothing, chair, or bed. A charge of battery can be made even if the contact does not actually cause physical harm to the person. The criterion is that the contact took place without the plaintiff's consent.

Sometimes nonconsensual physical contact can be justified. For example, health professionals may use physical force to subdue mentally ill patients or those under the influence of alcohol or drugs if their actions endanger their own safety or that of others. However, documentation must show that the situation required the degree of restraint that was used. Excessive force is never appropriate when less would have been just as effective. When recording information about these types of situations, it is essential to describe the behavior and the response of the patient when lesser forms of restraint were used first.

To protect health care workers from being charged with battery, adult patients are asked to sign a general permission for care and treatment at the time of admission (Fig. 3-1) and additional written consent forms for special tests, procedures, or surgery. Consent must be obtained from a parent or guardian in cases where the patient is a minor, mentally retarded, or mentally incompetent. In an emergency, consent can be implied. In other words, it is assumed that in life-threatening circumstances, if a patient was able to understand the risks, consent for treatment would be given.

False Imprisonment

A charge of false imprisonment can be made if a nurse interferes with a person's freedom to move about at will without legal authority to do so. Forced confinement may be legal if there is a judicial restraining order, court-ordered commitment, or medical order. Otherwise, a nurse cannot detain a competent patient from leaving the hospital or other type of health care agency. It is customary to request that a patient who intends to leave without being medically discharged sign a form indicating personal responsibility for leaving against medical advice (Fig. 3-2). The purpose of the form is to ensure protection from future allegations of negligence or malpractice.

Physical Restraints. Restraints are devices or methods that restrict movement. Examples include cloth limb restraints, bed rails, chairs with locking lap trays, and even drugs that are intended to subdue a patient's activity. The unnecessary or unprescribed application of physical restraints creates a potential liability for charges of false imprisonment or battery, or both.

The Nursing Home Reform Act of the Omnibus Budget Reconciliation Act (OBRA), passed in 1987 and implemented in 1990, mandates that residents in nursing homes have "the right to be free of and the facility must ensure freedom from any restraints imposed or psychoactive drug administered for purposes of discipline or convenience, and not required to treat the residents' medical symptoms." This is not to say that restraints cannot be used. Their use, however, should be the last resort taken, rather than the initial intervention. Furthermore, their use must be justified and accompanied by informed consent from the patient or responsible relative.

The best legal advice is first to implement alternative measures for protecting the wandering patient, reducing the potential for falls (see Chap. 19), and ensuring that the patient does not jeopardize medical treatment by pulling out feeding tubes or other therapeutic devices. However, if less restraining alternatives are unsuccessful, it is essential that the nurse obtain a medical order before each and every instance in which restraints are used. Once they are applied, charting must indicate that the patient was assessed frequently, offered fluids and nourishment, given an opportunity for bowel and bladder elimination, and released from the restraints for a trial period to justify their continued use. Once the patient is no longer a danger to himself or herself or others, the restraints must be removed.

Invasion of Privacy

The law holds that law-abiding people have the right to expect that they and their property will be left alone. Failure to do so, without a person's consent, constitutes an invasion of privacy. Torts of a nonmedical nature usually involve allegations of trespassing, illegal search and seizure, wiretapping, and revealing personal information about someone, even if the information is true.

Medical instances where privacy laws may be violated include photographing a patient without consent, revealing a patient's name in a public report, or allowing an unauthorized person to observe the patient's care. To ensure and protect patients' rights to privacy, medical records and information are kept confidential, personal names and identities are concealed or obliterated in case studies or research, privacy curtains are used during care, and permission is obtained if a nursing or medical student will be present as an observer during a procedure.

THREE RIVERS AREA HOSPITAL
THREE RIVERS, MICHIGAN 49093

CONSENT FOR INPATIENT, OUTPATIENT, MEDICAL AND / OR SURGICAL TREATMENT

PATIENT'S NAME: _____

DATE & TIME: _____

I, the undersigned, knowing that I have a condition requiring hospital and medical treatment, do hereby voluntarily consent to such routine diagnostic procedures and hospital care by Dr. _____ _____ , his assistants or his designees, including such hospital personnel as he deems necessary.

I am aware that the practice of medicine is not an exact science and I acknowledge that no guarantees have been made to me as to the results of said outpatient care which I have hereby authorized.

If applicable, I hereby authorize Three Rivers Area Hospital to retain, preserve, and use of scientific or teaching purposes, or otherwise dispose of, at their convenience, any specimens, tissues, parts or organs taken from my (or patient's) body, as a result of the procedure or procedures authorized above.

I understand that the physician is not an employee or agent of Three Rivers Area Hospital but that as a practicing physician in the State of Michigan, he is granted the privilege to utilize the facilities of care at this hospital.

This notice is to inform you that Michigan law allows this hospital to test your blood for the presence of antibodies which may indicate you have been exposed to HIV (AIDS). This test is permitted by Michigan law and may be done without your permission if any hospital personnel are exposed to blood and body fluids in the course of care for you. This is for your protection as well as for the course of care for you. This is for your protection as well as for the protection of the physicians, nurses and other associates of this hospital.

This form has been fully explained to me and I certify that I understand its contents.

_____   _____
Patient's Signature   Date

_____   _____
Witness   Date

If patient is unable to sign or is a minor, complete the following:
Patient is a minor, _____ years of age, and/or is unable to sign because:

_____

_____   _____
Signature (Closest Relative or Legal Guardian)   Date

_____   _____
Relationship to patient   Witness

FIGURE 3-1
Consent for treatment form. (Scherer JC, Timby BK. Introductory Medical–Surgical Nursing. 6th ed, p 29. Philadelphia: JB Lippincott, 1995.)

Defamation

Defamation is an act in which *untrue* information harms a person's reputation. If the character attack is uttered orally in the presence of others, it is called **slander**. If the damaging statement is written and read by others, it is called **libel**. Nurses must avoid offering unfounded or exaggerated negative opinions about clients, the expertise of physicians, or other coworkers. Injury is felt to occur because the derogatory remarks attack a person's character and good name.

UNINTENTIONAL TORTS

Unintentional torts involve situations that result in an injury, although the person responsible did not purposely mean to cause harm. Cases of unintentional torts involve allegations of negligence or malpractice.

THREE RIVERS HOSPITAL
THREE RIVERS, MICHIGAN 49093

Release from Responsibility for Discharge

Date: _____   Time: _____   A.M.
                                                                      P.M.

PATIENT: _____

This is to certify that I _____, a patient in
the _____ Hospital am being discharged
against the advice of the attending physician and the hospital administration. I acknowledge that I have
been informed of the risk involved and hereby release the attending physician and the hospital from all
responsibility for any ill effects which may result from such discharge.

Witnesses:

_____

                                                    (Signature of Patient)

_____

                                        (To be signed by the legal
                                        representative in case of a
                                        minor or of a patient who
                                        is not mentally competent,
                                        otherwise by the patient.)

FIGURE 3-2
Release form for discharging oneself against medical advice. (Scherer JC, Timby BK. Introductory Medical–Surgical Nursing. 6th ed, p 30. Philadelphia: JB Lippincott, 1995.)

Negligence

Negligence may be charged when a person claims to have been harmed because an individual did not act *reasonably* (eg, acted carelessly). In negligence cases, a jury decides if any other prudent person would have acted differently than the defendant given the same set of circumstances. Take, for example, a situation in which a person's car breaks down on the highway and the driver pulls the car to the side of the road, raises the hood, and activates the emergency flashing lights. If the disabled car is struck by another vehicle and the driver of the second car sues, the disabled car owner's guilt or innocence hinges on whether the jury feels the car owner's action was reasonable. *Reasonableness is based on the jury's opinion of what constitutes good common sense.*

Malpractice

Malpractice is a lawsuit alleging a professional's negligence. It differs from simple negligence in that it holds professionals to a higher standard of accountability. Rather than being held accountable for acting as an ordinary, reasonable lay person, in a malpractice case, the court would determine if a nurse or other health care worker acted in a manner comparable to that of his or her peers. There are four elements that must be proven to win a malpractice lawsuit; they include duty, breach of duty, causation, and injury (Display 3-2).

Because the jury may be unfamiliar with the scope of nursing practice, other resources may be presented in court to prove breach of duty. Some examples include the employing agency's standards for care, written policies and procedures, standardized care plans, and the testimony of expert witnesses.

Malpractice Lawsuits. The best protection from malpractice lawsuits is competent nursing. Competency can be demonstrated by participating in continuing education programs, taking nursing courses at a college or university, and becoming certified. Defensive nursing practice also involves thorough and objective documentation (see Chap. 9).

Probably the best defense against a lawsuit is to administer care compassionately. The "golden rule" of doing unto others as you would have them do unto you is a good principle to follow. Patients who per-

DISPLAY 3-2. *Elements in a Malpractice Case*

Duty

An obligation existed to provide care for the person who claims to have been injured or harmed

Breach of Duty

Failure to provide appropriate care, or the care that was provided was done so in a negligent manner, that is, in a manner that conflicts with how others with similar education would have acted given the same set of circumstances

Causation

The professional's action, or lack of it, caused the plaintiff harm

Injury

Physical, psychological, or financial harm occurred

---

ceive the nurse as caring and concerned tend to be satisfied with their care. These techniques communicate a caring attitude:

- Smile.
- Introduce yourself by name.
- Call the patient by the name he or she prefers.
- Touch the patient appropriately to demonstrate concern.
- Respond quickly to the call light.
- Communicate the time you will be leaving the unit, how long you will be detained, and inform the patient of your return.
- Provide the name of the person to whom you have delegated the patient's care in your absence.
- Spend time with the patient other than performing required care.
- Be a good listener.
- Explain everything so a patient can understand it.
- Be a good host or hostess; offer visitors extra chairs, snacks and beverages, directions for the restrooms and parking areas.
- Accept justifiable criticism without becoming defensive.
- Say "I'm sorry."

The patient can sense when the nurse really wants to do a good job rather than just do a job. A positive relationship is apt to reduce the potential for a lawsuit, even if harm occurs.

Professional Liability

Currently, all professionals, including nurses, are held responsible and accountable for providing safe, appropriate care. Because nurses possess specialized knowledge and work closely with patients, they have a primary role in protecting those entrusted to their care from preventable or reversible complications.

The number of lawsuits involving nurses is increasing. Therefore, it is to every nurse's advantage to obtain liability insurance and to become familiar with legal mechanisms, such as Good Samaritan laws and statutes of limitations, that may prevent or relieve culpability, as well as with strategies for providing a sound legal defense, such as written incident reports and anecdotal records.

LIABILITY INSURANCE

Liability insurance is a contract between an individual or corporation and a company that is willing to provide legal services and financial assistance when its policy holder is involved in a malpractice lawsuit. Although many agencies that employ nurses have liability insurance with an umbrella clause that includes its employees, it is recommended that nurses obtain their own personal liability insurance. This practice then enables nurses to have a separate attorney working on his or her sole behalf. Because the damages sought in malpractice lawsuits are so costly, the attorneys hired by the hospital are sometimes more committed to defending the hospital against liability and negative publicity, rather than an employed nurse whom they also are being paid to represent.

Student nurses are held accountable for their actions during clinical practice and should also carry liability insurance. Liability insurance is available through the National Federation for Licensed Practical Nurses (NFLPN), the National Student Nurses Association, the American Nurses Association (ANA), and other private insurance companies.

REDUCING LIABILITY

It is unrealistic to think that lawsuits can be totally avoided. There are, nevertheless, some avenues that protect nurses and other health care workers from being sued or that provide a foundation for a sound legal defense. It is essential for nurses to be aware of how Good Samaritan laws, statutes of limitations, incident reports, and anecdotal records can limit or reduce liability.

Good Samaritan Laws

Good Samaritan laws, a name based on the Biblical story of the person who gave aid to a beaten stranger along a roadside, have been enacted in many states. In essence, these laws provide legal immunity for passers-by who provide emergency first aid to accident victims.

None of the Good Samaritan laws, however, provide absolute exemption from prosecution in the event of an injury. Paramedics, ambulance personnel, physicians, and nurses who stop to provide assistance are still held to a higher standard of care because they supposedly have training above and beyond that of average lay people.

Statute of Limitations

When it comes to civil laws, each state establishes a statute of limitations (Fig. 3-3). A **statute of limitations** is a designated amount of time within which a person can file a lawsuit. The time is usually calculated from the time the incident occurred. However, when the injured party is a minor, the statute of limitations sometimes does not commence until the victim reaches adulthood. Once the time period expires, an injured party can no longer sue even if their claim is legitimate.

Incident Reports

An **incident report** is a written account of an unusual event involving a patient, employee, or visitor that has the potential for being injurious (Fig. 3-4). Incident reports, which are kept separate from the medical record, serve two purposes. Primarily, they are used to determine how hazardous situations can be prevented; and secondarily, they are used as a reference in case of any future litigation. Incident reports

must include five important pieces of information: (1) when the incident occurred, (2) where it took place, (3) who was involved, (4) what happened exactly, and (5) what actions were taken at the time. All witnesses are identified by name. Any pertinent statements made by the injured person, before or after the incident, are quoted. Accurate and detailed documentation can often help prove that the nurse acted reasonably or appropriately in a particular set of circumstances.

Anecdotal Records

An **anecdotal record** is a personal, handwritten account of an incident. Anecdotal notations are not recorded on any official form nor filed with administrative records. The information is retained by the nurse. The notation is safeguarded and may be used later to refresh the nurse's memory if a lawsuit develops. Anecdotal notes can be used in court on advice of an attorney.

Malpractice Litigation

A successful outcome in a malpractice lawsuit depends on many variables such as the physical evidence and the expertise of one's lawyer. However, the appearance, demeanor, and conduct of the nurse defendant inside and outside the courtroom can contribute or damage the case as well. The suggestions in Display 3-3 may be helpful should a nurse become involved in malpractice litigation.

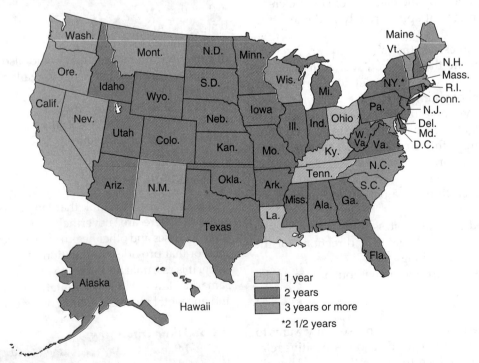

FIGURE 3-3
A guide to statutes of limitation on a state-by-state basis.

THREE RIVERS AREA HOSPITAL INCIDENT REPORT

Confidential - DO NOT DUPLICATE

Forward to Risk Management within 48 hours

Identification	Sex	Age	Incident Date	Time	Shift	Department
__Inpatient	__M	__	__/__/__	__:__	__1st	
__Outpatient	__F				__2nd	_____
__Visitor					__3rd	

Addressograph

Reason for hospitalization/presence on premises: _____

I.   Location of Incident
  __Patient Room #_____
  __Patient Bathroom
  __Corridor
  __Other _____

II. Type of Incident
  __Fall   __Treatment/Procedure
  __Medication   __Equipment
  __Infusion   __Needle/Sponge Count
  __Lost/Found   __Other_____
  __Burn

III. Description of Incident _____
_____
_____

IV. Nature of Incident
  A. **Falls:**

Activity Order:	Pt. Condition Prior to:	Fall Involved:	Patient/Visitor was:
__Restraints	__Weak, unsteady	__Chair, W/C	__Lying
__Bedrest only	__Alert, oriented	__Stretcher	__Standing
__BRP	__Disoriented/confused	__Tub/Shower	__Getting on/off
__Up w/asst.	__Senile	__Toilet	__Sitting
__Up AD LIB	__Unconscious	__Floor Condition(below)	__Ambulating
	__Medicated/Sedated	__Bed	__Other_____
	Med. Name _____	__Side Rails Up	_____
	Last Dose _____	__Side Rails Down	_____

  B. **Medications:**
Incident Involved:
  __Wrong Med, Tx, Procedure   __Adverse Reaction   __Patient I.D. Not Checked
  __Wrong Patient   __Infiltration   __Transcription
  __Wrong Time   __Other_____   __Labeling
  __Omission   _____   __Physician orders not clear
  __Incorrect Dose   _____   __Physician orders not checked
  __Incorrect Method of   _____   __Misread label/dose
    Administration   __Charting
                                                            __Wrong Med from Pharmacy
                                                            __Defective equipment
                                                            __Communications
                                                            __Other_____

  C. **Other:**
  __Loss of Property   __Equipment malfunction   __Patient ID
  __Struck by object, equipment   __Anesthesia   __Other_____

V.   Nature of Injury (Injury sustained as a result of incident):
  __Asphyxia, Strangulation,   __Fracture or dislocation __Burn or Scald
    Inhalation   __Viscera Injury   __Chemical Burn
  __Head Injury   __Sprain or strain   __No injury
  __Contagious or infectious   __Contusion, Cut,   __No apparent injury
    Disease Exposure   Laceration   __Other_____

VI. Action Taken:
  Physician __Yes   PT/Visitor seen by MD/T&EC   MD Name
  Notified   __No   __Yes   __No   _____
  Physician's Findings: _____   Time :__
  _____

  Other follow up: ___No __Yes - Specify_____

_____	__/__/__	_____	__/__/__
Name of Person Reporting	Date	Department Director	Date
_____	__/__/__	_____	__/__/__
Supervisor	Date	Risk Management	Date

8311-109

FIGURE 3-4

An incident report form. (Scherer JC, Timby BK. Introductory Medical–Surgical Nursing. 6th ed, p 35. Philadelphia: JB Lippincott, 1995.)

DISPLAY 3-3. *Legal Advice*

1. Notify the claims agent of your professional liability insurance company.
2. Contact the National Nurses Claims Data Base through the American Nurses Association. This confidential service provides information that supports nurses involved in litigation.
3. Discuss the particulars of the case only with your attorney.
4. Tell your attorney everything.
5. Avoid giving public statements.
6. Reread the patient's record, incident sheet, and your anecdotal note before testifying.
7. Ask to reread information again in court if it will help to refresh your memory.
8. Dress conservatively, in a businesslike manner. Avoid excesses in makeup, hairstyle, or jewelry.
9. Look directly at whomever asks a question.
10. Speak in a modulated but audible voice that can be heard easily by the jury and others in the court.
11. Tell the truth.
12. Use language you are comfortable with. Do not try to impress the court with legal or medical terms.
13. Say as little as possible in court under cross-examination.
14. Answer the prosecuting lawyer's questions with "Yes" or "No"; limit answers to only the questions that are asked.
15. If you do not know or cannot remember information, say so.
16. Wait to expand on information if asked by your defense attorney.
17. Remain calm, objective, and cooperative.

ETHICS

The word "ethics" comes from the Greek word *ethos*, meaning customs or modes of conduct. **Ethics** refers to moral or philosophical principles that define actions as being either right or wrong. Various organizations, such as those representing nurses, have identified standards for ethical practice, known as a code of ethics, for members within their discipline.

Codes of Ethics

A **code of ethics** is a list of written statements describing ideal behavior. The National Association for Practical Nurse Education and Services (NAPNES), the NFLPN, and the International Council of Nurses (ICN) are examples of organizations that have composed codes of ethics. Display 3-4 is a current code of ethics that was revised in 1985 by the ANA. Because of rapidly changing technology, no code of ethics is ever specific enough to provide answers to every dilemma that nurses may face.

ETHICAL DILEMMAS

Ethical dilemmas occur when individual values and laws conflict. This is especially true in relation to health care. From time to time, nurses find themselves in situations that may be considered legal, yet personally unethical; or ethical, but illegal. Take, for example, the issue of abortion. Abortion is legal, but there are some who believe it is unethical. Assisted suicide, on the other hand, is illegal, but some believe it is ethical.

Some guidelines that may be helpful in resolving an ethical dilemma include the following:

- Make sure that whatever is done is in the patient's best interest.
- Preserve and support the Patient's Bill of Rights (Display 3-5).
- Work cooperatively with the patient and other health care practitioners.
- Follow written policies, codes of ethics, and laws.
- Follow your conscience.

Ethics Committees

Ethical decisions are complex, especially when they affect the lives of patients. Because making a substituted judgment for another is a weighty responsibility, ethics committees have been established in many health agencies. Ethics committees are composed of professionals and nonprofessionals who represent a broad cross-section of people within the community, with varying viewpoints. Their diversity encourages

DISPLAY 3-4. *Code for Nurses*

1. The nurse provides services with respect for human dignity and the uniqueness of the client, unrestricted by considerations of social or economic status, personal attributes, or the nature of health problems.
2. The nurse safeguards the client's right to privacy by judiciously protecting information of a confidential nature.
3. The nurse acts to safeguard the client and the public when health care and safety are affected by incompetent, unethical, or illegal practice by any person.
4. The nurse assumes responsibility and accountability for individual nursing judgments and actions.
5. The nurse maintains competence in nursing.
6. The nurse exercises informed judgment and uses individual competency and qualifications as criteria in seeking consultation, accepting responsibilities, and delegating nursing activities.
7. The nurse participates in activities that contribute to the ongoing development of the profession's body of knowledge.
8. The nurse participates in the profession's efforts to implement and improve standards of nursing.
9. The nurse participates in the profession's efforts to establish and maintain conditions of employment conducive to high-quality nursing care.
10. The nurse participates in the profession's effort to protect the public from misinformation and misrepresentation and to maintain the integrity of nursing.
11. The nurse collaborates with members of the health professions and other citizens in promoting community and national efforts to meet the health needs of the public.

Reprinted with permission from Code for Nurses With Interpretive Statements. Kansas City, American Nurses Association, 1985.

healthy debate of ethical issues. Ethics committees are best used in a policy-making capacity before any specific dilemma occurs. However, ethics committees also may be called on to offer advice to protect a patient's best interests and to avoid legal battles.

Ethical Issues

There are several ethical issues that recur in nursing practice. Some common examples include telling the truth, maintaining confidentiality, withholding or withdrawing medical treatment, advocating for the most ethical allocation of scarce resources, and protecting vulnerable individuals from unsafe practices or practitioners.

TELLING THE TRUTH

Truth telling involves respecting the right of all patients to have information that is necessary for making their own health care decisions. This right implies that physicians and nurses have a duty to tell patients the truth about matters concerning their health. Therefore, in matters involving medical treatment, patients have the right to be told the status of their health problem, the benefits of treatment, alternative forms of treatment, and consequences if the treatment is not administered.

It is the physician's responsibility to inform patients. Conflict centers on whether (1) the patient has been given full information, (2) the facts have been misrepresented, and (3) the patient has understood the information correctly. In some cases a physician may be reluctant to talk honestly with patients, or the proposed treatment may be presented in a biased manner. The nurse is often forced to choose between remaining silent in allegiance to the physician or providing truthful information to the patient. Either action may have frustrating consequences.

CONFIDENTIALITY

The foundation of any patient relationship is trust. One way of ensuring trust is to protect the patient's right to confidentiality. **Confidentiality** involves safeguarding an individual's personal health information from public disclosure. Health information that the patient confides must not be divulged to unauthorized

DISPLAY 3-5. *A Patient's Bill of Rights*

1. The patient has the right to considerate and respectful care.

2. The patient has the right to and is encouraged to obtain from physicians and other direct caregivers relevant, current, and understandable information concerning diagnosis, treatment, and prognosis.

3. The patient has the right to make decisions about the plan of care prior to and during the course of treatment and to refuse a recommended treatment or plan of care to the extent permitted by law and hospital policy and to be informed of the medical consequences of this action.

4. The patient has the right to have an advance directive (such as a living will, health care proxy, or durable power of attorney for health care) concerning treatment or designating a surrogate decision maker with the expectation that the hospital will honor the intent of that directive to the extent permitted by law and hospital policy.

5. The patient has the right to every consideration of privacy. Case discussion, consultation, examination, and treatment should be conducted so as to protect each patient's privacy.

6. The patient has the right to expect that all communications and records pertaining to his or her care will be treated as confidential by the hospital, except in cases such as suspected abuse and public health hazards when reporting is permitted or required by law.

7. The patient has the right to review the records pertaining to his or her medical care and to have the information explained or interpreted as necessary, except when restricted by law.

8. The patient has the right to expect that, within its capacity and policies, a hospital will make reasonable response to the request of a patient for appropriate and medically indicated care and services. The hospital must provide evaluation, service, and/or referral as indicated by the urgency of the case.

9. The patient has the right to ask and be informed of the existence of business relationships among the hospital, educational institutions, other health care providers, or payers that may influence the patient's treatment and care.

10. The patient has the right to consent to or decline to participate in proposed research studies or human experimentation affecting care and treatment or requiring direct patient involvement, and to have those studies fully explained prior to consent.

11. The patient has the right to expect reasonable continuity of care when appropriate and to be informed by physicians and other caregivers of available and realistic patient care options when hospital care is no longer appropriate.

12. The patient has the right to be informed of hospital policies and practices that relate to patient care, treatment, and responsibilities.

© 1992 with permission of the American Hospital Association.

people without the patient's written permission. Even providing medical information to a patient's health insurance company requires a signed release.

Consequently, nurses must use discretion when sharing information verbally so that it is not overheard indiscriminately. Now that vast amounts of information about patients are stored and retrieved with computers, the duty to protect confidentiality extends to safeguarding written and electronic data as well.

WITHHOLDING AND WITHDRAWING TREATMENT

Because of the existence of sophisticated technology, it was often the practice to prolong life at all costs. Consequently, life-sustaining techniques were used beyond the point at which anyone could justify their benefits. Decisions involving life and death may in some cases continue to circumvent patients, which is clearly a violation of ethical principles.

There is now legislation that makes it mandatory to discuss the issue of terminal care with certain patients. Since the Patient Self-Determination Act was approved by Congress in 1990, health care agencies that are reimbursed through Medicare funds must ask elderly patients if they have executed an advance directive. An **advance directive** is a written statement identifying a competent person's wishes concerning his or her terminal care. In some cases, the advance directive may legally appoint another person with the power to make a proxy decision on their behalf (see Chap. 38).

Advanced directives are not reserved only for the elderly; they can be completed by any competent adult. They are best composed before a health crisis develops. Therefore, it is important that nurses inform all patients about their right to self-determination, encourage them to compose an advanced directive, and advocate and support the decisions they make.

ALLOCATION OF SCARCE RESOURCES

Allocation of scarce resources refers to the process of deciding how to distribute limited life-saving equipment or procedures among several who could benefit. In effect, what this means is that those who receive the resource will live and those who do not will die prematurely. Benefiting some results in harm to others.

Ethicists use various strategies to make this type of hard decision. They may elect a "first come/first serve" approach, or the choice may be made by trying to project which recipient if saved would result in the most good for the most number of people.

WHISTLE-BLOWING

Whistle-blowing refers to reporting incompetent or unethical practices. As the name implies, a person calls attention to an unsafe or potentially harmful situation within the institution where he or she is employed. For instance, a nurse may report another nurse or physician who cares for patients while under the influence of controlled substances such as alcohol or cocaine.

Usually, the first step is to report the situation to an immediate supervisor. However, if no action is taken, the reporter is faced with an ethical dilemma as to what further steps should be taken. Eventually, it may become necessary to go beyond the administrative hierarchy and make public revelations.

The decision to "blow the whistle" involves personal risks and may result in grave consequences such as character assassination, retribution in the form of crimes against one's person or property, negative evaluations, demotions, or being ostracized from the group. Nevertheless, the ethical priority is to protect patients in general and the community at large.

KEY CONCEPTS

- There are three types of laws: administrative, criminal, and civil.
- Administrative laws empower federal and state governments with legal authority to ensure the health and safety of citizens.
- Criminal laws protect the public's welfare; civil laws are statutes that protect personal freedoms and rights of individuals.
- Nurse practice acts are a type of state administrative law that defines the unique role of the nurse and differentiates it from those of other health care practitioners.
- Each state's board of nursing is the regulatory agency for managing the provision of its nurse practice act.
- In violations of criminal laws, the state prosecutes individuals for misdemeanors, which are minor offenses, or felonies, which are more serious.
- Violations of civil laws include intentional and unintentional torts.
- In an intentional tort, a private citizen sues another for a deliberately aggressive act.
- In unintentional torts, the lawsuit charges that harm occurred because of a person's negligence even though no harm was intended.
- Negligence lawsuits allege that a person's actions, or lack thereof, caused harm. The defendant is held to a standard expected of any other reasonable person.
- In the case of malpractice, the plaintiff alleges that a professional's actions, or lack thereof, caused harm. The defendant is held to the standard expected of others with similar knowledge and education.
- In a malpractice case, the prosecution must prove that the defendant (1) had a duty to the plaintiff, (2) the defendant breached that duty, (3) the breach of duty was the direct cause for harm, and (4) injury occurred.
- Liability for malpractice may be limited or reduced by the language within Good Samaritan laws, expiration of the statute of limitations, a timely and well written incident report, or a privately composed anecdotal record.
- Ethics refers to moral or philosophical principles that define actions as being right or wrong.
- A code of ethics is a written statement that describes ideal behavior for members belonging to a particular discipline.
- Some common ethical issues that nurses encounter in everyday practice include telling the truth, protecting patients' confidentiality, ensuring that patients' wishes for withholding and withdrawing treatment are followed, advocating for the nondiscriminatory allocation of scarce resources, and reporting incompetent or unethical practices.

CRITICAL THINKING EXERCISES

- Discuss the legal and ethical implications of falsifying narcotic medication records to steal controlled substances.
- A confused patient occasionally leaves the nursing home and has been found wandering outside the nursing home where he is a resident. What actions would you take to protect yourself from being sued?
- A heart becomes available for transplant. The tissue matches an adolescent and middle-aged patient who both are in need of the organ. What criteria might be used to decide which patient receives the organ transplant?

SUGGESTED READINGS

Bosek MD. Whistle blowing: an act of advocacy. MEDSURG Nursing December 1993;2:480–482.

Carson W. Nurses and professional boundaries: legal barriers to practice. American Nurse January 1993;25:26.

Coleman EA. Physical restraint use in nursing home patients with dementia. Journal of the American Medical Association November 3, 1993;17:2114–2115.

Data bank will track misbehaving health pros. American Journal of Nursing March 1989;89:418.

Grant A. Questions of life and death. Canadian Nurse May 1993; 13:31–34.

Haddad AM, Kapp MB. Legal implications of withholding and withdrawing medical treatment. Caring September 1991;10: 14–19.

Huntington SR. New provider responsibilities under the patient self-determination act. Caring September 1991;10:20–25.

Kallmann SL, Denine-Flynn M, Blackburn DM. Comfort, safety, and independence: restraint release and its challenges. Geriatric Nursing May–June 1992;13:142–148.

Post SG. To care but never to prolong? Caring June 1992;11:40–43.

Press MM. Restraints: protection or abuse? Canadian Nurse December 1991;11:29–30.

Sanchez-Sweatman L. What is informed consent? Canadian Nurse October 1993;89:49–50.

Varone L, Tappen RM, Dixon-Antonio E, Gonzales I, Glussman B. To restrain or not to restrain? The decision-making dilemma for nursing staff. Geriatric Nursing September–October 1992;13: 269–272.

CHAPTER 4

Health and Illness

Key Terms

Acute Illness	Morbidity
Case Method	Mortality
Chronic Illness	Nurse-managed Care
Congenital Disorder	Nursing Team
Continuity of Care	Primary Care
Exacerbation	Primary Illness
Extended Care	Primary Nursing
Functional Method	Remission
Health	Secondary Care
Health Care System	Secondary Illness
Health Care Team	Sequelae
Hereditary Condition	Team Nursing
Holism	Terminal Illness
Idiopathic Illness	Tertiary Care
Illness	

Learning Objectives

An understanding of the content within this chapter will be evidenced by the student's ability to:

• Describe how the World Health Organization (WHO) defines health

• Discuss the difference between values and beliefs
• List three health beliefs that are common among Americans
• Explain the concept of holism
• Identify five levels of human needs
• Define illness
• Explain the meaning of terms used to describe illnesses such as morbidity, mortality, acute, chronic, terminal, primary, secondary, remission, exacerbation, hereditary, congenital, and idiopathic
• Differentiate between primary, secondary, tertiary, and extended care
• Identify three national health goals targeted for the year 2000
• Discuss five patterns for administering patient care

Neither health nor illness is an absolute state; rather, there may be fluctuations along a continuum from time to time (Fig. 4-1). Because it is impossible to be well and stay well, or get well and remain well forever, nurses are committed to helping people prevent illness and restore or improve their health.

HEALTH

In the preamble of its constitution, the World Health Organization (WHO) defines **health** as "a state of complete physical, mental, and social well-being and not merely the absence of disease or infirmity." However, how each person perceives and defines health is varied and personal. It is important to respect individual differences rather than impose standards that may be personally unrealistic.

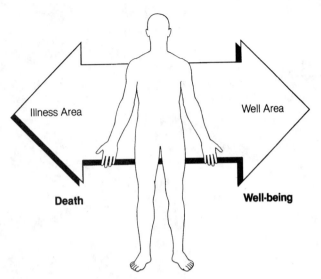

FIGURE 4-1
The health continuum.

Health Values and Beliefs

Health behaviors usually are an outcome of a person's values and belief system. Values are those ideals that a person feels are honorable attributes. Some examples include honesty, fidelity, dependability, and punctuality. Values guide a person's actions; they lead to behaviors that demonstrate or affirm the values that are prized. Thus, if someone values punctuality, he or she will strive to keep appointments on time. People who value health tend to act in ways to preserve it.

Beliefs are concepts that people hold to be true. When it comes to health, most Americans believe that health is a resource, a right, and a personal responsibility.

HEALTH—A LIMITED RESOURCE

A resource is a possession that is valuable because its supply is limited and it has no substitute. Given that definition, health is considered a resource. People often say, "as long as you have your health, you have everything," and "health is wealth."

HEALTH—A RIGHT

This country was established on the principle that all people are equal and entitled to life, liberty, and the pursuit of happiness. If this premise is accepted, then it would seem that everyone, regardless of age, gender, ethnic origin, social position, or wealth, is entitled to equal services for sustaining health. Unfortunately, as is discussed later in Chapter 6, there are disparities in the availability or quality of health care among various groups within the United States.

If all are equally deserving of health, it follows that the nation, in general, and nurses, in particular, have a duty to protect and preserve the health of those who may be unable to assert this right for themselves.

HEALTH—A PERSONAL RESPONSIBILITY

Health requires continuous personal effort. There is as much potential for illness as there is for health. Each person is instrumental in the outcome. Pilch (1981) said, "No one can do wellness to or for another; you alone do it, but you don't do it alone." Nurses stand ready to provide assistance and advocate on behalf of others.

WELLNESS

Wellness is a full and balanced integration of physical, emotional, social, and spiritual health. Physical health exists when body organs function normally. Emotional health results when one feels safe and capable of handling disappointments. Social health is an outcome of feeling accepted and useful, and spiritual health is characterized as feeling one's life is purposeful.

Holism

How "whole" or well an individual feels is the sum of his or her physical, emotional, social, and spiritual health, a concept referred to as **holism** (Fig. 4-2). Any change in one component—positive or negative—automatically causes similar repercussions in the others. Take, for example, the person who has a heart attack. There is an obvious and immediate impairment in the person's physical health. However, emotional, social, and spiritual health also are affected by the psycholog-

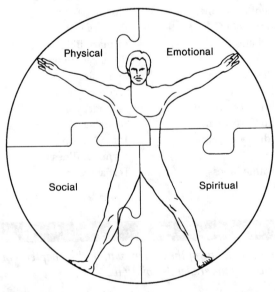

FIGURE 4-2
This diagram illustrates the concept of holism.

ical significance associated with the health change, the temporary or permanent alterations in social roles, and the philosophical issues that develop as the patient ponders the potential for death. Nurses, therefore, profess to be holistic practitioners because they are committed to restoring balance in each of the four spheres that affect health.

Hierarchy of Human Needs

In the 1960s, Abraham Maslow, a psychologist, identified various human needs that motivate behavior. He proposed that there are five levels of human needs (Fig. 4-3). He grouped them in tiers, or a sequential hierarchy, according to their significance: physiologic needs (first level), safety and security needs (second level), needs for love and belonging (third level), needs for esteem and self-esteem (fourth level), and self-actualization needs (fifth level).

The first-level needs, which are physiologic, are the most important. They are the activities that are needed to sustain life, like breathing and eating. Each higher level represents one of lesser importance to human existence than the ones previous to it. Maslow believed that until the physiologic needs are satisfied, humans could not or would not seek to fulfill needs less crucial to life. However, by progressively satisfying needs at each subsequent level, people can realize their maximum potential for health and well-being. Nurses have adopted Maslow's hierarchy as a tool for setting priorities for patient care.

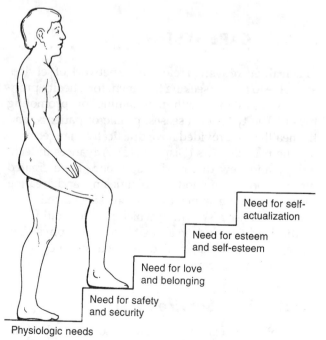

Need for self-actualization

Need for esteem and self-esteem

Need for love and belonging

Need for safety and security

Physiologic needs

FIGURE 4-3
Maslow's hierarchy of human needs.

ILLNESS

Illness is a state of discomfort that results when a person's health becomes impaired through disease, stress, or an accident or injury. There are several terms, including morbidity and mortality; acute, chronic, and terminal; primary and secondary; remission and exacerbation; and hereditary, congenital, and idiopathic, that are used when referring to illnesses.

Morbidity and Mortality

Morbidity refers to the incidence of a specific disease, disorder, or injury. The morbidity rate refers to the numbers of people affected. Statistics may be compiled on the basis of age, gender, or per 1,000 people within the population.

Mortality refers to death. The mortality rate of a given condition is the number of deaths per unit of population. Usually, mortality rates are calculated on the basis of 1,000 people (or some larger number). A list of the 10 leading causes of death among Americans and their rate of mortality is shown in Figure 4-4.

Acute, Chronic, and Terminal Illnesses

An **acute illness** is one that comes on suddenly and lasts a relatively short time. Influenza is an example of an acute illness. Although many acute illnesses can be cured, some lead to long-term problems because of their sequelae. **Sequelae** are ill effects that result from permanent or progressive organ damage caused by a disease or its treatment.

A **chronic illness** is one that comes on slowly and lasts a relatively long time. Arthritis, a joint disease, is an example of a chronic disease. As humans age, the incidence of chronic illnesses increases, causing many older adults to live with persistent health problems and disabilities.

A **terminal illness** is one in which there is no potential for cure. The terminal stage of an illness is one in which a person is approaching death.

Primary and Secondary Illnesses

A **primary illness** is one that has developed independently of any other disease. Any subsequent disorder that develops from a pre-existing condition is referred to as a **secondary illness**. For example, acquiring a pulmonary disease from smoking would be considered a primary illness. If heart failure developed, it would be considered a secondary problem due to the strain placed on the heart as a result of the pre-established respiratory condition. In essence, the heart failure was caused by the pulmonary disease and may not have occurred had the primary disease not been acquired.

While deaths from AIDS are more numerous than ever, lower death rates
from other major diseases mean Americans are living longer.
The average U.S. life expectancy is now 75.8 years

Rank	Cause of Death	1992 Age-adjusted death rate*	% change, 1979 to 1992
1	Heart Disease	144.3	−27.7 ↓
2	Cancer	133.1	1.8 ↑
3	Brain diseases	26.2	−37.0 ↓
4	Chronic lung diseases	19.9	36.3 ↑
5	Accidents	29.4	−31.5 ↓
	Motor-vehicle	15.8	−31.9 ↓
	All other	13.7	−30.1 ↓
6	Pneumonia and influenza	12.7	13.4 ↑
7	Diabetes	11.9	21.4 ↑
8	HIV infection	12.6	—
9	Suicide	11.1	−5.1 ↓
10	Homicide	10.5	2.9 ↑

*Per 100,00 population, age adjusted to the 1940 U.S. population

FIGURE 4-4
Top ten causes of death. (Centers for Disease Control and Prevention. Advance report of final mortality statistics, 1992 Monthly Vital Statistics Report, December 8, 1994;43:7.)

Remission and Exacerbation

The term **remission** refers to the disappearance of signs and symptoms associated with a particular disease. Although this may resemble a cured state, more often than not, the relief is only temporary. An **exacerbation** refers to the time when the disorder becomes reactivated or reverts from a chronic to an acute state.

Hereditary, Congenital, and Idiopathic Illnesses

A **hereditary condition** is one that is acquired from the genetic codes of one or both parents. Cystic fibrosis, a lung disease, and Huntington's chorea, a neurologic disorder, are examples of inherited illnesses. Hereditary diseases may be manifested immediately at birth or develop at some time later in life.

Congenital disorders are those that are present at birth and result from faulty embryonic development. Maternal illness, such as rubella (German measles) or exposure to toxic chemicals or drugs, especially during the first 3 months of pregnancy, often predispose the fetus to congenital disorders. There was much notoriety several decades ago when pregnant women who took the drug, thalidomide, gave birth to infants with missing arms and legs. Currently, there is a great deal of concern about the role of alcohol in producing fetal alcohol syndrome, a permanent, yet preventable, form of retardation, and the possible effects from exposure to other environmental toxins. Although the etiologies

for some congenital disorders have been well established, it is also possible for congenital disorders to occur randomly.

An **idiopathic illness** is one for which there is no known explanation for its development. Treatment of idiopathic illnesses usually focuses on relieving the signs and symptoms of the disease because the **etiology**, or cause of the disease, is unknown.

HEALTH CARE SYSTEM

The **health care system** refers to the network of services available to people seeking treatment for a health problem, or assistance with maintaining or promoting health. The types of diseases, profile of patients, and the health care provided have drastically changed during the past 25 years (Display 4-1). Advances in technology and new discoveries in science have created more elaborate methods of diagnosing and treating disease, creating a need for more specialized care. What was once a system in which people would seek medical advice and treatment from one physician, clinic, or hospital has now developed into a complex system for health care.

Health Care Services

Types of health care vary according to the needs of the patient. They may seek or be referred to resources that provide primary, secondary, tertiary, or extended care.

DISPLAY 4-1. *Trends in Health and Health Care*

- Increased older adult population
- Greater ethnically diverse groups
- More chronic, yet preventable, illnesses
- Growing numbers of older adults with cognitive disorders like Alzheimer's disease
- Higher incidence of drug-resistant infections
- Rising incidence of terminally ill infants and young adults infected by the virus causing acquired immunodeficiency syndrome (AIDS)
- Expanding application of genetic engineering (treating diseases by altering genetic codes)
- Greater success in organ transplantation
- Escalating costs for health care
- Major efforts at cost containment
- Fewer insured and more underinsured citizens
- More outpatient or ambulatory (1-day stays) care
- Shorter hospitalizations
- Use of less invasive forms of treatment
- Shift to more home care
- Greater focus on disease prevention, health promotion, and health maintenance
- Movement toward more self-care and self-testing
- More previously controlled drugs being approved for nonprescription use
- Nationally linked computer information systems
- Computerized medical record systems
- Shift to criterion-based treatment (eg, patients must meet established criteria to justify treatment measures)
- Increased litigation against health professionals

PRIMARY CARE

Primary care refers to the health services provided by the first health care professional or agency a person contacts. The initial consultation often is with a family practice physician in an office or clinic. However, in the future, cost-effective health care reforms are likely to provide opportunities for nurses to become more actively involved in primary health care.

SECONDARY CARE

Secondary care pertains to the health services to which primary caregivers refer patients for consultation and additional testing, such as at a cardiac catheterization laboratory.

TERTIARY CARE

Tertiary care takes place in a hospital, where complex technology and specialists are available. There is a growing trend to provide as many secondary and tertiary care services as possible on an outpatient or short-term basis, requiring less than 24 hours of care.

EXTENDED CARE

Extended care involves meeting the health needs of patients who no longer require hospitalization, but continue to require health services. Extended care may be provided through a home health care agency or community health service such as hospice care. Long-term, extended care also is provided in special facilities or rehabilitation units in which patients need prolonged health maintenance or restorative services, such as nursing homes.

NATIONAL HEALTH GOALS

A recent national effort identified goals and strategies for improving the nation's health by preventing major chronic illnesses, injuries, and infectious diseases by the year 2000 (Display 4-2). The results reflect the combined expertise of individuals in the Public Health Service, representatives from each state's health department, delegates from national health organizations, members of the Institute of Medicine of the National Academy of Sciences, and selected members of the public at large. To meet the nation's goals, health care workers, both public and private, are being challenged to implement strategies to improve the overall health of people living in the United States.

HEALTH CARE TEAM

The **health care team** is a group of specially trained personnel who work together to assist people with attaining, maintaining, or regaining health. The team may include several types of professionals, such as physicians, nurses, dietitians, pharmacists, and social workers, as well as allied health care workers with special training, like respiratory therapists, physical therapists, nursing assistants, and technicians. The group of nursing personnel who work together to provide direct patient care is called the **nursing team** (Fig. 4-5).

Hospitals are not the only places within the health care system where nurses work. Because nurses possess skills that assist the healthy or dying and all those at stages in between, there are many opportunities for providing the nursing skills and services that patients need. Nurses work in health maintenance organizations, physical fitness centers, diet clinics, public health

DISPLAY 4-2. *National Health Promotion and Disease Prevention Objectives*

Goals

- Increase the span of healthy life for Americans
- Reduce disparities among Americans
- Achieve access to preventive services for all Americans

Strategies

- Increase physical activity and fitness
- Improve nutrition
- Reduce tobacco, alcohol, and drug use
- Improve family planning
- Improve mental health and prevent mental disorders
- Reduce violent and abusive behavior
- Enhance educational and community-based programs
- Reduce unintentional injuries
- Improve occupational safety and health
- Improve environmental health
- Ensure food and drug safety
- Improve oral health
- Improve maternal and infant health
- Reduce heart disease and stroke
- Prevent and control cancer
- Reduce diabetes and chronic disabling conditions
- Prevent and control HIV (human immuno-deficiency virus) infections
- Reduce sexually transmitted diseases
- Increase immunizations and prevent infectious diseases
- Expand access and use of clinical preventive services
- Improve surveillance and data systems.

Healthy People 2000, U.S. Department of Health and Human Services, 1990

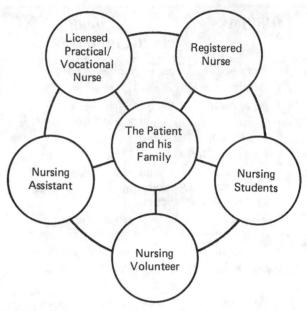

FIGURE 4-5
The nursing team.

departments, home health agencies, and hospices, to name but a few.

Patterns for Administering Patient Care

When nursing personnel work together, one of several methods may be used to promote efficiency in providing patient care. Each method—functional nursing, case method, team nursing, primary nursing, and managed care—has advantages and disadvantages. A critical pathway, also known as a recovery pathway, typically accompanies the managed care approach (Fig. 4-6). Students may encounter one or all of these methods while acquiring clinical experience.

FUNCTIONAL NURSING

One method for administering nursing care is the **functional method**. When this approach is used, each nurse on a patient unit is assigned specific tasks. For example, one is assigned to give the medications to the patients and another is assigned to do the treatments. This pattern is becoming the least used because its focus tends to be more on completing the task rather than treating the patient.

CASE METHOD

Providing nursing care by the **case method** involves assigning one nurse to administer all the care a patient needs for a designated period of time. The case method is most often used in home health and public health nursing.

TEAM NURSING

In **team nursing**, many nursing personnel divide the patient care and all work until it is completed. The personnel are organized and directed by a nurse called the team leader. The team leader may assist with, but usu-

(text continues on page 51)

RECOVERY PATHWAY TOTAL HIP   ADDRESSOGRAPH

DRG 209: (81.51)
Exp. LOS: 6 days
M.D.:

(Recovery Pathways do not represent a standard of care. They are guidelines for consideration which may be modified according to the individual patient's need.)

	DATE: Pre-Admit	DAY OF WK: DATE: DAY 1 (OR Day)	DAY OF WK: DATE: DAY 2- 1st PostOp	DAY OF WK: DATE: DAY 3- 2nd PostOp	DAY OF WK: DATE: DAY 4- 3rd PostOp	DAY OF WK: DATE: DAY 5- 4th PostOp	DAY OF WK: DATE: DAY 6- 5th PostOp
Diagnostic Studies	Auto Blood Y N Pre-op Lab, EKG, CXR	X-ray Joint PACU Y N	CBC Y N PT/PTT (INR) Y N	CBC Y N	CBC Y N		
Treatments		- Waffle - Foley - TED Hose - in OR Y N - SCD in OR Y N - Drain Y N - IS	- TED Hose Y N - SCD Y N - Drain Y N - IS - Foley (consider D/C) Y N	- SCD Y N - IS (pt doing own) Y N - Drain D/C Y N - Foley D/C 0700 Y N	- SCD Y N - IS - Consider IV out Y N	→	→
Therapy PT (one time/day unless specified)	Pre-Op teaching Y N OT safety checklist	Total Hip protocol WB per M.D. (PT & OT) (Evaluation & Treatment) Y N	- Gait training 10-20' Y N - Total Hip precautions given Y N - OT - Precaution instruction Y N	- Gait training 20-25' as tol. Y N - THR exercise x 10 rep with min Asst Y N - Understand total hip precautions Y N - Supine→sit w/ __ asst Y N - Sit→stand w/ __ asst Y N - OT: Pt participation as tol with LE dressing/bathing with equipment Y N	- Gait training 25-40' as tol Y N - Transfer sit ⇄ stand minimal asst Y N - Exercise 10-15 reps Y N - Begin ↕ stairs Y N - OT: Transfer training - tub/ toilet/auto Y N	- Gait training 40-50' as tol Y N - Transfer sit ⇄ stand - in ⇄ OOB independently Y N - Exercise 15-20 reps Y N - ↕ stairs Y N - OT: Refining/ reviewing prior instruction with home safety, task simplification Y N	- Gait training 50-60' as tol Y N - ↕steps independently YN - Independent with 15-20 reps of exercise Y N - Discharge Instructions
Multi-disciplinary Consults	SW Screen Medical Evaluation	Other MD consults			Consider Home Health Assessment Y N		
Medications	Physician preference	Antibiotics Analgesics	Antibiotics Analgesics	Antibiotics D/C Y N Analgesics (push po) Y N	Analgesics (po) Y N	Analgesics (po) Y N	Rx Written Analgesics
Nutrition	NPO after midnight	Clear liquids → DAT	Clear liquids → DAT	DAT GI function Y N	DAT	DAT	DAT

	DATE: Pre-Admit	DAY OF WK: ___ DATE: ___ DAY 1 (OR Day)	DAY OF WK: ___ DATE: ___ DAY 2- 1st PostOp	DAY OF WK: ___ DATE: ___ DAY 3- 2nd PostOp	DAY OF WK: ___ DATE: ___ DAY 4- 3rd PostOp	DAY OF WK: ___ DATE: ___ DAY 5- 4th PostOp	DAY OF WK: ___ DATE: ___ DAY 6- 5th PostOp
Activity	Pre-Op Teaching	- BR w/position ∆ q2° - Maintain Abduction Y N - Dorsiplantar Flex q2° Y N - DB Y N - If early a.m. surgery - ↑ chair Y N	- Chair Y N - Dorsiplantar Flex q4° Y N - DB Y N	- Chair/Up in room, Hall as tol Y N - Dorsiplantar Flex q4° Y N - DB Y N	- Chair/up in room/hall Y N - Dorsiplantar Flex q4° Y N - DB Y N	- Chair/Up in room/Hall Independent Y N - Dorsiplantar Flex q4° Y N - DB Y N	- Chair/Up in room/Hall Independent Y N - Dorsiplantar flex q4° Y N - DB Y N
Teaching	- Video Education - Pain Mgmt - Lt supper/ suppository	- Reinforce pre-op education Y N - Hip Precautions Y N - Pain Scale (0-10) Y N	Continue to reinforce	Continue to reinforce: - Ted Hose Y N - Gait training/transfers Y N - Hip Precautions Y N	Continue to reinforce	- Coumadin (if going home on) Y N - Continue to reinforce	Discharge Instructions Follow-up appointments
Discharge Planning	Patient to bring pre-op instuctions with them	SS- meet with family - Develop initial plan Y N	SS - Monitor progress	- Assess rehab potential vs. ECF Y N	- Assess rehab potential vs. ECF Y N - Identify equipment needs (for home) Y N - Clarify plan with patient/ family Y N	- Assess rehab potential vs. ECF Y N - Order Equipment Y N - Clarify plan with patient/ family Y N - Coordinate discharge home (home health/ equipment needs) Y N	DC to home or ECF Home Health liaison to finalize HH involvement Y N
Expected Patient Outcomes	Patient states his responsibility/role in recovery Y N	Patient understands treatment rationale Y N	- Patient actively participates in care Y N - Verbalizes understanding of care Y N	- Verbalize hip precautions Y N	Verbalizes/ Demonstrates: - hip precautions Y N - discharge plans Y N - Discharge to Rehab Y N	- Patient/family demonstrates independence w/ADLs Y N Discharge to - ECF Y N - rehab Y N - Home Y N	Patient/family understands discharge instructions and is confident in ability to care for self. Y N - Discharge to home Y N

Signatures: _____ _____ _____ _____ _____

MR-

Page 2

Rev. 3/1/94

FIGURE 4-6

Example of recovery pathway in managed care. (Courtesy of Elkhart General Hospital, Elkhart, IN.)

ally supervises, the care that other team members provide. All team members report the outcomes of their care to the team leader. It is the responsibility of the team leader to evaluate whether the goals of patient care are being met.

Conferences are an important part of team nursing. Conferences may cover a variety of subjects, but they are planned with certain goals in mind. Examples of goals include determining the best approaches to each patient's health problems, increasing the team members' knowledge, and promoting a cooperative spirit among nursing personnel.

PRIMARY NURSING

Primary nursing is a method in which the admitting nurse assumes responsibility for planning patient care and evaluating the progress of the patient. The primary nurse may delegate the patient's care, but is consulted when new problems develop or the plan for care requires modifications. The primary nurse continues to remain responsible and accountable for specific patients throughout their care.

MANAGED CARE

A new type of nursing care delivery system is being implemented in several areas of the United States. It is called **nurse-managed care** by some, and case management by others.

This innovative system was developed in response to several crises affecting the delivery of health care today, such as the need to balance the costs of medical care within limited reimbursement systems. Nurse-managed care relies on principles similar to those practiced by successful businesses. In the business world, corporations pay executives to forecast trends and facilitate the best strategies for making profits. In nurse-managed care, a professional nurse plans the nursing care of patients based on their type of case, or medical diagnosis. Predictable outcomes are forecast and evaluated on a daily basis. By meeting the outcomes in a timely manner, the patient is ready for discharge before or by the time designated by prospective payment systems.

Pilot studies indicate that this approach ensures that standards of care are met with greater efficiency and cost savings. Hospitals that are adopting case-managed care report that they are operating within their budgets and decreasing their financial losses.

CONTINUITY OF HEALTH CARE

Continuity of care refers to a continuum of health care. The goal is to avoid causing a patient, whether healthy or ill, to feel isolated, fragmented, or abandoned dur-

ing the transfer from one type of health care service to another. All too often, this occurs when one health practitioner fails to consult or communicate with others involved in the patient's care.

Chapters 9 and 10 provide examples of how nurses communicate among themselves and with personnel in other institutions so that the patient's care is both continuous and goal directed.

KEY CONCEPTS

- The WHO defines **health** as "a state of complete physical, mental, and social well-being and not merely the absence of disease or infirmity."
- Values are those ideals that a person feels are honorable attributes. Beliefs are concepts that people hold to be true.
- When it comes to health, most Americans believe that health is a resource, a right, and a personal responsibility.
- How "whole" or well a person feels is the sum of his or her physical, emotional, social, and spiritual health, a concept referred to as holism. Any change in one component—positive or negative—automatically causes similar repercussions in the others.
- There are five levels of human needs: physiologic needs (first level), safety and security needs (second level), needs for love and belonging (third level), needs for esteem and self-esteem (fourth level), and self-actualization needs (fifth level). By progressively satisfying needs at each subsequent level, people can realize their maximum potential for health and well-being.
- Illness is a state of discomfort that results when a person's health becomes impaired through disease, stress, or an accident or injury.
- Morbidity refers to the incidence of a specific disease, disorder, or injury, whereas mortality refers to the incidence of death associated with a specific condition.
- An acute illness is one that comes on suddenly and lasts a relatively short time. A chronic illness is one that comes on slowly and lasts a relatively long time. A terminal illness is one in which there is no potential for cure.
- A primary illness is one that has developed independently of any other disease. Any subsequent disorder that develops from a pre-existing condition is referred to as a secondary illness.
- The term "remission" refers to the disappearance of signs and symptoms associated with a particular disease. An exacerbation refers to the time when the disorder becomes reactivated or reverts from a chronic to an acute state.

- A hereditary condition is one that is acquired from the genetic codes of one or both parents. Congenital disorders are those that are present at birth and result from faulty embryonic development. An idiopathic illness is one for which there is no known explanation for its development.
- Primary care refers to the health services provided by the first health care professional or agency a person contacts. Secondary care pertains to the health services to which primary caregivers refer patients for consultation and additional testing, such as at a cardiac catheterization laboratory. Tertiary care takes place in a hospital, where complex technology and specialists are available. Extended care involves meeting the health needs of patients who no longer require hospitalization, but continue to need health services.
- There are three national health goals that have been targeted for the year 2000. They are: (1) to increase the span of healthy life for Americans, (2) to reduce health care disparities among Americans, and (3) to achieve access to preventive health services for all Americans.
- One of several patterns may be used when providing nursing care for patients. Functional nursing refers to a practice in which each nurse on a patient unit is assigned specific tasks involving patient care. The case method involves assigning one nurse to administer all the care a patient needs for a designated period of time. In team nursing, many nursing personnel divide the patient care and all work until it is completed. Primary nursing is a method in which the admitting nurse assumes responsibility for planning patient care and evaluating the progress of the patient. In managed care, a nurse manager plans the nursing care of patients based on their type of case or medical diagnosis, and evaluates patient progress so that each patient is ready for discharge before or by the time designated by prospective payment systems.

CRITICAL THINKING EXERCISES

- A friend confides that she has been having frequent bouts with indigestion. To whom might this person be referred for primary, secondary, and tertiary care?
- Discuss health strategies that would be appropriate for ensuring the health of children and young, middle-aged, and older adults.
- Which pattern for administering patient care seems to be most advantageous for nurses? Which pattern might patients prefer? Give reasons for your selections.

SUGGESTED READINGS

A prescription for cutting health care costs. Caring November 1992;11:10–14.

Betts VT. Reforming health care, transforming nursing. American Nurse January 1993;25:5.

Caserta JE. A case for universal access. Home Healthcare Nurse November–December 1991;9:5.

Ceslowitz SB. Managed care: controlling costs and changing practice. MEDSURG Nursing October 1993;2:359–366.

Huey FL. Is everything everyone's job? American Journal of Nursing September 1992;92:7.

Hurst K. Changes in nursing practice 1984–1992. Nursing Times March 18–24, 1992;88:54.

Kelly LY. The Nursing Experience: Trends, Challenges, and Transitions. 2nd ed. New York: Macmillan, 1992.

Lindeman CA. Nursing & technology: moving into the 21st century. Caring September 1992;11:5, 7–10.

Merker L. Meet the challenge: health care in the 1990s. Journal of Practical Nursing September 1991;41:32–33.

Perkins CB, Perkins KC. Uncompensated care: the millstone around the neck of U.S. health care. Nursing and Health Care January 1992;13:20–23.

Pilch JJ. Your Invitation to Full Life. Minneapolis, MN: Winston Press, 1981.

United States Department of Health and Human Services. Healthy People 2000: National Health Promotion and Disease Prevention Objectives. Boston: Jones and Bartlett, 1992.

CHAPTER 5

Homeostasis, Adaptation, and Stress

Key Terms

Adaptation   Homeostasis
Coping Mechanisms   Stress
General Adaptation   Stressor
Syndrome

Learning Objectives

An understanding of the content within this chapter will be evidenced by the student's ability to:

- Explain homeostasis
- List four categories of stressors that affect homeostasis
- Identify two beliefs that are based on the philosophic concept of holism
- Explain the purpose underlying adaptation and identify two possible outcomes of unsuccessful adaptation
- Trace the structures through which adaptive changes take place
- Differentiate between sympathetic and parasympathetic adaptive responses
- Define stress

- List 10 factors that affect the stress response
- Discuss the three stages of the general adaptation syndrome and the consequences that result
- Explain how psychological adaptation occurs and two possible outcomes that may result
- List eight nursing activities that are helpful when managing the care of stress-prone patients
- List four approaches for preventing, reducing, or eliminating a stress response

Health is a tenuous state. To sustain it, the body continuously adapts to changes, or **stressors**, acting on it. As long as the stressors are minor, the response is negligible and comes about quite unnoticed. However, there are circumstances when a more powerful response is required. The effort to restore balance sometimes results in uncomfortable signs and symptoms that many call "stress." If stress is prolonged, stress-related disorders and even death may occur.

HOMEOSTASIS

Homeostasis is the term used to describe a relatively stable state of physiologic equilibrium (balance). It literally means "staying the same." Although it sounds contradictory, staying the same requires constant physiologic activity.

Holism

Although homeostasis tends to be associated with a person's physical status, it is also affected by emotional, social, and spiritual components as well. This philosophic concept of interrelatedness is referred to as

TABLE 5-1. *Common Stressors*			
Physiologic	Psychological	Social	Spiritual
Prematurity	Fear	Gender, racial, age	Guilt
Aging	Powerlessness	discrimination	Doubt
Injury	Jealousy	Isolation	Hopelessness
Infection	Rivalry	Abandonment	Conflict in values
Malnutrition	Bitterness	Poverty	Pressure to join, abandon, or
Obesity	Hatred	Conflict in relationships	change religions
Surgery	Insecurity	Political instability	Religious discrimination
Pain		Denial of human rights	
Fever		Threats to safety	
Fatigue		Illiteracy	
Pollution		Infertility	

holism (see Chap. 4). Holism implies that multiple entities contribute to the *whole* of a human.

Based on the principles of holism, stressors may be physiologic, psychological, social, or spiritual in nature (Table 5-1).

Holism leads to two commonly held beliefs: (1) that humans are directly influenced by both the mind and body, and (2) that the relationship between the mind and body has a potential for sustaining health as well as causing illness. Consequently, it is helpful to understand how the mind perceives information and makes adaptive responses.

ADAPTATION

Adaptation refers to the manner in which an organism responds to change. Every system of the body has self-protective properties and mechanisms for regulating homeostasis. However, orchestrating homeostatic adaptive responses requires communication between the brain and its various organ systems. Human adaptation takes place through the coordinated efforts of the central nervous system, autonomic nervous system, and endocrine system.

The Central Nervous System

The central nervous system is composed of the brain and spinal cord. The brain can be divided into the cortex and the structures that make up the subcortex (Fig. 5-1).

THE CORTEX

The cortex is considered the higher functioning portion of the brain because it allows humans to think abstractly, use and understand language, accumulate and store memories, and make decisions about information it receives. The cortex also influences other, more primitive areas of the brain located in the subcortex.

THE SUBCORTEX

The subcortex consists of the structures in the midbrain and brain stem. The midbrain, which lies between the cortex and the brain stem, includes the basal ganglia, thalamus, and hypothalamus. The brain stem, so named because it resembles a stalk, contains the cerebellum, medulla, and pons.

The subcortical structures are primarily responsible for regulating and maintaining physiologic activities that promote survival. These include the regulation of breathing, heart contraction, blood pressure, body temperature, sleeping, appetite, and a variety of other organ functions, including the stimulation and inhibition of hormone production.

THE RETICULAR ACTIVATING SYSTEM

The reticular activating system (RAS), an area of the brain through which a network of nerves passes, is the

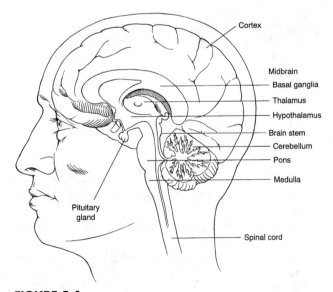

FIGURE 5-1
Central nervous system structures.

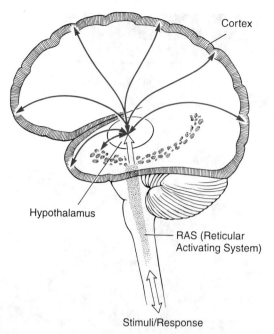

FIGURE 5-2
The reticular activating system is the link in the mind–body connection.

communicative link between the body and the mind. Information about a person's internal and external environment is funneled through the RAS to the cortex on both a conscious and unconscious level (Fig. 5-2). The cortex processes the information and generates behavioral and physiologic responses through activation of the hypothalamus. The hypothalamus influences the autonomic nervous system and endocrine functions (Fig. 5-3).

The Autonomic Nervous System

The autonomic nervous system, which is subdivided into the sympathetic and parasympathetic nervous systems, is composed of peripheral nerves that affect physiologic functions that are largely automatic and beyond voluntary control.

Organs throughout the body are supplied with nerve pathways from both the sympathetic and parasympathetic divisions of the autonomic nervous system. Each division takes its turn at being functionally dominant depending on which physiologic response is appropriate. For example, when there is a need for an increased heart rate, the sympathetic nervous system assumes dominance; when there is a need to slow the heart rate, the parasympathetic nervous system takes over.

THE SYMPATHETIC NERVOUS SYSTEM

When confronted with a situation that the mind perceives to be dangerous, the sympathetic nervous system prepares the body for *fight or flight*. It accelerates those physiologic functions that ensure survival through strength or a rapid escape. The person becomes active, aroused, and emotionally charged.

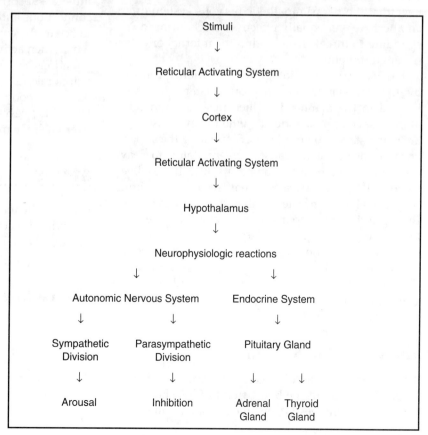

FIGURE 5-3
Homeostatic adaptive pathways.

TABLE 5-2. *Sympathetic and Parasympathetic Effects*

Target Structure	Sympathetic Effect	Parasympathetic Effect
Iris of the eye	Dilates pupils	Constricts pupils
Sweat glands	Increases perspiration	None
Salivary glands	Inhibits salivation	Increases salivation
Digestive glands	Inhibits secretions	Stimulates secretions
Heart	Increases rate and force of contraction	Decreases rate and force of contraction
Blood vessels in skin	Constrict, causing pale appearance	Dilate, causing blush or flushed appearance
Skeletal muscles	Increased tone	Decreased tone
Bronchial muscles	Relaxed (bronchodilation)	Contracted (broncho-constriction)
Digestive motility (peristalsis)	Decreased	Increased
Kidney	Decreased filtration	None
Bladder muscle (detrusor)	Inhibited (suppressed urination)	Stimulated (urge to urinate)
Liver	Release of glucose	None
Adrenal medulla	Stimulated	None

THE PARASYMPATHETIC NERVOUS SYSTEM

The parasympathetic nervous system tends to restore equilibrium after the danger is no longer apparent. It does so by inhibiting the physiologic stimulation created by its counterpart, the sympathetic nervous system.

However, the parasympathetic nervous system does not produce an opposite reaction for every sympathetic effect (Table 5-2). This fact has led some to believe that the parasympathetic nervous system offers an alternate, yet equally effective, mechanism for responding to threats from within the internal or external environment.

For example, physiologic deceleration, produced by the parasympathetic nervous system, has been likened to the manner in which possums and other animal species "play dead" when they sense they are being stalked by predators. Simulating the appearance of death often causes the predator to leave the animal alone, thus saving its life. It has been proposed that humans, too, may respond to stimuli they perceive as threatening by either slowing down their physiologic responses or by speeding them up (Nuernberger, 1981).

Thus, the autonomic nervous system provides the initial and immediate response to a perceived threat either through sympathetic or parasympathetic pathways. But, to sustain the response, the endocrine system becomes involved.

The Endocrine System

The endocrine system is a collective group of glands, located throughout the body, that produce hormones (Fig. 5-4). Hormones are chemicals that are manufactured in one part of the body, but whose actions have physiologic effects elsewhere. Homeostasis is maintained when hormones are released as they are needed or inhibited when an adequate amount is present. The pituitary gland, which is located in the brain, is considered the master gland because it produces hormones that influence other endocrine glands.

The pituitary gland is connected to the hypothalamus, a subcortical structure, through both vascular connections and nerve endings. For pituitary function to occur, the cortex first stimulates the hypothalamus, which then activates the pituitary gland.

As long as the demands on the central nervous system, autonomic nervous system, and endocrine system are within the body's adaptive capacity, homeostasis is maintained. However, when the internal or external changes overwhelm homeostatic adaptation, stress results.

STRESS

Stress is the term used to describe the physiologic and behavioral reactions that occur when the body's equilibrium is disturbed (Table 5-3).

The Nature of Stress

Although humans have the capacity to adapt, not everyone responds to a similar stressor in exactly the same way. Differences may vary according to:

- The intensity of the stressor
- The number of stressors
- The duration of the stressor

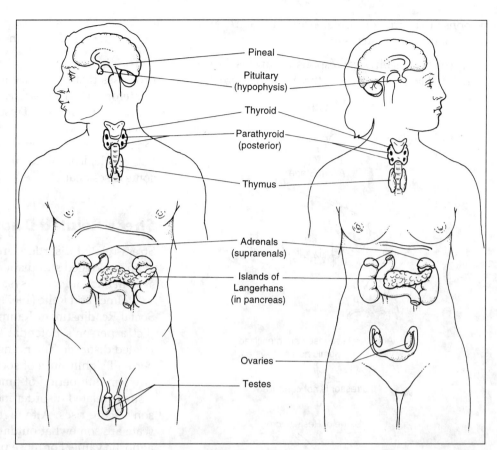

FIGURE 5-4
Endocrine glands. (Scherer JC, Timby BK: Introductory Medical–Surgical Nursing. 6th ed, p 768. Philadelphia: JB Lippincott, 1995.)

- Physical status
- Life experiences
- Coping strategies
- Social support
- Personal beliefs
- Attitudes
- Values

Because of unique differences, the outcomes may be adaptive or maladaptive, depending on each person's stress response.

The Stress Response

Hans Selye, a gifted physician in Canada during the early 20th century, devoted much of his life to researching the physiology of the stress response, which he called the general adaptation syndrome.

THE GENERAL ADAPTATION SYNDROME

The **general adaptation syndrome** (GAS) refers to the collective physiologic processes that take place in

TABLE 5-3. *Common Signs and Symptoms of Stress*

Physical	Emotional	Cognitive
Rapid heart rate	Irritability	Impaired attention and
Rapid breathing	Angry outbursts	concentration
Increased blood	Hypercritical	Forgetfulness
pressure	Verbal abuse	Preoccupation
Difficulty falling asleep,	Withdrawal	Poor judgment
or excessive sleep	Depression	
Loss of appetite, or excessive eating		
Stiff muscles		
Hyperactivity or inactivity		
Dry mouth		
Constipation or diarrhea		
Lack of interest in sex		

response to a stressor. Selye observed that, regardless of the nature of the stressor:

1. The body's physical response is always the same.
2. It follows a one-, two-, or three-stage pattern that he

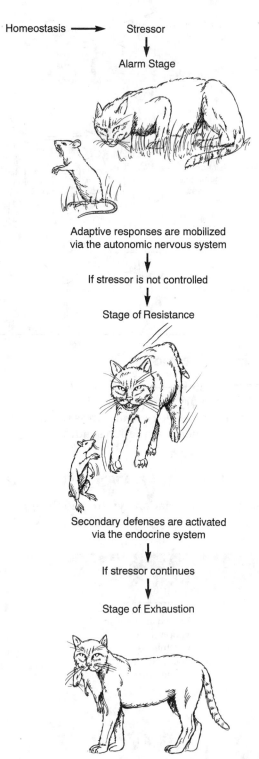

Homeostasis ——→ Stressor

Alarm Stage

Adaptive responses are mobilized
via the autonomic nervous system

If stressor is not controlled

Stage of Resistance

Secondary defenses are activated
via the endocrine system

If stressor continues

Stage of Exhaustion

Adaptation is unsuccessful and death ensues

FIGURE 5-5
Stages of the general adaptation syndrome.

identified as the *alarm stage*, the *stage of resistance*, and in some cases, the *stage of exhaustion* (Fig. 5-5).

The first two stages of the GAS parallel the same processes that take place in maintaining homeostasis. Therefore, brief stress responses generally result in adaptive outcomes and restoration of equilibrium. But, when the second stage, the stage of resistance, is prolonged, the process tends to become maladaptive and-pathologic, leading to stress related-disorders, and in some cases death.

Stress-Related Disorders

Stress-related disorders are those diseases that result from prolonged stimulation of the autonomic nervous system and endocrine system (Display 5-1).

Holmes and Rahe (1967) developed a tool, called the Social Readjustment Rating Scale, that is used to predict a person's potential for developing of a stress-related disorder. The rating scale is based on the number and significance of social stressors experienced in any 6-month period of time (Display 5-2). The risk for a stress-related disorder increases as the sum of a person's score rises. Although some of the items on the scale are somewhat outdated, it continues to have diagnostic value. For those people who are experiencing severe or cumulative stressors, appropriate interventions may be offered to minimize or relieve their stress and thus avoid a stress-related illness.

DISPLAY 5-1. *Stress-Related Disorders*

- Hypertension
- Headaches
- Gastritis
- Ulcerative colitis
- Asthma
- Rheumatoid arthritis
- Skin disorders
- Hyper/hypoinsulinism
- Hyper/hypothyroidism
- Depressive disorders
- Cancer
- Low back pain
- Irritable bowel syndrome
- Allergies
- Anxiety disorders
- Infertility
- Impotence
- Bruxism (tooth grinding)

DISPLAY 5-2. *The Social Readjustment Rating Scale*

Rank	Life Event	LCU Value
1	Death of spouse	100
2	Divorce	73
3	Marital separation	65
4	Jail term	63
5	Death of close family member	63
6	Personal injury or illness	53
7	Marriage	50
8	Fired at work	47
9	Marital reconciliation	45
10	Retirement	45
11	Change in health of family member	44
12	Pregnancy	40
13	Sex difficulties	39
14	Gain of new family member	39
15	Business readjustment	39
16	Change in financial state	38
17	Death of close friend	37
18	Change to different line of work	36
19	Change in number of arguments with spouse	35
20	Mortgage over $10,000	31
21	Foreclosure of mortgage or loan	30
22	Change in responsibilities at work	29
23	Son or daughter leaving home	29
24	Trouble with in-laws	29
25	Outstanding personal achievement	28
26	Wife begins or stops work	26
27	Begin or end school	26
28	Change in living conditions	25
29	Revision of personal habits	24
30	Trouble with boss	23
31	Change in work hours or conditions	20
32	Change in residence	20
33	Change in schools	20
34	Change in recreation	19
35	Change in church activities	19
36	Change in social activities	18
37	Mortgage or loan less than $10,000	17
38	Change in sleeping habits	16
39	Change in number of family get-togethers	15
40	Change in eating habits	15
41	Vacation	13
42	Christmas	12
43	Minor violations of the law	11

Social events are ranked from most stressful to least stressful. Each event is assigned a life change unit (LCU) that correlates with the severity of the stressor. The sum of LCUs over the past 6 months is calculated. A score of less than 150 LCUs is considered low risk, a score between 150 to 199 is an indication of mild risk, moderate risk is associated with a score between 200 to 299, and a score over 300 places the person at major risk.

Holmes TH, Rahe RH. The Social Readjustment Rating Scale. Journal of Psychosomatic Research. August 1967;11:216. Copyright © 1967, Pergamon Press, Ltd.

Psychological Adaptation

Just as the physical body adapts to stressors, the psyche (mind) maneuvers another set of defenses as well. It was Sigmund Freud (1937) who explained that humans unconsciously use coping mechanisms to protect themselves from feeling less than adequate.

COPING MECHANISMS

Coping mechanisms are unconscious tactics used to protect the psyche (Table 5-4). These techniques temporarily manipulate reality—they are a sort of psychological first aid. They allow people momentarily to avoid the emotional impact of a stressful situation. When used appropriately and in moderation, coping mechanisms enable people to maintain their mental equilibrium. Given the benefit of psychological adaptation, the person usually acquires insight, gains confidence to confront reality, and is able to implement additional adaptive strategies leading to emotional growth.

MALADAPTIVE COPING

If coping mechanisms are overused or used over a long span of time, however, they may have a pathologic effect. They may distort reality to such an extent that the person fails to recognize and correct his or her weaknesses. Consequently, the person may avoid responsibility for solving personal psychosocial problems. Alcoholics, for example, use denial as a coping mechanism to avoid admitting a drinking problem. Until the denial is abandoned, the alcoholic usually resists treatment.

NURSING IMPLICATIONS

Nurses must be aware of potential stressors that particularly affect patients because they add to the cumulative effect of other stressful life events. One research study ranked the unique stressors experienced by patients, according to their perspective, in a hierarchical list modeled after the Social Readjustment Rating Scale (Display 5-3). By being aware of how an illness or hospitalization affects people, nurses can be instrumental in supporting patients who are especially vulnerable.

When a patient is experiencing a stressor, nurses do one or several of the following:

- Identify stressors
- Assess the patient's response to stressors
- Eliminate or reduce the stressors
- Prevent additional stressors from occurring
- Promote the patient's physiologic adaptive responses

TABLE 5-4. *Coping Mechanisms*

Mechanism	Explanation	Example
Repression	Forgetting about the stressor	Wiping the experience of being sexually abused from conscious memory
Suppression	Purposely avoiding thinking about a stressor	Resolving to "sleep on a problem" or turn the problem over to a higher power like God
Denial	Rejecting information	Refusing to believe something like a life-threatening diagnosis
Rationalization	Relieving oneself of personal accountability by attributing responsibility to someone or something else	Blaming failure on a test to the manner in which the test was constructed
Displacement	Taking anger out on something or someone else who is less likely to retaliate	Kicking the wastebasket after being reprimanded by the boss
Regression	Behaving in a manner that is characteristic of a much younger age	Wanting to be bottle-fed like a newborn sibling
Projection	Attributing that which is unacceptable in oneself onto another	Accusing a person of another race of being prejudiced
Somatization	Manifesting emotional stress through a physical disorder	Developing diarrhea that conveniently excuses one from going to work
Compensation	Excelling at something to make up for a weakness of another kind	Becoming a motivational speaker although physically handicapped
Sublimation	Channeling one's energies into an acceptable alternative	Turning to sportscasting when an athletic career is not realistic
Reaction formation	Acting just the opposite of one's feelings	Being extremely nice to someone who is intensely disliked
Identification	Taking on the characteristics of another	Imitating the style of dress or speech of an actor or musician

DISPLAY 5-3. *Patient-Related Stressors*

Thinking you might lose your sight
Thinking you might have cancer
Thinking you might lose a kidney or some other organ
Knowing you have a serious illness
Thinking you might lose your hearing
Not being told what your diagnosis is
Not knowing for sure what illness you have
Not getting pain medication when you need it
Not knowing the results or reasons for your treatments
Not getting relief from pain medications
Being fed through tubes
Missing your spouse
Not having your questions answered by the staff
Not having enough insurance to pay for your hospitalization
Not having your call light answered
Having a sudden hospitalization you weren't planning to have
Being hospitalized far from home
Knowing you have to have an operation
Not having family visit you
Feeling you are getting dependent on medications
Having nurses or doctors talk too fast or use words you can't understand
Having medications cause you discomfort
Thinking about losing income because of your illness
Having the staff be in too much of a hurry
Not knowing when to expect things will be done to you
Being put in the hospital because of an accident
Being cared for by an unfamiliar doctor
Not being able to call family or friends on the phone
Having to eat cold or tasteless food
Worrying about your spouse being away from you
Thinking you might have pain because of surgery or test procedures
Being in the hospital during holidays or special family occasions
Thinking your appearance might be changed after your hospitalization
Being in a room that is too cold or too hot
Not having friends visit you
Having a roommate who is unfriendly
Having to be assisted with a bedpan
Having a roommate who is seriously ill or cannot talk with you
Being aware of unusual smells around you
Having to stay in bed or the same room all day
Having a roommate who has too many visitors
Not being able to get newspapers, radio, or TV when you want them
Having to be assisted with bathing
Being awakened in the night by the nurse
Having strange machines around
Having to wear a hospital gown
Having to sleep in a strange bed
Having to eat at different times than you usually do
Having strangers sleep in the same room with you

The events in this list are arranged in order of their perceived significance as a stressor. The first event is the most stressful, and the rest follow in descending order.

TABLE 5-5. *Interventions for Stress Management*

Intervention	Explanation
Modeling	Promotes the ability to learn an adaptive response by exposing a person to someone who demonstrates a positive attitude or behavior
Progressive relaxation	Eases tense muscles by clearing the mind of stressful thoughts and focusing on consciously relaxing specific muscle groups
Imagery	Uses the mind to visualize calming, pleasurable, positive experiences
Biofeedback	Alters autonomic nervous system functions by responding to electronically displayed physiologic data
Yoga	Reduces physical and emotional tension through postural changes, muscular stretching, and focused concentration
Meditation and prayer	Reduces physiologic activation by placing one's trust in a higher power
Placebo effect	Alters a negative physiologic response through the power of suggestion

- Support the patient's psychological coping strategies
- Assist in maintaining a network of social support
- Implement stress reduction and stress management techniques

Stress Reduction Techniques

Stress reduction techniques are methods that promote physiologic comfort and emotional well-being. Some general interventions that are appropriate during the care of any patient include providing adequate explanations in understandable language, keeping the patient and family informed, demonstrating confidence and expertise when providing nursing care, remaining calm during crises, being available to the patient, responding promptly to the patient's signal for assistance, encouraging family interaction, advocating on behalf of the patient, and referring the patient and family to organizations or people that provide post-discharge assistance.

People who are susceptible to intense stressors or who are likely to experience stressors over a long period of time may benefit from additional stress management approaches.

Stress Management

Stress management refers to therapeutic activities that are used for the specific purpose of reestablishing balance between the sympathetic and parasympathetic systems (Table 5-5). Techniques that counter sympathetic stimulation are characterized by a calming effect. Stimulating tactics counterbalance parasympathetic dominance.

Physical and emotional responses to stress may also be mediated by interventions that cause the release of endorphins or through manipulation of sensory stimuli.

ENDORPHINS

Endorphins are natural body chemicals that produce effects similar to those of opiate drugs, like morphine. Besides decreasing the sensation of pain, these chemicals promote a sense of pleasure, tranquility, and well-being.

Endorphins are manufactured in the pituitary gland, but they are present in the blood and other tissues (Porth, 1994). Some believe that certain activities, like massage, sustained aerobic exercise, and laughter, trigger the release of endorphins. Once released, endorphins attach themselves to receptor sites in the brain, perhaps in the limbic system, the center where emotions are experienced.

SENSORY MANIPULATION

Sensory manipulation involves altering moods, feelings, and physiologic responses by stimulating pleasure centers in the brain using sensory stimuli. Research is being conducted on the stress-reducing effects of certain colors, full-spectrum lighting in the home and workplace, music, and specific aromas that conjure up pleasant associations—like the smell of baking bread.

KEY CONCEPTS

- Homeostasis refers to a relatively stable state of physiologic equilibrium.
- Homeostasis is affected by physiologic, psychological, social, and spiritual stressors.
- The philosophic concept of holism leads to two commonly held beliefs: (1) that humans are directly influenced by both the mind and body, and (2) that the relationship between the mind and body has a potential for sustaining health as well as causing illness.

- Adaptation refers to the manner in which an organism responds to change. If done successfully, it is the key to maintaining and preserving homeostasis. Unsuccessful adaptation leads to illness and death.
- Adaptive changes occur through the cortex, which communicates with and through the RAS, the hypothalamus, the autonomic nervous system, and pituitary gland, along with other endocrine glands under its control.
- The sympathetic nervous system, a division of the autonomic nervous system, accelerates those physiologic functions that ensure survival through strength or a rapid escape (fight or flight response).
- The parasympathetic nervous system, a second division of the autonomic nervous system, inhibits physiologic stimulation, which restores homeostasis and provides an alternative mechanism for dealing with stressors.
- Stress consists of the physiologic and behavioral reactions that occur when the body's equilibrium is disturbed.
- People vary in their response to stressors depending on the intensity of the stressor, the number of stressors being experienced at any given time, the duration of the stressor, and the person's physical status, life experiences, coping strategies, social support system, personal beliefs, attitudes, and values.
- The general adaptation syndrome, a physiologic stress response described by Hans Selye, consists of the alarm stage, the stage of resistance, and the stage of exhaustion.
- In most cases the alarm stage and the stage of resistance lead to a restoration of homeostasis. However, when the stage of resistance is prolonged, adaptive resources are overwhelmed and the person enters the stage of exhaustion, which is characterized by stress-related disorders and, in some cases, death.
- Psychological adaptation occurs through the unconscious use of coping mechanisms.
- The healthy use of coping mechanisms allows people momentarily to avoid the emotional impact of a stressful situation, eventually deal with reality, and grow emotionally.
- Unhealthy use of coping mechanisms tends to distort reality to such an extent that the person fails to see or correct his or her weaknesses.
- The nursing care of patients includes identifying stressors, assessing the patient's response to stressors, eliminating or reducing stressors, preventing additional stressors, promoting adaptive responses, supporting coping strategies, maintaining a patient's network of support, and implementing stress reduction and stress management techniques.
- Four methods for preventing, reducing, or eliminating a stress response include using stress reduction techniques (such as providing adequate explanations in understandable language), implementing stress management interventions (such as progressive relaxation), promoting the release of endorphins (through massage, for example), and manipulating sensory stimuli, as might be done with aromatherapy.

CRITICAL THINKING EXERCISES

- Develop a list of stressors that are unique to students or student nurses using the Social Readjustment Rating Scale and the list of Patient-Related Stressors as models.
- Identify at least five interventions that would be both realistic and helpful in reducing the stressors associated with being a student.
- Which stress management technique from among those in Table 5-5 is best? Explain the reasons for your choice.

SUGGESTED READINGS

Freud S. The Ego and the Mechanisms of Defense. London: Hogarth Press, 1937.

Harrison L, Skinner R. Relax for health. Nursing Times December 1992;88:46–47.

Hawranik P. Preventing health problems after the age of 65. Journal of Gerontologic Nursing November 1991;17:20–25.

Holmes TH, Rahe RH. The Social Readjustment Rating Scale. Journal of Psychosomatic Research August 1967;11:216.

Kolanowski AM. The clinical importance of environmental lighting to the elderly. Journal of Gerontological Nursing January 1992; 18:10–13.

Memmler RL, Cohen BJ, Wood DL. The Human Body in Health and Disease. 7th ed. Philadelphia: JB Lippincott, 1992.

Nuernberger P. Freedom From Stress. Honesdale, PA: The Himalayan International Institute of Yoga Science and Philosophy, 1981.

Pearson M. The nurse, the elderly caregiver, and stress. Caring January 1993;12:14–17.

Peddicord K. Strategies for promoting stress reduction and relaxation. Nursing Clinics of North America December 1991;26:867–874.

Pelletier. Mind as Healer, Mind as Slayer. New York: Dell, 1977.

Porth CM. Pathophysiology: Concepts of Altered Health States. Philadelphia: JB Lippincott, 1994.

Selye H. The Stress of Life. New York: McGraw-Hill, 1956.

Tattam A. The gentle touch . . . aromatherapy for seriously ill or dying patients. Nursing Times August 5–11, 1992;88:16–17.

Weinberger R. Teaching the elderly stress reduction. Journal of Gerontological Nursing October 1991;17:23–27.

CHAPTER 6
Culture and Ethnicity

 NURSING GUIDELINES

Communicating With Non–English-Speaking Patients

Key Terms

Bilingual	Folk Medicine
Culture	Race
Culture Shock	Stereotype
Culturally Sensitive Care	Subculture
Ethnicity	Transcultural Nursing
Ethnocentrism	

Learning Objectives

An understanding of the content within this chapter will be evidenced by the student's ability to:

- Differentiate between culture, race, and ethnicity
- Discuss two factors that interfere with perceiving others who are dissimilar as individuals
- Explain why the American culture is described as being Anglicized
- List at least five characteristics of Anglo-American culture
- Define the term "subculture" and list four major subcultures in the United States
- List five ways in which people from subcultural groups may differ from Anglo-Americans
- Describe three characteristics of culturally sensitive care
- List at least five ways of demonstrating cultural sensitivity

Nurses have always cared for patients with differences of one kind or another. Patients vary according to their age, gender, race, health status, education, religion, occupation, and economic level. Culture, which is the focus of this chapter, is yet another characteristic that can be added to the list.

Despite the fact that differences exist, the tendency has been to treat patients as though there were none. Although equal treatment may be politically correct, many nurses now feel that denying differences contradicts what is in the best interest of patients. Consequently, there is a movement toward eliminating *acultural* nursing care, that which avoids concern for cultural differences, and promoting that which is *culturally sensitive*—that which respects and is compatible with each patient's culture.

CULTURE

Culture refers to the "values, beliefs, and practices of a particular group" (Giger and Davidhizar, 1991, p. 4). Cultural attitudes and customs are learned by socialization and passed on from one generation to the next.

Culture Shock

When the cultures of two people differ, one or the other, or both may experience culture shock. **Culture shock** is the bewilderment a person experiences when exposed to behavior that is culturally atypical. Therefore, unfamiliarity with other cultures may be problematic for both nurses and patients.

RACE

Race is a term that refers to biologic variations. The term is used to describe groups of people with genetically shared physical characteristics. Some examples include skin color, eye shape, and hair texture. Despite wide ranges in physical variations, skin color has been the chief, albeit imprecise, method for categorizing races. One could argue that there is very little racial purity at this time in history, and that skin color is just the inherited result of:

- the quantity of melanin, a dark brown pigment synthesized and deposited within skin cells,
- the degree to which oxygenated hemoglobin is reflected through the skin, which produces red hues, and
- the amount of bile and carotene skin pigments, which cause yellow hues (Irwin, 1991).

It is essential that nurses not equate skin color with culture. To do so leads to two possible misassumptions: (1) that all people of similar color share essentially the same culture, and (2) that all people of color have cultural values, beliefs, and practices that are different from those of white Americans.

ETHNICITY

Ethnicity is the bond or kinship a person feels with his or her country of birth or place of ancestral origin. Ethnicity may exist regardless of whether a person has ever lived or visited there.

Pride in one's ethnicity may be demonstrated by valuing certain physical characteristics, giving one's children ethnic names, wearing unique items of clothing (Fig. 6-1), appreciating folk music and dance (Fig. 6-2), and eating native food.

Because cultural characteristics and ethnic pride represent the norm in a homogeneous group, they tend to go unnoticed. However, when two or more cultural groups mix, as they often do at the borders of various countries or through the process of immigration, their unique differences become more obvious. Consequently, many ethnic groups have been victimized as a result of bigotry, which is based on stereotypical assumptions and ethnocentrism.

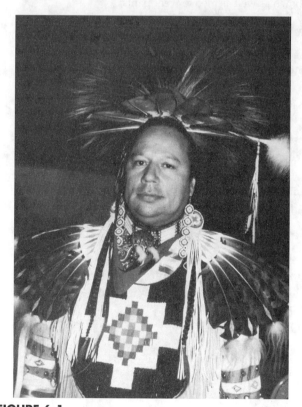

FIGURE 6-1
A Native American in tribal dress during an Indian powwow. (Courtesy of Ken Timby.)

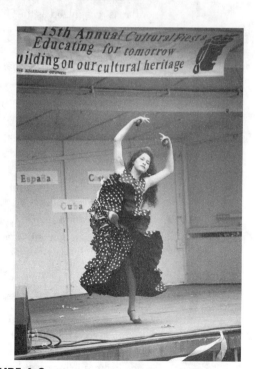

FIGURE 6-2
Latin American ethnicity is celebrated at a festival that includes folk dancing and music. (Courtesy of Ken Timby.)

Stereotyping

A **stereotype** is a fixed attitude about all people who share a common characteristic, like age, gender, race, or ethnicity. Because stereotypes are preconceived ideas that are usually unsupported by facts, they tend to be neither real nor accurate. In fact, they can be dangerous because they interfere with accepting others as unique individuals.

Ethnocentrism

Ethnocentrism is the belief that one's own ethnicity is superior to all others. Consequently, anyone who is different is considered deviant and undesirable. Ethno-centrism was the basis for the Holocaust, during which the Nazis attempted to carry out genocide, the planned extinction of an entire ethnic group—the Jews.

ANGLO-AMERICAN CULTURE

The American culture can be described as *Anglicized*, or English-based, because it evolved primarily from America's early English settlers. Display 6-1 provides an overview of some common characteristics of the American culture. It would be foolhardy, however, to suggest that all people who live in America necessarily embrace the totality of its culture.

DISPLAY 6-1. *Examples of American Cultural Characteristics*

- English is the language of communication.
- The pronunciation or meaning of some words vary according to regions within the United States.
- The customary greeting is a handshake.
- A distance of 4 to 12 feet is customary when interacting with strangers or doing business (Giger and Davidhizar, 1990).
- In casual situations, it is acceptable for women as well as men to wear pants; blue jeans are a common mode of dress.
- Most Americans are Christians.
- Sunday is recognized as the Sabbath.
- Government is expected to remain separate from religion.
- Guilt or innocence for alleged crimes is decided by a jury of one's peers.
- Selection of a marriage partner is an individual's choice.
- Legally, men and women are equals.
- Marriage is monogamous (only one spouse); fidelity is expected.
- Divorce and subsequent remarriages are common.
- Parents are responsible for their minor children.
- Aging adults live separately from their children.
- Status is related to occupation, wealth, and education.
- Common beliefs are that everyone has the potential for success and that hard work leads to prosperity.
- Daily bathing and use of a deodorant are standard hygiene practices.
- Anglo-American women shave the hair from their legs and underarms; most men shave their faces daily.
- Health care is provided by licensed practitioners.
- Drugs and surgery are the traditional forms of medical treatment.
- Americans tend to value technology and equate it with quality.
- As a whole, Americans are time oriented, and therefore rigidly schedule their activities according to clock hours.
- Forks, knives, and spoons are used, except when eating "fast foods," for which using the fingers is appropriate.

Multiculturalism

In the past, history books described the United States as a "melting pot"—implying that culturally diverse groups became assimilated and abandoned their native cultures. Publicly, that may have occurred in some cases, especially when to be different meant facing certain oppression. Privately, however, many foreign-born citizens cherished and tried to sustain their unique cultural heritage.

In the United States today, cultural diversity tends to be the rule rather than the exception. There are many geographic pockets where groups of people who share a common cultural background are located. Some examples include the area of Detroit known as Hamtramack, where people of Polish descent have settled; the Amish regions of Ohio and Pennsylvania; the districts of New York City called Harlem and Spanish Harlem; the section of Miami known as "Little Cuba"; the French quarter in New Orleans; the Indian reservations in the Southwest; and the Chinatowns of Chicago and San Francisco.

AMERICAN SUBCULTURES

A **subculture** is a unique cultural group that co-exists within the dominant culture. Although it is a grossly oversimplified classification, one can identify four major subcultures within the United States. In addition to Anglo-Americans, there are African Americans, Latinos, Asian Americans, and Native Americans.

The term *African American* is used here to refer to black Americans because it alludes to ancestral origin rather than skin color. The term *Latino* refers to those who trace their ethnic origin to South America. Collectively, this includes Puerto Ricans, Cubans, Mexicans, and those from South and Central America. Sometimes the term *Hispanic* is used when referring to people of Spanish descent; *Chicano* is a term used to denote people from Mexico. *Asian Americans* come from China, Japan, Korea, the Philippines, Thailand, Indochina, and Vietnam. People from the Philippines are currently the fastest-growing Asian American minority in the United States (Manio and Hall, 1987). *Native Americans* comprise all the Indian nations and tribes found in North America, including the Eskimos and Aleuts. Currently there are approximately 270 Indian tribes in the United States, with the Navajos being the largest surviving group (Wilson, 1983).

Although Anglo-American culture predominates in the United States, those who trace their ancestry to the United Kingdom and western European countries are gradually becoming the minority. The Bureau of the Census predicts that by the middle of the 21st century, the majority of American citizens will be of African, Asian, Hispanic, or Arabic descent (Kavanaugh, 1993). As a result, the richly diverse population in America today will become even more so. Therefore, the time has come—perhaps late, but better than never—to promote transcultural nursing.

TRANSCULTURAL NURSING

Transcultural nursing, a term coined by Madeline Leininger in the 1970s, refers to providing nursing care within the context of another's culture. **Culturally sensitive care** requires acceptance of each patient as an individual, knowledge of health problems that affect particular cultural groups, and planning care within the patient's health belief system to achieve the best health outcomes. To provide culturally sensitive care, nurses must become skilled at managing language differences, understanding biologic and physiologic variations, promoting health teaching that will reduce prevalent diseases, and respecting alternative health beliefs or health practices.

Some forewarning about generalizations is in order at this time. After learning about differences among cultural groups, nurses may, themselves, fall into the trap of stereotyping. It is always wrong to assume that all people who affiliate themselves with a particular group behave or believe exactly alike. There is, of course, diversity even within cultural groups.

DIVERSITY AND NURSING CARE

Language

Because language is the primary way in which information is gathered and shared, the inability to communicate may be one of the biggest deterrents to providing culturally sensitive care. Foreign travelers and many residents in the United States do not speak English, or have learned it as their second language, and do not speak it well. Even those who can communicate in English may prefer to speak in their primary language, especially when they are under stress.

If the nurse is not **bilingual**, that is, able to speak a second language, an alternate method for communicating must be used. Some options that may be helpful are listed in the guidelines that follow.

NURSING GUIDELINES FOR COMMUNICATING WITH NON–ENGLISH-SPEAKING PATIENTS

- Greet the patient or say words and phrases in the patient's language, even if it is not possible to carry on a conversation.
  Rationale: Indicates a desire to communicate with the patient, even if the nurse lacks the expertise to do so.
- Refer to an English–foreign language dictionary, like *Taber's Cyclopedic Medical Dictionary*.
  Rationale: Provides a list of medical words and phrases that may help in obtaining pertinent information
- Compile a loose-leaf folder or file cards of medical words in one or more languages spoken by patients in the community, and place it where other reference books are located on the nursing unit.
  Rationale: Provides a readily available language resource for communicating with others in the local area
- Call ethnic organizations or church pastors to obtain a list of people who speak the patient's language and may be willing to act as translators.
  Rationale: Develops a network of fluent translators for obtaining necessary information and explaining proposed treatments
- Contact an international telephone operator if there is no other option for communicating with a patient.
  Rationale: Provides a resource for communication in an emergency, however, their main responsibility is the job for which they were hired
- When it is possible to choose from several translators, select one who is the same gender as the patient and approximately the same age.
  Rationale: Reduces embarrassment when relating personal information
- Look at the patient, not the translator, when asking questions and listening for a response.
  Rationale: Indicates that the patient is the primary focus of the interaction and facilitates interpretation of nonverbal clues
- If the patient speaks some English, speak slowly—not loudly—using simple words and short sentences
  Rationale: Enhances communication with someone who is not skilled in the spoken language
- Avoid using technical terms, slang, or phrases with a double or colloquial meaning.
  Rationale: Promotes understanding
- Ask questions that can be answered by a "yes" or "no."
  Rationale: Avoids the need to provide an elaborate response in English words.

- If the patient appears confused by a question, repeat it without changing the words
  Rationale: Avoids having to translate yet another group of unfamiliar words.
- Give the patient sufficient time to respond.
  Rationale: Facilitates the process of interpreting what has been said in English and then converting their response into English
- Use nonverbal communication or pantomime.
  Rationale: Enhances verbal communication
- Be patient.
  Rationale: Reduces anxiety and frustration
- Show the patient written English words.
  Rationale: Accommodates reading skills, which are usually better than other skills in a second language
- Work with the health agency's records committee to obtain consent forms, authorization for health insurance benefits, and copies of patients' rights that are written in languages other than English.
  Rationale: Protects legal rights
- Develop or obtain foreign translations describing common procedures, routine care, and health promotion. One resource is the *Patient Education Resource Center* in San Francisco, which provides publications in many languages on numerous health topics.
  Rationale: Provides explanations and educational services to which all patients are entitled

Communication Styles

Even when people from different nationalities speak the same language, the manner in which they do so may cause conflicts and miscommunication. What may be an accepted pattern during verbal interactions for one may be unusual, rude, or offensive to another. Therefore, understanding some unique cultural characteristics involving verbal as well as nonverbal aspects of communication may facilitate the transition toward culturally sensitive care.

VERBAL DIFFERENCES

Anglo-Americans are comfortable with asking and answering personal questions. Yet, some cultural groups feel ill at ease in verbally disclosing information about themselves. For instance, Native Americans tend to be rather private people and may be hesitant to share much personal information with a stranger. Questioning may be interpreted as prying or meddling. Also, because Native Americans traditionally preserved their heritage through oral rather than written history, they may be skeptical of Anglo-American nurses who write down what they say.

How close a nurse sits to a person and how questions are asked are two more factors that influence intercultural communication. Although there are always exceptions, African Americans seem to prefer answering open-ended questions, those that require discussion, rather than direct questions that solicit specific information. People from the Latino culture are characterized as feeling more comfortable sitting close to the interviewer and letting the interview slowly unfold, rather than being asked one direct question after another. On the other hand, many Asian Americans are described as feeling more comfortable when positioned further than an arm's length from the interviewer.

Anglo-American nurses may find data collection difficult when caring for Asian Americans, who may respond to questions with brief, factual answers and very little elaboration. This characteristic may be the result, in part, of the Asian value for simplicity, meditation, and introspection. Consequently, they may view Anglo-American attempts at friendly conversation to be idle chatter and mindless nonsense. Also, because of their respect for harmony, Asian Americans may not openly disagree with authoritarian figures, which include nurses and physicians. Their reticence to be assertive may conceal a potential for noncompliance when a particular therapeutic regimen is unacceptable from their perspective.

There also may be cultural differences in how family members play a role in the patient's care and treatment. The Navajos feel that no person has the right to speak for another, and they may refuse to comment on a family member's health problems. On the other hand, Latino men are generally protective and authoritarian. They may expect to be consulted in decision-making when a family member is the patient.

NONVERBAL DIFFERENCES

Although it may be natural for Anglo-Americans to look directly at a person while speaking, it may offend Asian Americans or Native Americans, who are more likely to feel that lingering eye contact is an invasion of privacy. Even the Anglo-American custom of a strong handshake can be interpreted as offensive among some Native Americans, who may be more comfortable with just a light passing of the hands.

Anglo-Americans, in general, express their feelings, both positive and negative. Asian Americans, however, tend to control their emotions and the expression of physical discomfort (Zborowski, 1952, 1969), especially when among people with whom they are unfamiliar. Similarly, Latino men may not demonstrate their feelings or readily discuss their symptoms because it may be interpreted as less than manly (Boyle and Andrews, 1989). The Latino cultural response can be attributed to *machismo*, a belief that virile men are physically strong

and must deal with their emotions in private. Because this type of behavior is somewhat atypical from an Anglo-American perspective, nurses are more apt to overlook the emotional and physical needs of people from these cultural groups.

Biologic Variations

The biologic characteristics that are of primary importance to nurses are those that involve the skin and hair.

SKIN CHARACTERISTICS

The skin assessment techniques that are commonly taught are biased in favor of Caucasians, who are light skinned. To provide culturally sensitive care, nurses must modify their assessment techniques to obtain accurate data from dark-skinned patients.

The best technique for observing baseline skin color in dark-skinned cultural groups is to use natural or bright artificial light. Because the palms of the hands, feet, and abdomen contain the least amount of pigmentation and are less likely to have been tanned from exposure to the sun, they are often the best areas to inspect.

According to Giger and Davidhizar (1991), all skin, regardless of a person's ethnic origin, contains an underlying red tone. Its absence or lighter appearance is indicative of pallor, a characteristic of anemia or inadequate oxygenation. The lips and nailbeds, common sites for assessing cyanosis in Caucasians, may be highly pigmented among culturally diverse patients, and normal findings may be misinterpreted. The conjunctiva and oral mucous membranes are likely to provide more accurate data. The sclera or the hard palate, rather than the skin, are the better locations for assessing jaundice. However, the sclera of some non-Caucasians may have a yellow cast because of carotene and fatty deposits, and this should not be misconstrued as jaundice (Spector, 1991).

Rashes, bruising, and inflammation may not be as obvious among people with darker skin. Palpating for variations in texture, warmth, and tenderness is a better assessment technique than inspection. Keloids, irregular, elevated, thick scars, are common among dark-skinned ethnic groups (Fig. 6-3). It is believed that keloids form because of a genetic tendency to produce excessive amounts of transforming growth factor-β (TGFβ), a substance that promotes fibroblast proliferation during tissue repair.

Some Anglo-American nurses misinterpret the brown discoloration on a washcloth while bathing a dark-skinned patient as a sign of poor hygiene. In reality, the appearance is caused by a normal shedding of dead skin cells, which retain their pigmentation, and not a disregard for regular bathing.

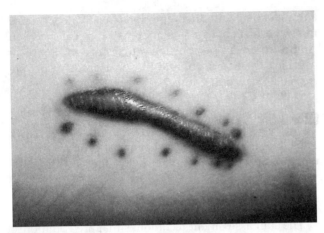

FIGURE 6-3
Keloids are raised, thick scars. (Jackson DB, Saunders R. Child Health Nursing: A Comprehensive Approach to the Care of Children and Their Families. Philadelphia, JB Lippincott, 1993)

Hypopigmentation and Hyperpigmentation

Hypopigmentation and hyperpigmentation are conditions in which the skin is not a uniform color.

Hypopigmentation may result when skin becomes damaged. Regardless of ethnic origin, damaged skin characteristically manifests temporary redness that fades to a lighter hue; on dark-skinned patients, the effect is much more obvious. Vitiligo, a disease that affects whites as well as those with darker skin, produces irregular white patches on the skin from the absence of melanin. Other than hypopigmentation, there are no physical symptoms, but the cosmetic effects may create emotional distress. Patients who are concerned about the irregularity of their skin color may choose to use a pigmented cream as a skin cover to disguise areas that are noticeable.

Mongolian spots are an example of hyperpigmentation. Mongolian spots, dark blue areas on the lower back of darkly pigmented infants and children (Fig. 6-4), are rare among Caucasians. They tend to fade by the time a child is 5 years old. Mongolian spots can be mistaken as a sign of physical abuse or injury by nurses who are unfamiliar with ethnic differences. One method for differentiating the two is to press the pigmented area. Mongolian spots will not produce pain when pressure is applied.

HAIR CHARACTERISTICS

Hair color and texture are also biologic variants. Darker-pigmented people usually have dark brown or black hair. Hair texture, also an inherited characteristic, is the result of the amount of protein molecules within the hair. Variations may range from straight to very curly hair.

The curlier the hair, the more difficult it is to comb. In general, using wide-toothed combs or picks, wetting the hair with water before combing, or applying a moisturizing cream makes hair grooming more manageable. Some patients with very curly hair prefer to arrange it in small, tightly braided sections.

Physiologic Variations

There are three inherited enzymatic variations that are prevalent among people from various subcultures in the United States. They include absence or insufficiency of the enzymes lactase, glucose-6-phosphate dehydrogenase (G-6-PD), and alcohol dehydrogenase (ADH).

LACTASE DEFICIENCY

Lactase is a digestive enzyme that converts lactose, the sugar in milk, into simpler sugars, glucose and galactose. A lactase deficiency causes an intolerance to dairy products. Without lactase, people experience cramps, intestinal gas, and diarrhea approximately 30 minutes after ingesting milk or foods that contain milk. The symptoms may continue for up to 2 hours (Dudek, 1993). The discomfort may be prevented by eliminating or reducing sources of lactose in the diet. Liquid tube feeding formulas and those used for bottle-fed infants also can be prepared with milk substitutes.

Because milk is a good source of calcium, which is necessary for health, affected people are taught to obtain calcium from other sources such as calcium supplements, green leafy vegetables, dates, prunes, canned

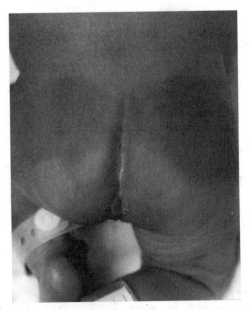

FIGURE 6-4
Mongolian spots are blue discolorations that are common in dark-skinned infants. (Courtesy of Ken Timby.)

PATIENT TEACHING FOR REDUCING OR ELIMINATING LACTOSE

Teach the patient or the family to do the following:

- Avoid milk and dairy products, and packaged foods that list dry milk solids or whey among their ingredients; these may include bread, cereals, puddings, gravy mixes, and caramels and chocolate.
- Use nondairy creamers, which are lactose free, in lieu of cream
- Consume only small amounts of milk or dairy products at a time.

- Substitute milk that has been cultured with the *Acidophilus* organism, which changes lactose into lactic acid.
- Drink LactAid, a commercial product, in which the lactose has been preconverted into other absorbable sugars.
- Use Kosher foods, which are prepared without milk, and identifiable by the word *pareve* on the label.

sardines and salmon with bones, egg yolk, whole grains, and dried peas and beans.

GLUCOSE-6-PHOSPHATE DEHYDROGENASE DEFICIENCY

Glucose-6-phosphate dehydrogenase is an enzyme that assists red blood cells to metabolize glucose. African Americans and those who come from Mediterranean countries commonly lack this enzyme. The disorder is manifested by men because the gene is sex linked, but women can carry and transmit the faulty gene.

A G-6-PD deficiency makes red blood cells vulnerable during stress, when metabolic needs are increased. When this happens, red blood cells are destroyed at a much greater rate than in unaffected populations. If the production of new red blood cells cannot match the rate of current destruction, anemia develops.

There are several drugs that can precipitate the anemic process (Table 6-1). It is therefore important that nurses intervene if these drugs, or those that depress red cell production, are prescribed for ethnic patients who are at greatest risk. Or, at the very least, nurses must monitor susceptible patients and advocate for laboratory tests, like red blood cell count and hemoglobin levels, that will indicate if adverse effects are occurring.

ALCOHOL METABOLISM

When alcohol is consumed, it is eventually broken down into acetic acid and carbon dioxide through a process of chemical reactions involving enzymes, one of which is ADH. Asian Americans and Native Americans often metabolize alcohol at a different rate because of physiologic variations in their enzyme system. The result is that affected people experience dramatic vascular effects, like flushing and rapid heart rate, soon after consuming alcohol. In addition, middle metabolites of alcohol (those that are formed before acetic acid) remain unchanged for a prolonged period of time. Many scientists believe that the middle metabolites, like acetaldehyde, are extremely toxic and subsequently play the primary role in causing organ damage. This theory may explain why cirrhosis accounts for three times more deaths among Native Americans than in the general population.

Disease Prevalence

There are several diseases, like sickle cell anemia, hypertension, diabetes, and stroke, that occur with much greater frequency among ethnic subcultures than in the general population. The incidence of chronic illness affects mortality rates differently as well (Table 6-2).

TABLE 6-1. *Drugs That Precipitate Glucose 6-Phosphate Dehydrogenase Anemia*

Drug Category	Example	Use
Quinine compounds	Primaquine phosphate	Prevention and treatment of malaria
Urocosurics	Probenecid (Benemid)	Treatment of gout
Sulfonamides	Sulfasalazine (Azulfidine)	Treatment of urinary infections

TABLE 6-2. *Leading Causes of Death Among U.S. Cultural Groups*

Rank	All Americans*	African Americans†	Latinos‡	Native Americans§	Asian Americans‖
1	Heart disease	Heart disease	Heart disease	Heart disease	Heart disease
2	Cancer	Cancer	Cancer	Cancer	Cancer
3	Stroke	Stroke	Injuries	Injuries	Stroke
4	Chronic lung disease	Injuries	Stroke	Stroke	Injuries
5	Injuires	Homicide	Homicide	Liver disease	Pneumonia/influenza
6	Pneumonia/influenza	Diabetes	Liver disease	Diabetes	Chronic lung disease
7	Diabetes	Pneumonia/influenza	Pneunomia/influenza	Pneumonia/influenza	Suicide
8	HIV infection	Perinatal conditions	Diabetes	Suicide	Diabetes
9	Suicide	Chronic lung disease	HIV infection	Homicide	Perinatal conditions
10	Homicide	HIV infection	Perinatal conditions	Chronic lung disease	Liver disease

HIV, human immunodeficiency virus.
*Leading causes of death, U.S. population, 1989, National Center for Health Statistics (CDC).
†Leading causes of death for blacks, 1987, National Center for Health Statistics (CDC).
‡Leading causes of deaths for Hispanics in 18 states and District of Columbia, 1987, Monthly Vital Statistics Report, Supplement, September 26, 1989 (national death rate unavailable).
§Leading causes of death for American Indians in Reservation States, 1987, Indian Service and National Center for Health Statistics (CDC).
‖Leading causes of deaths for Asians and Pacific Islanders in California, 1987, California State Department of Health and Asian American Health Forum.

The incidence of some chronic diseases and their complications may be the result, in part, of variations in social factors like poverty. Minority cultural groups tend to be less affluent. Consequently, their access to expensive health care is often limited. Without preventive health care, early detection, and treatment, higher death rates are bound to occur. The United States has, therefore, committed itself to reducing the disparity in health care among all Americans (see National Health Promotion and Disease Prevention Objectives, Chap. 4).

With the knowledge that special populations are at higher risk for chronic diseases, culturally sensitive nurses focus heavily on health teaching, participate in community health screening, and campaign for more equitable health services.

Health Beliefs and Practices

There are many differences in health beliefs among subcultures living in the United States. They exist and are perpetuated because of strong ethnic influences. Health beliefs, in turn, affect health practices (Table 6-3).

The health practices that are unique to a particular group of people are sometimes referred to as **folk medicine**. Folk medicine has come to mean those methods of disease prevention or treatment that are outside the mainstream of conventional practices. Folk medicine is often provided by lay rather than formally educated and licensed people.

However, just because a health belief or practice is different, does not make it wrong. It is up to culturally

TABLE 6-3. *Common Health Beliefs and Practices*

Cultural Group	Health Belief	Health Practices
Anglo-Americans	Illness is caused by infectious microorganisms, organ degeneration, and unhealthy lifestyles.	Physicians are consulted for diagnosis and treatment; nurses provide physical care.
African Americans	Supernatural forces can cause disease and influence recovery.	Individual and group prayer is used to speed recovery.
Asian Americans	Health is the result of a balance between *yin* and *yang* energy; illness results when equilibrium is disturbed.	Acupuncture, acupressure, food, and herbs are used to restore balance.
Latinos	Illness and misfortune occur as a punishment from God, referred to as *castigo de Dios*, or they are caused by an imbalance of "hot" or "cold" forces within the body.	Prayer and penance are performed to receive forgiveness; the services of lay practitioners who are believed to possess spiritual healing power are used; foods that are "hot" or "cold" are consumed to restore balance.
Native Americans	Illness occurs when the harmony of nature (Mother Earth) is disturbed.	A *shaman*, or medicine man, who has both spiritual and healing power, is consulted to restore harmony.

sensitive nurses to respect the patient's belief system and integrate scientifically based treatment along with folk medicine practices.

DEMONSTRATING CULTURAL SENSITIVITY

Just accepting that Americans are multicultural is a beginning step toward transcultural nursing. In addition, the following recommendations are offered for demonstrating culturally sensitive nursing care:

- Learn to speak a second language.
- Use techniques for facilitating interactions, like sitting within the patient's comfort zone and making appropriate eye contact.
- Become familiar with physical differences among ethnic groups.
- Perform physical assessments, especially of the skin, using techniques that will provide accurate data.
- Learn or ask patients about their cultural beliefs concerning health, illness, and techniques for healing.
- Consult the patient on ways to solve health problems.
- Never ridicule a cultural belief or practice, verbally or nonverbally.
- Integrate cultural practices that are helpful or harmless within the plan of care.
- Modify or gradually change practices that are unsafe.
- Avoid removing religious medals or clothing that hold symbolic meaning for the patient; but if this must be done, keep them safe and replace them as soon as possible.
- Provide food that is customarily eaten.
- Advocate that patients be routinely screened for diseases to which they are genetically or culturally prone.
- Facilitate rituals by whomever the patient identifies as a healer within his or her belief system.
- Apologize if cultural traditions or beliefs are violated.

KEY CONCEPTS

- Culture refers to the values, beliefs, and practices of a particular group. Race refers to biologic variations. Ethnicity is the bond or kinship a person feels with his or her country of birth or place of ancestral origin.
- Two factors that interfere with perceiving others as individuals are stereotyping, which involves ascribing fixed beliefs about people based on some general

characteristic, and ethnocentrism, the belief that one's own ethnicity is superior to all others.

- The American culture is said to be Anglicized because many of the values, beliefs, and practices evolved from the early settlers, who were English.
- Some examples of Anglo-American culture include speaking English; valuing work, time, and technology; holding parents responsible for the health care, behavior, and education of minor children; keeping government separate from religion; and, when health care is necessary, seeking the assistance of licensed practitioners.
- A subculture is a unique cultural group that coexists within the dominant culture. There are four major subcultures living within the United States: African Americans, Latinos, Asian Americans, and Native Americans.
- Subcultural groups differ from Anglo-Americans in one or more of the following ways: language, communication style, biologic and physiologic variations, prevalence of diseases, and health beliefs and practices.
- There are three characteristics of culturally sensitive nursing care. They are (1) acceptance of each patient as an individual, (2) knowledge of health problems that affect particular cultural groups, and (3) planning care within the patient's health belief system to achieve the best health outcomes.
- Some ways that nurses can demonstrate cultural sensitivity include learning a second language, performing physical assessments and care according to the patient's unique biologic differences, consulting with each patient as to his or her cultural preferences, advocating for modifications in diet and dress according to the patient's customs, and allowing patients to continue to rely on cultural health practices that are not harmful.

CRITICAL THINKING EXERCISES

- During the war in Vietnam, nurses cared for both military casualties as well as sick and wounded Vietnamese. Discuss how both American nurses and their non-American patients may have experienced culture shock during this time.
- A nurse who is employed by a home health agency is assigned to the home care of a non–English-speaking patient from Pakistan. Discuss how a culturally sensitive nurse might prepare for this patient's care.
- A pregnant Haitian woman explains to a nurse that she is wearing a chicken bone about her neck to protect her unborn child from birth defects. Discuss how best to respond to this woman from a culturally sensitive perspective.

SUGGESTED READINGS

Blackburn JA. Achieving a multicultural service orientation: adaptive models in service delivery and race and culture training. Caring April 1992;11:22–26.

Boyle JS, Andrews MM. Transcultural Concepts in Nursing Care. Glenview, IL: Scott, Foresman/Little, Brown College Division, 1989.

Cerny L. Ethnocentric nursing. Canadian Nurse June 1991;87:10.

Chinn PL. Diversity: what does it mean? Nursing Outlook March–April 1992;40:54.

Dudek SG. Nutrition Handbook for Nursing Practice, 2nd ed. Philadelphia: JB Lippincott, 1993.

Giger JN, Davidhizar R. Transcultural nursing assessment: a method for advancing nursing practice. International Nursing Review January–February 1990;37:199–202.

Giger JN, Davidhizar RE. Transcultural Nursing: Assessment and Intervention. St. Louis: Mosby, 1991.

Irwin MJ. Assessing color changes for dark skinned patients. Advancing Clinical Care November–December 1991;6:8–10.

Kavanaugh KH. Transcultural nursing: facing the challenges of advocacy and diversity/universality. Journal of Transcultural Nursing Summer 1993;5:4–13.

Leininger MM. Leininger's theory of nursing: Cultural care diversity and universality. Nursing Science Quarterly May 1988;152–160.

Manio EB, Hall RR. Asian family traditions and their influence in transcultural health care delivery. Children's Health Care Winter 1987;3:172–177.

Outlaw FH. A reformulation of the meaning of culture and ethnicity for nurses delivering care. MEDSURG Nursing April 1994;3:108–111.

Robertson MHB. Defining cultural and ethnic differences to adapt to a changing patient population. American Nurse September 1993;25:6.

Rosenbaum JN. A cultural assessment guide: learning cultural sensitivity. Canadian Nurse April 1991;87:32–33.

Sheridan DR, Zimbler E. Nursing Management Skills. Module IV: Transcultural Nursing. New York: National League for Nursing, 1993.

Spector RE. Cultural Diversity in Health and Illness. 3rd ed. Norwalk, CT: Appleton & Lange, 1991.

Wilson UM. Nursing care of American Indian patients. Ethnic Nursing Care: A Multicultural Approach. MS Orgue, B Block, and LSA Monrroy, Editors. St. Louis: Mosby, 1983, 271–295.

Zborowski M. Cultural components in responses to pain. Journal of Social Issues 1952;8:16–30.

Zborowski M. People in Pain. San Francisco: Jossey Bass, 1969.

UNIT III

Fostering Communication

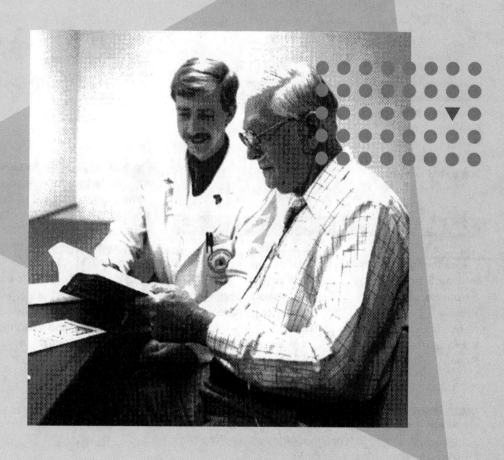

CHAPTER 7

The Nurse–Patient Relationship

Key Terms

Affective Touch	Public Space
Communication	Relationship
Intimate Space	Social Space
Introductory Phase	Task-related Touch
Kinesics	Terminating Phase
Nonverbal Communication	Touch
Paralanguage	Verbal Communication
Personal Space	Working Phase

Learning Objectives

An understanding of the content within this chapter will be evidenced by the student's ability to:

- Describe the current role expectations for patients
- List at least five principles that underlie a nurse–patient relationship
- Identify three phases of a nurse–patient relationship
- Differentiate between communication and therapeutic communication
- Give five examples of therapeutic and nontherapeutic communication techniques
- List at least five factors that affect oral communication
- Describe three forms of nonverbal communication
- Differentiate task-related touch from affective touch
- List at least five situations in which affective touch may be appropriate

Nurses provide services, or skills, that assist people, called patients or clients, to resolve health problems that are beyond their own capabilities or to cope with those that will not improve. There are several differences between the services that nurses provide and those provided by other caring individuals (Display 7-1).

An intangible factor that helps hold nurses in high regard is the relationship that develops between nurses and patients. And, one of the primary keys to establishing and maintaining a positive nurse–patient relationship is the manner and style of a nurse's communication.

THE NURSE–PATIENT RELATIONSHIP

The word **relationship** refers to an association between two people. During the time when nursing services are provided, a relationship is established between the nurse and patient. The nurse–patient relationship could also be called a therapeutic relationship because the desired outcome of the association is almost always one of moving toward a goal of restored health.

The relationship between nurses and patients has gradually changed. In the past, patients were expected to play a passive role, allow others to make decisions for them, and submit to treatments without question or protest. Nurses now encourage and expect people for whom they care to become actively involved, to communicate, to question, to assist in planning their care,

Timby BK: *Fundamental Skills and Concepts in Patient Care, Sixth Edition* © 1996 Lippincott-Raven Publishers

DISPLAY 7-1. *Differentiating Caring Acts From Nursing Acts*

Caring Acts	Nursing Acts
Prompted by observing a person in distress	Prompted by a concern for the well-being of everyone
Motivated by sympathy	Motivated by altruism
Spontaneous	Planned
Goal is to relieve crisis	Goal is to promote self-reliance
Outcomes are short-term	Outcomes are long-term
Assume major responsibility for resolving the person's problem	Expect mutual cooperation in resolving health problems
Experience-based	Knowledge-based
Modeled on a personal moral code	Modeled on a formal code of ethics
Guided by common sense	Legally defined
Accountability based on acting reasonably prudent	Accountability based on meeting professional standards

and, overall, retain as much independence as possible (Display 7-2).

Underlying Principles

A therapeutic nurse–patient relationship is more likely to develop when the nurse:

- Treats each patient as a unique person
- Respects the patient's feelings
- Strives to promote the patient's physical, emotional, social, and spiritual well-being
- Encourages the patient to participate in problem-solving and decision-making
- Accepts that a patient has the potential for growth and change
- Communicates using terms and language that the patient understands
- Uses the nursing process to individualize the patient's care
- Incorporates those people to whom the patient turns to for support, such as family and friends, when providing care
- Implements health care techniques that are compatible with the patient's value system and cultural heritage.

Phases of the Nurse–Patient Relationship

Nurse–patient relationships ordinarily are brief. They begin when patients seek services that will maintain or restore health, or prevent disease. They end when patients can independently achieve their health-related goals. This type of relationship is usually described as having three phases: the introductory phase, the working phase, and the terminating phase.

THE INTRODUCTORY PHASE

The relationship between the patient and the nurse begins with the **introductory phase**, or the period of getting acquainted. Each person usually brings preconceived ideas about the other to the initial interaction. These assumptions are eventually either confirmed or dismissed.

The patient initiates the relationship by identifying one or more health problems for which help is being sought. It is important for the nurse to demonstrate courtesy, active listening, empathy, competency, and appropriate communication skills to ensure that the relationship begins positively.

THE WORKING PHASE

The **working phase** involves mutually planning the patient's care and putting the plan into action. Both the nurse and the patient participate. Each shares in performing those tasks that will lead to the desired outcomes identified by the patient. During the working phase, the nurse tries not to retard the patient's independence. Doing too much can be as harmful as doing too little.

THE TERMINATING PHASE

The nurse–patient relationship is self-limiting. The **terminating phase** occurs when there is mutual agree-

DISPLAY 7-2. *Responsibilities Within the Nurse–Patient Relationship*

Nursing Responsibilities	Patient Responsibilities
Possess current knowledge	Identify current problem
Be aware of unique age-related differences	Describe desired outcomes
Perform technical skills safely	Answer questions honestly
Be committed to patient care	Provide accurate historical and subjective data
Be available and courteous	Particpate to fullest extent possible
Allow participation in decisions	Be open and flexible to alternatives
Remain objective	Comply with the plan for care
Advocate on the patient's behalf	Keep appointments for follow-up care
Provide explanations in language that is easily understood	
Promote independence	

ment that the patient's immediate health problems have improved. The nurse uses a caring attitude and compassion in facilitating the patient's transition of care to other health care services or independent living.

COMMUNICATION

Communication is an exchange of information. It involves both sending and receiving messages between two or more individuals. It is followed by feedback indicating that the information was understood or requires further clarification (Fig. 7-1).

Communication takes place simultaneously on a verbal and nonverbal level. Because no relationship can exist without verbal and nonverbal communication, it is essential that the nurse develop skills that enhance therapeutic interactions with patients.

Verbal Communication

Verbal communication is communication that uses words. It includes speaking, reading, and writing. Verbal communication is used by both the nurse and patient to gather facts. It is also used to instruct, clarify, and exchange ideas.

The ability to communicate orally or through a written medium is affected by:

- Attention and concentration
- Language compatibility
- Verbal skills
- Hearing and visual acuity
- Motor functions involving the throat, tongue, and teeth

- Noise and distracting activity
- Interpersonal attitudes
- Literacy
- Cultural similarities

Therapeutic Communication

Communication can take place on a social or therapeutic level. **Therapeutic communication** refers to using words and gestures to accomplish a particular objective. The ability of the nurse to encourage communication is extremely important, especially when exploring problems with the patient or encouraging the expression of feelings. Techniques that the nurse may find helpful are described in Table 7-1.

In situations where patients are quiet and noncommunicative, the nurse must never assume that it indicates the patient is problem-free or understands everything. It

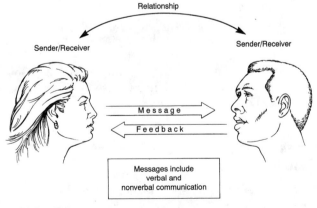

FIGURE 7-1

Communication is a two-way process between a sender and a receiver.

TABLE 7-1. *Therapeutic Communication Techniques*

Technique	Use	Example
Broad openings	Relieves tension before getting to the real purpose of the interaction	"Wonderful weather we're having."
Giving information	Provides facts	"Your surgery is scheduled at noon."
Direct questioning	Acquires specific information	"Do you have any allergies?"
Open-ended questioning	Encourages the patient to elaborate	"How are you feeling?"
Reflecting	Confirms that the conversation is being followed	Patient: "I haven't been sleeping well." Nurse: "You haven't been sleeping well."
Paraphrasing	Restates what the patient has said to demonstrate listening	Patient: "After every meal, I feel like I will throw up." Nurse: "Eating makes you nauseous, but you don't actually vomit."
Verbalizing what has been implied	Shares how a statement has been interpreted	Patient: "All the nurses are so busy." Nurse: "You're feeling that you shouldn't ask for help."
Structuring	Defines a purpose and sets limits	"I have 15 minutes. If your pain is relieved, I could go over how your test will be done."
Giving general leads	Encourages the patient to continue	"Uh, huh," or "Go on."
Sharing perceptions	Shows empathy for how the patient is feeling	"You seem depressed."
Clarifying	Avoids misinterpretation	"I'm afraid I don't quite understand what you're asking."
Confronting	Calls attention to manipulation, inconsistencies, or lack of responsibility	"You're concerned about your weight loss, but you didn't eat any breakfast."
Summarizing	Reviews information that has been discussed	"You've asked me to check on increasing your pain medication and getting your diet changed."
Silence	Allows time for considering how to proceed; or, arouses the patient's anxiety to the point that it stimulates more verbalization	

is never appropriate to probe and pry; rather, it may be advantageous to wait and be patient. It is not unusual for reticent patients to share their feelings and concerns after they feel that the nurse is sincere and trustworthy.

On the other hand, the response of the nurse to a very vocal and emotional patient must also be handled delicately. For instance, when patients are angry or cry, the best nursing approach is to allow them to express their emotions. Allowing patients to display their feelings without fear of retaliation or censure contributes to a therapeutic relationship.

Although nurses often have the best intentions of interacting therapeutically with patients, some fall into traps that block or hinder verbal communication. Table 7-2 lists common examples of nontherapeutic communication.

Listening

Listening is as important during communication as speaking. Giving attention to what patients say provides a stimulus for meaningful interaction. It is important for the nurse to avoid giving signals that indicate boredom, impatience, or the pretense of listening. For example, looking out a window, interrupting a comment, or looking distant or away are signs of a lack of interest. When communicating with most Americans, it is best to position oneself at the person's level and make frequent eye contact (see Chap. 6 for cultural exceptions). Nodding and encouraging the patient to continue with comments like "Yes, I see," conveys full involvement in what is being said.

Silence

Silence plays an important role in communication. **Silence** involves intentionally withholding verbal commentary. At first glance, it may seem contradictory to include silence as a form of verbal communication. However, one of its uses is actually to encourage participation in verbal discussions. Other therapeutic uses for silence are to relieve a patient's anxiety just by providing a personal presence and to provide a brief period of time during which patients can process information or respond to a question.

Patients may use silence to camouflage their fears or to express contentment. Silence also may be used for introspection when exploring feelings or when praying. Interrupting silence, when someone is deep in concentration, disturbs the thinking process. A common obstacle to effective communication is ignoring the importance of silence and talking excessively.

TABLE 7-2. *Nontherapeutic Communication Techniques*

Technique and Consequence	Example	Improvement
Giving False Reassurance Trivializes the unique feelings of the patient and discourages further discussion	"You've got nothing to worry about. Everything will work out just fine."	"Tell me about your specific concerns."
Using Clichés Provides worthless advice and curtails exploring alternatives	"Keep a stiff upper lip."	"It must be difficult for you right now."
Giving Approval or Disapproval Holds the patient to a rigid standard; implies that future deviation may lead to subsequent rejection or disfavor	"I'm glad you're exercising so regularly." "You should be testing your blood sugar each morning."	"Are you having any difficulty fitting regular exercise into your schedule?" "Let's explore some ways that will help you test your blood sugar each morning."
Agreeing Does not allow the patient flexibility to change his or her mind	"You're right about needing surgery immediately."	"Having surgery immediately is one possibility. What others have you considered?"
Disagreeing Intimidates the patient; makes the patient feel foolish or inadequate	"That's not true! Where did you get an idea like that?"	"Maybe I can help clarify that for you."
Demanding an Explanation Puts the patient on the defensive; the patient may be tempted to make up an excuse rather than risk disapproval for an honest answer	"Why didn't you keep your appointment last week?"	"I see you couldn't keep your appointment last week."
Giving Advice Discourages independent problem-solving and decision-making; provides a biased view that may prejudice the patient's choice	"If I were you, I'd try drug therapy before having surgery."	"Share with me the advantages and disadvantages of your options as you see them."
Defending Indicates such a strong allegiance that any disagreement to the contrary is not acceptable	"Ms. Johnson is my best nursing assistant. She wouldn't have let your light go unanswered that long."	"I'm sorry you had to wait so long."
Belittling Disregards how the patient is responding as an individual	"Lots of people learn to give themselves insulin."	"You're finding it especially difficult to stick yourself with a needle."
Patronizing Treats the patient in a condescending manner as less than capable of making an independent decision	"Are *we* ready for *our* bath yet?"	"Would you like your bath now, or should I check with you later?"
Changing the Subject Alters the direction of the discussion to a topic that is safer or more comfortable	Patient: "I'm so scared that a mammogram will show I have cancer." Nurse: "Tell me more about your family."	"It is a serious disease. What concerns you the most?"

Nonverbal Communication

Nonverbal communication is the exchange of information without using words. It is what is *not* said. The manner in which verbal information is conveyed affects its meaning. A person has less control over nonverbal than verbal communication. Words can be chosen with care, but a facial expression is harder to control. As a result, messages are often communicated more accurately through nonverbal communication.

People communicate nonverbally through techniques described as kinesics, paralanguage, proxemics, and touch.

KINESICS

Kinesics refers to body language, or those collective nonverbal techniques like facial expressions, posture, gestures, and body movements. Some add that clothing style and accessories like jewelry also affect the context of communication.

PARALANGUAGE

Paralanguage is vocal sounds that are not actually words, but communicate a message. Some examples include drawing in a deep breath to indicate surprise, clucking the tongue to indicate disappointment, whistling to get someone's attention. Vocal inflections, volume, pitch, and rate of speech also add another dimension to communication. Crying, laughing, and moaning are additional forms of paralanguage.

PROXEMICS

Proxemics is the use and relationship of space to communication. In general, there are four zones that are observed among interactions between Americans (Hall, 1959, 1963, 1966). They include an **intimate space**, **personal space**, **social space**, and **public space** (Table 7-3).

Most Americans comfortably tolerate strangers up to a 2- to 3-foot area. Venturing closer within that boundary may cause some to feel anxious. Understanding the range of a person's comfort zone helps the nurse know how spatial relationships affect nonverbal communication.

Closeness is common in nursing because of the many times nurses and patients are in direct physical contact. Therefore, physical nearness and touching within intimate and personal spaces can be misinterpreted as having sexual connotations. Approaches that may prevent a misunderstanding of a nurse's intentions include explaining how a nursing procedure will be performed beforehand, ensuring that the patient is properly draped, and asking that another staff person of the patient's gender be present during an examination or procedure.

TOUCH

Touch is a tactile stimulus produced by making personal contact with another person or object. In the course of caring for patients, touch can be either task-oriented, affective, or both (Brady and Nesbitt, 1991; Burnside, 1988). **Task-oriented touch** involves the personal contact that is required when performing nursing procedures (Fig. 7-2). **Affective touch** is used to demonstrate concern or affection (Fig. 7-3).

Affective touch has different meanings to different people, depending on how they were raised and their cultural background. Because nursing care involves a high degree of touching, the nurse must be sensitive to how it is perceived. Most people respond positively to being touched. However, there may be a great deal of variation among individuals. Therefore, affective

TABLE 7-3. *Communication Zones*		
Zone	Distance	Purpose
Intimate space	Within 6 inches	• Lovemaking • Confiding secrets • Sharing confidential information
Personal space	6 inches to 4 feet	• Interviewing • Physical assessment • Therapeutic interventions involving touch • Private conversations • Teaching one-on-one
Social space	4 to 12 feet	• Group interactions • Lecturing • Conversations that are not intended to be private
Public space	12 or more feet	• Giving speeches • Gatherings of strangers

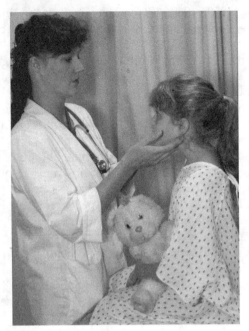

FIGURE 7-2
Examining a patient involves task-oriented touch. (Courtesy of Ken Timby.)

touching must be used cautiously, even though its intention is to communicate caring and support. In general, affective touch may be used therapeutically when a patient is:

- Lonesome
- Uncomfortable
- Near death
- Anxious, insecure, or frightened
- Disoriented
- Disfigured
- Semiconscious or comatose
- Visually impaired
- Sensory deprived

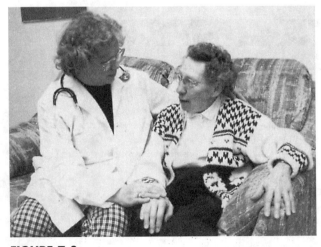

FIGURE 7-3
This nurse uses affective touch as she talks with her home-bound patient. (Courtesy of Ken Timby.)

 FOCUS ON OLDER ADULTS

- To show genuine respect, older adults are always called by their title and surname (eg, Mr. Wentworth) until it has been determined by which name they preferred to be called.
- In spite of functional deficits, older adults are never treated as if they are children.
- Older adults tend to cling to their world through the sense of touch; touching may be more important than talking (Brady and Nesbitt, 1991).
- It is important to let older adults control decisions and make choices as much as possible. Dependence is often difficult for older adults to accept. Being allowed to maintain independence maintains their self-esteem and dignity.
- Older adults are allowed to pace their own care. This requires more time, but rushing an older patient often results in frustration, anger, and resentment.
- A useful technique for facilitating communication with older adults is to encourage reminiscing. Giving older adults an opportunity to talk about experiences and events that took place during an earlier time of their lives reinforces their value and unique identity.

KEY CONCEPTS

- The current patient role expectations are that he or she becomes actively involved, communicates, asks questions, assists in planning his or her care, and, overall, retains as much independence as possible
- Some principles that underlie a therapeutic nurse–patient relationship include (1) treating each patient as a unique person, (2) respecting the patient's feelings, (3) striving to promote the patient's physical, emotional, social, and spiritual well-being, (4) encouraging the patient to participate in problem-solving and decision-making, and (5) accepting that a patient has the potential for growth and change.
- A nurse–patient relationship usually spans three phases: the introductory phase, the working phase, and the terminating stage.
- Communication involves sending and receiving messages between two or more individuals, followed by feedback indicating that the information was understood or requires further clarification. Therapeutic communication refers to using words and gestures to accomplish a particular objective.
- Examples of therapeutic communication techniques include questioning, reflecting, paraphrasing, sharing

perceptions, and clarifying. Examples of nontherapeutic communication techniques include giving false reassurance, using clichés, giving approval or disapproval, demanding an explanation, and giving advice.
- Some factors that may affect oral communication include language compatibility; verbal skills; hearing and visual acuity; motor functions involving the throat, tongue, and teeth; noise and activity; and interpersonal attitudes.
- There are three forms of nonverbal communication. Kinesics refers to body language; paralanguage involves vocal sounds; and proxemics relates to how space is used in communication.
- Task-related touch involves the personal contact that takes place when performing nursing procedures. Affective touch is used to demonstrate concern or affection.
- There are many situations in which affective touch may be appropriate, such as when caring for patients who are lonesome, uncomfortable, near death, anxious, and sensory deprived.

CRITICAL THINKING EXERCISES

- Because nursing is a service-oriented profession, describe specific services a person might expect from a nurse that would be different from those expected from a physician.
- Discuss why older adults may not be touched with the same frequency as patients in other age groups.

SUGGESTED READINGS

Brady BA, Nesbitt SN. Using the right touch. Nursing May 1991;21: 46–47.
Burnside I. Nursing and the Aged. 3rd ed. St. Louis: CV Mosby, 1988.
Hall ET. A system for the notation of proxemic behavior. American Anthropologist May 1963;65:1003–1026.
Hall ET. The Hidden Dimension. New York: Doubleday, 1966.
Hall ET. The Silent Language. New York: Fawcett, 1959.
Marquis BL, Huston CJ. Leadership Roles and Management Functions in Nursing. Philadelphia: JB Lippincott, 1992.
McFarland GK, Thomas MD. Psychiatric Mental Health Nursing. Philadelphia: JB Lippincott, 1991.

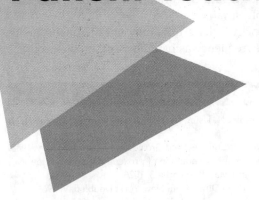

CHAPTER 8
Patient Teaching

Key Terms

Affective Domain
Androgogy
Cognitive Domain
Functionally Illiterate
Gerogogy

Illiterate
Literacy
Pedagogy
Psychomotor Domain

Learning Objectives

An understanding of the content within this chapter will be evidenced by the student's ability to:

* Describe three learning styles
* Discuss three age-related categories of learners
* Discuss at least three characteristics that are unique to older adult learners
* Identify four factors that are assessed before teaching patients

One of the most important uses for communication in nursing is patient teaching. Health teaching promotes the patient's independent ability to meet his or her own health needs. An old proverb that reinforces how education promotes self-sufficiency says, "Give a man a fish and he will eat for a day; teach a man to fish and he will eat for a lifetime."

PATIENT TEACHING

Health teaching is no longer an optional nursing activity. Many state nurse practice acts legally require it. Nurses have been sued when discharged patients are readmitted or harmed because they were uninformed or failed to understand the information that was taught. Medical records must show what has been taught and the evidence that learning took place. Limited hospitalization time has demanded that nurses begin teaching as soon as possible after admission rather than waiting until discharge.

Learning Styles

There are three styles of learning. They include the cognitive, affective, and psychomotor domains. The **cognitive domain** involves processing information by listening to or reading facts and descriptions (Fig. 8-1). The **affective domain** refers to learning that appeals to a person's feelings, beliefs, or values. The **psychomotor domain** involves learning by doing. Display 8-1 lists the types of activities that are associated with each of the learning domains.

People tend to prefer one domain for learning. One way to determine which method is preferred is to ask, "When you learned to add fractions, what helped you most: hearing the teacher's explanation or reading about it in a mathematics book, recognizing the value of the exercise, or actually working sample problems?"

Concepts in Patient Care, Sixth Edition © 1996 Lippincott-Raven Publishers

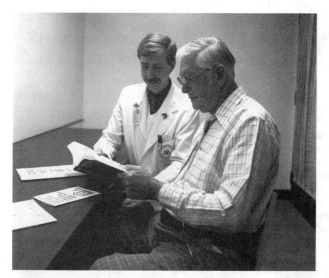

FIGURE 8-1
Teaching via the cognitive domain. (Courtesy of McLaren Regional Medical Center, Flint, MI.)

Although most favor one domain, learning tends to be optimized by presenting information through a combination of teaching approaches. This is evidenced by the fact that "learners retain 10% of what they read, 20% of what they hear, 30% of what they see, 50% of what they see and hear, 70% of what they teach/talk, and 90% of what they talk/do" (Heinrich et al., 1992; Rega, 1993).

Age-Related Differences

Educators emphasize that learning takes place differently depending on a person's developmental level. **Pedagogy** refers to the science of teaching children. **Androgogy** refers to principles that affect adult learners. Recently, a distinction has been made between learners at the early and later ends of the adult spectrum, and a separate set of principles, referred to as **gerogogy**, concerns approaches that enhance learning among older adults.

Teaching tends to be more effective when it is designed to accommodate unique age-related differences. Therefore, nurses and anyone else who provides instruction must be aware of the learning characteristics of child, adult, and older adult learners (Table 8-1).

Assessing the Learner

Besides determining which style of learning a patient prefers and the patient's developmental stage, the nurse must consider many other variables, such as the capacity to learn, motivation for learning, and readiness to learn.

ASSESSING THE CAPACITY TO LEARN

For the mind to receive, remember, analyze, and apply new information, a certain amount of intellectual ability must exist. Illiteracy, sensory deficits, and a shortened attention span may require special adaptations when implementing health teaching.

Literacy

Literacy refers to the ability to read and write. There are approximately 27 million **illiterate** Americans who can do neither (Lynch, 1992). There are an additional 35 million Americans who are considered **functionally illiterate** (Kozol, 1985), which means they can sign their name, perform simple mathematical tasks (like making change), and read at or below a ninth grade level. Functional illiteracy may be the consequence of a learning disability, not a below-average intellectual capacity.

Because many illiterate or functionally illiterate people are not apt to volunteer this information, literacy may be difficult to assess. Those who are illiterate and functionally illiterate usually develop elaborate mechanisms to disguise or compensate for their learning deficits. To protect the patient's self-esteem, the nurse may ask, "How do you learn best?", and plan accordingly. Some approaches that may be useful when teaching illiterate or semiliterate patients include:

- Using verbal and visual modes for instruction
- Repeating directions several times in the same sequence each time so the patient can memorize the required information
- Providing pictures, diagrams, or audiotapes for future review

DISPLAY 8-1. _Activities That Promote Learning_		
Cognitive Domain	**Psychomotor Domain**	**Affective Domain**
Listing	Assembling	Advocating
Identifying	Changing	Supporting
Locating	Emptying	Accepting
Labeling	Filling	Promoting
Summarizing	Adding	Refusing
Selecting	Removing	Defending

TABLE 8-1. Age-Related Differences Among Learners*

Pedagogic Learners	Andragogic Learners	Gerogogic Learners
Physically immature	Physically mature	Undergoing degenerative changes
Lacks experience	Building experience	Vast experience
Compulsory learners	Voluntary learners	Crisis learners
Passive	Active	Passive/active
Needs direction and supervision	Self-directed and independent	Needs structure and encouragement
Motivated to learn by potential rewards or punishment	Seeks knowledge for its own sake or personal interest	Motivated by a personal need or goal
Learning is subject-centered	Learning is problem-centered	Learning is self-centered
Short attention span	Longer attention span	Attention affected by low energy level, fatigue, and anxiety
Convergent thinkers (unidirectional; eg, see one application for new information)	Divergent thinkers (process multiple applications for new information)	Practical thinkers (process new information as it applies to a unique personal problem)
Needs immediate feedback	Can postpone feedback	Responds to frequent feedback
Rote learning	Analytical learning	Experiential learning
Short-term retention	Long-term retention	Short-term unless reinforced by immediate use
Task oriented	Goal oriented	Outcome oriented
Thinks concretely	Thinks abstractly	Concrete/abstract
Responds to competition	Responds to collaboration	Responds to family encouragement

*Each learner is unique and may demonstrate characteristics associated with other age groups.

Sensory Deficits

The abilities to see and hear are essential to almost every learning situation. Older adults tend to have visual and auditory deficits, although they are not exclusive to older adult learners. Some techniques for teaching a sensory-impaired patient follow.

 NURSING GUIDELINES FOR TEACHING SENSORY-IMPAIRED PATIENTS

- Make sure the patient who is visually impaired is wearing prescription eyeglasses, and the hearing-impaired patient is wearing a hearing aid, if available
  Rationale: Maximizes the ability to perceive sensory stimuli.
- Speak in a normal tone of voice to a visually impaired patient.
  Rationale: Dispels the myth that one sense becomes more acute than another
- Use at least a 75- to 100-watt light source, preferably in a lamp that shines over the patient's shoulder.
  Rationale: Concentrates light on a small area where the patient needs to focus
- Avoid standing in front of a window through which bright sunlight is shining.
  Rationale: Reduces distracting glare

- Provide a magnifying glass for reading.
  Rationale: Enlarges standard or small print to a size that is comfortable to read
- Obtain pamphlets in large print size (12- to 16-point) and serif lettering, which has horizontal lines at the bottom and top of each letter (Fig. 8-2).
  Rationale: Promotes visual discrimination
- Avoid using materials that are printed on glossy paper.
  Rationale: Decreases glare that makes reading uncomfortable
- Select black print on white paper.
  Rationale: Provides maximum contrast and makes the letters more legible

For the Hearing-Impaired Patient
- Use a magic slate, chalkboard, flash cards, and writing pads to communicate.
  Rationale: Provides visual alternatives
- Lower the voice pitch.
  Rationale: Accommodates for hearing loss that is usually in the higher pitch ranges
- Try to select words that do not begin with "f," "s," "k," and "sh."
  Rationale: Avoids using letters that are formed with high-pitched sounds and therefore difficult to discriminate.
- Rephrase rather than repeat when the patient does not understand.
  Rationale: Provides additional visual or auditory clues to facilitate the patient's understanding

- Insert a stethoscope into a patient's ears and speak into the bell with a low voice.
  Rationale: Acts like a primitive hearing aid. It directs sounds directly to the ears and reduces background noise

Cultural Differences

Because teaching and learning involve language, the nurse must modify teaching approaches if the patient cannot speak English or English is a second language (see Chap. 6, Nursing Guidelines for Communicating With Non–English-Speaking Patients). However, language barriers do not justify omitting health teaching. In most cases, if neither the nurse nor the patient speak a compatible language, a family member, friend, health care worker, or resident within the community may be asked to act as a translator.

Attention and Concentration

The patient's attention and concentration affect the choice of teaching methods that may be used, as well as the duration and delivery of the information to be presented. Some approaches that may be helpful include:

- Observing and implementing health teaching when the patient is most alert and comfortable
- Keeping the teaching session short
- Using the patient's name frequently throughout the instructional period because this refocuses the patient's attention
- Showing enthusiasm, which is likely to be communicated to the patient
- Using colorful brochures and gestures to stimulate the patient visually
- Involving the patient in an active way

12 pt. Times

Aa Bb Cc Dd Ee Ff Gg Hh Ii Jj Kk Ll
Oo Pp Qq Rr Ss Tt Uu Vv Ww Xx Yy

14 pt. Times

Aa Bb Cc Dd Ee Ff Gg Hh Ii Jj Kk
Oo Pp Qq Rr Ss Tt Uu Vv Ww Xx

16 pt. Times

Aa Bb Cc Dd Ee Ff
Oo Pp Qq Rr Ss Tt

FIGURE 8-2
Selecting printed materials with 12- to 16-point size type, black print on white paper, and serif lettering helps to improve visual clarity.

- Varying the tone and pitch of voice to stimulate the patient aurally

ASSESSING MOTIVATION

Optimum learning takes place when a person has a purpose for acquiring new information. The relevance of learning is also an individual variable. The patient's reasons for new learning may include satisfying intellectual curiosity, restoring independence, preventing complications, or facilitating discharge and return to the comfort of home. Other, less desirable reasons for learning are to please others and to avoid criticism.

ASSESSING READINESS

When the capacity and motivation for learning exist, learning readiness must be determined. Readiness refers to the patient's physical and psychological well-being. For example, a person who is in pain, uncomfortably warm or cold, having difficulty breathing, or feeling depressed or fearful is not in the best condition for learning. In these situations, it is best to restore comfort and then attend to teaching.

ASSESSING LEARNING NEEDS

The best teaching and learning takes place when it is individualized. To be most efficient and personalized, the nurse needs to gather pertinent information from the patient.

The following are questions the nurse can ask to assess the patient's learning needs:

- What does being healthy mean to you?
- What things in your life interfere with being healthy?
- What don't you understand as fully as you would like to?
- What activities do you need help with?
- What do you hope to accomplish before being discharged?
- How can I help you at this time?

Informal and Formal Teaching

Informal teaching is unplanned and occurs spontaneously at the patient's bedside. Formal teaching requires a plan; without a plan, teaching becomes haphazard. The potential for reaching goals, providing adequate information, and ensuring the patient's comprehension is jeopardized unless there is some organization of time and content. Potential teaching needs are usually identified at the time of a patient's admission, but may be amended as the patient's care and treatment progress.

A student nurse may work with a staff nurse or instructor in developing a teaching plan. Usually one or more nurses carry out certain specific parts of a teaching plan (Fig. 8-3). This is the most desirable approach because the patient is not overwhelmed with processing volumes of new information or learning skills that are difficult for a novice to perform.

The nursing guidelines that follow can be used as a model when teaching an adult patient. For unique approaches that may be more appropriate to use for older adults, refer to the Focus on Older Adults display.

NURSING GUIDELINES FOR TEACHING ADULT PATIENTS

- Find out what the patient wants to know.
  Rationale: Facilitates learning by addressing personal interests.
- Determine what the patient should know if he or she is to remain healthy.
  Rationale: Identifies priorities
- Collaborate with the patient on establishing content, goals, and a realistic time for accomplishing the task.
  Rationale: Promotes collaboration and active involvement in the learning process.
- Develop a written plan that builds from simple to complex, familiar to unfamiliar, normal to abnormal.

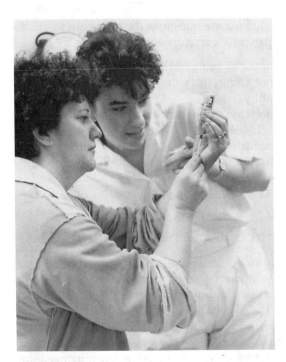

FIGURE 8-3
The nurse promotes multisensory stimulation by giving the patient verbal explanations and encouraging her to look at and hold the insulin bottle and syringe. (Courtesy of Ken Timby.)

Rationale: Improves learning by applying information from the adult's present level of knowledge or past experiences.
- Divide the information into manageable amounts.
  Rationale: Avoids overwhelming learners
- Select teaching methods and resources that are compatible with the patient's preferred style for learning.
  Rationale: Facilitates learning
- Use a variety of instructional methods from the cognitive, affective, and psychomotor domains.
  Rationale: Promotes retention when a variety of instructional techniques are used
- Teach when the patient appears interested and physically and emotionally ready to learn, if that is possible.
  Rationale: Hastens learning when the patient can focus on the task at hand
- Select an environment that is quiet, well lighted, and a comfortable temperature
  Rationale: Avoids distractions, interruptions, and discomfort that may interfere with concentration
- Identify how long the teaching session will last.
  Rationale: Prepares the patient for the demands on his or her time and attention
- Review previously taught information briefly.
  Rationale: Increases retention of information
- Use vocabulary that is within the patient's level of understanding, neither beneath nor above it.
  Rationale: Preserves personal dignity and ensures that the patient comprehends what is being taught
- Involve the patient actively by encouraging feedback and handling of equipment.
  Rationale: Appeals to an active learning style
- Stimulate as many of the senses as possible.
  Rationale: Enhances learning
- Use equipment similar to or an exact duplicate of what the patient will use at home.
  Rationale: Prepares the patient for self-care in the home environment
- Allow time for questions and answers.
  Rationale: Provides an opportunity for clarifying information and preventing misunderstanding
- Summarize the key points that were covered during the current period of teaching.
  Rationale: Reinforces important concepts
- Ask the patient to recall or apply information or demonstrate skills being taught
  Rationale: Provides evidence that short term learning took place
- Identify the time, place, and content for the next teaching session.
  Rationale: Gives a time frame during which the patient may review and practice what has been taught
- Arrange an opportunity for the patient to use or apply the new information as soon as possible after it was taught.

Rationale: Reinforces learning and promotes long-term retention
- Document the information that was taught and the evidence that demonstrates the patient's understanding.
Rationale: Provides a written record of the patient's progress and prevents omissions or duplications during future teaching sessions

 FOCUS ON OLDER ADULTS

When caring for older adults, it is important to:

- Identify the value of or purpose for learning new information
- Make sure an older adult is wearing glasses or using a hearing aid, if they are needed
- Reduce noise and distractions in the environment
- Sit at eye level and face the patient
- Use short sentences of 10 words or less
- Avoid speaking rapidly
- Keep technical terms and medical jargon to a minimum
- Use simple words that a seventh to ninth grader would understand
- Present one but no more than three new ideas at each teaching session
- Review frequently
- Use the active form of the verb rather than passive (eg, "Wipe straight down the center of the incision," rather than "The incision should be wiped down the center")
- Use examples with which the older adult can identify
- Relate new information to prior learning
- Build in some type of learner performance evaluation, such as asking the patient to repeat or paraphrase prior information, demonstrate a skill, or apply the information to a hypothetical situation, such as "What would you do if. . . ."
- Cut teaching short if the patient cannot remain attentive

When providing printed materials for an older adult, it is helpful to:

- Pick material written at a fifth- to eighth-grade reading level
- Choose material that features older adults in a positive manner
- Avoid illustrations that are cluttered with extensive amounts of information

- Review the progress toward reaching goals with the patient.
Rationale: Keeps the patient focused on expected outcomes
- Evaluate the need for further teaching.
Rationale: Allows for revising the teaching plan

KEY CONCEPTS

- There are three main styles of learning. The cognitive domain refers to processing information that usually is provided in oral or written forms, the affective domain refers to learning information that appeals to a person's feelings, beliefs, or values, and the psychomotor domain involves learning by doing.
- The three categories of learners are organized according to age: pedagogic learners (children), androgogic learners (young and middle-aged adults), and gerogogic learners (older adults).
- Characteristics unique to the gerogogic learner are (1) they are motivated to learn by a personal need, (2) they may be experiencing degenerative physical changes, and (3) they can draw on a vast repertoire of past experiences.
- Before teaching a patient, the nurse assesses the patient's capacity to learn, motivation, learning readiness, and learning needs.

CRITICAL THINKING EXERCISES

- How would the technique for tooth brushing be taught differently if the person were a child versus an older adult?
- What teaching strategies could be used to teach tooth brushing from the standpoints of the cognitive, affective, and psychomotor domains of learning?
- Give two examples of how you could determine if the information you selected to teach, such as tooth brushing, was actually learned.

SUGGESTED READINGS

Heinrich R, Molenda M, Russell JD. Instructional Media and the New Technologies of Instruction. 4th ed. New York: Macmillan, 1992.
Kozol J. Illiterate American. Garden City: Anchor Press, 1985.
Lynch ME. When the patient is illiterate: how nurses can help. Journal of Practical Nursing March 1992;42:41–42.
Rega MD. A model approach for patient education. MEDSURG Nursing December 1993;2:477–479, 495.
Weinrich SP, Boyd M. Education in the elderly: adapting and evaluating teaching tools. Journal of Gerontological Nursing January 1992;18:15–20.
Weinrich SP, Boyd M, Nussbaum J. Continuing education: adapting strategies to teach the elderly. Journal of Gerontological Nursing November 1989;15:17–21.

CHAPTER 9

Recording and Reporting

 ## NURSING GUIDELINES

Making Entries in a Patient's Record

Key Terms

Auditors
Change of Shift Report
Chart
Charting (Synonyms: Documenting, Recording)
Charting by Exception
Checklist
Computerized Charting
Flow Sheet
Focus Charting
Kardex

Medical Records
Military Time
Narrative Charting
Nursing Care Plan
PIE Charting
Problem-oriented Records
Quality Assurance
Rounds
SOAP Charting
Source-oriented Records

Learning Objectives

An understanding of the content within this chapter will be evidenced by the student's ability to:

• Identify seven uses for medical records
• List six components that are usually found in any patient's medical record

• Differentiate between source-oriented records and problem-oriented records
• Identify six methods of charting
• List four aspects of documentation that are required in the medical records of all patients cared for in acute care settings
• Discuss why it is important to use only approved abbreviations when charting
• Explain how to convert traditional time to military time.
• List at least 10 guidelines that apply to charting
• Identify four written forms used for communicating information about patients
• List five examples of ways patient information is exchanged among health care workers other than by reading the medical record

Nurses must be able to communicate health care information clearly, concisely, and accurately, both in writing and when speaking. This chapter describes various written and spoken forms of communication and nursing responsibilities for record keeping and reporting.

MEDICAL RECORDS

Medical records, also referred to as health records or patient records, contain information about a person's health problems and the care provided by health practitioners. Medical records consist of many different printed forms. The collection of forms is usually placed in a binder or folder referred to as the patient's **chart**. The process of writing information on chart forms is called **recording, charting,** or **documenting**.

Timby BK: *Fundamental Skills and Concepts in Patient Care, Sixth Edition* © 1996 Lippincott-Raven Publishers

Uses for Medical Records

A medical record primarily serves as a permanent account of a person's health problems, care, and progress. In addition, the chart provides a means for sharing information among health care workers, thus ensuring safety and continuity of patient care. From time to time, medical records are also used to investigate the quality of care within a health agency, demonstrate compliance with national accreditation standards, promote reimbursement from insurance companies, facilitate health research, and provide evidence during the course of a malpractice lawsuit.

PERMANENT ACCOUNT

The patient's medical record is a chronologically written account of a person's illness or injury and health care from the onset of the problem through discharge. The record is filed when care is terminated, and safeguarded for future reference. Previous health records are often requested during subsequent admissions so that specific information about the patient's health history can be reviewed.

SHARING INFORMATION

Because it is impossible for all health care workers to meet and exchange information on a personal basis at the same time, the written record becomes central to sharing information among personnel. The documentation serves as a reference for informing others about the current status of the patient and plan for care.

Sharing information prevents duplication of care and helps reduce the chance of error or omission. For example, if a patient requests medication for pain, the nurse checks the patient's chart to determine when the last pain-relieving drug was administered. Accurate and timely documentation prevents the chance that the medication will be administered too frequently or unnecessarily withheld. Maintaining immunization records is an example of how documentation promotes continuity. The record ensures that subsequent immunizations are administered according to an appropriate schedule from one appointment to the next.

QUALITY ASSURANCE

To maintain a high level of care, hospitals and other health care agencies maintain quality assurance programs. **Quality assurance** is a peer review process conducted by a committee of staff nurses and physicians within a particular health care institution. The committee's mission is to evaluate if the documented care reflects established agency standards. If significant deficiencies are identified, the committee makes recommendations for improvement and reevaluates the outcomes at a later date.

ACCREDITATION

The Joint Commission on Accreditation of Health Organizations (JCAHO) is a private association that has established criteria that reflect high standards for institutional health care. Representatives of this agency periodically inspect health care agencies to determine if the agency demonstrates evidence of high-quality care.

The documentation within randomly selected medical records is just one of the components that is examined during an accreditation visit. In the 1991 Accreditation Manual for Hospitals, the JCAHO identified six items that nurses must document to qualify for accreditation. They include:

* The initial patient assessment and reassessments
* Identification of nursing diagnoses and patient care needs
* The interventions that have been planned to meet the patient's nursing care needs
* The nursing care that is provided
* The patient's response to, and the outcome of, the care provided, and
* The abilities of the patient or significant other(s) to manage the patient's needs for continuing care after discharge

If the documentation is substandard, accreditation may be withdrawn or withheld.

REIMBURSEMENT

The costs of most patients' hospital and home care are billed to third-party payers such as Medicare, Medicaid, and private insurance companies. **Auditors**, inspectors who examine patient records, survey medical records to determine if the care that was provided meets established criteria for reimbursement. Undocumented, incomplete, or inconsistent documentation of care may result in a denial for payment.

RESEARCH

Patient records contain an abundance of information. Some types of clinical research are difficult to conduct because there may not be enough participants or test facilities may be limited; hence, information from medical records may be an alternative source of data.

However, only authorized persons are allowed access to patient records. Formal permission must be obtained from the health agency's administrator or other authority whenever a patient's record is used for a purpose other than record keeping.

LEGAL EVIDENCE

The chart is considered a legal document. It may be subpoenaed as evidence by the defense or prosecuting attorney to prove or disprove allegations of malpractice. Therefore, it is essential that written entries in medical records follow legally defensible criteria (Display 9-1).

Each person who writes in the patient's medical record is responsible for the information he or she records and may be called as a witness to testify concerning what has been written. Any writing that cannot be clearly read, or is vague, scribbled through, whited out, written over, or erased makes for a poor legal defense.

Patient Access to Records

Historically, patients were not allowed to see their medical record. However, health agencies today are more flexible on this issue. The Patient's Bill of Rights, described in Chapter 3, specifically states that patients have a right to read their medical records. Consequently, many institutions have written policies that describe the guidelines by which patients may read their own medical records. Policies range from complete, unrestricted access on the patient's written request, to arranging access to their record in the presence of the patient's physician or the hospital administrator. Nurses must follow whatever policies have been established.

Components of a Medical Record

The patient's health care record is maintained in such a manner that information can be accessed quickly and easily. Various paper forms within the chart may be color coded or separated by tabbed sheets.

All charts usually contain:

- An information sheet identifying the patient's name, address, nearest relative, marital status, religion, and insurance company
- Medical information
- A plan for care
- Nursing documentation
- Medication administration records, and
- Laboratory and diagnostic test results

DISPLAY 9-1. *Criteria for Legally Defensible Charting*

When making an entry on a patient's medical record, the nurse should:
- Never chart for someone else.
- Ensure that the information is permanent by making notations with an ink or ballpoint pen, or using a computer.
- Date and time each entry.
- Make entries in chronologic order.
- Chart assessment findings frequently.
- Identify documentation that is out of chronologic sequence with the words "late entry."
- Write or print legibly.
- Reflect the plan for care.
- Describe the outcomes of care.
- Record relevant details.
- Use only approved abbreviations.
- Never obliterate what has been written.
- Record facts, not interpretations.
- Quote verbal comments.
- Never imply criticism of another's care.
- Document the circumstances for notifying a physician, the specific data that were reported, and the physician's recommendations.
- Identify specific information provided when teaching a patient and the evidence that indicates the patient has understood the instructions.
- Sign each entry by name and title.

Creighton H. Legal significance of charting: part I. Nursing Management September 1987;18:17–22; Part II, October 1987;18:14–15.

TABLE 9-1. *Common Components in a Source-Oriented Record*

Component	Description
History and physical examination	Summarizes the patient's current and past health and describes normal and abnormal physical findings
Physician's order sheet	Lists diagnostic tests, prescribed medications, diet orders, and special care for the patient
Physician's progress notes	Describes the current status and outcomes of medical treatment
Admission nursing assessment	Summarizes biologic, psychological, social, and cultural patterns that affect the patient's health and describes the results of a head-to-toe physical examination
Nursing care plan	Contains a list of the patient's problems, goals, and directions for patient care
Nursing notes	Identifies ongoing assessment data, nursing interventions, and the patient's response to nursing care

Types of Patient Records

Although health records in most agencies contain similar information, the record is usually organized in one of two ways. Health care agencies may adopt either a source-oriented or problem-oriented format.

SOURCE-ORIENTED RECORDS

Source-oriented records, which are the most traditional type of patient record, are organized according to the source of information. That is, there are separate forms on which physicians, nurses, dietitians, physical therapists, and so on, make written entries about their activities with regard to the patient's care. Some common components that are included in most source-oriented records are listed in Table 9-1.

One of the criticisms of source-oriented records is that it is difficult to demonstrate that there is a unified, cooperative approach among caregivers for resolving the patient's problems. More often than not, the fragmented documentation gives the impression that each professional is working independently of the others.

PROBLEM-ORIENTED RECORDS

Problem-oriented records, sometimes abbreviated *POR*, are organized according to the patient's health problems. There are four major parts to a POR: the data base, the problem list, the initial plan, and progress notes (Table 9-2). People using a POR find that the information is compiled and arranged so as to emphasize goal-directed care, promote recording of pertinent information, and facilitate communication among health care professionals.

METHODS OF CHARTING

There are a variety of styles used to record information on the patient's record. Examples of charting methods include narrative notes, SOAP charting, focus charting, PIE charting, charting by exception, and computerized charting.

Narrative Charting

Narrative charting, the style usually used in source-oriented records, involves writing information about the patient and patient care in chronologic order. There

TABLE 9-2. *Common Components in a Problem-Oriented Record*

Component	Description
Data base	Contains initial health information
Problem list	Consists of a numeric list of the patient's health problems
Initial plan	Identifies methods for solving each identified health problem
Progress notes	Describes the patient's responses to what has been done and revisions to the initial plan

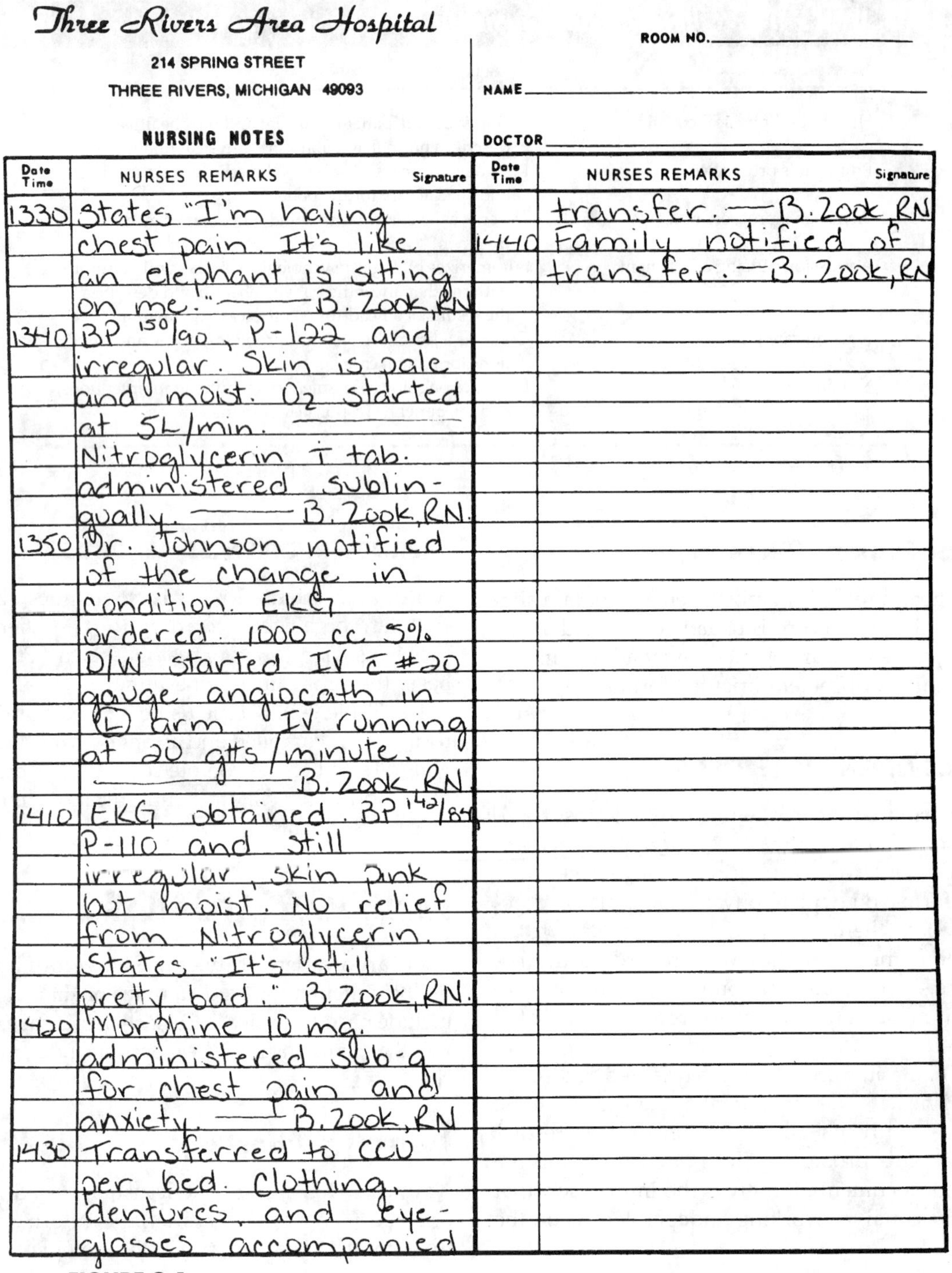

Three Rivers Area Hospital

214 SPRING STREET
THREE RIVERS, MICHIGAN 49093

ROOM NO._____

NAME_____

NURSING NOTES

DOCTOR_____

Date Time	NURSES REMARKS Signature	Date Time	NURSES REMARKS Signature
1330	States "I'm having chest pain. It's like an elephant is sitting on me." ——— B. Zook, RN		transfer. ——— B. Zook RN
		1440	Family notified of transfer. —B. Zook, RN
1340	BP 150/90, P-122 and irregular. Skin is pale and moist. O$_2$ started at 5L/min. Nitroglycerin I tab. administered sublingually. ——— B. Zook, RN		
1350	Dr. Johnson notified of the change in condition. EKG ordered. 1000 cc 5% D/W started IV c̄ #20 gauge angiocath in (L) arm. IV running at 20 gtts/minute. ——— B. Zook, RN		
1410	EKG obtained. BP 142/84, P-110 and still irregular. Skin pink but moist. No relief from Nitroglycerin. States "It's still pretty bad." B. Zook, RN.		
1420	Morphine 10 mg. administered sub-q for chest pain and anxiety. ——— B. Zook, RN		
1430	Transferred to CCU per bed. Clothing, dentures, and eyeglasses accompanied		

FIGURE 9-1

Sample of narrative charting. (Courtesy of Three Rivers Area Hospital, Three Rivers, MI.)

is no established format for narrative notations; the content resembles a log or journal (Fig. 9-1).

One criticism of narrative charting is that it is time consuming; there are other disadvantages as well. For example, it is difficult to read through the lengthy narration to find specific information that correlates the patient's problems with care and progress. Depending on the skill of the person who is doing the narrative charting, pertinent documentation may be omitted, or insignificant information may be included.

SOAP Charting

SOAP charting is a documentation style that is more likely to be used in a POR record. The SOAP format refers to the four essential components addressed by all caregivers in a progress note:

S = subjective data,
O = objective data,
A = analysis of the data, and
P = plan for care.

TABLE 9-3. *SOAPIER Charting Format*

Letter	Explanation	Example of Recording
S = Subjective information	Information reported by the patient	S—"I don't feel well."
O = Objective information	Observations made by the nurse	O—Temperature 102.4°F.
A = Analysis	Problem identification	A—Fever
P = Plan	Proposed treatment	P—Offer extra fluids and monitor body temperature
I = Implementation	Care provided	I—750 mL of fluid intake in 8 hours; temperature assessed every 4 hours
E = Evaluation	Outcome of treatment	E—Temperature reduced to 101°F
R = Revision	Changes in treatment	R—Increase fluid intake to 1,000 mL per shift until temperature is ≤100°F

In some agencies, the SOAP format has been expanded to the SOAPIE or SOAPIER arrangements, with the additions of *I* = interventions, *E* = evaluation, and *R* = revision to the plan for care (Table 9-3).

Any one of the variations in the SOAP format tends to keep the documentation focused on pertinent information. SOAP charting also tends to demonstrate interdisciplinary cooperation because all professionals involved in the care of a patient make entries in the same location within the chart.

Focus Charting

Focus charting is a modified form of SOAP charting. It substitutes "focus" rather than "problem," which, for some, carries negative connotations. A focus can refer to a patient's current or changed behavior, significant events in the patient's care, or even a North American Nursing Diagnosis Association (NANDA) nursing diagnosis category. Instead of making entries using the SOAP format, a DAR framework, which stands for *Data, Action,* and *Response* is used. DAR notations tend to reflect the steps in the nursing process.

PIE Charting

PIE charting is another method of recording that promotes documentation of the patient's progress. The PIE letters stand for *Problem, Intervention,* and *Evaluation,* which prompts the nurse to address specific content in a charted progress note.

When the PIE method is used, assessments are documented on a separate form and the patient's problems are given a corresponding number. The number is subsequently used in the progress notes when referring to the interventions and patient's responses (Fig. 9-2).

Charting by Exception

Charting by exception is a documentation method that eliminates recording normal assessment findings and routine care. The content that is addressed includes only patient assessments that are abnormal and nursing care that deviates from written standards (eg, the exceptions to what is normal and usual). Besides being time efficient, those who chart by exception say this method provides quick access to abnormal findings because normal and routine information is not described.

Computerized Charting

Computerized charting refers to documenting patient information electronically. This technology is most advantageous to nursing when it is available at the point of care or bedside of the patient (Fig. 9-3). Computer terminals located at nursing stations are less desirable, primarily because they take the nurse away from the source of the data. Centralized computer terminals are connected to large information systems that facilitate communication between and among various departments within the institution, such as the pharmacy, laboratory, admissions office, accounting, and therefore are less specific for nursing use.

Although each computer system varies, computerized charting is usually done by touching the monitor screen with a finger or using an electronic device like a light pen to select from among a list of menu options. A few require entering data by using a keyboard, as a typist would do, or a combination of keyboarding and touch-screen technology. Data entry by voice activation is on the horizon. A single keystroke saves the information displayed on the monitor to the patient's record (Fig. 9-4).

Computerized charting has many advantages:

- The information is always legible.
- The date and exact time of the documentation is automatically recorded.
- The abbreviations and terms are consistent with agency-approved lists.
- Trivia are eliminated.
- There are fewer omissions because the computer prompts the nurse to enter specific information.

NURSING NOTES

Date Time	NURSES REMARKS	Signature
6/19 0750	P#1 Crackles heard on inspiration in the bases of R and L lungs. ——— I#1 Incision splinted with pillow. Instructed to breathe deeply, open mouth, and cough at the end of expiration ——— E#1 Lungs clear with coughing. ——— a. Walker, LPN	

FIGURE 9-2
Sample of PIE charting.

- Computerized charting saves at least a half-hour of time previously spent in handwritten documentation (Meyer, 1992).
- Electronic data entry reduces the costs in overtime directly attributed to uncompleted end-of-shift charting (Meyer, 1992).
- Electronic data takes up less storage space and can be retrieved very quickly.

The major disadvantages include the initial expense of purchasing a computer system and training personnel to use it. In addition, there may be times when

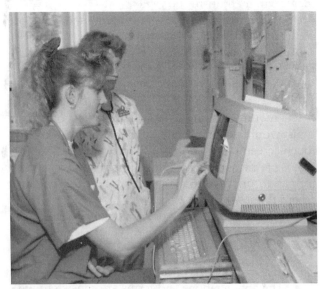

FIGURE 9-3
Using a bedside computer for charting. (Scherer JC, Timby BK: Introductory Medical-Surgical Nursing, 6th ed, p 7. Philadelphia, JB Lippincott, 1995)

nurses have to resort to written documentation, such as during a power failure or equipment malfunction.

Besides charting, there are other computer applications that benefit nursing. Computers are being used to generate nursing care plans, develop staffing patterns that meet the current patient census and acuity levels, analyze numeric assessment data from monitoring equipment, call attention to drugs that have not been administered, and alert the nurse to incompatibilities between or contraindications to prescribed drugs.

PROTECTING COMPUTERIZED RECORDS

With the advent of computerized record keeping, maintaining confidentiality has become somewhat more difficult. Because electronically stored data can be accessed by multiple individuals who enter and retrieve information from computer files, it has been difficult to monitor or limit access to specific authorized individuals only.

Health agencies are adopting methods to ensure protection of computerized patient records. Some techniques include:

- Automatic saving or storage of information on a monitor screen and a return to a menu if the data have been displayed for a period of time
- Assigning an access password to authorized personnel; the password is kept secret and is changed frequently
- Issuing a plastic card or key that is used by authorized personnel to retrieve information
- Locking out patient information except to those who have been authorized through a fingerprint or voice-activation device
- Blocking the type of information that can be retrieved by personnel in various departments. In other words, laboratory employees may obtain information from the medical orders but are prevented from viewing information in the patient's personal history.
- Identifying the time and location from which the patient's record is accessed

DOCUMENTING INFORMATION

Each health agency sets its own documentation policies. In addition to identifying the method for charting, the policy usually indicates the type of information that is recorded on each chart form, who is responsible for charting, and the frequency with which entries are made on the record. The content that nurses are generally required to document is listed in Display 9-2. Current JCAHO standards require that the steps of the nursing process—assessment, problem identification, planning, implementation, and evaluation of out-

Washington Hospital Center

- -

Requested by   Page — 1

RoutneNurseCare
- - - - - - - - - - -

- -

DATE (1990)	6/18	6/19		6/20	6/21		
TIME	2200	0400	1300	2200	0200	2000	2310
Bath Care	Complt	None	Partl	Complt	Partl	Complt	None
Oral Care	q4h	q8h	q4h	q2h	q4h	q4h	q4h
Skin Care	Yes	Yes	Yes	Yes	Yes	Yes	Yes
Freq. Turned	q2h	q2h	q2h	q2h	q2h	q2h	q2h
ROMq4	Ys-Act	No	Ys-Act	Ys-Pas	Ys-Pas	Ys-Pas	
Decubitus care	None	None	None			None	None
Foly/Texs Care	Yes	Yes	Yes	Yes	Yes	Yes	Yes
Line Dressing	Ok	Ok	Ok	None	None	Ok	Ok
IV tubing	Ok	Ok	Chnged	Ok	Chnged	Chnged	Chnged
HeprinLk Flush	None	None		Yes	None		None
OOB	Assist	Bedrst	Assist			Assist	Bedrst
OOB-hrs	>1hr		>2hr			>1hr	
Slept-hrs	1–4hr	>4hr	1–4hr			<1hr	>4hr
Nares Care	q8h	q8h		q8h	q8h	q8h	q8h
ET/Trach Care	q8h	q8h	q8h	q8h	q8h	q4h	q8h
Chest PT	q6h	q6h		q6h	q6h	q6h	q6h
Restr.check q2		Yes	None				
Pulse check q8	Palp	Palp	Palp	Palp	Palp	Palp	Palp
NG/Dobpatentq4	Yes	Yes	Yes	Yes	Yes	Yes	Yes
BowelSounds q8	Normal	Normal	Normal	Normal	Normal	Normal	Normal
Wound Dressing						Ok	
Daily Wght (kg)			66.1	65.5			
Alrmlmitchk q4	Yes	Yes	Yes	Yes	Yes	Yes	Yes
Stop cock chk					No	Yes	
CXR done			No	No	No		Yes
12 Lead EKG			No	No	No		
Pt.Clasificati	B	B	B	B	B	B	B

- -

- -

Critical Care Data	Date: 6/22/90	Patient : Hosp. No.:
RoutneNurseCare		Location : 4G08

FIGURE 9-4
Sample of computerized charting.

comes—must be identified in the medical record of patients cared for in acute care agencies such as a hospital.

Because consistency in charting is important legally, it is essential that nurses follow the documentation policy of the particular health agency where they are employed. Deviation from an agency's charting policy increases legal risks if the record is subpoenaed.

Using Abbreviations

Use of abbreviations shortens what is written and thereby limits the volume of paper that must be filed and stored. Brevity, however, never takes priority over complete and accurate documentation. It is better to write at length than to omit information or make entries that are vague.

DISPLAY 9-2. *Content of Nursing Documentation*

Nurses are usually responsible for documenting:
- Assessment data*
- Patient care needs
- Routine care, such as hygiene measures
- Safety precautions that have been used
- Nursing interventions described in the care plan
- Medical treatments prescribed by the physician
- Outcomes of treatment and nursing interventions
- Patient activity
- Medication administration
- Percentage of food consumed at each meal
- Visits or consults by physicians or other health professionals
- Reasons for contacting the physician and the outcome of the communication
- Transportation to other departments, like the radiography department, for specialized care or diagnostic tests, and time of return
- Patient teaching and discharge instructions
- Referrals to other health care agencies

In acute care settings, a registered nurse is required by JCAHO to document the admission nursing assessment findings and develop the initial plan for care. Some aspects of the initial data collection may be delegated to the practical or vocational nurse.

Many abbreviations have common meanings; however, nurses cannot assume that *all* abbreviations will be interpreted the same way universally. Some may have one meaning in one locale or agency, and may mean something different or be unfamiliar in another. To avoid confusion and misinterpretation, each health agency provides a written list of approved abbreviations and their meanings. When documenting, nurses are careful to use only those abbreviations on the agency's approved list. Some common abbreviations are listed in Table 9-4; more can be found in Appendix A.

Indicating Documentation Time

Each entry on a medical record is dated and timed. Some hospitals use traditional time and identify the hours from 1:00 to 12:00 and minutes from 1 to 59, followed by A.M. or P.M. Other agencies use military time.

Military time is based on a 24-hour clock (Fig. 9-5). When military time is used, a different four-digit number is identified for each hour and minute of the day. The first two of the four digits indicate the hour within the 24-hour period; the last two digits indicate the minutes. This avoids confusion because no number is ever duplicated. It also eliminates the need to always add the labels A.M., P.M., midnight, and noon.

Military time begins at midnight, which is identified as 2400 by some, or 0000 by others. One minute after midnight is 0001. A zero is placed before the hours of 1 through 9 in the morning to provide a number that consistently contains four digits. For example, 0700 refers to seven o'clock in the morning, and would be stated as "0-seven hundred." After noon, 12 is added to each hour; therefore, 1:00 P.M. is identified as 1300. The minutes in military time are identified in numbers from 1 to 59. Table 9-5 gives examples of traditional time converted to military time.

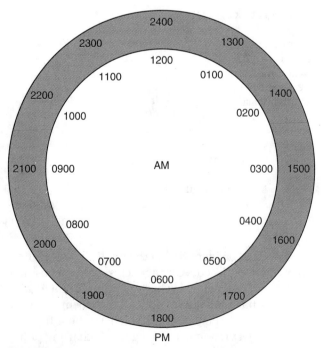

FIGURE 9-5
Military time is based on a 24-hour numbering system.

◄ NURSING GUIDELINES FOR MAKING ENTRIES IN A PATIENT'S RECORD

- Make sure the patient's name is identified on the form.
  Rationale: Ensures that the chart form will be reinserted into the appropriate record
- Use a pen to make entries; use the color of ink indicated by agency policy.
  Rationale: Ensures permanence and enhances photocopying
- Write or print information so it can be read with ease.
  Rationale: Promotes legibility
- Record the date and time of each entry.
  Rationale: Provides a chronologic reference
- Make entries in the chart as promptly as possible after performing a procedure or obtaining assessment data.
  Rationale: Avoids the potential for inaccuracies or omissions
- Fill all the space on each line of the form or draw a line through the blank space on an unfilled line.
  Rationale: Prevents the possibility that someone else may add information to what appears to be the original documentation
- Never chart nursing activities before they have been performed.
  Rationale: Causes legal problems, especially if the patient's condition suddenly changes
- Follow the agency's policy for the minimum interval between entries.
  Rationale: Validates that the patient has been observed and attended to at reasonable periods of time
- Indicate the current time when charting a late entry (documentation of information that occurred earlier but was accidentally omitted), and identify the time within the notation that the omitted data took place.
  Rationale: Identifies the time of actual events; promotes logic and order when evaluating the patient's progress
- Delete words such as "a," "an," or "the."
  Rationale: Avoids adding length to the entry
- Omit stating the patient's name or use of *pt.* as an abbreviation.
  Rationale: Avoids unnecessary documentation because it is understood that all the entries refer to the patient identified on the chart form.
- Use agency-approved abbreviations and symbols.
  Rationale: Promotes consistent interpretation
- Never use ditto marks.
  Rationale: Promotes clarity
- Identify actual or approximate sizes when describing assessment data rather than using relative descriptions such as "large," "moderate," or "small."
  Rationale: Avoids nonspecific estimations that are subject to wide interpretation.
- Draw a line through a mistake rather than scribbling through or in any other way obscuring the originally written words. Put the word *error* followed with a date and initials next to the entry and immediately enter the corrected information.
  Rationale: Maintains legibility and complies with legal principles
- Document information clearly and accurately without any subjective interpretation. Quote the patient, if a statement is pertinent.
  Rationale: Provides facts, not opinions
- Avoid phrases such as "appears to be" or "seems to be."
  Rationale: Suggests uncertainty if used
- Record adverse reactions and include the measures used to manage them.
  Rationale: Helps document that the nurse acted reasonably and that the care was not substandard
- Identify the specific information that is taught and the evidence of the patient's learning.
  Rationale: Ensures continuity in preparing the patient for discharge
- Sign each entry with a first initial, last name, and title.
  Rationale: Demonstrates accountability for what has been written.

WRITTEN FORMS OF COMMUNICATION

In addition to the patient's record, written forms of communication include the nursing care plan and the nursing Kardex.

Nursing Care Plans

A **nursing care plan** is used to identify patient problems, establish a time frame for improving, controlling, or resolving the problem, and order nursing interventions necessary for accomplishing the plan (Locher, 1992). The principles and style for writing a diagnostic statement, goals, and nursing orders are described in Chapter 2.

At the present time, JCAHO's documentation standards require that the medical record show evidence of a plan for care; JCAHO does *not* specify that the plan for care must be identified separately. Standard N.C.1.3.5. states that "Nursing care data related to patient assessments, *the nursing care planned*, nursing interventions, and patient outcome are permanently integrated into the clinical information system" (eg, the medical record). Nevertheless, many agencies require a separate nursing care plan as a means of demonstrating compliance with the JCAHO standard.

TABLE 9-4. *Commonly Used Abbreviations**

Abbreviation	Meaning	Abbreviation	Meaning
abd.	abdomen	OB	obstetrics
a.c.	before meals	OD	right eye
ad lib	as desired	OOB	out of bed
AMA	against medical advice	OR	operating room
amt.	amount	OS	left eye
approx.	approximately	OU	both eyes
b.i.d.	twice a day	per	by or through
BM	bowel movement	P	pulse
BP	blood pressure	p.c.	after meals
bpm	beats per minute	p.o.	by mouth
BRP	bathroom privileges	postop.	postoperative
$\bar{c}$	with	preop.	preoperative
C	Centigrade	pt.	patient
cc	cubic centimeter	PT	physical therapy
CCU	coronary care unit	q	every
c/o	complains of	q.d.	every day
dc	discontinue	q.i.d.	four times a day
ED	emergency department	q.o.d.	every other day
et	and	q.s.	quantity sufficient
H_2O	water	R, Rt, or R	right
HS	hour of sleep, bedtime	R	respirations
I & O	intake and output	$\bar{s}$	without
IM	intramuscular	ss	one half
IV	intravenous	SS	soap suds
kg	kilogram	stat	immediately
L, Lt, or L	left	t.i.d.	three times a day
L	liter	TPR	temperature, pulse, respirations
lb	pound	UA	urinalysis
NKA	no known allergies	via	by way of
NPO	nothing by mouth	WC	wheelchair
NSS	normal saline solution	WNL	within normal limits
O_2	oxygen	Wt.	weight

*For more abbreviations, see Appendix A at the end of the book.

The plan for care is kept current by revising it as the patient's condition changes.

Most nursing care plans are handwritten on a form developed by the health agency (Fig. 9-6). However, some agencies use preprinted care plans, computer-generated care plans, standards of care, or cite the plan for care within progress notes.

Because the nursing care plan is a part of the permanent record, and thus a legal document, it is compiled and maintained following documentation principles. All entries and revisions are dated. The written components are clear, concise, and legible. Information must not be obliterated. Only approved abbreviations are used. Each addition or revision to the plan is signed.

Nursing Kardex

The nursing **Kardex** is a quick reference for current information about the patient and the patient's care (Fig. 9-7). The Kardex forms for all patients are kept collectively in a folder that allows flipping from one to another. The Kardex may be used to:

- Locate patients by name and room number
- Identify each patient's physician and medical diagnosis
- Serve as a reference for a change-of-shift report
- Serve as a guide for making nursing assignments
- Provide a rapid resource for current medical orders on each patient
- Check quickly on a patient's type of diet
- Alert nursing personnel to a patient's scheduled tests or test preparations
- Inform staff of a patient's current level of activity
- Identify comfort or assistive measures a patient may require
- Provide a tool for estimating the personnel-to-patient ratio for a nursing unit

The information within the Kardex changes frequently, sometimes daily or even several times in one day. The Kardex form is not a part of the permanent record. Therefore, information can be written in pencil or erased.

TABLE 9-5. *Military Time Conversions*

Traditional Time	Military Time
12:00 midnight	0000 or 2400
12:01 A.M.	0001
1:30 A.M.	0130
12:00 noon	1200
1:00 P.M.	1300
3:15 P.M.	1515
7:59 P.M.	1959
10:47 P.M.	2247

Checklists

A **checklist** is a form of documentation in which the nurse marks pertinent information with a check mark rather than writing a narrative note. Checklists are used primarily to document routine types of care that are repetitious, such as bathing and mouth care. This charting technique is especially helpful when the care is similar each day and the patient's condition does not differ much for extended periods of time.

DISCHARGE GOALS:

Pt will be discharged home with approximated incision, pain within tolerable level, normal vital signs, voiding well able to eat sufficient food, clear lungs, and active bowel sounds

DIRECTIONS: Each entry must be signed with nurse's name and title.

DATE	PATIENT PROBLEM/NURSING DIAGNOSIS	GOAL/EXPECTED OUTCOMES	GOAL REVIEWED WITH PT./S.O.	NURSING ORDER/ACTIONS	DATE RESOLVED
1/7	Risk for infection related to impaired skin integrity 2° to surgical incision	Pt. will remain free of infection as evidenced by absence of redness, swelling, drainage from wound and afebrile for length of stay	1/7	1. Observe appropriate handwashing before and after patient care. 2. Keep dressing dry and intact. 3. Provide aseptic wound care. D. Miller, LPN	
1/7	Risk for ineffective breathing pattern related to abdominal incisional pain	Pt.'s respiratory rate will remain within normal limits (16-20/min) for length of stay.	1/7	1. Give analgesic for pain rated >5 on a scale of 1-10. 2. Instruct to splint incision when turning and deep breathing. D. Miller, LPN	

FIGURE 9-6
Sample nursing care plan.

BATH:	DIET:	BOWEL/BLADDER:	PHYSICAL TRAITS:
_____ Complete	_____ NPO	_____ Catheter	_____ Left handed
_____ Partial	_____ Hold Brkfst	_____ Commode	_____ Right handed
_____ Self	_____ Feed	_____ Incontinent	_____ Paraplegic
_____ Tub	_____ Liquid	_____ Ostomy	_____ Hemiplegic
_____ Shower	_____ Soft	Type: _____	L ___ R ___
	_____ General		_____ Blind
ACTIVITY:	_____ Special	SAFETY MEASURES:	L ___ R ___
_____ Bed Rest		_____ Siderails	_____ Deaf
_____ BRP only	FLUIDS:	_____ Restraints	L ___ R ___
_____ Dangle	_____ I & O	Jacket: _____	_____ Speech Imp.
_____ Ambulate	_____ Restrict to:	Wrist: _____	_____ Other (list)
_____ Change pos.	_____	Ankles: _____	_____
_____ Up as tol.	_____ Increase to:	Constant: _____	
	_____	When OOB: _____	ALLERGIES (in red) If
HYGIENE:	_____ IV	Night only _____	none, so state:
_____ Dentures		_____ Supervise	_____
_____ Oral Care	VITAL SIGNS:	Smoking	_____
_____ Special	_____ TPR	_____ Other (list)	_____
_____	_____ BP	_____	

DIAGNOSIS: _____   OPERATION: _____   DATE: _____   RELIGION: _____

ROOM: _____   NAME: _____   AGE: _____   DOCTOR: _____

FIGURE 9-7
Sample of a Kardex form. (Courtesy of Fairview Medical Care Facility, Centreville, MI.)

Flow Sheets

A **flow sheet** is a chart form that contains sections for recording frequently repeated assessments. Flow sheets often provide room for recording numbers or brief descriptions. They enable nurses to evaluate trends because similar information is located on one form.

INTERPERSONAL COMMUNICATION

In addition to using the chart as a source for exchanging information, health professionals communicate with each other throughout the day (Fig. 9-8), during change-of-shift reports, when making patient care assignments, during team conferences, while participating in patient rounds, and when using the telephone.

Change-of-Shift Report

A **change-of-shift report** is a discussion between a nursing spokesperson from the shift that is ending with personnel who will be relieving the current staff (Fig. 9-9). The report includes a summary of each patient's condition and current status of care (Display 9-3).

To facilitate a change-of-shift report, it is important to:

- Be prompt so that the report can start and end on time
- Come prepared with a pen and paper or clipboard
- Avoid socializing during reporting sessions
- Take notes on the information that is reported
- Clarify information that is not clear
- Ask questions about pertinent information that may have been omitted

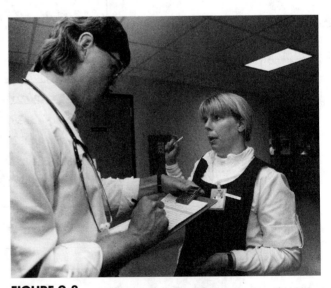

FIGURE 9-8
A staff nurse discusses patient care with a student nurse. (Courtesy of Suzanne Weaver/Bay Health Systems.)

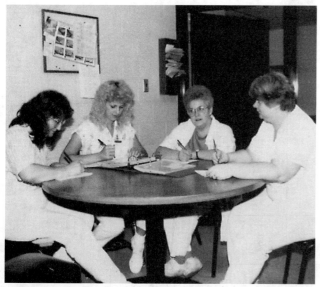

FIGURE 9-9
Nurses begin their shift by receiving a report on their patients.

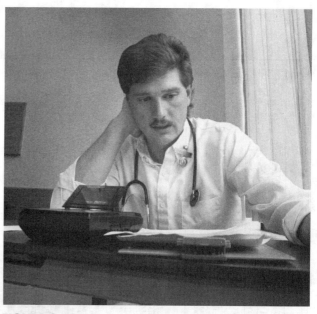

FIGURE 9-10
Some agencies use a tape-recorded end-of-shift report. (Courtesy of Suzanne Weaver/Bay Health Systems.)

In some agencies the report is tape recorded (Fig. 9-10). A taped report saves time because there are no interruptions or digressions during the report. The tape can be replayed if there is a need to have information repeated. The greatest disadvantage is that it does not permit direct communication and clarification with the person giving the report.

Patient Care Assignments

Patient care assignments are made at the beginning of each shift. Assignments may be posted, discussed verbally with team members, or written on a work sheet

---

DISPLAY 9-3. *Change-of-Shift Report*

A change-of-shift report usually includes:
- Name of the patient, age, and room number
- Name of physician
- Medical diagnosis or surgical procedure and date
- Range in vital signs
- Abnormal assessment data
- Characteristics of pain, medication, amount, time last administered, and outcome achieved
- Type of diet and percentage consumed at each meal
- Special body position and level of activity, if applicable
- Scheduled diagnostic tests
- Test results, including those performed by the nurse, such as blood sugar levels
- Changes in medical orders, including newly prescribed drugs
- Intake and output totals
- Type and rate of infusing intravenous fluid
- Amount of intravenous fluid that remains
- Settings on electronic equipment, such as amount of suction
- Condition of incision and dressing, if applicable
- Color and amount of wound or suction drainage

NURSING ASSIGNMENT SHEET

TEAM MEMBER Jane Doe L.P.N. BREAK 9:15 A.M. CONFERENCE 10:30 A.M. LUNCH 12:00 N. DATE:

TEAM LEADER Mary Black RN ASSIGNMENT Filling and distributing water carafes on the Northwing

ROOM	PATIENT	BATH	ACTIVITY	DIET	FLUIDS	TO BE CHECKED	TREATMENTS	SPECIMEN	COMMENTS
296¹	Flora Brown Duodenal Ulcer	BED SELF * SHOWER TUB SITZ	BED DANGLE B R P B R P · HELP AMB AMB · HELP WALKER CRUTCHES W C	REGULAR SOFT SURG LIQ FULL LIQ SPECIAL Bland III FASTING TUBE FEEDING	FORCE N P O LIMIT SIPS WATER ICE CHIPS I V DIST WATER	BLOOD PRESSURE 8A T P R 8A TEST URINE A C & HS SLIDING SCALE I & O LEVIN TUBE CHEST TUBE FOLEY OXYGEN	ENEMA DOUCHE PERI CARE · LIGHT WEIGH ORAL HYGIENE SPECIAL BACK CARE PREPARE FOR SURG PREPARE FOR X-RAY O T · P T · E C T	STOOL OB URINE SPUTUM BLOOD CULTURE TISSUE	
296²	Mary Green Coronary	BED SELF * SHOWER TUB SITZ	BED DANGLE B R P B R P HELP AMB AMB · HELP WALKER CRUTCHES W C	REGULAR SOFT SURG LIQ FULL LIQ SPECIAL 2Gm Na FASTING TUBE FEEDING	FORCE N P O LIMIT SIPS WATER ICE CHIPS I V DIST WATER	BLOOD PRESSURE 8-12 T P R 8-12 TEST URINE A C & HS SLIDING SCALE I & O LEVIN TUBE CHEST TUBE FOLEY OXYGEN 4L/M - 1hr pc × III	ENEMA DOUCHE PERI CARE · LIGHT WEIGH · 8A ORAL HYGIENE SPECIAL BACK CARE PREPARE FOR SURG PREPARE FOR X-RAY O T · P T · E C T	STOOL URINE SPUTUM BLOOD CULTURE TISSUE	
298¹	John Snapp C.O.P.D.	BED SELF * SHOWER TUB SITZ	BED DANGLE B R P B R P · HELP AMB c̄ O2 AMB · HELP WALKER CRUTCHES W C	REGULAR SOFT SURG LIQ FULL LIQ SPECIAL FASTING TUBE FEEDING	FORCE N P O LIMIT SIPS WATER ICE CHIPS I V DIST WATER	BLOOD PRESSURE T P R TEST URINE A C & HS SLIDING SCALE I & O LEVIN TUBE CHEST TUBE FOLEY OXYGEN 1L/M CONT.	ENEMA Fleets DOUCHE PERI CARE · LIGHT WEIGH ORAL HYGIENE SPECIAL BACK CARE PREPARE FOR SURG PREPARE FOR X-RAY O T · P T · E C T	STOOL URINE SPUTUM BLOOD CULTURE TISSUE	1000cc 5% D/W c̄ 500mg Aminophyllin @ 100cc/hr CONT.
298²	Tom Henry C.H.F.	BED SELF * SHOWER TUB SITZ	BED DANGLE B R P B R P HELP AMB AMB HELP WALKER CRUTCHES W C	REGULAR SOFT SURG LIQ FULL LIQ SPECIAL ½Gm Na FASTING TUBE FEEDING	FORCE N P O LIMIT · 300/8h SIPS WATER ICE CHIPS I V DIST WATER	BLOOD PRESSURE q2h T P R q2h TEST URINE A C & HS SLIDING SCALE I & O LEVIN TUBE CHEST TUBE FOLEY OXYGEN 4L/M Cont.	ENEMA DOUCHE PERI CARE · LIGHT WEIGH 8 ORAL HYGIENE 8-12 SPECIAL BACK CARE PREPARE FOR SURG PREPARE FOR X-RAY O T · P T · E C T	STOOL URINE SPUTUM BLOOD CULTURE TISSUE	Change position q 2hr.
299	Jim Smith Diabetes Mellitus	BED SELF * SHOWER TUB SITZ	BED DANGLE B R P B R P · HELP AMB AMB · HELP WALKER CRUTCHES W C	REGULAR SOFT SURG LIQ FULL LIQ SPECIAL 1800 Cal Diabetic FASTING TUBE FEEDING	FORCE N P O LIMIT SIPS WATER ICE CHIPS I V DIST WATER	BLOOD PRESSURE T P R 8 TEST URINE A C & HS SLIDING SCALE I & O LEVIN TUBE CHEST TUBE FOLEY OXYGEN	ENEMA DOUCHE PERI CARE · LIGHT WEIGH ORAL HYGIENE SPECIAL BACK CARE PREPARE FOR SURG PREPARE FOR X-RAY O T · P T · E C T	STOOL URINE SPUTUM BLOOD CULTURE TISSUE	
		BED SELF * SHOWER TUB SITZ	BED DANGLE B R P B R P HELP AMB AMB HELP WALKER CRUTCHES W C	REGULAR SOFT SURG LIQ FULL LIQ SPECIAL FASTING TUBE FEEDING	FORCE N P O LIMIT SIPS WATER ICE CHIPS I V DIST WATER	BLOOD PRESSURE T P R TEST URINE A C & HS SLIDING SCALE I & O LEVIN TUBE CHEST TUBE FOLEY OXYGEN	ENEMA DOUCHE PERI CARE · LIGHT WEIGH ORAL HYGIENE SPECIAL BACK CARE PREPARE FOR SURG PREPARE FOR X-RAY O T · P T · E C T	STOOL URINE SPUTUM BLOOD CULTURE TISSUE	
		BED SELF * SHOWER TUB SITZ	BED DANGLE B R P B R P HELP AMB AMB · HELP WALKER CRUTCHES W C	REGULAR SOFT SURG LIQ FULL LIQ SPECIAL FASTING TUBE FEEDING	FORCE N P O LIMIT SIPS WATER ICE CHIPS I V DIST WATER	BLOOD PRESSURE T P R TEST URINE A C & HS SLIDING SCALE I & O LEVIN TUBE CHEST TUBE FOLEY OXYGEN	ENEMA DOUCHE PERI CARE · LIGHT WEIGH ORAL HYGIENE SPECIAL BACK CARE PREPARE FOR SURG PREPARE FOR X-RAY O T · P T · E C T	STOOL URINE SPUTUM BLOOD CULTURE TISSUE	
		BED SELF * SHOWER TUB SITZ	BED DANGLE B R P B R P HELP AMB AMB HELP WALKER CRUTCHES W C	REGULAR SOFT SURG LIQ FULL LIQ SPECIAL FASTING TUBE FEEDING	FORCE N P O LIMIT SIPS WATER ICE CHIPS I V DIST WATER	BLOOD PRESSURE T P R TEST URINE A C & HS SLIDING SCALE I & O LEVIN TUBE CHEST TUBE FOLEY OXYGEN	ENEMA DOUCHE PERI CARE · LIGHT WEIGH ORAL HYGIENE SPECIAL BACK CARE PREPARE FOR SURG PREPARE FOR X-RAY O T · P T · E C T	STOOL URINE SPUTUM BLOOD CULTURE TISSUE	

CODE * You wash back and legs
B R P Bathroom privileges
AMB Ambulatory
I & O Intake and output
W C Wheelchair
B P Blood pressure
N P O Nothing by mouth
DIST Distilled water
E C T . Electrical Convulsive Therapy
O T . Occupational Therapy
P T . Physical Therapy

FIGURE 9-11
Sample of a nursing assignment sheet.

(Fig. 9-11). Each assignment identifies the patients for whom the staff person will be responsible and a description of the care that is needed. Meal times and break times may also be scheduled, as well as special tasks such as checking and restocking supplies. Near the end of the shift the charge nurse seeks out each staff person for a summary report on the status of their assigned patients.

Team Conferences

Conferences are commonly used for exchanging information. Topics include patient care problems, personnel conflicts, new equipment or treatment methods, and changes in policies or procedures.

Team conferences may include nursing staff, hospital staff from other departments who are involved in patient care, physicians, social workers, personnel from community agencies, and, in some cases, patients and their significant others. Usually one person organizes and directs the conference. Responsibilities for certain outcomes that result from the team conference may be delegated to various staff who attend the meeting.

Patient Rounds

Rounds involve visiting individual patients singularly or as a group. Rounds are used as a means of learning first-hand about patients. The patient is a witness to and often active participant in the interaction.

Some nurses use walking rounds as a method for giving a change-of-shift report. Giving report in the patient's presence provides new staff with an opportunity for personally surveying the patient's condition and determining the status of equipment used in the patient's care. It also tends to boost the patient's confidence and security in the transition of care.

Telephone

The telephone may be used to exchange information when it is difficult for people to get together or when information must be communicated quickly (Fig. 9-12). When using the telephone, it is important to:

- Answer the telephone as promptly as possible
- Speak in a normal tone of voice
- Identify yourself by name, title, and nursing unit
- Obtain or state the reason for the call
- Carefully identify the patient being discussed
- Spell the patient's name if there is any chance of confusion
- Converse in a courteous and businesslike manner
- Repeat information to make sure it has been heard accurately

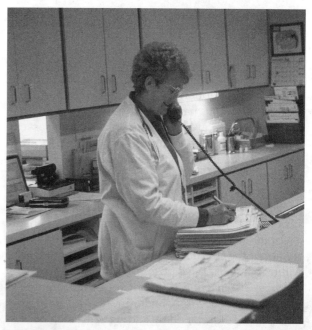

FIGURE 9-12
Nurses frequently report information to the physician and other departments involved in patient care. (Courtesy of Ken Timby.)

When notifying a physician about a change in a patient's condition, document the information that was reported and the instructions that were received in the patient's record. If the nurse feels that the physician has not responded in a safe manner to the information that was given, the nursing supervisor or head of the medical department may be notified.

KEY CONCEPTS

- Medical records are used (1) as a permanent account of a patient's health problems, care, and progress, (2) for sharing information among health care personnel, (3) as a self-study resource for investigating the quality of care within an institution, (4) to acquire and maintain JCAHO accreditation, (5) to obtain reimbursement for billed services and products, (6) for conducting research, and (7) as legal evidence in malpractice cases.
- In general, all medical records contain a patient information sheet, medical information, a plan for care, nursing documentation, medication administration records, and laboratory and diagnostic test results.
- Health care agencies may organize the information in the medical record using either a source-oriented format or a problem-oriented format. Source-oriented records categorize the information according to the source reporting the information, whereas problem-oriented records are organized according to the pa-

tient's health problems, regardless of who is doing the documentation.

- Information may be documented within the medical record using one of the following methods: narrative charting, SOAP charting, focus charting, PIE charting, charting by exception, and computerized charting.
- Regardless of the charting style, all documentation in an acute health care agency includes ongoing assessment data, problem identification, a plan for care, a record of the care that has been implemented, and the outcomes of the implemented care.
- Agency-approved abbreviations are used when documenting information to promote clarity in communication among health professionals and to ensure accurate interpretation of the documented information if the chart is subpoenaed as legal evidence.
- Military time is based on a 24-hour clock. When military time is used, a different four-digit number is identified for each hour and minute of the day. After noon, time is identified by adding 12 to each hour.
- When charting, some of the principles that apply include making sure the documentation form identifies the patient, using a pen, printing or writing legibly, recording the time of each entry, filling all the space on a line, using approved abbreviations, describing information objectively, providing precise measurements when possible, avoiding any obliteration of the information, and signing each entry by name and title.
- Other written forms of communication include the nursing care plan, nursing Kardex, checklists, and flow sheets.
- Besides the written record, information is exchanged among the health care team during change-of-shift reports, when making patient care assignments, during team conferences, while participating in patient rounds, and when using the telephone.

CRITICAL THINKING EXERCISES

- Implement the Nursing Guidelines for Making Entries in a Patient's Record to document the scenario that follows. Use the current date, military time, and abbreviations approved by a health agency used for your clinical experience. Select either narrative charting or SOAP format, or the style adopted in an agency your school uses for clinical experience.

Scenario: A 67-year-old woman is transferred from a nursing home to the hospital for unexplained weight loss. At the time of admission, her weight is 103 pounds. Her nursing home record indicates that she weighed 120 pounds 1 month ago. She tells the admitting nurse that she has no appetite and feels uncomfortably full after eating a meal.

- Use the information that follows, to simulate a change-of-shift report:

Assume Mrs. Anna Raposi is the patient of Dr. Campbell in the first scenario. She has been admitted with a tentative diagnosis of possible abdominal tumor. The plan is to weigh her each morning, obtain a urine specimen and blood for routine laboratory tests, and schedule her for a lower gastrointestinal x-ray. There are no dietary or activity restrictions at this time.

SUGGESTED READINGS

Carpenito LJ. Has JCAHO eliminated care plans? American Nurse June 1991;23:6.

Carr P. Putting it together: care and documentation. Home Healthcare Nurse November–December 1991;9:46–49.

Computer charting: minimizing legal risks. Nursing May 1993;23:86.

Eggland ET. Documentation do's and don'ts. Nursing August 1993;23:30.

Grant AE. Documenting by computer. Canadian Nurse September 1993;89;53.

Joint Commission on Accreditation of Healthcare Organizations (JCAHO). Accreditation Manual for Hospitals: Volume 1, Standards. Oak Terrace, IL: JCAHO, 1991.

Locher CJ. How to make the most of your charting. Journal of Practical Nursing June 1992;42:35–39, 43.

Locher CJ. Myths and facts . . . about charting: *part 1*. Nursing February 1993;23:70.

Locher CJ. Myths and facts . . . about charting: *part 2*. Nursing March 1993;23:25.

Meyer C. Bedside computer charting: inching toward tomorrow. American Journal of Nursing April 1992;92:38–42, 44.

Schaffer CL. Documenting special legal situations. Nursing May 1992;22:32C–32D.

Stephan A. Notifying the doctor by phone. Nursing November 1993;23:20.

Walker D. A-ND-I-O: linking nursing notes and care plans. Nursing Management August 1993;24:58–59.

Worthy MK, Siegrist-Mueller L. Integrating a "plan of care" into documentation systems. Nursing Management October 1992;23:68–70, 72.

Wright BA, Fishman N. Telephone reporting to physicians. Geriatric Nursing September–October 1992;13:279–280.

Fundamental Nursing Skills

UNIT IV
Performing Assessment and Evaluation

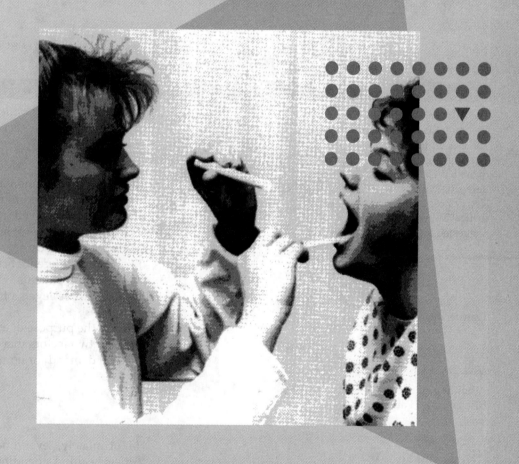

CHAPTER 10

Admission, Discharge, Transfer, and Referrals

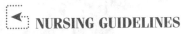
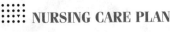
Learning Objectives

An understanding of the content within this chapter will be evidenced by the student's ability to:

- List four major steps involved in the admission process
- Identify four common responses that may occur when patients are admitted to a health agency
- List the steps involved in the discharge process
- Give three examples of how transfers are used in the course of patient care
- Explain the difference between transferring patients and referring patients
- Describe three levels of care provided by nursing homes
- Discuss the purpose of a Minimum Data Set
- Identify two factors that have contributed to the increased demand for home health care

Unfortunately, everyone experiences changes in their health. Depending on the seriousness of the condition, there are several levels of available health care (see Chap. 4). Some people may be able to recover with self-treatment or by following health instructions from a nurse or other member of the health team. However, others who become seriously ill, are injured, or have chronic health problems may require admission and temporary or long-term care within a hospital or nursing home.

This chapter addresses the nursing skills involved in admitting sick people to health care institutions, and their subsequent discharge, transfer, or referral to other agencies that provide health care.

Timby BK: *Fundamental Skills and Concepts in Patient Care, Sixth Edition* © 1996 Lippincott-Raven Publishers

THE ADMISSION PROCESS

Admission is a process that takes place when a person enters a health care agency for more than 24 hours of care and treatment. The process involves (1) obtaining medical authorization, (2) compiling billing information, (3) completing nursing admission activities, and (4) fulfilling mandated medical responsibilities.

Medical Authorization

Before patients are admitted, a physician determines that their condition requires special tests, technical care, or treatment that cannot be provided other than in a hospital or other health care agency. Some patients may be scheduled for nonurgent care, like certain types of surgery, at a date and time that is mutually agreeable. However, most patients are seen just before their admission by a primary care or emergency room physician. The physician advises both the patient and nursing staff to proceed with the admission process.

The Admitting Department

In the admitting department, clerical personnel begin to gather information from the prospective patient or a family member. The medical record is initiated with data obtained at this time. A form is prepared with the patient's address, place of employment, insurance company and policy numbers, and other personal data. This information is used primarily by the hospital's business office for record keeping and future billing.

Those patients who are extremely unstable or in severe discomfort may bypass the fact-finding that takes place in the admitting department and be transported directly to the nursing unit. Someone from the family is eventually directed to the admitting department on the patient's behalf, or personnel are sent to the patient's bedside to obtain needed information.

The admissions clerk usually prepares an identification bracelet for the patient. The identification bracelet gives the patient's name, identification number, the name of the patient's physician, and the patient's room number. The bracelet is usually applied by someone in the admitting department or by the admitting nurse (Fig. 10-1). For the patient's safety, it is important that the bracelet remain on throughout the duration of the patient's care. Apart from asking a patient's name, the bracelet is the single most important method for identifying the patient. If the identification bracelet is missing or has been removed, the nurse is responsible for replacing it as soon as possible.

Once the preliminary data have been collected, the nursing unit is notified and the patient is escorted to the location where he or she will receive care. The form initiated in the admitting department is delivered to the

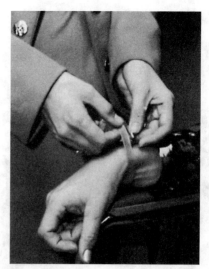

FIGURE 10-1
Applying an identification bracelet.

nursing unit along with a plastic card, called an addressograph plate. The card is used to identify all future pages within the patient's medical record.

Nursing Admission Activities
PREPARING THE PATIENT'S ROOM

When the nurse is informed by the admissions department that the patient is about to be escorted to the unit, the room is checked to make sure that it is clean and completely stocked with basic equipment for initial care.

WELCOMING THE PATIENT

One of the most important steps in the admission process is to make the patient feel welcome. Therefore, on arrival, it is appropriate to greet the patient warmly with a smile and a handshake (Fig. 10-2) and introduce oneself. Being treated in a friendly manner helps put the patient at ease. If the patient feels unexpected or unwanted, it is likely to make a rude, and lasting, first impression.

ORIENTING THE PATIENT

Orientation is the act of helping a person become familiar with a new environment (or role) to facilitate adaptation. When orienting a patient, the nurse points out the location of the nursing station, the toilet, the shower or bathing area, and lounge that may be used by the patient and family.

The nurse also explains how to use equipment within the room and the daily routine and activities that affect patient care. For example, the nurse shows the patient how to operate the television, electric bed,

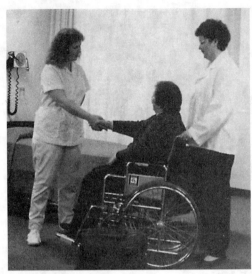

FIGURE 10-2
Greeting a new patient.

and signal cord or intercommunication system. In addition, the policy regarding phone calls, the times for meals, when the doctor may be expected, when surgery is scheduled, and when laboratory tests or x-rays may be performed are explained.

Because many patients are anxious when they are admitted, and do not remember much of the verbal information, some hospitals provide printed booklets with much of the same general information. The booklet reinforces what has been previously explained. However, booklets should never take the place of the nurse's explanations.

SAFEGUARDING VALUABLES AND CLOTHING

It is preferable that certain items such as prescription and nonprescription medications, valuable jewelry, and money be given to family members to take home. If this is not possible, *the agency's policies must be carefully observed.* Some institutions allow patients' valuables to be placed temporarily in the hospital's safe. A notation is made in the medical record identifying the type of valuables and the manner in which they were safeguarded. It is best to be as descriptive as possible. For example, rather than indicating that a ring was placed in the safe, it is better to describe the type of metal and stones in the ring.

Losing a patient's personal items can have serious legal implications for both the nurse and the health care agency. The patient may sue, claiming his or her belongings were lost or stolen because they were handled carelessly. Therefore, it is best to have a second nurse, supervisor, or security personnel present when assuming responsibility for safeguarding valuables.

Making an inventory list is one method of avoiding discrepancies between the items that were entrusted to the nurse and what is eventually returned (Fig. 10-3). When this approach is used, the nurse and the patient co-sign the inventory. One copy is given to the patient, and another is attached to the chart. When items are returned, the list is revised and the patient signs the new inventory. Problems with theft or loss may still occur if other items are brought in without subsequent documentation.

It is best to identify patient-owned equipment, such as a walker or wheelchair, with a large label that is easily read. Labeling personal equipment may help prevent it from being confused with hospital property.

Most agencies have facilities in the patient's room for the storage of street clothing. However, because eyeglasses and dentures may be removed from time to time, there is always the possibility that they may be lost or broken. The health care agency usually will assume responsibility for replacing these items in the event they were accidentally damaged or lost through the negligence of staff.

HELPING THE PATIENT UNDRESS

To facilitate a physical examination, the patient must undress. There will be times, however, when a patient is unable to undress without the nurse's help. Methods for helping the patient are as follows:

- Provide privacy.
- Have the patient sit on the edge of the bed, which has already been lowered.
- Remove the patient's shoes.
- Gather each stocking, sliding it down the leg and over the foot.
- Assist the patient to turn on the bed and assume a lying position if weak or tired.
- Release fasteners, such as zippers and buttons, and remove the item of clothing from the patient in whatever manner is most comfortable and least disturbing. For example, fold or gather a garment and work it up and over the body. Have the patient lift his or her hips to slide clothes up or down.
- Lift the patient's head so garments can be guided over the head.
- Roll the patient from side to side to remove clothes that fasten up the front or back.
- Cover the patient with a bath blanket after removing the outer clothing or put a hospital gown on the patient.

COMPILING THE NURSING DATA BASE

At the time of admission, the nurse begins assessing the patient and collecting information for the data base (see Chap. 2). Although the registered nurse is responsi-

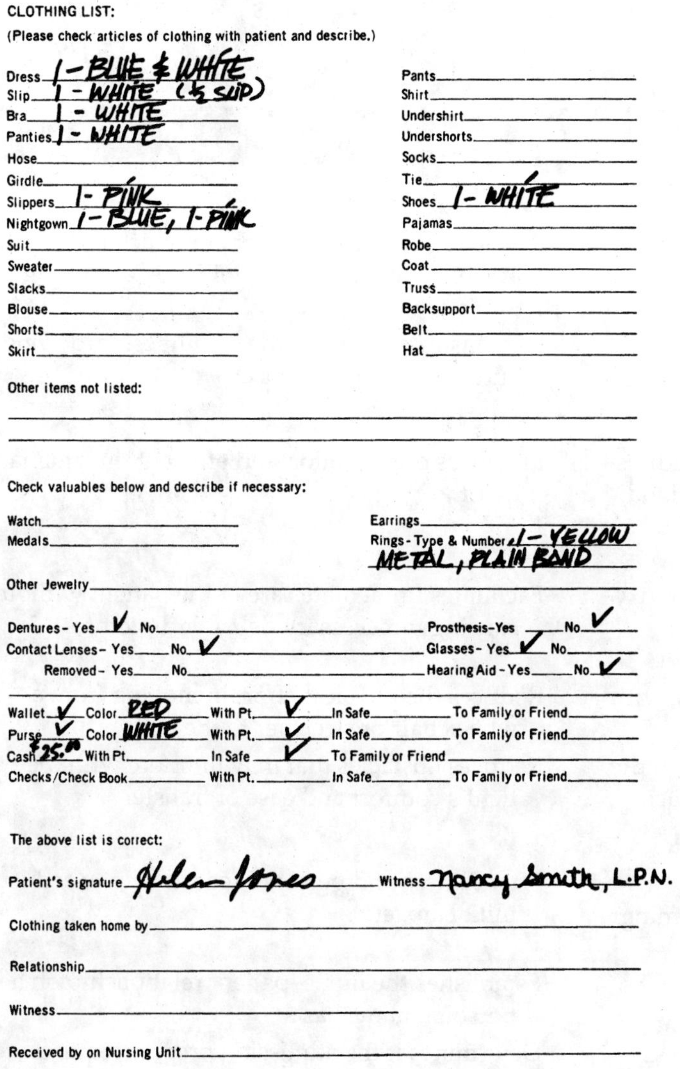

CLOTHING LIST:

(Please check articles of clothing with patient and describe.)

Dress	*1 - BLUE & WHITE*	Pants	
Slip	*1 - WHITE (& SLIP)*	Shirt	
Bra	*1 - WHITE*	Undershirt	
Panties	*1 - WHITE*	Undershorts	
Hose		Socks	
Girdle		Tie	
Slippers	*1 - PINK*	Shoes	*1 - WHITE*
Nightgown	*1 - BLUE, 1 - PINK*	Pajamas	
Suit		Robe	
Sweater		Coat	
Slacks		Truss	
Blouse		Backsupport	
Shorts		Belt	
Skirt		Hat	

Other items not listed:

_____

_____

Check valuables below and describe if necessary:

Watch_____   Earrings_____

Medals_____   Rings - Type & Number *1 - YELLOW METAL, PLAIN BAND*

Other Jewelry_____

Dentures – Yes ✔ No____   Prosthesis – Yes____ No ✔

Contact Lenses – Yes____ No ✔   Glasses – Yes ✔ No____

Removed – Yes____ No____   Hearing Aid – Yes____ No ✔

Wallet ✔ Color *RED* With Pt. ✔ In Safe____ To Family or Friend____

Purse ✔ Color *WHITE* With Pt. ✔ In Safe____ To Family or Friend____

Cash *$25.⁰⁰* With Pt. ✔ In Safe____ To Family or Friend____

Checks/Check Book____ With Pt.____ In Safe____ To Family or Friend____

The above list is correct:

Patient's signature *Helen Jones*   Witness *Nancy Smith, L.P.N.*

Clothing taken home by_____

Relationship_____

Witness_____

Received by on Nursing Unit_____

FIGURE 10-3

Inventory of the patient's personal belongings.

---

ble for the admission assessment, some aspects may be delegated to the practical nurse or other ancillary staff. Physical assessment skills, which include taking vital signs, are discussed in more depth in Chapters 11 and 12.

Skill 10-1 describes the basic steps in admitting a patient. Additions or modifications in the procedure depend largely on the patient's condition and agency policies. Once the admission assessment has been performed, the registered nurse is responsible for identifying the patient's problems and developing the initial plan for nursing care.

Medical Admission Responsibilities

After the nursing data are collected, the patient's physician is notified for the purpose of obtaining medical orders. The physician is also obligated to obtain a medical history and perform a physical examination, which must be documented within 24 hours of admission. This task may in turn be delegated to some other mem-

ber of the medical team such as a medical student, intern, or resident.

In general, the medical history and physical examination includes the following information: (1) identifying data, (2) the patient's chief complaint, (3) history of present illness, (4) personal history, (5) past health history, (6) family history, (7) a review of body systems, and (8) conclusions (Display 10-1). If the physician is unsure of the actual medical diagnosis, the term *rule out*, or the abbreviation *R/O*, is used to indicate that the condition is suspected as a cause of the patient's symptoms, but additional diagnostic data must be obtained before it can be confirmed.

Regardless of how many times nurses and physicians have admitted patients, it is a unique and emotionally traumatic experience for each patient. Leaving the security of home and entering the unfamiliar environment of a health facility compounds the stress of physical illness and contributes to emotional and social problems.

SKILL 10-1
Admitting a Patient

Suggested Action	Reason for Action
Assessment	
Obtain the name, admitting diagnosis, condition of the patient, and the room to which the patient has been assigned.	Provides preliminary data from which to plan the activities that may be involved in admitting the patient
Check the appearance of the room and presence of basic supplies.	Demonstrates concern for cleanliness, orderliness, and patient convenience
Planning	
Assemble equipment that will be needed: admission assessment form(s), thermometer, blood pressure cuff (if not wall-mounted), stethoscope, scale, urine specimen container.	Enhances organization and efficient time management
Obtain special equipment, like an IV pole or oxygen, that may be needed according to the unique needs of the patient.	Facilitates immediate care of the patient without causing unnecessary delay or discomfort
Arrange the height of the bed to coordinate with the expected mode of arrival.	Reduces the physical effort in moving from a wheelchair or stretcher to the bed
Fold the top linen to the bottom of the bed, if the patient will be immediately confined to bed.	Reduces obstacles that may interfere with the patient's comfort and ease of transfer
Implementation	
Greet the patient by name and demonstrate a friendly smile; extend a hand as a welcoming gesture.	Friendliness and personal regard help to reduce initial anxiety
Introduce yourself to the patient and those who have accompanied the patient.	Establishes the nurse–patient relationship on a personal name basis
Observe the patient for signs of acute distress.	Determines if the admission process requires modification
Attend to urgent needs for comfort and breathing.	Demonstrates concern for the patient's well-being
Introduce the patient to his or her roommate, if there is one, and anyone else who enters the room.	Familiarity relieves social awkwardness and demonstrates a concern for the patient's emotional comfort
Offer the patient a chair unless the patient requires immediate bed rest.	Demonstrates concern for the patient's physical comfort
Check the patient's identification bracelet.	Safety depends on being able to identify the patient accurately
Orient the patient to the physical environment of the room and the nursing unit.	Aids in adapting to unfamiliar surroundings
Demonstrate the equipment in the room, such as the adjustments for the bed, how to signal for a nurse, and use of the telephone and television.	Promotes comfort, self-reliance, and ensures safety
Explain the general routines and schedules that are followed for visiting hours, meals, and care.	Reduces uncertainty about when to expect activities
Explain the need to examine the patient and ask personal health questions.	Prepares the patient for what will follow next

(continued)

SKILL 10-1
Admitting a Patient *(Continued)*

Suggested Action	Reason for Action
Inquire as to whether the patient would like family members to leave or remain	Promotes a sense of control over decisions and their outcomes
Make provisions for privacy.	Demonstrates respect for the patient's dignity
Request that the patient undress and don a patient gown; assist as necessary	Facilitates physical assessment
Ask the patient about the need to urinate at the present time, and explain that a urine specimen will be needed whenever there is an opportunity for the patient to do so.	Shows concern for the patient's immediate comfort, promotes cooperation in obtaining a voided urine specimen, and facilitates physical assessment of the abdomen
Weigh the patient before helping him or her into bed.	Avoids disturbing the patient once settled in bed
Assist the patient to a comfortable position in bed.	Shows concern for the patient's comfort and facilitates the examination
Take care of the patient's clothing and valuables according to agency policy.	Safeguards the patient's personal possessions
Ask the patient to identify allergies to food, drugs, or other substances and describe the type of symptoms that accompany a typical allergic reaction.	Aids in preventing a potential allergic reaction during care; prepares staff for the manner in which the patient reacts to the allergen
Wash hands thoroughly.	Reduces the direct transmission of microorganisms from the nurse's hands to the patient (see Chap. 21)
Obtain the patient's temperature, pulse, respiratory rate, and blood pressure (see Chap. 11).	Contributes to the initial data base assessment
Place the signal cord where it can be conveniently reached.	Reduces the potential for accidents by ensuring that the patient can make his or her needs known
Make sure the bed is in low position and follow agency policy about raising the side rails on the bed.	Side rails are considered a form of physical restraint; their use may require written permission from the patient
Remove the urine specimen, if obtained at this time, attach a laboratory request form, and place it in the refrigerator or take it to the laboratory.	Ensures proper identification of the specimen, identifies the test that is to be performed, and prevents deterioration that may affect test results
Wash hands thoroughly.	Removes microorganisms acquired from contact with the patient or handling the urine specimen
Report the progress of the patient's admission to the registered nurse, who may perform the nursing interview and physical assessment or delegate components at this time.	Complies with Joint Commission on Accreditation of Health Organizations (JCAHO) standards; the entire admission assessment must be completed within 24 hours; parts of the assessment may be performed at periodic intervals.
Inform family or friends that they may resume visiting the patient when the nursing activities are completed.	

(continued)

SKILL 10-1
Admitting a Patient (Continued)

Suggested Action	Reason for Action

Evaluation

- Patient is comfortable and oriented to room and routines
- Safety measures are implemented
- Data base assessments are initiated
- Status and progress are communicated to nursing team

Document

- Date and time of admission
- Age and gender of patient
- Overall appearance
- Mode of arrival to the unit
- Room number where patient is located
- Initial vital signs and weight
- List of allergies, if any; quote the patient's description of a typical reaction, or indicate if the patient has no allergies by using the abbreviation NKA (no known allergies) or whatever abbreviation is acceptable
- Disposition of urine specimen
- The present condition of the patient

*Sample Documentation**

Date and Time   68-year-old female admitted to Room 258^2 by wheelchair from admitting dept. with moderate dyspnea. O_2 running at 2 L per nasal cannula. Weighs 173 lbs. on bed scale wearing only a patient gown. T—98.4°, P—92, R—32, BP 146/68 in R. arm while sitting up. Unable to void at the present time. Allergic to penicillin which causes "hives and difficulty breathing." In high Fowler's position at this time with a respiratory rate of 24 at rest. _____ **Signature, Title**

* See Appendix A for explanations of abbreviations and the Glossary for terms that may be unfamiliar.

COMMON RESPONSES TO ADMISSION

Although the specific responses to admission are unique to each person, some common reactions include anxiety, loneliness, decreased privacy, and loss of identity. In addition, the nurse may identify one or more nursing diagnoses that develop as a consequence of an admission to a health care agency.

Anxiety

Anxiety is an uncomfortable feeling caused by insecurity. It has been defined by the North American Nursing Diagnosis Association (1992) as "a vague uneasy feeling whose source is often nonspecific or unknown to the individual."

Many adults do not manifest their anxiety in obvious ways. Observant nurses may note that adults appear sad or worried, are restless, have a reduced appetite, or have trouble sleeping (see Chap. 5). Because adults have a greater capacity to process information than children, it may be helpful to acknowledge their uneasiness, and provide explanations and instructions before any new experience occurs. The Nursing Care Plan for Anxiety provides an example of how the nursing process is used when planning the care of a patient with anxiety.

Loneliness

Loneliness occurs when admitted patients are not able to interact with family and friends. Although nurses can never replace those who are significant to a patient,

DISPLAY 10-1. *Components of a Medical History*

Identifying Data

The patient's age, gender, marital status, general appearance, circumstances under which the physician became involved in the patient's care, reliability of the patient as a historian, identification of others who have provided information relevant to the patient's history

Chief Complaint

The reason for seeking care from the patient's perspective

Present Illness

A chronologic description of the onset, frequency, and duration of current signs and symptoms; outcomes of earlier attempts at self-treatment and medical treatment

Personal History

The patient's occupation; highest level of education; religious affiliation; place of residence; country of origin; primary language; military service; date, location, and length of foreign travel or residence

Past Health History

A summary of childhood diseases; physical injuries; major illnesses; previous medical or psychiatric hospitalizations; surgical procedures; drug history; use of alcohol and tobacco; allergy history

Family History

Health problems among immediate family members, both living and dead, longevity and cause of death among deceased blood relatives—especially parents and grandparents

Review of Body Systems

Findings obtained after examining the patient

Conclusions

A primary diagnosis based on the patient's chief complaint and physical examination findings; secondary diagnoses that may reflect conditions that are stable and existed before the current medical problem, but that nevertheless affect the patient's treatment

 APPLICABLE NURSING DIAGNOSES

- Anxiety
- Fear
- Decisional Conflict
- Self-Esteem Disturbance
- Powerlessness
- Social Isolation

they may act as temporary surrogates. Making frequent contact and being available and interested in the patient may substitute somewhat for those who cannot be physically near.

To help combat loneliness, many hospitals and nursing homes have adopted liberal visiting hours to accommodate the varied schedules of potential visitors. Age restrictions are also being lifted to allow more contact between children and their sick relatives.

Decreased Privacy

Privacy in most health agencies is at a premium. Very few patients, for example, have a private room. In fact, most patients have little more than the few feet around them. Combine that with the fact that patients often share a room with a total stranger, that their room doors are open most of the time, and that many people pass by at all hours of the day and night, and it is easy to understand how privacy is compromised.

To compensate for these situations, it is important to demonstrate respect for and ensure protection of each patient's right to privacy. For instance, patients must always be protected from the view of others when personal care is given. Furthermore, if a patient's door is closed or the curtains are pulled, it is a common courtesy to knock or ask permission to enter. If there is a place within the health agency where patients may retreat and find solitude, like a chapel or reading room, the information should be included in the admission orientation.

Loss of Identity

Becoming a patient may temporarily deprive a person of his or her personal identity. For example, when patients are required to wear institutional gowns, they may all look somewhat the same. Consequently, patients may be treated in an impersonal manner—simply as a face or warm body with no name. This attitude makes patients feel like they are receiving care, but no caring.

NURSING CARE PLAN:
Anxiety

Assessment	**Subjective Data** States, "Ever since my doctor told me I had to come to the hospital for this test, I've felt like a rubberband that's stretched to the limit." **Objective Data** 35-year-old woman admitted for heart catheterization. Heart rate 105, flushed, pacing about room. Twists hair with fingers. Asks that admission questions be repeated. Stares out window. Crying off and on during interview.
Diagnosis	Anxiety related to change in health status.
Plan	**Goal** The patient will report a reduction in anxiety by 4/17. **Orders:** 4/14 1. Sit calmly with patient at least t.i.d. 2. Reinforce that most people have similar feelings in these circumstances. 3. Explore the specific problems associated with hospitalization. 4. Do not discourage crying if it occurs. _____ S. FRIEDMAN, RN
Implementation 4/14 *(Documentation)*	1115 Spent ½ hr talking. Shared that anxiety is a common feeling among patients. Asked to identify the most distressing aspect of this experience. States, "I don't have any health insurance." Asked if she would like to see a social worker to discuss a partial payment schedule. _____ C. SKINNER, SN
Evaluation *(Documentation)*	1115 Stated, "Oh yes. I didn't know that was possible. I'm so relieved. I thought I'd have to sell my car." No crying. Ate most of lunch. _____ C. SKINNER, SN

Therefore, it is important to learn and call all patients by name. However, first names are used only if a patient requests it. Patients also may be encouraged to display family pictures or other small personal objects that reaffirm their unique life and personality. In long-term care facilities, many patients are urged to dress in their own clothing and invited to furnish their rooms with personal items from home.

Regardless of where patients are admitted and for whatever reason, the goal is to keep the admission as brief as possible and to discharge patients back to their homes as soon as possible.

THE DISCHARGE PROCESS

Discharge is a process that occurs when a patient leaves a health agency. It consists of: (1) obtaining a written medical order for discharge, (2) completing discharge instructions, (3) notifying the business office, (4) helping the patient leave the health agency, (5) writing a summary of the patient's condition at the time

of discharge, and (6) requesting that the room be cleaned.

Authorization for Medical Discharge

The physician determines when the patient is well enough to be discharged. The physician usually waits to write the medical order until after examining the patient. Before leaving the nursing unit, the physician writes the discharge order, provides written prescriptions for the patient, and indicates when and where a follow-up appointment should take place.

LEAVING AGAINST MEDICAL ADVICE

Leaving against medical advice (AMA) is a term that applies to situations in which the patient leaves the health agency before the physician authorizes the discharge. Often, the situation arises because the patient is disgruntled with some aspect of his or her care or treatment. In some cases, the nurse may successfully negotiate a compromise or persuade the patient temporarily to delay taking such action. In the meantime, the nurse informs the physician and nursing supervisor of the patient's wish to leave.

If the patient remains undaunted and he or she is determined to leave, the nurse asks the patient to sign a special form (see Chap. 3). The signed form releases the physician and health agency from future responsibility for any complications that may occur. If the patient refuses to sign the form, he or she cannot be detained from leaving. The fact that the form was presented and subsequently refused is, however, noted in the patient's medical record.

When a patient's discharge takes place under more amicable circumstances, the nurse's next responsibility is to provide discharge instructions.

Providing Discharge Instructions

Planning for discharge actually begins when patients are admitted. Shortly after admission, the nurse identifies the anticipated knowledge and skills that each patient will need to maintain a safe level of self-care. One planning technique involves using the acronym METHOD as a guide (Table 10-1). The actual patient teaching identified in the discharge plan is provided periodically throughout the patient's length of stay (see Chap. 8).

Once again before the patient leaves, the nurse reviews the teaching that has been provided, gives the patient prescriptions to fill, and advises the patient to make an office appointment for the date specified by the physician. Usually a written summary of discharge instructions is provided. The patient signs one sheet, and a carbon copy is attached to the patient's medical record.

Notifying the Business Office

Before the patient leaves the health agency, the business office is notified. At that time, clerical personnel verify that all insurance information is complete and that the patient has signed a consent form authorizing the release of medical information to the insurance carrier. If records are incomplete, or if the patient has no health insurance, it may be necessary for the patient to make future financial arrangements before being discharged.

Discharging a Patient

When all of the preliminary business has been completed, patients are helped to gather their belongings, plan for transportation, and actually leave the health agency. For a step-by-step description of the discharge process from beginning to end, refer to Skill 10-2.

GATHERING BELONGINGS

Patients are assisted, if necessary, with repacking all of the personal items they brought to the health agency. If a valuables or inventory list is available, it should be used to ensure that nothing has been lost or forgotten. Because most hospitals dispose of the plastic utensils kept at the bedside, the nurse can offer the basin, bed pan, urinal, and the like to the patient. If the patient has no use for these items, they are discarded in receptacles in the soiled utility room. A cart with wheels may be helpful when transporting all of the patient's belongings at the time of discharge.

ARRANGING TRANSPORTATION

To expedite arranging transportation, it may be helpful to inform patients if there is a particular time before which they can avoid being charged for another full day in the health agency. In most cases, the patient contacts a family member or friend for assistance. If no transportation is available, the patient may choose to call a taxicab. Van transportation may be available for

(text continues on page 122)

TABLE 10-1. *The Method Discharge Planning Guide*		
Topic	Nursing Activity	Example
M—Medications	Instruct the patient about drugs that will be self-administered.	Insulin
E —Environment	Explore how the home environment can be modified to ensure the patient's safety.	Remove scatter rugs
T —Treatments	Demonstrate how to perform skills involved in self-care and provide opportunities for returning the demonstration.	Dressing changes
H—Health teaching	Identify information that is necessary for maintaining or improving health.	Signs and symptoms of complications
O—Outpatient referral	Explain what community services are available that may ease the patient's transition to independent living.	Physical therapy
D—Diet	Arrange for the dietitian to provide verbal and written instructions on modifying or restricting certain foods or suggestions for altering their methods of preparation.	Low-fat diet

SKILL 10-2
Discharging a Patient

Suggested Action	Reason for Action
Assessment	
Determine that a medical order has been written.	Provides authorization for discharging the patient
Check for written prescriptions and other medical discharge instructions.	Enables the patient to continue self-care
Note if there are any new medical orders that must be carried out before the patient's discharge.	Ensures that the patient will leave in the best possible condition
Review the nursing discharge plan.	Determines if more health teaching is needed or if the instructions have been completed
*Planning**	
Discuss the patient's time frame for leaving the hospital.	Helps in coordinating nursing activities within the patient's schedule
Determine the patient's mode of transportation.	Clarifies if the services of a cab company or other resource may be needed
*Notify the business office of the patient's impending discharge.	Allows times for the clerical department to review the patient's billing information and determine the necessity for further actions
*Inform the housekeeping department that the patient will be leaving.	Prepares cleaning staff for the fact that the patient unit will need terminal cleaning
*Cancel any meals that the patient will miss after discharge.	Avoids preparing food that will be wasted
*Notify the pharmacy of the approximate time of discharge.	Eliminates preparation of drugs that will go unused
Plan to provide hygiene and medical treatments early.	Prevents delays in the patient's departure
Implementation	
Wash hands.	Reduces the transmission of microorganisms.
Provide for hygiene, but omit changing the bed linen.	Eliminates unnecessary work
Complete medical treatment and nursing interventions according to the plan for care.	Promotes continuation of nursing care up through the time of discharge
Help the patient dress in clothing that will be worn home.	Demonstrates concern for the patient's appearance in public
Review discharge instructions and complete health teaching.	Promotes safe self-care
Have the patient sign the discharge instruction sheet and paraphrase the information it contains.	Validates if the patient has understood instructions for maintaining health
Assist the patient with packing personal items; if appropriate, have the patient sign the clothing inventory or valuables list.	Reduces claims that personal items were lost or stolen; signing a clothing inventory or valuables list is more likely to apply when a patient is discharged from a nursing home or rehabilitation center

Starred activities may be delegated to a clerk.

(continued)

SKILL 10-2
Discharging a Patient *(Continued)*

Suggested Action	Reason for Action
Obtain a cart for the patient's personal belongings.	Eases the work of transporting multiple or heavy items
Assist the patient into a wheelchair when transportation is available.	Reduces the potential for a fall if the patient is weak or unsteady
Stop, if necessary, at the business office.	Complies with billing procedures
Escort the patient to the awaiting vehicle.	Promotes safety while still within the hospital
Return any forms from the business office.	Confirms that the patient has left the hospital
Replace the wheelchair in its proper location on the nursing unit.	Makes equipment available for others to use
Wash hands.	Reduces the transmission of microorganisms
Complete a discharge summary in the medical record.	Closes the medical record for this particular admission

Evaluation

- Health condition is stable (if being transferred in unstable condition, is accompanied by qualified personnel who have the knowledge and skills to intervene in emergencies)
- Able to paraphrase discharge instructions accurately
- Business office indicates that billing records are in order
- No injuries during transport from room to vehicle

Document

- Date and time of discharge
- Condition at the time of discharge
- Summary of discharge instructions
- Mode of transportation
- Identity of person(s) who accompanied patient

Sample Documentation*

Date and Time	No fever or wound tenderness at this time. Sutures removed. Abdominal incision is intact. No dressing applied. Given prescription for Keflex. Able to repeat how many capsules to self-administer per dose, the appropriate times for administration, and possible side effects. Repeated signs and symptoms of infection and the need to report them immediately. Instructed to shower as usual and temporarily avoid lifting objects over 10 lbs. Informed to make follow-up appointment in 1 week with physician as indicated on discharge instruction sheet. Given patient's copy of written discharge instructions. Escorted to business office in wheelchair accompanied by spouse. Assisted into private car without any unusual events. _____ **Signature, Title**

* See Appendix A for explanations of abbreviations and the Glossary for terms that may be unfamiliar.

older adults through the local Commission on Aging agency, but scheduling usually requires notification 24 hours in advance.

ESCORTING THE PATIENT

When the patient is ready, he or she is taken to the door in a wheelchair or allowed to walk there with assistance. In some hospitals the patient may choose to have discharge prescriptions filled at the hospital's pharmacy before leaving. The nurse usually remains with the patient until he or she is safely inside a vehicle.

Writing a Discharge Summary

Once the patient has left the health agency, the nurse documents a summary of the discharge activities (see information to document in Skill 10-2).

Terminal Cleaning

Except in unusual circumstances, the housekeeping personnel prepare the vacated room for the next admission. The bed is stripped of linen and cleaned with a disinfectant and the bedside cabinet is restocked with basic equipment. When the job is complete, the admitting department is notified that the room is ready. This prevents assigning a patient to a room that still requires cleaning.

TRANSFERRING PATIENTS

A transfer involves discharging a patient from one unit or agency and admitting him or her to another without going home in the interim. A transfer may take place when a patient's condition changes for better or worse.

In general, a transfer has some advantage for the patient. For example, it may facilitate more specialized care in a life-threatening situation (Fig. 10-4). Or, it may reduce health care costs because the patient can improve with a different type of care, like going from a hospital to a nursing home or one unit of a hospital to another. Many hospitals are creating what are called **step-down units** or **progressive care units**. The patients in these nursing units were once in critical condition, but have recovered sufficiently to require less intensive nursing care.

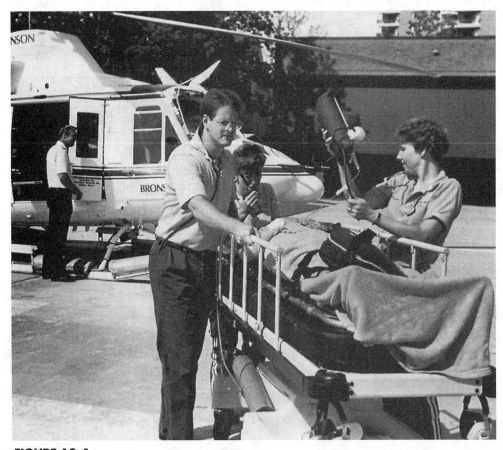

FIGURE 10-4
Transferring a patient rapidly may be a lifesaving measure. (Courtesy of Bronson Methodist Hospital, Kalamazoo, MI.)

Facilitating a Transfer

When an admitted patient is transferred to a nursing home or other health care facility, the transfer is conducted similarly to a discharge. The patient is discharged from acute care and then readmitted after arriving at the transfer facility. Use the following recommended nursing guidelines when transferring a patient.

◄ NURSING GUIDELINES FOR TRANSFERRING A PATIENT

- Be sure that the patient and family are informed of the need for a transfer as early as possible.
  Rationale: Promotes cooperation when anticipating a change
- If time permits, and the patient or family have some choice in the matter, encourage the family to investigate and collaborate on which facility they prefer.
  Rationale: Allows participation in decision making
- Communicate with the agency or unit where the patient will be transferred.
  Rationale: Provides time to plan and prepare for the patient's arrival
- Make a photocopy of the medical record if the patient has given written permission and is being transferred to a different health facility. (If the patient is being transferred to a unit within the same health agency, the original chart accompanies the patient.)
  Rationale: Aids in continuity of care and avoids duplicating services
- Provide a brief verbal or written summary (Fig. 10-5) of the patient's condition, treatment, and care. For a verbal report, follow the format for a change-of-shift report identified in Chapter 9.
  Rationale: Prepares new personnel for the patient's care
- Collect all of the patient's belongings.
  Rationale: Avoids loss of the patient's clothing or valuables and the inconvenience in returning them
- Accompany emergency medical staff or paramedics to the patient's room.
  Rationale: Reduces the patient's anxiety
- Help transfer the patient onto the stretcher or into a wheelchair.
  Rationale: Reduces the efforts and demands on the patient
- Place the copy of the medical record in a sealed folder and give it to the transfer personnel.
  Rationale: Protects the patient's confidentiality and prevents losing parts of the record

- Complete the original medical record by adding a summary of the patient's discharge.
  Rationale: Terminates the current record
- Send the completed chart to the medical records department.
  Rationale: Maintains the chart for future reference
- Notify the business office, admitting office, and housekeeping department of the patient's transfer.
  Rationale: Alerts each department to complete its responsibilities, which are similar to those that apply when a patient is discharged

---

Older adults in particular may be transferred directly from an acute care hospital to a facility that provides extended care (Table 10-2).

EXTENDED CARE FACILITIES

Extended care facilities are institutions that provide care for people who are unable to care for themselves, but who do not require hospitalization. Although there are several examples that may fit this description, like group homes for assisted living, adult day care centers, and senior residential communities, long-term care is usually provided in nursing homes.

Nursing Homes

Nursing homes are classified as being either skilled nursing facilities, intermediate facilities, or basic care facilities.

SKILLED NURSING FACILITIES

Skilled nursing facilities (SNF) are those that provide 24-hour nursing care under the direction of a registered nurse. To qualify as a skilled care patient, the person must be referred by a physician and require specific technical nursing skills, such as:

- Observation during an acute or unstable phase of an illness
- Administration of enteral feedings or intravenous fluids
- Bowel or bladder retraining
- Administration of injectable medications
- Changing sterile dressings

Skilled care is provided from a multidisciplinary perspective. Besides a 24-hour team of nurses, a skilled nursing facility must provide rehabilitative services such as physical therapy and occupational therapy, pharmaceutical services, dietary services, diversional and therapeutic activities, and routine and emergency

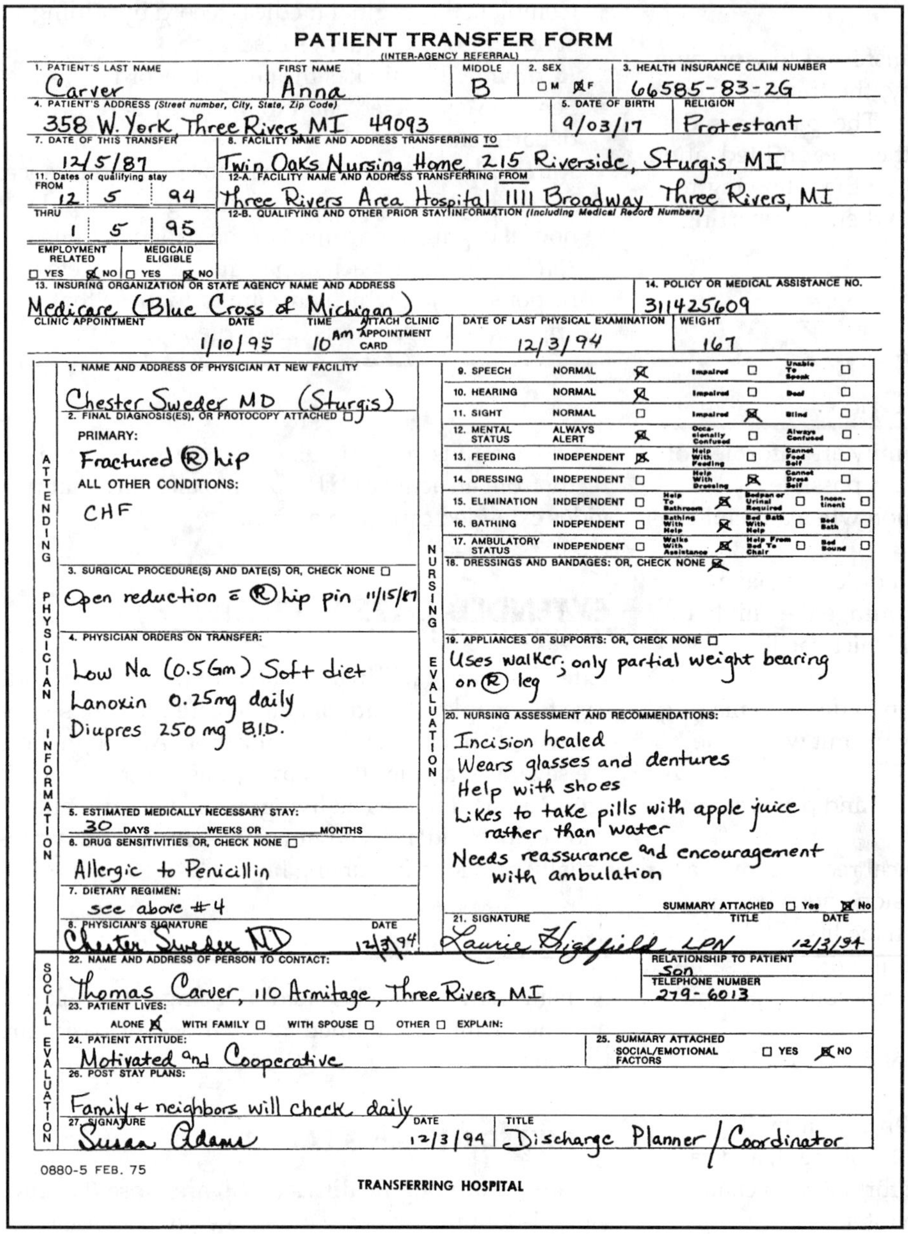

PATIENT TRANSFER FORM
(INTER-AGENCY REFERRAL)

1. PATIENT'S LAST NAME: Carver
FIRST NAME: Anna
MIDDLE: B
2. SEX: ☒ F
3. HEALTH INSURANCE CLAIM NUMBER: 66585-83-2G

4. PATIENT'S ADDRESS (Street number, City, State, Zip Code): 358 W. York Three Rivers MI 49093
5. DATE OF BIRTH: 9/03/17
RELIGION: Protestant

7. DATE OF THIS TRANSFER: 12/5/87
7. FACILITY NAME AND ADDRESS TRANSFERRING TO: Twin Oaks Nursing Home 215 Riverside, Sturgis, MI

11. Dates of qualifying stay FROM: 12 5 94
12-A. FACILITY NAME AND ADDRESS TRANSFERRING FROM: Three Rivers Area Hospital 1111 Broadway Three Rivers, MI
THRU: 1 5 95
12-B. QUALIFYING AND OTHER PRIOR STAY INFORMATION (Including Medical Record Numbers):

EMPLOYMENT RELATED: ☐ YES ☒ NO
MEDICAID ELIGIBLE: ☐ YES ☐ NO

13. INSURING ORGANIZATION OR STATE AGENCY NAME AND ADDRESS: Medicare (Blue Cross of Michigan)
14. POLICY OR MEDICAL ASSISTANCE NO.: 311425609

CLINIC APPOINTMENT DATE: 1/10/95   TIME: 10 Am   ATTACH CLINIC APPOINTMENT CARD
DATE OF LAST PHYSICAL EXAMINATION: 12/3/94   WEIGHT: 167

ATTENDING PHYSICIAN INFORMATION

1. NAME AND ADDRESS OF PHYSICIAN AT NEW FACILITY: Chester Sweder MD (Sturgis)

2. FINAL DIAGNOSIS(ES), OR PROTOCOPY ATTACHED ☐
PRIMARY: Fractured ℞ hip
ALL OTHER CONDITIONS: CHF

3. SURGICAL PROCEDURE(S) AND DATE(S) OR, CHECK NONE ☐: Open reduction c ℞ hip pin 11/15/87

4. PHYSICIAN ORDERS ON TRANSFER:
Low Na (0.5Gm) Soft diet
Lanoxin 0.25mg daily
Diupres 250 mg B.I.D.

5. ESTIMATED MEDICALLY NECESSARY STAY: 30 DAYS ___ WEEKS OR ___ MONTHS

6. DRUG SENSITIVITIES OR, CHECK NONE ☐: Allergic to Penicillin

7. DIETARY REGIMEN: see above #4

8. PHYSICIAN'S SIGNATURE: Chester Sweder MD   DATE: 12/3/94

NURSING EVALUATION

9. SPEECH   NORMAL ☒   Impaired ☐   Unable To Speak ☐
10. HEARING   NORMAL ☒   Impaired ☐   Deaf ☐
11. SIGHT   NORMAL ☐   Impaired ☒   Blind ☐
12. MENTAL STATUS   ALWAYS ALERT ☒   Occasionally Confused ☐   Always Confused ☐
13. FEEDING   INDEPENDENT ☒   Help With Feeding ☐   Cannot Feed Self ☐
14. DRESSING   INDEPENDENT ☐   Help With Dressing ☒   Cannot Dress Self ☐
15. ELIMINATION   INDEPENDENT ☒   Help To Bathroom ☐   Bedpan or Urinal Required ☐   Incontinent ☐
16. BATHING   INDEPENDENT ☐   Bathing With Help ☒   Bed Bath With Help ☐   Bed Bath ☐
17. AMBULATORY STATUS   INDEPENDENT ☐   Walks With Assistance ☒   Help From Bed To Chair ☐   Bed Bound ☐
18. DRESSINGS AND BANDAGES: OR, CHECK NONE ☒

19. APPLIANCES OR SUPPORTS: OR, CHECK NONE ☐
Uses walker; only partial weight bearing on ℞ leg

20. NURSING ASSESSMENT AND RECOMMENDATIONS:
Incision healed
Wears glasses and dentures
Help with shoes
Likes to take pills with apple juice rather than water
Needs reassurance and encouragement with ambulation

SUMMARY ATTACHED ☐ Yes ☒ No

21. SIGNATURE: Laurie Highfield   TITLE: LPN   DATE: 12/3/94

SOCIAL EVALUATION

22. NAME AND ADDRESS OF PERSON TO CONTACT: Thomas Carver, 110 Armitage, Three Rivers, MI
RELATIONSHIP TO PATIENT: Son
TELEPHONE NUMBER: 279-6013

23. PATIENT LIVES:
ALONE ☒   WITH FAMILY ☐   WITH SPOUSE ☐   OTHER ☐   EXPLAIN:

24. PATIENT ATTITUDE: Motivated and Cooperative
25. SUMMARY ATTACHED SOCIAL/EMOTIONAL FACTORS ☐ YES ☒ NO

26. POST STAY PLANS: Family + neighbors will check daily

27. SIGNATURE: Susan Adams   DATE: 12/3/94   TITLE: Discharge Planner / Coordinator

0880-5 FEB. 75   TRANSFERRING HOSPITAL

FIGURE 10-5
A transfer form provides information that promotes continuity of care.

dental services. Many of the latter services are provided by qualified personnel on a contractual basis rather than through full-time employment at the agency.

Those who are enrolled in Medicare are entitled to 20 days of full coverage and 80 days of partial coverage per year for skilled care. Some older adults have private insurance policies that assist with

TABLE 10-2. *Discharge Outcomes of Hospitalized Older Adults*

Age Range (years)	Discharged Home	Referred to Home Care Programs	Transferred to Nursing Homes	Discharged to Rehabilitation Facilities
65–74	85.7%	6.7%	3.9%	1.1%
75 and older	69.2%	12.3%	15.9%	1.5%

Source: Densen PM. Tracing the Elderly Through the Health Care System: An Update. Rockville, MD: Agency for Health Care Policy and Research, U.S. Department of Health and Human Services, January 1991.

Medicare copayments. If that is not the case, or if patients continue to require skilled care beyond 100 days, they must bear the cost personally until they are considered indigent. Once patients have exhausted their own financial resources and those of their spouse, they may apply to their respective state for Medicaid or its equivalent.

INTERMEDIATE CARE FACILITIES

Intermediate care facilities (ICF) provide health-related care and services to people who because of their mental or physical condition require institutional care, but not 24-hour nursing care. Patients who require intermediate care may need supervision because they tend to wander or are confused. For this reason they need assistance with medications, bathing, dressing, toileting, and mobility.

Medicare does not provide reimbursement for intermediate care. The costs must be assumed personally or through state welfare programs, like Medicaid, for impoverished residents. To make matters even worse, some nursing homes do not accept Medicaid patients because the fees for reimbursement are fixed by the state at much lower dollar amounts than Medicare and private insurance provides.

BASIC CARE FACILITIES

Basic care facilities (BCF) provide custodial care. The emphasis is on providing shelter, food, and laundry services in a group setting. Basic care patients may assume much of the responsibility for their own activities of daily living, such as hygiene and dressing,

preparing for sleep, joining others at meal time, and so on. Intermediate and basic care may be provided within a skilled nursing facility, but patients are segregated in separate wings for appropriate management of their care.

DETERMINING THE LEVEL OF CARE

The level of care is determined at the time of the patient's admission to a nursing home. Each patient is assessed using a standardized form developed by the Health Care Financing Association called a **Minimum Data Set** (MDS) for Nursing Home Resident Assessment and Care Screening. By federal law, the MDS is repeated at 3-month intervals or whenever a patient's condition changes. The MDS requires assessment of:

- Cognitive patterns
- Communication/hearing patterns
- Vision patterns
- Physical functioning and structural problems
- Continence patterns in the last 14 days
- Psychosocial well-being
- Mood and behavior patterns
- Activity pursuit patterns
- Disease diagnoses
- Health conditions
- Oral/nutritional status
- Oral/dental status
- Skin condition
- Medication use
- Special treatment and procedures

Problems that are identified on the MDS are then reflected in the nursing plan for care.

 PATIENT TEACHING FOR SELECTING A NURSING HOME

Teach the patient or family to do the following:

- Find out the levels of care (skilled, intermediate, or basic) for which the nursing home is licensed to provide.
- Review inspection reports on the nursing homes that are being considered; this information is available on a fee-per-page basis from the state's Department of Public Health.
- Ask others in the community, including the family physician, for recommendations.
- Visit nursing homes with, and again without, a prior appointment; go at least once during a mealtime.
- Note the appearance of current residents and the manner in which staff respond to their needs.
- Observe the cleanliness of the surroundings and presence of unpleasant odors.
- Request brochures that identify medical care, nursing services, rehabilitation therapy, social services, activities programs, religious observances, rights, and privileges.
- Clarify charges and billing procedures.
- Analyze if your overall impression of the agency is positive or negative.

TABLE 10-3. *Common Community Services*

Organization	Service
Commission on Aging	Assists older adults with transportation to medical appointments, outpatient therapy, and community meal sites
Hospice	Supports the family and terminally ill patients who choose to stay at home
Visiting Nurses' Association	Offers intermittent nursing care to home-bound patients
Meals on Wheels	Provides one or two hot meals per day, delivered either at home or at a community meal site
Homemaker Services	Sends adults to the home to assist in shopping, meal preparation, and light housekeeping
Home-Health Aid	Assists with bathing, hygiene, and medications
Adult Protective Services	Makes social, legal, and accounting services available to incompetent adults who may be victimized by others
Respite Care	Provides short-term, temporary relief to full-time caregivers of homebound patients
Older Americans' Ombudsman	Investigates and resolves complaints made by, or on behalf of, nursing home residents; at least one full-time ombudsman is mandated for each state

SELECTING A NURSING HOME

Unfortunately, when the need arises, family members are often ill prepared for selecting a nursing home. Various brochures on choosing a nursing home are available from the American Association of Retired Persons (AARP), the Commission on Aging, or the state's public health and welfare departments. The nurse also may offer the patient teaching guidelines that follow.

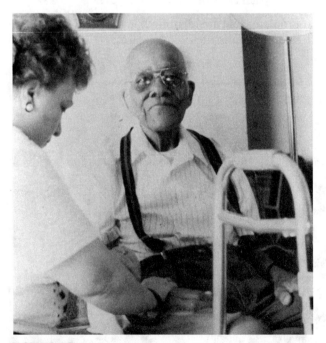

FIGURE 10-6
Home health care assessment. (Courtesy of the Visiting Nurse Association of Southwest Michigan.)

REFERRING PATIENTS

A **referral** is the process of sending someone to another person or agency for special services. In general, referrals are offered to patients who are being discharged to their homes. Referrals may be made to private practitioners or particular agencies. Table 10-3 lists some common community services to which people with declining health, physical disabilities, or special needs, may be referred.

Thinking about a referral is a part of good discharge planning. Because planning, coordinating, and communicating take time, referrals are initiated as soon as possible once the need is identified. Early planning helps ensure that **continuity of care** is maintained. This term means that the patient's care remains uninterrupted despite the change in caregivers, thus avoiding any loss in the progress that has already been made.

Home Health Care

Home health care refers to the care provided in the home by an employee of a home health agency (Fig. 10-6). Home health agencies may be public, that is, administered through a regional, state, or federal agency such as the public health department, or privately administered.

Between 1981 and 1987, there was a 98% increase in the number of home health agencies (Kent & Hanley, 1990), and the numbers continue to rise. The growth in home care is in part an outcome of the limitations imposed by Medicare and insurance companies on the number of hospital and nursing home days for which

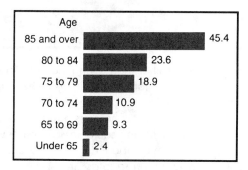

FIGURE 10-7

Percentage of people needing assistance with everyday activities by age. (U.S. Bureau of the Census. The Need for Personal Assistance With Everyday Activities: Recipients and Caregivers. Table B. Current Population Reports, Series P-70, No. 19. Washington, DC: U.S. Government Printing Office, 1990.

care is reimbursed. Another factor is the growing number of older adults in the population who are chronically ill and in need of assistance (Fig. 10-7).

Home care nursing services help shorten the time spent recovering in the hospital as well as prevent admissions to acute care and long-term care facilities. Display 10-2 identifies the responsibilities assumed by home health nurses who provide community-based care.

DISPLAY 10-2. *Responsibilities of Home Health Nurses*

Home health nurses do the following:
- Assess the readiness of the patient and home environment
- Treat each patient with respect regardless of the person's standard of living
- Identify health or social problems that require nursing, allied health, or supportive care services
- Plan, coordinate, and monitor home care
- Give skilled care to patients requiring part-time nursing services
- Teach and supervise the patient in self-care activities and family members who participate in the patient's home care
- Assess the safety of health practices that are being used
- Observe, evaluate, and modify environmental and social factors that affect the patient's progress
- Evaluate the urgency and complexity of each patient's changing health needs
- Keep accurate written records and submit documentation to the agency for the purpose of reimbursement
- Arrange for referrals to other health care agencies
- Discharge patients who have reached a level of self-reliance

---

 FOCUS ON OLDER ADULTS

- Older adults may minimize their symptoms to avoid admission to a hospital or nursing home.
- Many older adults find dependence on others difficult to accept, even though they may recognize the need for it.
- There is a definite correlation between increasing age and increased disease, disability, and length of hospital stays (United States Bureau of the Census 1992).
- Older adults occupy more than 50% of the available adult hospital beds and use more than 70% of the available health care services, including institutional, home care, and ambulatory care services (Miller, 1990).
- When admitting, discharging, or transferring older adults, it is best to allow additional time because of compromises in their mobility, attention, and concentration.

- Single and widowed older adults may be very concerned on admission about the welfare of their pets, whose care has been entrusted to someone else.
- Although hospitalizations tend to be a few days longer for older clients, early discharge planning and appropriate use of community resources can return many older adults back to their own homes (see Table 10-2).
- Since the advent of diagnosis-related groups (DRGs), a method for controlling Medicare expenses by limiting hospital reimbursement according to a predetermined number of days per medical diagnosis, older adults tend to be discharged earlier and sicker. This factor alone has increased the need for extended care within the home and community.

(continued)

FOCUS ON OLDER ADULTS (*Continued*)

- To obtain Medicare reimbursement for home care, older adults must be homebound (eg, requiring significant effort to leave the home). For those older adults who meet this qualification, Medicare will pay for 9 weeks of nursing care without recertification (Reeves, 1993).
- Many older adults are extremely distressed by having to use their life savings, and in some cases impoverish a healthy spouse, to finance care in their final years.
- Adults older than 85 years of age are 18 times more likely to require nursing home care than those who are 65 to 74 years old (Carnevali & Patrick, 1993).
- It is best to advise family members to be honest about taking an older adult to a nursing home

- for admission rather than giving the older adult a dishonest explanation to gain his or her temporary cooperation.
- Admission to a nursing home is a major stressor for older adults; the social losses and new environment may compound physical changes, a phenomenon referred to as "transfer trauma."
- More than 1,000,000 nurses will be needed by the year 2000 to manage adequately the care of older adults requiring care in nursing homes (Carnevali & Patrick, 1993).
- About 42% of people admitted to a nursing home reenter an acute care hospital at least once in a year (Densen, 1991).

KEY CONCEPTS

- The process of admission involves obtaining authorization from a physician, obtaining billing information, completing nursing admission responsibilities like orienting the patient and obtaining a data base assessment, and fulfilling medical responsibilities like documenting the patient's history and results of a physical examination.
- Some common patient reactions to being admitted to a health care agency are anxiety, loneliness, a sense of decreased privacy, and loss of identity.
- The discharge process consists of obtaining a written medical order for discharge, completing discharge instructions, notifying the business office, helping the patient leave the health agency, writing a summary of the discharge in the medical record, and requesting that the room be cleaned.
- A transfer involves discharging a patient from one unit or agency and admitting him or her to another without going home in the interim. A referral involves sending someone who will be discharged home to another person or agency for special services.
- Nursing homes may provide skilled, intermediate, or basic care.
- To determine the level of care that a nursing home patient requires, federal law requires that licensed, long-term care facilities complete a Minimum Data Set assessment form on admission, every 3 months thereafter, or whenever the patient's condition changes.
- In addition to nursing home care, the demand for home health care services has increased due to the impact of diagnosis-related groups (DRGs) and the growing number of older adults in the population who are in need of health care assistance.

CRITICAL THINKING EXERCISES

- Discuss how the admission of a child might be different from that of an adult.
- Describe the similarities and differences between an admission to a hospital and one involving a nursing home.
- Besides being ready for a new patient and greeting the patient warmly, what other factors might help to make a good first impression on patients?

SUGGESTED READINGS

Carnevali DL, Patrick M. Nursing Management for the Elderly. 3rd ed. Philadelphia: JB Lippincott, 1993.

Carr P. Home care: beyond the hospital walls. American Journal of Nursing August 1993;93:14.

Densen PM. Tracing the Elderly Through the Health Care System: An Update. Rockville, MD: Agency for Health Care Policy and Research, U.S. Department of Health and Human Services, 1991.

Eliopoulos C. Gerontological Nursing. 3rd ed. Philadelphia: JB Lippincott, 1993.

Kent V, Hanley B. Home health care. Nursing and Health Care November 1990;11:234.

Matteson MA, McConnell ES. Gerontological Nursing: Concepts and Practice. Philadelphia: WB Saunders, 1988.

Miller CA. Nursing Care of Older Adults: Theory and Practice. Glenview, IL: Scott, Foresman and Company, 1990.

Reeves K. Bottom-line issues in home care. American Journal of Nursing November 1993;93:19.

Rice R. Home Health Nursing Practice: Concepts and Application. St. Louis: Mosby, 1992.

United States Bureau of the Census. Sixty-Five Plus in America. Washington, DC: U.S. Government Printing Office, 1992.

CHAPTER 11
Vital Signs

Learning Objectives

An understanding of the content within this chapter will be evidenced by the student's ability to:

*   List four physiologic components that are measured when assessing vital signs
*   Differentiate between shell and core body temperature
*   Identify two scales that are used to measure temperature and demonstrate how to convert each to an equivalent measurement

- List four temperature assessment sites and indicate the site that is considered the closest to core temperature
- Name three types of clinical thermometers
- Discuss the difference between a fever and hyperthermia
- Name the four phases of a fever
- List at least four signs or symptoms that accompany a fever
- Give two reasons for using a tympanic thermometer for measuring subnormal body temperature
- List at least four signs and symptoms that accompany a subnormal body temperature
- Identify three characteristics that are noted when assessing a patient's pulse
- Name the most commonly used site for pulse assessment and three alternative assessment techniques that may be used
- Explain the difference between respiration and ventilation
- Name and explain at least four terms used to describe abnormal breathing characteristics
- Discuss the physiologic data that can be inferred from a blood pressure assessment
- Explain the difference between systolic and diastolic blood pressure
- Name three pieces of equipment that are used for assessing blood pressure
- List the five phases of Korotkoff sounds and explain how each is characterized
- Identify two alternative techniques for assessing blood pressure besides listening to Korotkoff sounds
- Name three alternatives to an aneroid or mercury manometer that may be used to assess blood pressure

Body temperature, pulse rate, respiratory rate (TPR), and blood pressure (BP) are referred to as **vital signs**. Vital signs are objective data that indicate how well or poorly the body is functioning.

Because the body mechanisms that regulate vital signs are very sensitive to alterations in physiology, vital signs are measured at periodic intervals to monitor a patient's health status (Display 11-1). This chapter describes how to assess each specific component of vital signs and provides explanations for what the measurements may indicate.

BODY TEMPERATURE

"Body temperature," as used here, refers to the warmth of the human body. The body's **shell temperature**, or warmth at the skin surface, is usually lower than its

---

DISPLAY 11-1. *Recommendations for Measuring Vital Signs*

Vital signs may be taken:
- On admission when obtaining data base assessments
- According to written medical orders
- Once per day when patient is stable
- At least every 4 hours when one or more vital signs is abnormal
- Every 5 to 15 minutes when a patient is unstable or at risk for rapid physiologic changes, like after surgery
- Whenever a patient's condition appears to have changed
- A second time, or at more frequent intervals, when there is a significant difference from the previous measurement
- When a patient reports feeling unusual
- Before and after a blood transfusion
- Before administering medications that may affect any one of the vital signs, and afterward to monitor the drug's effect

---

core temperature, that near the center of the body, where vital organs are located. Therefore, core temperature is much more significant than shell temperature.

In healthy adults, shell temperature generally ranges between 96.6° to 99.3° Fahrenheit (F) or 35.8° to 37.4° centigrade (C) (Porth, 1994), whereas core body temperature has a narrower range, between 98°F to 99.5°F or 36.6°C to 37.5°C (Smeltzer & Bare, 1992). In recent research, Mackowiak and colleagues (1992) found that the mean oral temperature is 98.2°F (36.7°C), thus disputing the belief that 98.6°F (37°C), a long-held standard, is the norm. Both the Fahrenheit and centigrade temperature scales are explained later.

Body heat is produced primarily by exercise and by the body's metabolism of food. Heat is lost from the skin, the lungs, and the body's waste products through the processes of **radiation, conduction, convection**, and **evaporation** (Table 11-1).

Temperature Regulation

In healthy people, the hypothalamus, a structure within the brain, is the center for temperature regulation. When functioning properly, the hypothalamus maintains the core temperature **set point**, or optimum body temperature, within plus or minus 1°C by responding to ever-so-slight changes in skin surface and blood temperatures (Fig. 11-1).

TABLE 11-1. Mechanisms of Heat Exchange

Method	Description	Example
Radiation	Transfer of heat into the air space of the environment	Body heat warms the air within a sleeping bag
Conduction	Transfer of heat through contact with a solid substance	Heat from the hands warms an iced drink
Convection	Transfer of heat by moving it through air, gas, or liquid currents	Warmed air escapes during exhalation from the lungs
Evaporation	Transfer of heat by changing fluid to a vapor (moisture-filled air)	Warm body fluid in the form of perspiration leaves the skin as a vapor

Temperatures beyond 105.8°F (41°C) or 93.2°F (34°C) indicate that the hypothalamic regulatory center is impaired. According to Porth (1994), the upper limits of survival tend to diminish when body temperatures exceed 110°F (43.3°C) or fall below 84°F (28.8°C).

Factors Affecting Body Temperature

Several factors affect body temperature. They include:

Age. Infants and older adults have more difficulty in maintaining normal body temperature. Both have limited body fat, which would otherwise provide insulation and prevent heat loss. Their ability to shiver and perspire may also be inadequate, putting them at risk for abnormally low or high body temperatures.

There are additional thermoregulatory risk factors that are unique to the very young and old. Newborns and young infants tend to experience temperature fluctuations because they have a

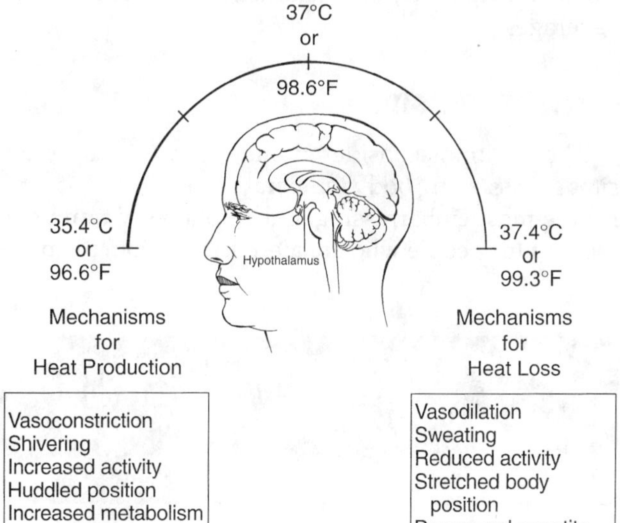

FIGURE 11-1
The hypothalamus is responsible for regulating body temperature.

metabolic rate (use of calories for sustaining body functions) twice that of adults. Older adults may be further compromised by impaired circulation, which interferes with losing or retaining heat through the dilation or constriction of blood vessels near the skin.

Gender. Women of reproductive age demonstrate a slight rise in body temperature when ovulating. This is most probably the result of hormonal changes affecting metabolism or tissue injury and repair after an ovum (egg) is released. The change in body temperature is so minor that most women are unaware of it unless they are monitoring their temperature on a daily basis.

Exercise and activity. Both exercise and activity involve muscle contraction, which produces body heat. To provide energy, the metabolic rate is also increased; this leads to the combustion of calories. The combination of the two increases heat production, which may raise body temperature if compensatory cooling mechanisms are inadequate or impaired.

Circadian rhythm. Circadian rhythms are physiologic changes, like fluctuations in body temperature and other vital signs, that cycle at 24-hour intervals. It has been demonstrated that body temperature fluctuates between 0.5°F to 2.0°F (0.28°C–1.1°C) during a 24-hour period. Body temperature tends to be lowest from midnight to dawn and highest in the late afternoon to early evening. People who routinely work at night and sleep during the day have temperature fluctuations that cycle in reverse.

Emotions. Emotions may affect metabolic rate by affecting hormonal changes through the sympathetic and parasympathetic pathways of the autonomic nervous system (see Chap. 5). People who tend to be consistently high-strung and emotional are likely to have higher-than-average body temperatures. Conversely, people who are apathetic and depressed are likely to have body temperatures in the lower ranges of normal.

Illness or Injury. Diseases, disorders, or injuries that affect the function of the hypothalamus may alter body temperature, sometimes quite dramatically. Some examples include tissue injury, infections, injury to the skin, impaired circulation, and head injury.

Drugs. Some drugs affect body temperature by increasing or decreasing the body's metabolic rate and energy requirements. Drugs like aspirin and acetaminophen (Tylenol) directly lower body temperature by acting on the hypothalamus itself. However, in the absence of a fever, their use does not lower body temperature to subnormal levels.

Temperature Scales

Body temperature is measured either in degrees centigrade, abbreviated °C, or in degrees Fahrenheit, abbreviated °F. The centigrade scale is used more often in scientific research and in countries where the metric system is used.

CENTIGRADE MEASUREMENT

The **centigrade scale**, also known as Celsius for the man who devised it, measures temperature in a range between 0°C to 100°C. Zero degrees centigrade is the temperature at which water freezes; 100°C is the temperature at which water boils.

FAHRENHEIT MEASUREMENT

The **Fahrenheit scale**, another method for measuring temperatures, is graduated differently from the centigrade scale. When the Fahrenheit scale is used, the temperature at which water freezes is 32°F, and boiling is 212°F. However, there is no actual difference in the temperature at which water crystallizes or boils–only a difference in the scale used to measure it. Therefore, nurses, who are required to use both scales from time to time, must be able to convert between the two measurements (Display 11-2).

Assessment Sites

Body temperature is usually assessed at the mouth, rectum, axilla, or ear. These areas are anatomically close to superficial arteries containing warm blood, or they are enclosed areas where heat loss is minimal, or both.

Temperature measurements vary slightly depending on the assessment site that is used (Table 11-2). To facilitate the evaluation of trends in body temperature, it is a good rule to identify the assessment site as "O" for oral, "R" for rectal, and "AX" for axillary when documenting the measurements, and to take the temperature by the same route each time.

DISPLAY 11-2. *Temperature Conversion Formulas*

To convert Fahrenheit to centigrade, use the formula:

$$(°F - 32) \times 5/9 = °C$$

Example: Step 1: 98.6°F − 32 = 66.6
Step 2: 66.6 × 5/9 = 37°C

To convert centigrade to Fahrenheit, use the formula:

$$(°C \times 9/5) + 32 = °F$$

Example: Step 1: 15°C × 9/5 = 27
Step 2: 27 + 32 = 59°F

THE ORAL SITE

The oral site, or mouth, which generally measures 0.5°F below core temperature, is a convenient assessment site. The area under the tongue is in direct proximity to the sublingual artery. As long as a patient keeps his or her mouth closed, the temperature of the tissue remains fairly consistent.

Unfortunately, this route is contraindicated for patients who have had oral surgery, those who are uncooperative or very young, unconscious patients, those prone to seizures, mouth breathers, and patients who continue to talk during temperature assessment. Oral temperature assessment must be delayed for at least 30 minutes if the person has been chewing gum, recently smoked a cigarette, or consumed hot or cold food or beverages.

THE RECTAL SITE

The rectum is considered one of the most accurate sites for assessing body temperature. However, it is by far the most embarrassing and emotionally traumatic method for people who are alert. In addition, the pres-

---

TABLE 11-2. *Equivalent Mercury Thermometer Measurements According to Site*

Assessment Site	Fahrenheit	Centigrade
Oral	98.6°	37°
Rectal equivalent	99.6°	37.5°
Axillary equivalent	97.6°	36.4°

ence of stool within the rectum has been shown to affect the accuracy of rectal temperature assessment.

THE AXILLARY SITE

The axilla, or underarm, is an alternative site for assessing body temperature. Temperature measurements from this site are approximately 1°F lower than those obtained at the oral site, and reflect shell rather than core temperature. The axillary site has several advantages: it is readily accessible in most instances; it is a safe site to use; there is less potential for spreading microorganisms compared to the oral or rectal sites; and it is less disturbing psychologically than using the rectal site. However, this route requires the longest assessment time, and temperature assessment may be invalid if the patient has recently bathed the area or rubbed it dry with a towel.

THE EAR

Research indicates that the temperature of the tympanic membrane within the ear has the closest correlation to core temperature (Tourangeau et al., 1993). This conclusion is based on the fact that the warm blood passing through branches of the internal and external carotid arteries travels through the tympanic membrane en route to the hypothalamus. For this reason, temperature assessment at this site is considered more reliable than those obtained from oral or axillary sites.

But, in random samples, Ward and coworkers (1988) found an extremely close correlation between tympanic and rectal temperatures. Refer to the discussion on tympanic thermometers for factors that affect accurate temperature assessments at this site.

Thermometers

A **thermometer** is an instrument used to measure temperature. A **clinical thermometer** is used to measure body temperature. Nurses may use a glass mercury thermometer, electronic thermometer, or tympanic (ear) thermometer when caring for patients (Table 11-3). There are other types of thermometers, such as disposable thermometers, which may be used in home care or as an inexpensive substitute for more complex equipment. There are also continuous monitoring devices, which are used in critical care areas.

GLASS MERCURY THERMOMETERS

A glass mercury thermometer, which may be calibrated in either the centigrade or Fahrenheit scale, has two parts, the bulb and the stem (Fig. 11-2).

The bulb, the tip that is inserted, may be long and slender or more bluntly rounded. The long, slender bulb provides a larger surface for contact with tissues, and is therefore preferred for taking oral (mouth) temperatures. The more rounded bulb is less fragile, and more appropriately used for placement within the rectum.

TABLE 11-3. *Types of Clinical Thermometers*

Type	Advantages	Disadvantages
Glass	Inexpensive Small	Breakable Must be cleaned before being used by another patient Cannot be sterilized using heat Use is time consuming High risk for injury if broken during use Mercury, if not properly disposed, is an environmental pollutant.
Electronic	Faster than glass Accurate Does not require sterilization or disinfection.	Expensive Must be recharged Probe needs to be held by the patient or nurse Holding the probe with one hand and the unit in the other interferes with simultaneously taking the patient's pulse.
Tympanic	Fastest type of recording device Closest approximation of core temperature Least invasive Most sanitary Does not require sterilization or disinfection	Expensive Battery must be recharged Improper placement and probe size affect accuracy. Actual ear and core temperature ranges are slightly different from those measured from oral, rectal, and axillary sites.

CENTIGRADE

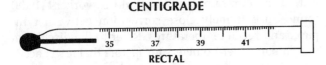

RECTAL

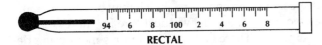

ORAL

FAHRENHEIT

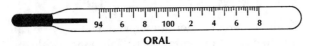

RECTAL

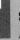

ORAL

FIGURE 11-2
Glass mercury thermometers.

The stem of a glass thermometer is a long tube that contains liquid mercury. When mercury is heated, it expands and moves upward through the space within the stem of the thermometer.

The stem of a glass thermometer is calibrated in whole and tenths of degrees. Body temperature is measured at the highest point to which the mercury rises in the stem. Temperatures that are less than a whole degree are recorded as decimals, such as 97.8°F. To assess body temperature using a glass mercury thermometer, follow the steps described in Skill 11-1.

Glass thermometers have largely been replaced by electronic devices in health agencies. However, almost every household has one thermometer which is usually glass. Because glass thermometers are not disposable, nurses must be prepared to teach the technique for cleaning them.

ELECTRONIC THERMOMETERS

An electronic thermometer consists of a temperature-sensitive probe, covered with a disposable sheath, which is attached to a display unit by a coiled, electronic wire. Although electronic thermometers are

(text continued on page 139)

SKILL 11-1
Assessing Body Temperature With a Mercury Thermometer

Suggested Action	Reason for Action
Oral Method	
Assessment	
Determine when and how frequently to monitor the patient's temperature (refer to Display 11-1).	Demonstrates accountability for making timely and appropriate assessments
Review the data collected in previously recorded temperature measurements.	Aids in identifying trends and analyzing significant patterns
Observe the patient's ability to support a thermometer within the mouth and breathe adequately through the nose with the mouth closed.	Shows consideration for accuracy
Read the patient's history for any reference to recent seizures or a seizure disorder.	Shows consideration for safety
Determine if the patient has been chewing gum, consumed any hot or cold substances, or has smoked within the past 30 minutes.	Shows consideration for accuracy
Planning	
Arrange the plan for care so as to take the patient's temperature as near to the scheduled routine as possible.	Ensures consistency and accuracy

(continued)

SKILL 11-1
Assessing Body Temperature With a Mercury Thermometer *(Continued)*

Suggested Action	Reason for Action
Gather supplies, which include a clean oral thermometer and a watch. Clean gloves are optional unless the patient is being cared for with specific communicable disease precautions (see Chap. 22) that require their use.*	Promotes efficiency, accuracy, and safety

Implementation

Suggested Action	Reason for Action
Introduce yourself to the patient if this has not been done during earlier contact.	Demonstrates responsibility and accountability
Explain the procedure to the patient.	Reduces apprehension and promotes cooperation
Wash your hands.	Reduces the spread of microorganisms
Grasp the thermometer at the stem and shake it with a snapping motion from the wrist until the mercury is well within the bulb.	Makes room for the mercury to expand and rise when exposed to heat
Place the bulb of the thermometer under the patient's tongue in the right or left posterior pocket.	Locates the bulb near the sublingual artery

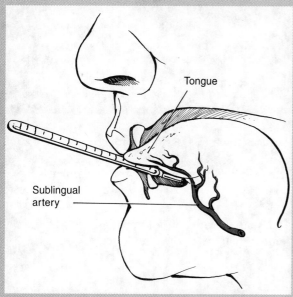

Assessing body temperature, using the oral method.

Suggested Action	Reason for Action
Leave the thermometer in place no less than 3 minutes if the patient is not feverish, or 5 minutes if the temperatures have been borderline or elevated above normal in previous measurements.	Ensures adequate time for the thermometer to reach the maximum measurement (Robinchaud-Ekstrand & Davies, 1989)

The use of gloves must be determined on an individual basis. The virus that causes AIDS has not been shown to be transmitted through contact with oral secretions unless they contain blood; thorough hand washing is always appropriate after any patient contact.

(continued)

SKILL 11-1
Assessing Body Temperature With a Mercury Thermometer (Continued)

Suggested Action	Reason for Action
Remove the thermometer and wipe it toward the bulb with a tissue, using a firm, twisting motion.	Removes mucus, making it easier to see the numeric markings
Read the thermometer by holding it horizontally at eye level and rotating it until the column of mercury can be seen.	Places the mercury and calibrations in a position at which they can be read most accurately

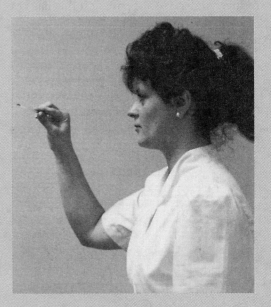

Reading the mercury thermometer. (Courtesy of Ken Timby.)

Follow agency policy for cleaning and disinfecting the thermometer; wash your hands.	Reduces the transmission of microorganisms
Record assessed measurement on the graphic sheet, flow sheet, or in the narrative nurses' notes.	Provides documentation for future comparisons
Verbally report elevated or subnormal temperatures.	Alerts others to monitor the patient closely and make changes in the plan for care

Evaluation
- Thermometer remained in place the appropriate length of time
- Level of temperature is consistent with accompanying signs and symptoms
- Thermometer and tissue remain intact

Document
- Date and time
- Degree of heat to the nearest tenth
- Temperature scale
- Site of assessment
- Accompanying signs and symptoms
- To whom abnormal information was reported and outcome of the communication

(continued)

SKILL 11-1
Assessing Body Temperature With a Mercury Thermometer *(Continued)*

Suggested Action	Reason for Action

Sample Documentation

Date and Time   T—100°F (O). States, "I feel cold." _____ **Signature, Title**

Rectal Method
Follow Assessment, Planning, Implementation, Evaluation, and Documentation Steps
as described for the oral method, with the following modifications:

Planning Gather rectal thermometer, lubricant, tissues, and clean gloves.	Promotes efficiency, accuracy, and safety
Implementation Provide privacy. Raise the height of the bed. Place the patient in a side-lying position. Wash your hands and don gloves. Spread at least 1 inch (2.5 cm) of lubricant at the bulb end of the thermometer. Instruct the patient to take deep breaths. Insert the thermometer approximately 1.5 inches (3.8 cm) in an adult, 1 inch (2.5 cm) in a child, and 0.5 (1.25 cm) in an infant.	Demonstrates respect for the patient's dignity Reduces musculoskeletal strain Facilitates access to the rectum Reduces the spread of microorganisms Reduces friction during insertion Relaxes the rectal sphincter and reduces discomfort during insertion Promotes appropriate placement according to anatomic dimensions

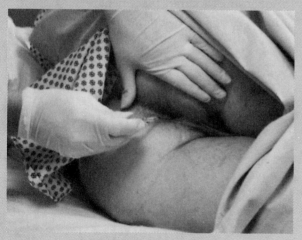

Assessing body temperature, using the rectal method.

Hold the thermometer in place for a minimum of 2 minutes or as specified by agency policy.	Allows sufficient time for accurate measurement and reduces the risk of injury
Remove the thermometer and place it on a paper tissue.	Confines microorganisms to a source that is easily disposed
Wipe lubricant and any stool from around the patient's rectum.	Demonstrates concern for the patient's comfort

(continued)

SKILL 11-1
Assessing Body Temperature With a Mercury Thermometer (Continued)

Suggested Action	Reason for Action
Wipe lubricant, mucus, and stool from the thermometer.	Facilitates examination of the calibrated marks
Read the thermometer, place it on a clean tissue, and remove gloves.	Ensures that the thermometer can be transported without actually touching it
Wash your hands.	Reduces the transmission of microorganisms
Restore the patient to a therapeutic position or one of comfort and lower the height of the bed.	Ensures comfort and safety
Enclose the thermometer within the tissue and transport it to the appropriate area for cleaning and disinfection.	Reduces the transmission of microorganisms
Document the recorded measurement and specify that it was obtained rectally.	Facilitates analysis and future comparisons

Axillary Method
Follow Assessment, Planning, Implementation, Evaluation, and Documentation Steps as described for the oral method, with the following modifications:

Planning

Follow agency policy as to whether an oral or rectal thermometer is used.	Ensures compliance with the agency's standards for care; oral thermometers provide maximum contact with skin folds, but they have a potential for injury if the elongated bulb is broken

Implementation

Provide privacy and arrange the patient's gown to expose the axilla.	Demonstrates concern for the patient's dignity and ensures accurate placement
Place the bulb of the thermometer well into the axilla and lower the patient's arm so as to enclose the thermometer between the two folds of skin.	Confines the tip of the thermometer within a warm body area

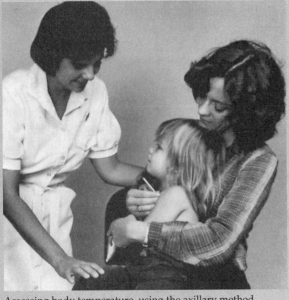

Assessing body temperature, using the axillary method.

(continued)

SKILL 11-1
Assessing Body Temperature With a Mercury Thermometer *(Continued)*

Suggested Action	Reason for Action
Hold the thermometer in place for at least 10 minutes.	Allows sufficient time to record an accurate temperature
Document the recorded measurement and specify that it was obtained in an axillary location	Facilitates analysis and future comparisons

portable, the unit is plugged into an electronic wall outlet to recharge the battery when it is not being used.

Electronic thermometers usually have two optional temperature probes that may be used for oral, axillary, or rectal use. Some offer both a centigrade or Fahrenheit measurement, which is accurately displayed in 60 seconds or less. However, because there is no established length of time for probe placement, the electronic unit senses when the temperature ceases to change and emits an audible beep. The signal alerts the nurse that the probe may be removed and the displayed numeric reading recorded.

The use of an electronic thermometer (Fig. 11-3) for assessing body temperature is described in Skill 11-2.

TYMPANIC THERMOMETERS

Tympanic thermometers are the newest type of electronic equipment for assessing body temperature. The device consists of a hand-held, covered probe that is inserted within the ear canal (Fig. 11-4). The probe contains an infrared sensor that detects radiated heat from the tympanic membrane (eardrum) and converts the warmth into a displayed temperature measurement in

2 to 5 seconds. The potential for transferring microorganisms from one patient to another is reduced because the probe is covered and because the ear does not contain mucoid secretions.

Despite its advantages, some researchers are finding that tympanic membrane thermometers may produce inaccurate measurements if the ear canal is not straightened appropriately, if the probe is too large for the ear canal (a problem with infants and small children), or if the sensor is directed at the ear canal rather than directly at the tympanic membrane (Tourangeau et al., 1993). Baird and colleagues (1992) also report that the first use of a tympanic thermometer after recharging is not always as accurate as a second reading. Another criticism of tympanic temperature measurement is that there is no standard for actual ear or core temperatures. Currently, tympanic thermometers use internally calculated **offsets**, or mathematical conversions for oral and rectal temperatures. However, the numeric offsets vary somewhat from manufacturer to manufacturer.

Refer to Skill 11-3 for a description of how to use a tympanic thermometer for assessing body temperature at this site.

PATIENT TEACHING FOR CLEANING GLASS THERMOMETERS

Teach the patient or the family to do the following:

- Don gloves if there is the potential for contact with blood or stool, as may be the case after rectal assessment.
- Hold the thermometer at the tip of the stem and keep the bulb lower than the stem.
- Wipe the soiled thermometer toward the bulb with a clean, soft tissue using a firm, twisting motion.

- Wash the thermometer with soap or detergent solution, again using friction.
- Rinse the thermometer under cold, running water.
- Dry the thermometer with a soft towel.
- Soak the thermometer in 70% to 90% isopropyl alcohol or 1:10 solution of household bleach (1 part bleach to 10 parts water).
- Rinse the thermometer after disinfecting it.
- Store the thermometer in a clean, dry container.

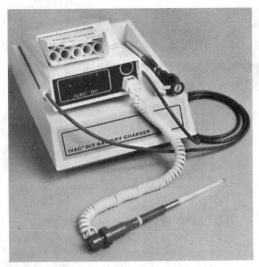

FIGURE 11-3
Electronic thermometer. (Photograph courtesy of the IVAC Corporation, San Diego, CA.)

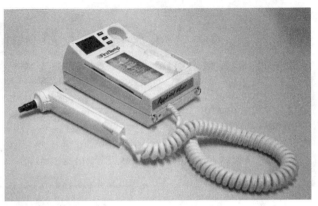

FIGURE 11-4
Tympanic thermometer. (Courtesy of Ken Timby.)

DISPOSABLE THERMOMETERS

There are various types of disposable thermometers. One example is a paper or plastic strip with chemically treated dots designed for a single use (Fig. 11-5). The temperature is determined by noting how many dots change color after the strip is held in the mouth.

Another type of disposable thermometer is made of a heat-sensitive tape or patch that is applied to the abdomen or forehead (Fig. 11-6). The tape or patch also changes color according to the body temperature. Heat-sensitive tapes and patches can be reused several times before being thrown away.

CONTINUOUS MONITORING DEVICES

Continuous temperature monitoring devices are used primarily in critical care areas. Body temperature by this method may be measured using probes inserted within the esophagus of anesthetized patients or by means of a thermistor attached to a pulmonary artery catheter. These measurements are required when caring for patients with extreme levels of hypothermia or hyperthermia. Warming or cooling blankets are usually used at the same time. The assessment aids in evaluating the effectiveness of these treatment devices.

Despite differences in assessment sites and thermometers, it is appropriate to report a patient's temperature that falls outside normal ranges, to continue to assess the temperature at frequent intervals, and implement nursing and medical interventions for restoring normal body temperature when they are appropriate.

Elevated Body Temperature

Body temperature is considered elevated when it exceeds 99.3°F (37.4°C). A **fever**, or state of **pyrexia**—a word derived from the Greek word for "fire," is a term used to describe a warmer-than-normal set point. A person with a fever is said to be **febrile**, as opposed to **afebrile**, which means without a fever.

(*text continues on page 144*)

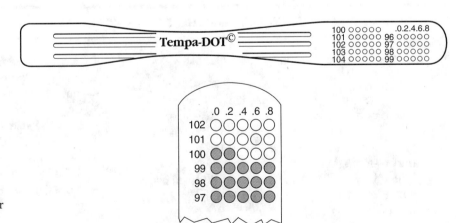

FIGURE 11-5
Chemically treated dots change color according to body temperature.

SKILL 11-2
Assessing Body Temperature With an Electronic Thermometer

Suggested Action	Reason for Action
Follow Assessment, Planning, Implementation, Evaluation, and Documentation Steps as described in Skill 11-1, with the following modifications:	

Planning

Gather the following equipment: electronic unit and disposable probe covers. Include lubricant paper tissues, and gloves if using the rectal site.	Ensures organization and efficient time management

Implementation

Remove the electronic unit from the charging base.	Promotes portability
Select the oral or rectal probe, depending on the intended site for assessment.	Ensures appropriate use
Insert the probe into a disposable cover until it locks into place.	Protects the probe from contamination with microorganisms

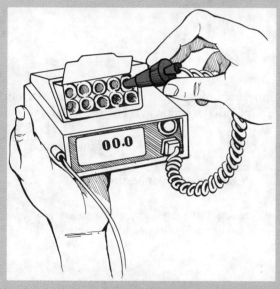

Inserting the probe into a disposable cover.

(continued)

Suggested Action	Reason for Action
Place the covered probe beneath the tongue or within the rectum, as described in Skill 11-1.	Follows established principles for accurate measurement

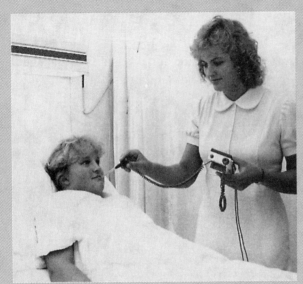

Maintaining the probe in position. (Courtesy of Ken Timby.)

Suggested Action	Reason for Action
Hold the probe in place.	Supports the probe so it does not drift away from its intended location and ensures valid data collection
Maintain the probe in position until an audible sound occurs.	Signals when the sensed temperature remains constant
Observe the numbers displayed on the electronic unit.	Indicates temperature measurement
Remove the probe and eject the probe cover into a lined receptacle.	Confines contaminated objects to an area for proper disposal without direct contact

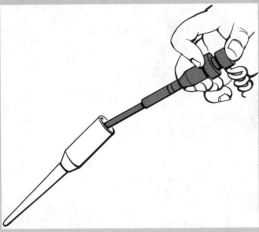

Releasing the probe cover.

Suggested Action	Reason for Action
Return the probe to its storage location within the electronic unit.	Prevents damage to the probe attachment
Return the electronic unit to its charging base.	Facilitates reuse

Suggested Action	Reason for Action
Follow Assessment, Planning, Implementation, Evaluation, and Documentation Steps as described in Skill 11-1, with the following modifications:	

Planning

Suggested Action	Reason for Action
Gather the following equipment: tympanic thermometer and disposable probe covers.	Ensures organization and efficient time management

Implementation

Suggested Action	Reason for Action
Explain the equipment and technique to the patient.	Informs patients who are unfamiliar with this new technology
Hold the probe in your dominant hand.	Improves motor skill and coordination
Rotate the head so as to access the same ear as the hand holding the probe.	Promotes proper probe placement; if the right hand is holding the probe, the right ear is assessed
Apply a disposable cover over the probe.	Reduces the transmission of microorganisms
Select the desired temperature mode. The rectal equivalent is recommended for children who are 3 years old or younger.	Programs the offset for converting the measured temperature
Wait for a "Ready" message to be displayed.	Indicates the offest has been programmed
Pull the external ear of adults up and back by grasping the external ear at its midpoint with your nondominant hand; for children 6 years old or younger, pull the ear down and back (see Chap. 12)	Straightens the ear canal
Insert the probe into the ear, advancing it with a gentle back-and-forth motion until it seals the ear canal.	Seats the tip of the probe within the ear canal and confines the radiated heat within the area of the probe
Point the tip of the probe in an imaginary line between the sideburn hair and the eyebrow on the opposite side of the face.	Positions the probe in alignment with the tympanic membrane

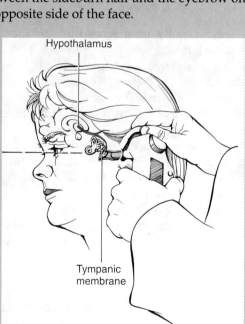

(continued)

SKILL 11-3
Assessing Body Temperature With a Tympanic Thermometer (Continued)

Suggested Action	Reason for Action
Press the button that activates the thermometer as soon as the probe is in position.	Initiates electronic sensing; for some models, this action must be done within 25 seconds of having removed the thermometer from its holding cradle
Keep the probe within the ear until the thermometer emits a sound or flashing light.	Indicates that the procedure is complete
Repeat the procedure if this is the first use of the tympanic thermometer since it was recharged.	Ensures accuracy with a second assessment
Read the temperature and release the probe cover into a lined receptacle.	Controls the transmission of microorganisms
Return the thermometer to its charging base.	Ensures that the thermometer is charged when needed again

Hyperthermia, on the other hand, is a state in which a person has an excessively high core temperature, usually exceeding 105.8°F (41°C). At this level, a person is at extremely high risk for brain damage or death from complications associated with increased metabolic demands.

The following are common signs and symptoms associated with a fever:

- Pinkish, red (flushed) skin that is warm to touch
- Restlessness or, in others, excessive sleepiness
- Irritability
- Poor appetite
- Glassy eyes and a sensitivity to light

- Increased perspiration
- Headache
- Above-normal pulse and respiratory rates
- Disorientation and confusion (when the temperature is high)
- Convulsions in infants and children (when the temperature is high)
- Fever blisters about the nose or lips in people who harbor the herpes simplex virus

PHASES OF A FEVER

A fever usually progresses through four distinct phases: (1) the *prodromal phase*, during which a person experiences nonspecific symptoms just before the temperature rises; (2) the *onset* or *invasion phase*, when mechanisms for increasing body temperature develop; (3) the *stationary phase*, during which the fever is sustained; and (4) the *resolution* or *defervescence phase*, when the temperature returns to normal (Fig. 11-7). If the fever suddenly drops to a normal temperature, it is referred to as a resolution by *crisis*; if it gradually descends, it is a resolution by *lysis*.

Fevers and the manner in which they subside may take a variety of courses. Common variations in fever patterns are described and illustrated in Table 11-4.

NURSING MANAGEMENT

A fever is considered an important body defense for destroying infectious microorganisms. Therefore, as long as the fever remains below 102°F (38.9°C) and the person does not have a chronic medical condition, providing fluids or rest may be all that is necessary.

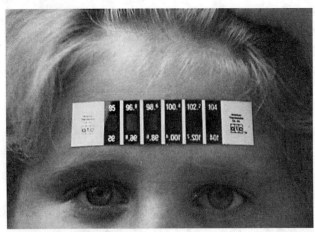

FIGURE 11-6
This type of disposable skin thermometer contains liquid crystals that change color according to body temperature. (Courtesy of Ken Timby.) (Taylor C, Lillis C, LeMone P: Fundamentals of Nursing: The Art and Science of Nursing Care, 2nd ed, p 392. Philadelphia, JB Lippincott, 1993)

Antipyretics, drugs that reduce fever, like aspirin or acetaminophen (Tylenol), may be helpful when the temperature climbs between 102°F and 104°F (38.9°C–40°C); physical cooling measures may be used for temperatures between 104°F and 105.8°F (40°C–40.6°C). If the temperature is higher than 105.8°F (40.6°C), or if a high temperature is unchanged after conventional interventions, more aggressive treatment may be warranted (Letizia & Janusek, 1994).

NURSING GUIDELINES FOR PATIENTS WITH A FEVER

- Cover patients during periods when shivering is evident.
  Rationale: Prevents heat loss and assists the hypothalamus in reaching a higher set point
- Keep patients in a warm, but not hot, environment.
  Rationale: Provides comfort while the body adapts to the new adjusted set point
- Remove blankets or heavy clothing once shivering subsides.
  Rationale: Facilitates heat loss from radiation and convection and maintains body temperature within the new set point
- Limit activity.
  Rationale: Reduces heat production
- Provide liberal amounts of oral fluids.
  Rationale: Replaces fluid lost because of perspiration and increased metabolism
- Provide light, but high-calorie nourishment.
  Rationale: Compensates for increased metabolic rate, delayed gastric emptying, and decreased intestinal motility (Letizia & Janusek, 1994)
- Administer fever-reducing drugs according to medical orders. (Note: aspirin is contraindicated for treating feverish children because its use has been associated with a complication called Reye's syndrome.)
  Rationale: Blocks the set point elevation in the hypothalamus
- Apply cool cloths or an ice bag to the forehead, behind the neck, and between the axillary and inguinal skin folds.
  Rationale: Cools blood that flows near the peripheral skin surface
- Promote room ventilation.
  Rationale: Increases heat loss through evaporation.
- Discontinue physical cooling measures if the patient begins to shiver
  Rationale: Reduces the potential for raising body temperature

- Apply an electronically regulated cooling pad beneath the patient as directed by a physician (see Chap. 28).
  Rationale: Increases heat loss through conduction

Subnormal Body Temperature

A core body temperature less than 95°F (35°C) is called **hypothermia**. A person is considered *mildly hypothermic* at temperatures between 95°F to 93.2°F (35°C–34°C); *moderately hypothermic* at temperatures of 93°F to 86°F (33.8°C–30°C); and *severely hypothermic* at temperatures below 86°F (30°C).

Cold body temperatures are best measured with a tympanic thermometer for two reasons. First, other clinical thermometers do not have the capacity to measure temperatures in hypothermic ranges. Second, the blood flow in the mouth, rectum, or axilla is usually so reduced that measurements taken from these sites are inaccurate.

The following are common signs and symptoms associated with hypothermia:

- Shivering until body temperature is extremely low
- Pale, cool skin
- Puffiness of the skin
- Impaired muscle coordination
- Listlessness
- Slow pulse and respiratory rates
- Irregular heart rhythm
- Decreased ability to think coherently and use good judgment
- Diminished ability to feel pain or other sensations.

There are some illnesses, like hypothyroidism and starvation, in which the patient typically has a subnormal temperature. Therefore, it is important to assess patients just as closely when the body temperature falls below normal ranges as when it is elevated.

Death usually occurs at severely hypothermic temperatures. However, cases of survival have been reported when body temperatures have fallen considerably low, as in cases of cold water drownings and exposure in extremely cold environments. This phenomenon has led to the saying among paramedics and emergency department personnel that "Patients aren't dead until they're warm and dead."

NURSING MANAGEMENT

There are various supportive measures that may be implemented when patients have subnormal body temperatures.

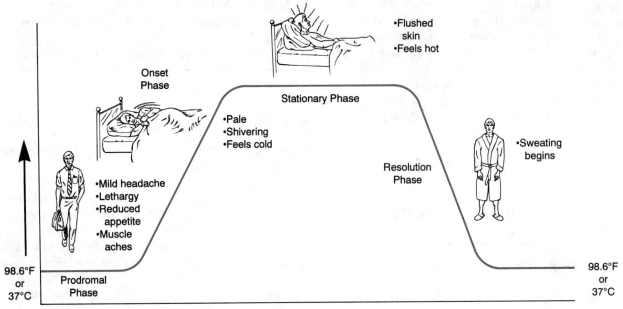

FIGURE 11-7
Curve showing the phases of a fever and common physiologic changes that occur at each phase.

NURSING GUIDELINES FOR PATIENTS WITH A SUBNORMAL TEMPERATURE

- Raise the environmental temperature in the room.
  Rationale: Warms the surface of the body
- Remove wet clothing.
  Rationale: Reduces heat loss
- Apply layers of dry clothing and loosely woven blankets.
  Rationale: Traps body heat next to the skin.
- Warm blankets and clothing in a warming oven or microwave if the body temperature is quite low.
  Rationale: Raises the temperature of woven fabrics above ambient (room) temperature
- Position the patient so that the arms are next to the chest and the legs are tucked toward the abdomen.
  Rationale: Prevents heat loss
- Cover the head with a cap or towel.
  Rationale: Reduces heat loss from exposed body areas
- Provide warm fluids.
  Rationale: Conducts heat to internal organs
- Massage the skin unless it is frostbitten.
  Rationale: Produces mechanical friction, which produces warmth
- Apply bags filled with warm water between areas of skin folds or place an electronic warming pad beneath the back and hips (see Chap. 28) according to medical orders.
  Rationale: Transfers heat to the blood as it circulates through the skin

PULSE

The **pulse** is a wave-like sensation that can be palpated in a peripheral artery. It is produced by the movement of blood during the heart's contraction. In most adults, the heart contracts 60 to 100 times a minute.

The **pulse rate** is the number of peripheral pulsations that are palpated in a minute. The pulse rate is counted by compressing a superficial artery against an underlying bone with the tips of the fingers.

Any factors that affect the rate of heart contraction also cause a comparable effect in the pulse rate. Because one depends on the other, the pulse rate can never be faster than the actual heart rate per minute.

Factors Affecting Heart and Pulse Rates

A variety of factors affect heart and pulse rates. Both may vary with:

Age. Some common rates are listed in Table 11-5.
Circadian rhythm. Rates tend to be lower in the morning and increase later in the day.
Gender. Men average approximately 60 to 65 beats per minute at rest, whereas the average rate for women is slightly faster, by about 7 to 8 beats per minute.
Body build. Tall, slender people usually have slower heart and pulse rates than short, stout people.
Exercise and activity. Rates increase with exercise and activity and decrease with rest. However, with regular aerobic exercise, a *training effect* can be ob-

TABLE 11-4. *Variations in Fever Patterns*

Type of Fever	Description	Illustration
Sustained fever	Remains elevated with very little fluctuation	
Remittent fever	Fluctuates several degrees, but never reaches normal between the fluctuations	
Intermittent fever	Cycles frequently between periods of normal or subnormal temperatures and spikes of fever	
Relapsing fever	Reoccurs after a brief but sustained period during which the temperature has been normal	

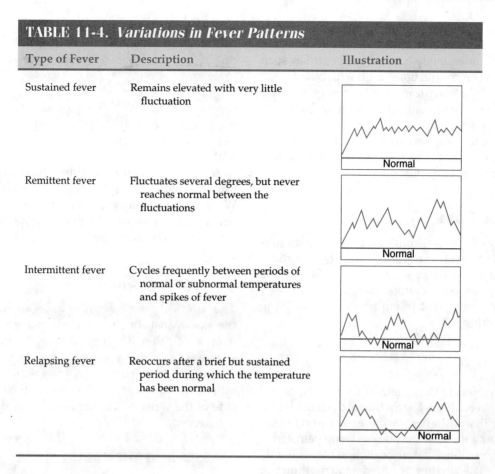

served. This means that the heart rate, and consequently the pulse rate, become consistently lower than average. The training effect occurs because the heart muscle becomes quite efficient at supplying body cells with a sufficient volume of oxygenated blood with fewer beats. Those who are physically fit exhibit slower pulse rates even during exercise.

Stress and emotions. Stimulation of the sympathetic nervous system and emotions like anger, fear, and excitement increase heart and pulse rates.

Pain, which is stressful—especially when it is moderate to severe—can trigger faster rates.

Body temperature. For every 1°F elevation, the heart and pulse rate increase 10 beats per minute; a similar increase in centigrade measurement causes a 15—beat-per-minute increase (Porth, 1994). With a fall in body temperature, an opposite effect occurs.

Blood volume. Excessive blood loss causes the heart and pulse rates to increase. When there are decreased red blood cells or inadequate hemoglobin to distribute oxygen to cells, the heart rate accelerates in an effort to keep cells adequately supplied.

Drugs. Certain drugs can slow or speed the rate of heart contraction. For example, digitalis preparations and sedatives typically slow the heart rate. Caffeine, nicotine, cocaine, thyroid replacement hormones, and epinephrine are some drugs that increase heart contractions and subsequently the pulse rate.

TABLE 11-5. *Normal Pulse Rates per Minute at Various Ages*

Age	Approximate Range	Approximate Average
Newborn	120–160	140
1–12 months	80–140	120
1–2 years	80–130	110
3–6 years	75–120	100
7–12 years	75–110	95
Adolescence	60–100	80
Adulthood	60–100	80

Rapid Pulse Rate

The pulse rate of adults is considered rapid if it exceeds 100 beats per minute at rest. **Tachycardia** is the term used to describe a fast heart rate. Heart and pulse rates can exceed 150 beats per minute. Rapid contraction, if sustained, tends to overwork the heart and may not oxygenate cells adequately because the heart has such little time between contractions to fill with blood.

The term **palpitation** means that the person is aware of his or her own heart contraction without having to feel the pulse. The pulse rate is usually rapid when palpitations are noted. Anyone with a rapid pulse rate is monitored closely and the results are reported and recorded according to agency policy.

Slow Pulse Rate

The pulse rate of adults is considered slower than normal if it falls below 60 beats per minute. **Bradycardia** is the term used to describe a slow heart rate. Slow pulse and heart rates are less common than rapid rates, but, when present, they merit prompt reporting and continued monitoring.

Pulse Rhythm

Pulse rhythm refers to the pattern of the pulsations and the pauses between them. The rhythm of the pulse is normally regular; that is, the beats and the pauses occur similarly throughout the time the pulse is being palpated.

An irregular pattern of heartbeats, and consequently an irregular pulse rhythm, is called an **arrhythmia** or **dysrhythmia**. Arrhythmias are reported promptly because some can indicate cardiac dysfunction that may warrant more sophisticated monitoring. Details about arrhythmias and their causes can be found in textbooks that discuss cardiac disorders.

Pulse Volume

Pulse volume refers to the quality of the pulsations that are felt. The volume of the pulse is usually related to the amount of blood pumped with each heart contraction.

A normal pulse is described as feeling *strong* when it can be felt with mild pressure over the artery. A *feeble, weak,* or *thready pulse* describes a pulse that is difficult to feel or, once felt, is easily obliterated with slight pressure. A patient with a thready pulse usually also has a rapid pulse. A rapid, thready pulse is a serious sign and is reported promptly. A *bounding* or *full pulse* produces a pronounced pulsation that does not easily disappear with pressure.

Another way to describe the volume or quality of the pulse is with corresponding numbers (Table 11-6). When documenting pulse volume, it is best to follow agency policy as to whether descriptive terms or a numbering system is used.

Assessment Sites

The arteries used for pulse assessment lie close to the skin. Most, but not all, are named for the bone over which they are located (Fig. 11-8). These pulse sites are collectively called *peripheral pulses* because they are distant from the heart. Of all the peripheral pulses, the radial artery, located on the inner (thumb) side of the wrist, is the site most often used for pulse assessment.

ASSESSING THE RADIAL PULSE

The actions described in Skill 11-4 may be used when assessing the rate, rhythm, and volume of the pulse at the radial artery.

Other Pulse Assessment Techniques

There are three alternative assessment techniques that may be used in lieu of, or in addition to, an assessment of a peripheral pulse. These techniques include counting the apical heart rate, obtaining an apical–radial rate, and using a Doppler ultrasound device.

TABLE 11-6. *Identifying Pulse Volume*

Number	Definition	Description
0	Absent pulse	No pulsation is felt despite extreme pressure.
1+	Thready pulse	Pulsation is not easily felt; slight pressure causes it to disappear.
2+	Weak pulse	Stronger than a thready pulse; light pressure causes it to disappear.
3+	Normal pulse	Pulsation is easily felt; moderate pressure causes it to disappear.
4+	Bounding pulse	The pulsation is strong and does not disappear with moderate pressure.

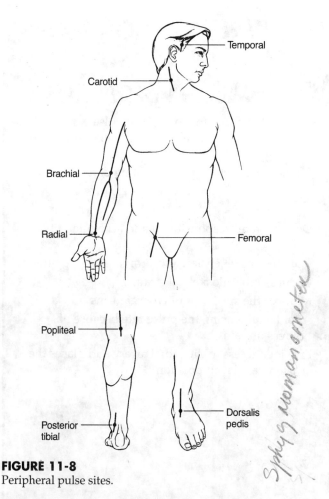

FIGURE 11-8
Peripheral pulse sites.

APICAL HEART RATE

The **apical heart rate** is the number of ventricular contractions that occur in a minute. The apical rate is considered more accurate than the radial pulse rate, but it is less convenient to obtain. It usually is assessed when a peripheral pulse is difficult or impossible to palpate, or if it is necessary to obtain an actual heart rate.

The apical heart rate is counted by listening at the chest with a stethoscope or by feeling the pulsations in the chest at an area called the *point of maximum impulse*. As the name suggests, the heartbeats are best heard, or felt, at the apex, or lower tip, of the heart. The apex in a healthy adult is slightly below the left nipple in line with the middle of the clavicle (Fig. 11-9).

When assessing the apical heart rate by listening—which is the more common technique—the nurse listens for the "lub/dub" sound. The "lub" sound is louder if the stethoscope has been correctly applied. These two sounds equal one pulsation at a peripheral pulse site. The apical heart rate is counted for 1 minute. The rhythm is also noted.

APICAL–RADIAL RATE

The **apical–radial rate** is the number of sounds heard at the heart's apex and the rate of the radial pulse during the same period of time. Each is counted by separate nurses using one watch or clock (Fig. 11-10).

(*text continues on page 152*)

SKILL 11-4
Assessing the Radial Pulse

Suggested Action	Reason for Action
Assessment	
Determine when and how frequently to monitor the patient's pulse (refer to Display 11-1).	Demonstrates accountability for making timely and appropriate assessments
Review the data collected in previously recorded assessments.	Aids in identifying trends and analyzing significant patterns
Read the patient's history for any reference to cardiac or vascular disorders.	Demonstrates an understanding of factors that may affect the pulse rate
Review the list of prescribed drugs for any that may have cardiac effects.	Helps in analyzing the results of assessment findings
Planning	
Arrange the plan for care so as to take the patient's pulse as near to the scheduled routine as possible.	Ensures consistency and accuracy
Make sure a watch or wall clock with a second hand is available.	Ensures accurate timing when counting pulsations

SKILL 11-4
Assessing the Radial Pulse (Continued)

Suggested Action	Reason for Action
Plan to assess the patient's pulse after a 5-minute period of inactivity.	Reflects the characteristics of the pulse at rest rather than data that may be influenced by activity.
Plan to use the right or left radial pulse site, unless it is inaccessible or difficult to palpate.	Provides consistency in evaluating data

Implementation

Introduce yourself to the patient if this has not been done during earlier contact.	Demonstrates responsibility and accountability
Explain the procedure to the patient.	Reduces apprehension and promotes cooperation
Raise the height of the bed.	Reduces musculoskeletal strain
Wash your hands.	Reduces the spread of microorganisms
Help the patient to a position of comfort.	Avoids influencing the pulse rate because of stress or pain
Rest or support the patient's forearm with the wrist extended.	Provides access to the radial artery and places the arm in a relaxed position

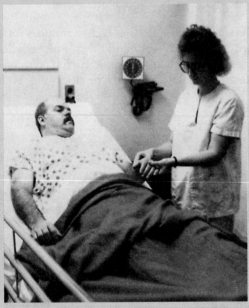

Supporting the patient's forearm.
(Courtesy of Ken Timby.)

Press the first, second, and third fingertips toward the radius while feeling for a recurrent pulsation.	Ensures accuracy because the nurse may feel his or her own pulse if the thumb is used; light palpation should not obliterate the pulse

(continued)

SKILL 11-4
Assessing the Radial Pulse

Suggested Action	Reason for Action
Palpate the rhythm and volume of the pulse once it is located.	Provides comprehensive assessment data

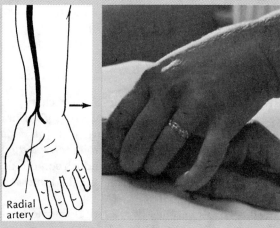

Locating the radial artery.

Suggested Action	Reason for Action
Note the position of the second hand on the clock or watch.	Identifies the point at which the assessment begins
Count the number of pulsations for 15 to 30 seconds and multiply the number by 4 or 2, respectively. If the pulse is irregular, count for a full minute.	Adjusts technique according to regularity or irregularity
Write down the pulse rate.	Ensures accurate documentation
Restore the patient to a therapeutic position or one that provides comfort, and lower the height of the bed.	Demonstrates responsibility for patient care, safety, and comfort
Record assessed measurement on the graphic sheet, flow sheet, or in the narrative nurses' notes.	Provides documentation for future comparisons
Verbally report rapid or slow pulse rates.	Alerts others to monitor the patient closely and make changes in the plan for care

Evaluation

- Pulse rate remained palpable throughout the period of assessment
- Pulse rate is consistent with the patient's condition

Document

- Date and time
- Assessment site
- Rate of pulsations per minute, pulse volume, and rhythm
- Accompanying signs and symptoms if appropriate
- To whom abnormal information was reported, and outcome of the interaction

Sample Documentation

Date and Time   Radial pulse 88 bpm, full, and regular. _____ **Signature, Title**

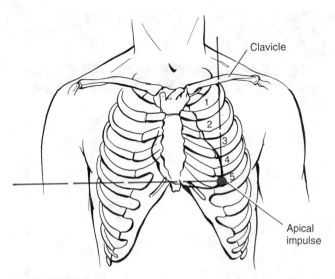

FIGURE 11-9
The apical heart rate is assessed to the left of the sternum at the interspace below the fifth rib in midline with the clavicle.

The apical and radial rate should be the same, but for some patients they are not. The difference between the apical and radial pulse rates is called the **pulse deficit**. If a significant difference is noted in the two rates—and the rates have been counted accurately—the findings are reported promptly and documented in the patient's medical record.

DOPPLER ULTRASOUND DEVICE

A Doppler ultrasound device is an electronic instrument that detects the movement of blood through peripheral blood vessels and converts the movement to an audible sound. This instrument is most helpful when slight pressure occludes pulsations or arterial blood flow is severely compromised.

When the device is used, conductive jelly is applied over the arterial site and the probe is moved at an angle over the skin until a pulsating sound is heard (Fig. 11-11). The pulsating sounds are counted to determine the rate. The documented findings include the assessment site and the rate, followed by the abbreviation "D" to indicate that it was obtained by using a Doppler device.

RESPIRATION

Respiration is a term that refers to the exchange of oxygen and carbon dioxide. The process of exchanging oxygen and carbon dioxide between the alveolar and capillary membranes is called *external respiration*. The process of exchanging oxygen and carbon dioxide between the blood and body cells is called *internal respiration* or *tissue respiration*.

Ventilation, on the other hand, is the movement of air in and out of the chest. *Inhalation*, or *inspiration*, is the act of breathing in; *exhalation*, or *expiration*, is the act of breathing out.

Ventilation is controlled by the medulla, which is the respiratory center in the brain. The medulla is sensitive to the amount of carbon dioxide in the blood and adapts the rate of ventilations accordingly. However, breathing can be voluntarily controlled to a certain extent.

Respiratory Rate

The **respiratory rate** is the number of ventilations that take place in 1 minute. Respiratory rates have been observed to vary considerably in healthy people. How-

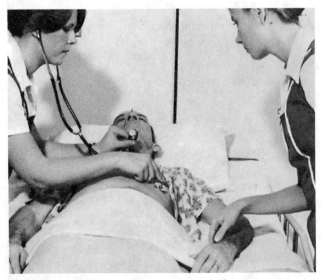

FIGURE 11-10
One nurse counts the radial pulse while the other counts the apical rate.

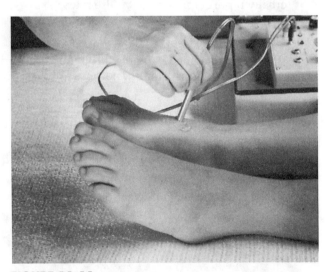

FIGURE 11-11
Using Doppler ultrasound device. (Courtesy of Ken Timby.)

ever, some normal ranges have been established (Table 11-7). Factors that influence the pulse rate usually also affect the respiratory rate. The faster the pulse rate, the faster the respiratory rate, and vice versa. The ratio of one respiration to approximately four or five heartbeats is fairly consistent in normal people.

RAPID RESPIRATORY RATE

Resting respiratory rates that exceed the standards for a patient's age are considered abnormal. **Tachypnea** is the term used to describe a rapid respiratory rate. Tachypnea may be observed with an elevated temperature or when diseases affect the cardiac and respiratory systems.

SLOW RESPIRATORY RATE

A slower-than-normal respiratory rate is referred to as **bradypnea**. Certain drugs, such as morphine sulfate, may slow the respiratory rate. Slow respirations may also be observed in patients with neurologic disorders or those experiencing hypothermia.

Breathing Patterns and Abnormal Characteristics

Various breathing patterns and abnormal characteristics may be identified when assessing respiratory rates. For example, *Cheyne-Stokes respiration* refers to a breathing pattern in which there is a gradual increase then decrease in the depth of respirations followed by a period when breathing stops briefly before resuming again.

Hyperventilation is a term that describes a respiratory rate that is rapid or deep, or both. **Hypoventilation** describes a state in which there is an insufficient volume of air entering and leaving the lungs.

Dyspnea is difficult or labored breathing. It is almost always accompanied by a rapid respiratory rate as patients work to improve the efficiency of their breathing. Dyspneic patients usually appear anxious and worried. The nostrils flare (widen) as the patient struggles to fill the lungs with air. Abdominal and neck

TABLE 11-7. *Normal Respiratory Rates at Various Ages*

Age	Average Range
Newborn	30–80
Early childhood	20–40
Late childhood	15–25
Adulthood	
Male	14–18
Female	16–20

muscles may be used to assist other muscles in the act of breathing. When observing the patient, it is important to note how much and what type of activity brings on dyspnea. For example, walking to the bathroom may bring on dyspnea in a patient who may not be distressed by sitting in a chair.

Orthopnea is a type of breathing that is facilitated by sitting up or standing. Dyspneic patients frequently find it easier to breathe in this manner. An upright position causes organs in the abdominal cavity to fall away from the diaphragm with gravity. This gives more room for the lungs to expand and take in more air with each breath.

Apnea refers to the absence of breathing. This is a serious situation if it lasts more than 4 to 6 minutes. Prolonged apnea can lead to brain damage or death.

Several terms are used to describe sounds that can be heard as a patient breathes. *Stertorous breathing* is a general term used to refer to noisy respirations. *Stridor* is a harsh, high-pitched sound that is heard on inspiration when there is a laryngeal obstruction. Infants and young children with croup often manifest stridor when breathing.

The nurse may listen to the sounds of air moving through the chest with a stethoscope. The technique and characteristics of lung sounds are described in Chapter 12.

Assessing the Respiratory Rate

Skill 11-5 suggests techniques to use when counting the respiratory rate.

BLOOD PRESSURE

Blood pressure is the force exerted by blood within the arteries. In healthy people, the arterial walls are elastic and easily stretch and recoil to accommodate for the changing volume of circulating blood. Measuring the blood pressure helps to assess the efficiency of the circulatory system. Its measurement reflects (1) the ability of the arteries to stretch, (2) the volume of circulating blood, and (3) the amount of resistance the heart must overcome when it pumps blood.

Pressure Measurements

When the blood pressure is assessed, both a systolic and diastolic pressure measurement is obtained. **Systolic pressure**, or the pressure within the arterial system when the heart contracts, is higher than **diastolic pressure**, or the pressure within the arterial system when the heart relaxes and fills with blood.

Blood pressure measurement is expressed as a fraction. The numerator is the systolic pressure and the de-

SKILL 11-5
Assessing the Respiratory Rate

Suggested Action	Reason for Action
Assessment	
Determine when and how frequently to monitor the patient's respiratory rate (refer to Display 11-1).	Demonstrates accountability for making timely and appropriate assessments
Review the data collected in previously recorded assessments of the respiratory rate and other vital signs.	Aids in identifying trends and analyzing significant patterns
Read the patient's history for any reference to respiratory, cardiac, or neurologic disorders.	Demonstrates an understanding of factors that may affect the respiratory rate
Review the list of prescribed drugs for any that may have respiratory or neurologic effects.	Helps in analyzing the results of assessment findings
Planning	
Arrange the plan for care so as to count the patient's respiratory rate as close to the scheduled routine as possible.	Ensures consistency and accuracy
Make sure a watch or wall clock with a second hand is available.	Ensures accurate timing
Plan to assess the patient's respiratory rate after a 5-minute period of inactivity.	Reflects the characteristics of respirations at rest rather than under the influence of activity
Implementation	
Introduce yourself to the patient if this has not been done during earlier contact.	Demonstrates responsibility and accountability
Explain the procedure to the patient.	Reduces apprehension and promotes cooperation
Raise the height of the bed.	Reduces musculoskeletal strain
Wash your hands.	Reduces the spread of microorganisms
Help the patient to a sitting or lying position.	Facilitates the ability to observe breathing
Note the position of the second hand on the clock or watch.	Identifies the point at which the assessment begins
Choose a time when the patient is unaware of being watched; it may be helpful to count the respiratory rate while appearing to count the pulse.	Discourages conscious control of breathing during the assessment
Observe the rise and fall of the patient's chest for a full minute, if breathing is unusual. If breathing appears noiseless and effortless, count the ventilations for a fractional portion of a minute and then multiply to calculate the rate.	Determines the respiratory rate per minute
Write down the respiratory rate.	Ensures accurate documentation
Restore the patient to a therapeutic position or one that provides comfort, and lower the height of the bed	Demonstrates responsibility for patient care, safety, and comfort
Record the respiratory rate on the graphic sheet, flow sheet, or in the narrative nurses' notes.	Provides documentation for future comparisons

(continued)

SKILL 11-5
Assessing the Respiratory Rate (Continued)

Suggested Action	Reason for Action
Verbally report rapid or slow respiratory rates or any other unusual breathing characteristics.	Alerts others to monitor the patient closely and make changes in the plan for care

Evaluation
- Respiratory rate is counted for an appropriate amount of time
- Respiratory rate is consistent with the patient's condition

Document
- Date and time
- Rate per minute
- Accompanying signs and symptoms, if appropriate
- To whom abnormal information was reported, and outcome of the communication

Sample Documentation

Date and Time   Respiratory rate of 20/min. at rest. Breathing is noiseless and effortless.

_____ **Signature, Title**

nominator is the diastolic pressure. The pressure is expressed in millimeters of mercury, abbreviated mm Hg. Thus, a recording of 140/80 means the systolic blood pressure was measured at 140 mm Hg and the diastolic blood pressure was measured at 80 mm Hg.

The difference between systolic and diastolic blood pressure measurements is called the **pulse pressure**. It is computed by subtracting the smaller figure from the larger. For example, when the blood pressure is 126/88 mm Hg, pulse pressure is 38. A pulse pressure between 30 and 50 is considered to be in a normal range, with 40 being a healthy average.

Blood pressure can fluctuate within a wide range and still be normal. Because individual differences can be considerable, it is important to analyze the usual ranges and patterns of blood pressure measurements for each person. A sudden rise or fall of 20 to 30 mm Hg is significant, even if the blood pressure is well within the generally accepted range for normal.

Factors Affecting Blood Pressure

Various factors can influence the blood pressure. They include:

Age. Blood pressure tends to rise with age because of *arteriosclerosis*, a process in which arteries lose their elasticity and become more rigid, and *atherosclerosis*, a process in which the arteries become narrowed with fat deposits. The rate at which these conditions occur depends on one's heredity and lifestyle habits, such as diet and exercise.

Circadian rhythm. Blood pressure tends to be lowest after midnight, begins rising at approximately 4 or 5 A.M., and reaches its peak during late morning or early afternoon.

Gender. Women tend to have lower blood pressure than men of the same age.

Exercise and activity. Blood pressure rises during periods of exercise and activity, when the heart pumps a greater volume of blood. Regular exercise, however, helps maintain the blood pressure within normal levels.

Emotions and pain. Strong emotional experiences and pain tend to cause blood pressure to rise from sympathetic nervous system stimulation.

Miscellaneous factors. As a rule, a person has a lower blood pressure when lying down than when sitting or standing, although the difference in most people may be insignificant. It has also been observed that blood pressure rises somewhat when the urinary bladder is full, when the legs are crossed, or when the person is cold. Drugs that stimulate the heart such as nicotine, caffeine, and cocaine also tend to constrict the arteries and raise blood pressure.

Assessment Sites

The blood pressure is most often assessed over the brachial artery at the inner aspect of the elbow area. However, in situations where both arms may be missing or inaccessible, the blood pressure may be measured over the popliteal artery behind the knee.

Equipment for Measuring Blood Pressure

Blood pressure is measured by listening for characteristic sounds with a stethoscope while pressure is released from a cuff attached to a pressure gauge. The pressure-monitoring device is called a **sphygmomanometer**.

SPHYGMOMANOMETER

A sphygmomanometer consists of a manometer, or instrument for measuring the pressure of a gas or liquid, and a cuff. The manometer may be either a mercury or aneroid gauge (Fig. 11-12). Some sphygmomanometers are portable, whereas others are wall mounted.

Mercury Gauge Manometer

A mercury gauge manometer contains liquid mercury within a column calibrated in millimeters. To ensure an accurate measurement, the mercury must be even with the zero level at the base of the calibrated column when not in use.

It also must be positioned vertically with the gauge at eye level. Positioning the gauge in this manner allows the nurse to observe more accurately the column of mercury, the top of which appears slightly curved (Fig. 11-13).

Aneroid Manometer

An aneroid manometer contains a gauge with a needle that moves about a dial calibrated in millimeters. The needle must be positioned initially at zero to ensure an accurate recording.

Either type of gauge, provided it is working properly and used correctly, can measure blood pressure accurately. The readings obtained with one type of gauge are comparable to those obtained with the other.

INFLATABLE CUFF

The cuff of a sphygmomanometer contains an inflatable bladder, to which two tubes are attached. One is connected to the manometer, which registers the pressure. The other is attached to a bulb, which is used to inflate the bladder with air. A screw valve on the bulb allows the nurse to fill and empty the bladder of air. As the air escapes, the pressure is measured.

Cuffs come in a variety of sizes. The nurse selects a cuff with an appropriate bladder size for each patient (Table 11-8). A common guide is to use a cuff whose bladder encircles at least two-thirds the limb at its midpoint (Solomon, 1993) and is at least as wide as 40% of mid-limb circumference (Fig. 11-14). If the cuff is too wide, the blood pressure reading will be falsely low. If the cuff is too narrow, the blood pressure reading will be falsely high.

STETHOSCOPE

A **stethoscope** is an instrument that carries sound to the ears. A stethoscope is composed of eartips, a brace and binaurals, and tubing leading to a chest piece that may be a bell, diaphragm, or both (Fig. 11-15).

The eartips are usually rubber or plastic. When the stethoscope is used, the eartips are positioned down-

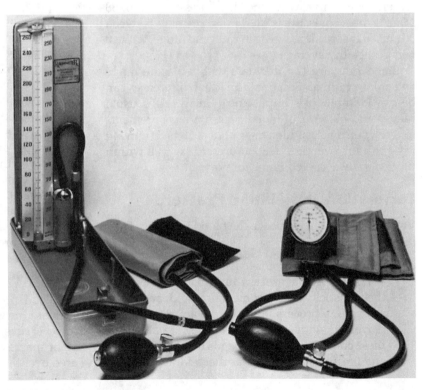

FIGURE 11-12
The sphygmomanometer on the left has a mercury gauge; the one on the right has an aneroid gauge.

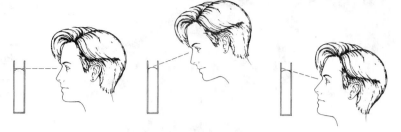

FIGURE 11-13
The illustration on the left indicates how to observe the column of mercury to avoid an inaccurate assessment.

ward and forward within the ears to produce the best sound perception. If stethoscopes are used by various people, the eartips are cleaned between uses with alcohol swabs. Individually owned stethoscopes also need periodic cleaning to keep the eartips free of ear wax and dirt.

The brace and binaurals are usually made of metal. They connect the eartips to the tubing and chest piece. The brace prevents the tubing from kinking and distorting the sound.

Stethoscope tubing may be rubber or plastic. The best length for good sound conduction is about 20 inches (50 cm).

The bell, or cup-shaped chest piece, is used for detecting low-pitched sounds, like those produced in blood vessels. The diaphragm, or disk-shaped chest piece, detects high-pitched sounds, like those in the lungs, heart, or abdomen. If the diaphragm becomes cracked, it must be replaced. When the bell is used, care is taken to position it lightly because pressure flattens the skin and creates the same effect as a diaphragm.

Measuring Blood Pressure

Most blood pressure recordings are obtained indirectly—that is, they are determined by applying a blood pressure cuff, briefly occluding arterial blood

flow, and listening for unique sounds, known as **Korotkoff sounds**. Korotkoff sounds are thought to be the result of vibrations in the arterial wall or changes in blood flow—which one exactly is uncertain. Whatever the cause, the blood pressure measurements are determined by correlating certain phases in Korotkoff sounds with the numbers on the gauge of the sphygmomanometer (Skill 11-6).

KOROTKOFF SOUNDS

Korotkoff sounds usually follow five unique phases (Fig. 11-16).

Phase I

Phase I begins with the first faint but clear tapping sound that follows a period of silence as pressure is released from the cuff. When the first sound occurs, it corresponds to the peak pressure in the arterial system during heart contraction, or systolic pressure measurement. It is recorded as the first number in the numeric fraction.

The first sound, which is heard for at least two consecutive beats and sometimes more, may be missed if the cuff pressure is not pumped high enough initially to occlude arterial blood flow. Palpating for the disappearance of a distal pulse when inflating the cuff

Arm Circumference at Midpoint* (cm)	Cuff Name	Bladder Width (cm)	Bladder Length (cm)
5–7.5	Newborn	3	5
7.5–13	Infant	5	8
13–20	Child	8	13
24–32	Adult	13	24
32–42	Wide adult	17	32
42–50†	Thigh	20	42

TABLE 11-8. *Recommended Bladder Dimensions for Blood Pressure Cuffs*

*Midpoint of arm is defined as half the distance from the acromion to olecranon processes.

†In people with very large limbs, indirect blood pressure should be measured in leg or forearm.

Reproduced with permission. Recommendations for Human Blood Pressure Determination by Sphygmomanometers, © American Heart Association, 1987.

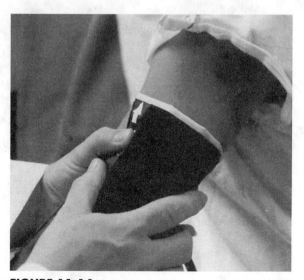

FIGURE 11-14
Selecting an appropriate-size blood pressure cuff. (Courtesy of Ken Timby.)

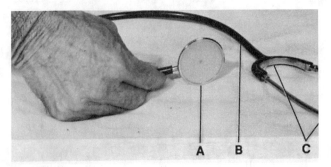

FIGURE 11-15
A stethoscope contains *(A)* a chest piece, *(B)* tubing, *(C)* brace and binaurals, and *(D)* eartips.

helps to ensure that the cuff pressure is above arterial pressure.

Phase I sounds may briefly disappear altogether, especially in people with blood pressures that are elevated above normal ranges, before they become reestablished. The period during which sound disappears is known as an **auscultatory gap**. The gap may cover a range of as much as 40 mm Hg. Failure to identify the first sound preceding an auscultatory gap results in an inaccurate blood pressure measurement.

150 mmHg → 120 mmHg		→ 80 mmHg	→ 0 mmHg	
Phase I	Phase II	Phase III	Phase IV	Phase V
Faint tapping	Swishing	Loud knocking	Muffled	Silence

FIGURE 11-16
Characteristics of Korotkoff sounds.

Phase II
Phase II is characterized by a change from the tapping sounds to swishing sounds. At this time the diameter of the artery is widening, allowing more arterial blood flow.

Phase III
Phase III is characterized by a change to sounds that are loud and distinct. They are described as crisp knocking sounds. During this phase, blood is flowing relatively freely through the artery once more.

Phase IV
Phase IV sounds are muffled and have a blowing quality. The sound change is the result of a loss in

(text continued on page 162)

SKILL 11-6
Assessing Blood Pressure

Suggested Action	Reason for Action
Assessment	
Determine when and how frequently to monitor the patient's pulse (refer to Display 11-1).	Demonstrates accountability for making timely and appropriate assessments
Review the data collected in previously recorded assessments.	Aids in identifying trends and analyzing significant patterns
Determine in which arm and in what position previous assessments were made.	Ensures consistency when evaluating data
Read the patient's history for any reference to cardiac or vascular disorders.	Demonstrates an understanding of factors that may affect the blood pressure
Review the list of prescribed drugs for any that may have cardiovascular effects.	Helps in analyzing the results of assessment findings
Planning	
Gather the necessary supplies: blood pressure cuff, sphygmomanometer, and stethoscope.	Promotes efficient time management
Select a cuff that is an appropriate size for the patient.	Ensures valid assessment findings
Arrange the plan for care so as to take the patient's blood pressure as near to the scheduled routine as possible.	Ensures consistency

SKILL 11-6
Assessing Blood Pressure (Continued)

Suggested Action	Reason for Action
Plan to assess the blood pressure after at least 3 minutes of inactivity, unless it is an emergency situation.	Reflects the blood pressure under resting conditions
Plan to use the right or left arm unless they are inaccessible.	Provides consistency in evaluating data
Implementation	
Introduce yourself to the patient if this has not been done during earlier contact.	Demonstrates responsibility and accountability
Explain the procedure to the patient.	Reduces apprehension and promotes cooperation
Raise the height of the bed.	Reduces musculoskeletal strain
Wash your hands	Reduces the spread of microorganisms
Help the patient to a position of comfort.	Relaxes the patient and reduces elevation in blood pressure due to stress or discomfort.
Support the patient's forearm at the level of the heart with the palm of the hand upward.	Ensures collecting accurate data and facilitates locating the brachial artery
Expose the inner aspect of the elbow by removing clothing or loosely rolling up a sleeve.	Facilitates application of the blood pressure cuff and optimum sound perception
Center the cuff bladder so that the lower edge is about 1 to 2 inches (2.5–5 cm) above the inner aspect of the elbow.	Places the cuff in the best position for occluding the blood flow through the brachial artery

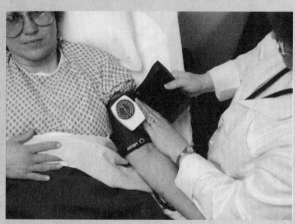

Applying the blood pressure cuff. (Courtesy of Ken Timby.)

Suggested Action	Reason for Action
Wrap the cuff snugly and uniformly about he circumference of the arm.	Ensures the application of even pressure during inflation
Position the mercury manometer on an even surface at eye level; make sure the aneroid gauge can be clearly seen.	Prevents errors when observing the gauge

(continued)

SKILL 11-6
Assessing Blood Pressure (Continued)

Suggested Action	Reason for Action
Palpate the brachial pulse.	Determines the most accurate location for assessment

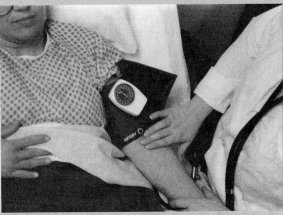

Palpating the brachial artery. (Courtesy of Ken Timby.)

Suggested Action	Reason for Action
Tighten the screw valve on the bulb.	Prevents loss of pumped air

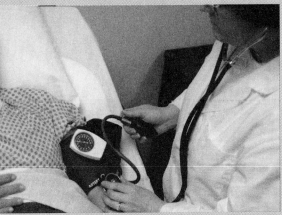

Tightening the screw valve. (Courtesy of Ken Timby.)

Suggested Action	Reason for Action
Compress the bulb until the pulsation within the artery stops.	Provides an estimation of systolic pressure
Deflate the cuff and wait 15 seconds.	Allows the return of normal blood flow

(continued)

Assessing Blood Pressure *(Continued)*

Suggested Action	Reason for Action
Place the eartips of the stethoscope within the ears and position the bell* of the stethoscope lightly over the location of the brachial artery.	Ensures an accurate assessment

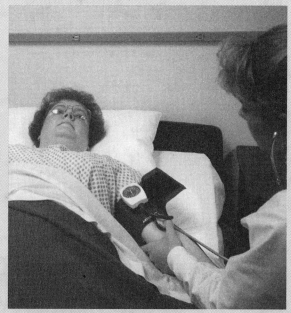

Placing the stethoscope. (Courtesy of Ken Timby.)

Suggested Action	Reason for Action
Keep the tubing free from contact with clothing.	Reduces sound distortion
Pump the cuff bladder to a pressure that is 30 mm Hg above the point where the pulse previously disappeared.	Facilitates identifying phase I of Korotkoff sounds

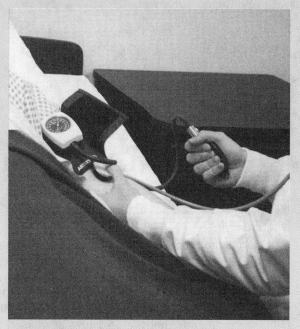

Pumping the bulb. (Courtesy of Ken Timby.)

(continued)

SKILL 11-6
Assessing Blood Pressure (Continued)

Suggested Action	Reason for Action
Loosen the screw on the valve.	Releases air from the cuff bladder
Control the release of air at a rate of approximately 2 to 3 mm Hg per second.	Ensures accurate assessment between the time when a sound is perceived and the numbers are noted on the gauge
Listen for the onset and changes in Korotkoff sounds.	Aids in determining the systolic and diastolic pressure measurements
Read the manometer gauge to the closest even number when phases I, IV, and V are noted.	Follows recommended standards
Release the air quickly when there has been silence for at least 10 to 20 mm Hg.	
Write down the blood pressure measurements.	Ensures accurate documentation
Restore the patient to a therapeutic position or one that provides comfort, and lower the height of the bed.	Demonstrates responsibility for patient care, safety, and comfort
Record assessed measurement on the graphic sheet, flow sheet, or in the narrative nurses' notes.	Provides documentation for future comparisons
Verbally report elevated or low blood pressure measurements.	Alerts others to monitor the patient closely and make changes in the plan for care

Evaluation

• Korotkoff sounds are heard clearly
• Blood pressure is consistent with the patient's condition

Document

• Date and time
• Systolic pressure measurement, first or second diastolic pressure measurement, or both
• Assessment site
• Position of the patient
• Accompanying signs and symptoms, if appropriate
• To whom abnormal information was reported, and outcome of the interaction

*Sample Documentation**

Date and Time   BP 136/72/68 in R. arm while in sitting position _____ **Signature, Title**

The diaphragm may be used, but it is not the preferred option (Hill & Grim, 1991).

transmission of pressure from the deflating cuff to the artery. The point at which the sound becomes muffled is considered the first diastolic pressure measurement. It is generally preferred when documenting the blood pressure measurements in children.

Phase V

Phase V is the point at which the last sound is heard, or the second diastolic pressure measurement. This is considered the best reflection of adult diastolic pressure because phase IV is often 7 to 10 mm Hg higher than direct diastolic pressure measurements. If only two numbers are used for recording adult blood pressure measurements, the American Heart Association (1987) recommends that the pressures at phase I and phase V be used.

To ensure accuracy and facilitate consistency in interpreting blood pressure assessments, some health agencies suggest documenting three numbers for adult blood pressure measurements: (1) the systolic pressure, (2) the first diastolic pressure, and (3) the second diastolic pressure. If this policy is followed, the blood pressure is recorded, for example, as 120/80/72. If sound is heard down to zero, the pressure is recorded as 120/80/0. If the first muffled sound is also the last sound heard, the blood pressure is recorded as 120/80/80.

INTENSIFYING KOROTKOFF SOUNDS

There are two techniques, either one of which may be used, for intensifying Korotkoff sounds that are difficult to hear:

- Have the patient elevate his or her arm before and during inflation of the cuff, and then lower the arm after it is fully inflated.
- Have the patient open and close his or her fist after the cuff has been inflated.

Assessment Errors

There are several variables that may result in inaccurate blood pressure measurements (Table 11-9).

Alternative Assessment Techniques

In situations when it is difficult to hear Korotkoff sounds no matter how conscientious the effort to augment them, the blood pressure may be assessed by palpation or by using a flush method.

PALPATING THE BLOOD PRESSURE

When palpating the blood pressure, the nurse applies a blood pressure cuff in the usual manner, but instead of using a stethoscope, the fingers are positioned over the artery as the cuff pressure is released. The point at which the first pulsation is felt corresponds to the systolic pressure. The diastolic pressure cannot be measured because there is no perceptible change in the quality of pulsations, as there is in the sounds. When recording a blood pressure taken in this manner, it is important to indicate that it was assessed using palpation.

FLUSH METHOD

The flush method, which is best performed with the assistance of another nurse, is used to obtain the blood pressure of infants. The principle is to reduce blood flow in the infant's hand or foot and observe the pressure at which flushing occurs. The flush pressure is comparable to the mean arterial pressure, that is, a pressure approximately between the systolic and diastolic pressures.

When the flush method is used, the nurse:

- Applies a newborn or infant blood pressure cuff above the wrist or ankle
- Raises the hand or foot to reduce blood volume within the extremity
- Wraps the exposed hand or foot with an elastic bandage from the fingers or toes to the edge of the cuff (Fig. 11-17)
- Inflates the cuff to 120 to 140 mm Hg
- Returns the wrapped extremity to its natural position
- Unwraps the elastic bandage (the hand or foot should appear white)
- Releases the air from the cuff at a rate of 2 to 3 mm Hg second
- Asks the assistant to indicate when the extremity becomes pink or flushes
- Notes the corresponding pressure on the manometer
- Records the pressure at which flushing occurred

TABLE 11-9. *Common Causes of Blood Pressure Assessment Errors*

Cause	Effect	Correction
Inaccurate manometer calibration	Inaccurate high or low readings	Recalibrate, repair, or replace gauge
Loosely applied cuff	High reading	Wrap snugly with equal pressure about extremity
Cuff too small for extremity	High reading	Select appropriate size
Cuff too large for extremity	Low reading	Select appropriate size
Cuff applied over clothing	Creates noises or interferes with sound perception	Remove arm from sleeve or don a patient gown
Tubing that leaks	Rapid loss of pressure	Replace or repair
Improper positioning of eartips	Poor sound conduction	Reposition and retake blood pressure
Impaired hearing	Altered sound perception	Use an alternative assessment technique or equipment
Loud environmental noise	Interferes with sound perception	Reduce noise and reassess
Impaired vision	Inaccurate observation of gauge	Correct vision; reposition gauge within adequate range
Rapid cuff deflation	Inaccurate observation of gauge	Reassess and deflate at 2 to 3 mm Hg/second

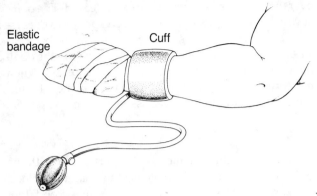

FIGURE 11-17
Using the flush method to obtain the blood pressure of infants.

Alternative Equipment

Sometimes the blood pressure may be measured with an electronic sphygmomanometer, an automatic blood pressure monitoring device, or a Doppler ultrasound device.

ELECTRONIC SPHYGMOMANOMETER

Electronic sphygmomanometers transform blood pressure measurements into audible sounds or a digital display of numbers, making a stethoscope unnecessary. They are helpful when it is difficult to hear Korotkoff sounds or when people without much technical experience wish to monitor their own blood pressure. However, because of their delicate instrumentation, electronic sphygmomanometers should be recalibrated more than once each year. People who use an electronic sphygmomanometer are advised to have their blood pressure checked periodically by health personnel. Periodic monitoring provides an opportunity for evaluating the data collected through self-monitoring and provides assistance with interpreting the results.

AUTOMATIC BLOOD PRESSURE MONITORING

An automatic blood pressure monitoring (ABPM) device consists of a blood pressure cuff attached to a microprocessing unit supported either at the shoulder or waist. ABPM is used to diagnose unusual fluctuations in blood pressure that are not identifiable during single or sporadic monitoring. When used, the device records an ambulatory patient's blood pressure every 10 to 30 minutes throughout a 24-hour period. The data are stored in the microprocessor's memory, printed after the test, and analyzed both electronically and by the consulting physician.

DOPPLER ULTRASOUND ASSESSMENT

A Doppler ultrasound device is used in lieu of a stethoscope to identify the peak pressure at which arterial blood flow resumes. Refer to the section on Other Pulse Assessment Techniques earlier in this chapter for a description of how the Doppler is used. When documenting the pressure measurement, a capital "D" is used to indicate that it was obtained with the use of a Doppler device.

Abnormal Blood Pressure Measurements

Blood pressures that exceed or fall below normal ranges may indicate significant health problems.

HIGH BLOOD PRESSURE

High blood pressure is called **hypertension**. It exists when the systolic pressure, or diastolic pressure, or both, is sustained above normal levels for a person's age. The Joint National Committee for the Detection, Evaluation, and Treatment of High Blood Pressure (1993) considers a systolic pressure of 140 mm Hg or greater in adults 18 years or older, and a diastolic pressure of 90 mm Hg or greater, to be abnormally high (Table 11-10).

An occasional elevation in blood pressure does not necessarily mean a person has hypertension, but it does mean that the blood pressure should be monitored at

TABLE 11-10. *Classification of Adult Blood Pressure Measurements*	
Blood Pressure (mm Hg)	**Category***
Diastolic	
<85	Normal blood pressure
85–89	High normal blood pressure
90–104	Mild hypertension
105–114	Moderate hypertension
≥115	Severe hypertension
Systolic when DBP < 90 mm Hg	
<140	Normal blood pressure
140–159	Borderline isolated systolic hypertension
≥160	Isolated systolic hypertension

*A classification of borderline isolated systolic hypertension (SBP 140–159 mm Hg) or isolated systolic hypertension (SBP ≥160 mm Hg) takes precedence over a classification of high normal blood pressure (DBP 85–89 mm Hg) when both occur in the same person. A classification of high normal blood pressure (DBP 85–89 mm Hg) takes precedence over a classification of normal blood pressure (SBP <140 mm Hg) when both occur in the same person.

Classification terms and measurements from the 1993 Joint National Committee Report on Detection, Evaluation, and Treatment of High Blood Pressure.

TABLE 11-11. *Recommendations for Follow-up Based on Initial Set of Blood Pressure Measurements for Adults Age 18 Years and Older*

Initial Screening Blood Pressure (mm Hg)*		
Systolic	Diastolic	Follow-up Recommended†
<130	<85	Recheck in 2 years
130–139	85–89	Recheck in 1 year‡
140–159	90–99	Confirm within 2 months
160–179	100–109	Evaluate or refer to source of care within 1 month
180–209	110–119	Evaluate or refer to source of care within 1 week
≥210	≥120	Evaluate or refer to source of care immediately

*If the systolic and diastolic categories are different, follow recommendation for the shorter time to follow-up (eg, 160/85 mm Hg should be evaluated or referred to source of care within 1 month).
†The scheduling of follow-up should be modified by reliable information about past blood pressure measurements, other cardiovascular risk factors, or target-organ disease.
‡Consider providing advice about lifestyle modifications. From the fifth report of the Joint National Committee for the Detection, Evaluation, and Treatment of High Blood Pressure, National Heart, Lung, and Blood Institute, National Institutes of Health, January 1993.)

various intervals depending on the significance of the pressure measurements (Table 11-11).

Hypertensive blood pressure measurements are often associated with:

- Anxiety
- Obesity
- Vascular diseases
- Stroke
- Heart failure
- Kidney diseases

LOW BLOOD PRESSURE

Low blood pressure is called **hypotension**. It exists when the blood pressure measurements are below the normal systolic values for the person's corresponding age. Having a sustained low pressure seems to cause no harm. In fact, low blood pressure is usually associated with efficient functioning of the heart and blood vessels. However, people with low blood pressure measurements should continue to be monitored to evaluate its significance.

Low blood pressure measurements may be an indication of:

- Shock
- Hemorrhage
- Side effects from drugs

POSTURAL HYPOTENSION

Postural or **orthostatic hypotension** is a sudden, but temporary, drop in blood pressure when rising from a reclining position. It is most common among those with circulatory problems, those who are dehydrated, or those who take diuretics or other drugs that lower the blood pressure. A consequence of a sudden drop in blood pressure is dizziness and even fainting.

Patients who are in high-risk categories or who become symptomatic during the course of care are assessed for postural hypotension using the following nursing guidelines.

NURSING GUIDELINES FOR ASSESSING POSTURAL HYPOTENSION

- Have the patient lie down for at least 3 minutes.
  Rationale: Allows for the blood pressure to stabilize
- Take the patient's blood pressure.
  Rationale: Establishes a baseline for comparison
- Assist the patient to a sitting or standing position.
  Rationale: Stimulates reflexes for maintaining blood flow to the brain
- Prepare to steady or assist patients who may become dizzy or faint.
  Rationale: Demonstrates an understanding of the relationship between the potential for hypotension and risk for injury
- Repeat the blood pressure assessment 30 seconds after the patient assumes an upright position (Hill & Grim, 1991).
  Rationale: Provides data for comparison
- Determine if the systolic blood pressure in the upright position is 15 mm Hg less than the reclining blood pressure.
  Rationale: Validates that the patient experiences postural hypotension (Carnevali & Patrick, 1993)

DOCUMENTING VITAL SIGNS

Once vital sign measurements are obtained, they are usually documented in the medical record on a graphic sheet to facilitate the analysis of patterns and trends (Fig. 11-18). However, vital sign measurements, along with any other subjective or objective data, may also be entered elsewhere in the patient's record, such as in the nursing notes.

THREE RIVERS AREA HOSPITAL
CLINICAL SHEET

SHIFT	N	D	E	N	D	E	N	D	E	N	D	E	N	D	E
TIME	24	4	8	12	16	20	24	4	8	12	16	20	24	4	8	12	16	20	24	4	8	12	16	20	24	4	8	12	16	20

TEMPERATURE (106, 105, 104, 103, 102, 101, 100, 99, 98.6, 98, 97, 96, 95, 94)

| PULSE | | | 104 | 100 | 96 | 94 | 94 | 98 | 94 | 90 | 88 | 88 | 80 | 82 | 80 | 82 | 80 | 82 | 84 | 80 | 76 | 76 | 78 | 78 | 82 |
| RESPIRATION | | | 26 | 24 | 24 | 22 | 20 | 22 | 24 | 22 | 20 | 18 | 18 | 20 | 20 | 18 | 18 | 20 | 20 | 18 | 16 | 16 | 18 | 18 | 20 |

DATE	7/15			7/16			7/17			7/18			7/19		
ADM. DAY / POST OP. DAY	1			2			3			4			5		
SHIFT	N	D	E	N	D	E	N	D	E	N	D	E	N	D	E
B/P AS NEEDED		136/84		132/80			130/80			128/78			128/80		
URINE		✓	✓	✓		✓	✓	✓	✓	✓			✓	✓	
STOOL						✓								✓	
SIDE RAILS		✓	✓	✓	✓	✓	✓	✓	✓	✓		✓	✓		
WEIGHT	134#														
SHIFT	D		E	D		E	D		E	D		E	D		E
APPETITE	P		P	P		F	F		G	G		G			
CARE	H.S.		C	H.S.		P	H.S.		S	H.S.		S			
ACTIVITY	BR		BRP	BRP		Ch	Amb		Up	Up		Up			
DR. VISITED	✓					✓				✓			✓		

NURSE'S SIGNATURE AND INITIALS
N — Fern Miller FM ... FM ... FM
D — Ane Roher AR ... AR ... AR
E — Sally Carpenter SC ... SC ... SC ... SC

APPETITE	ACTIVITY	CARE
NPO = O	Bedrest = BR	Complete = C
Good = G	Bathroom = BRP	Partial = P
Fair = F	Chair = Ch	Self = S
Poor = P	Ambulated = Amb	Refused = R
Ref. = R	Up ad lib = UP	Eve. Care = H.S.

FIGURE 11-18
Graphic recording of vital signs.

NURSING IMPLICATIONS

Vital sign assessment is part of every patient's care and forms the basis for identifying problems. Based on analysis of assessment data, the nurse may identify any one or more of the accompanying Applicable Nursing Diagnoses.

The Nursing Care Plan describes approaches that can be used for a patient with a nursing diagnosis of hyperthermia. Hyperthermia is defined in theNANDA Taxonomy (1992) as, "A state in which an individual's body temperature is elevated above his/her normal range." If the alteration is so severe that it requires medical interventions, it is considered a collaborative problem.

APPLICABLE NURSING DIAGNOSES

- Hyperthermia
- Hypothermia
- Ineffective Thermoregulation
- Decreased Cardiac Output
- Risk for Injury
- Ineffective Breathing Pattern

NURSING CARE PLAN:

Hyperthermia

Assessment	**Subjective Data**
	Daughter states, "Mother insists on working in her garden in this heat. Luckily the neighbors saw her faint, or who knows how long she would have lain there." Patient states, "I feel dizzy."

Objective Data

76-year-old woman. T—102.6 (O), P—104 thready and irregular, R—28, BP 106/52 in R. arm lying down. Skin is flushed, hot, and dry. Can identify daughter by name and relationship. Says this is summer, but cannot name the month or year. Knows she is in the hospital. Last meal and fluid consumed 6 hours ago. Not currently taking any type of medication.

Diagnosis   Hyperthermia related to overexertion in hot weather

Plan   **Goal**

The patient's body temperature will return to 98.6 ± 1° in 24 hours (1600 on 8/7).

Orders: 8/6

1. Assess vital signs q̄ 4 h while awake on even hours.
2. Use only hospital gown while temp. is elevated.
3. Cover with just one cotton sheet while temp. is elevated.
4. Maintain bed rest and siderails.
5. Provide 1500 mL oral intake before bedtime. Likes lemonade, apple juice, and ginger ale.
6. Record I & O
7. When stable, instruct to:
   * wear a wide brimmed hat when outside
   * garden before 9 A.M. or after 7 P.M.
   * limit sun exposure to no more than 30 min
   * increase fluid intake on hot days
   * sit in front of fan after coming inside. _____ S. EVANS, RN

Implementation   8/6   1800   T—100.4 (O), P—100 weak and irregular, R—20 s̄ effort. BP 108/60 R. arm
(Documentation)   while lying down. Dress, undergarments, and stockings removed and given to daughter. Wearing hospital gown covered with top sheet. Bed is in low position with siderails up. Feels "dizzy" when head is elevated. BP 104/60 R. arm lying; BP 90/50 3 minutes after assuming a sitting position. Bed rest maintained. _____ A. WHITE, LPN

Evaluation   2000   T—100 (O), P—96 full but irregular, R—20. BP 110/64 R. arm lying down. Skin
(Documentation)   is pink, dry, and cool. Drinking oral liquids. Urinating comparable amounts. Urine has changed from dark yellow to light yellow. Can identify current year correctly. No further dizziness experienced. Teaching postponed at this time._____ A. WHITE, LPN

KEY CONCEPTS

* Vital signs include assessments of a patient's temperature, pulse, respirations, and blood pressure.
* The body's shell temperature is its warmth at the skin surface, whereas core temperature is that near the center of the body.
* Temperature may be measured using the centigrade or Fahrenheit scale.

* The mouth, rectum, axilla, or ear are sites used for assessing body temperature; the temperature of the tympanic membrane within the ear is the closest approximation of core temperature.
* A glass mercury thermometer, electronic thermometer, or tympanic thermometer is used clinically to assess body temperature.
* A fever exists when a patient has a body temperature that exceeds 99.3°F (37.4°C); hyperthermia, on the

other hand, is a life-threatening condition character-ized by a body temperature that exceeds 105.8°F (41°C).

- A fever usually follows four phases: the prodromal phase, the onset or invasion phase, the stationary phase, and the resolution or defervescence phase.
- A fever may be accompanied by chills, flushed skin, irritability, and headache, as well as several other signs and symptoms.
- A tympanic thermometer is the best assessment tool for measuring subnormal temperatures because glass and electronic thermometers do not have the capacity to measure temperatures in hypothermic ranges, and the blood flow in the mouth, rectum, or axilla is usually so reduced that measurements taken from these sites are inaccurate.
- Subnormal temperatures may be accompanied by shivering, pale skin, listlessness, and impaired mus-cle coordination, as well as several other signs and symptoms.
- A pulse assessment includes the rate per minute, its rhythm, and volume.
- The radial artery is the most common pulse assess-ment site; however, similar data may be obtained by assessing the apical heart rate, the apical–radial rate, or by using a Doppler ultrasound device.
- Respiration refers to the exchange of oxygen and car-bon dioxide. Ventilation is the movement of air in and out of the chest. The rate of ventilations is as-sessed when obtaining vital signs.
- Several abnormal breathing characteristics may be noted. Some include tachypnea (rapid breathing), bradypnea (slow breathing), dyspnea (labored breath-ing), and apnea (absence of breathing).
- Blood pressure measurements reflect the ability of the arteries to stretch, the volume of circulating blood, and the amount of resistance the heart must overcome to pump blood.
- Systolic pressure is the pressure within the arterial system when the heart contracts. Diastolic pressure is the pressure within the arterial system when the heart relaxes and fills with blood.
- A stethoscope, inflatable cuff, and sphygmomanometer are usually required for measuring blood pressure.
- During blood pressure assessment five distinct sounds, called Korotkoff sounds, are heard. Phase I is characterized by faint tapping sounds; in phase II, the sounds are swishing; in phase III, the sounds are loud and crisp; in phase IV, the sound becomes sud-denly muffled; followed by phase V, in which there is one last sound followed by silence.
- The systolic blood pressure may also be measured by palpating the brachial pulse while releasing the air from the cuff bladder, and by using the flush method, a technique in which skin color is assessed.

 FOCUS ON OLDER ADULTS

- Older adults may not generate fevers in ranges that reflect the seriousness of an infec-tious condition.
- Older adults living in inadequately heated homes or apartments are particularly vulnera-ble to hypothermia (Porth, 1994).
- To avoid "white coat" or "office" hyperten-sion, a phenomenon in which blood pressure readings exhibit a transitory rise by as much as 20% above the usual measurement when taken by a uniformed professional (Van Buskirk and Gradman, 1993), it may be helpful to recommend that older adults ob-tain regular blood pressure assessments at locations in the community where they feel more comfortable, such as at a community meal site.
- Older adults have a high incidence of chronic cardiovascular disorders, which affect pulse rate and blood pressure measurement.
- Hypertension accounts for a significant inci-dence of heart attacks, heart failure, kidney failure, and strokes among older adults.
- Older adults may manifest more profound ef-fects when given drugs to control their heart rate or blood pressure.
- Respiratory reserves decrease in older adults, resulting in faster-than-normal respiratory rates (Matteson and McConnell, 1988).
- Older adults who experience more than a 20 mm Hg drop in blood pressure with pos-tural changes may be helped by wearing elas-tic stockings, which prevent pooling of blood in the extremities (Carnevali and Patrick, 1993).
- It may be helpful to obtain blood pressure measurements in each arm when collecting baseline assessments and documenting subse-quent trends.
- Older adults, like their younger counterparts, do not often experience symptoms associated with hypertension, known as the "silent killer." However, they may be observed to have an unsteady gait, memory deficits, and chest pain during activity, which are suggestive of vascular problems and elevated blood pressure.
- The pulse pressure of older adults tends to widen with age because of a rising systolic pressure that exceeds the rate of diastolic ele-vation (Carnevali and Patrick, 1993).

• In addition to mercury and aneroid manometers, blood pressure may be measured with an electronic sphygmomanometer that provides a digital display of the pressure measurements, an automatic blood pressure monitoring device that uses computerized microprocessing equipment, and a Doppler ultrasound device that converts arterial blood flow into an audible sound.

CRITICAL THINKING EXERCISES

• If a neighbor with no medical experience asks how to tell if her child, who is 4 years old, has a fever, what information would you provide?
• An 80-year-old patient explains that as an economy measure during winter she keeps her thermostat set at 65°F. What health information would be appropriate considering this woman's age?
• While participating in a community health assessment, you discover a person with a blood pressure that measures 190/110. What action(s) would be appropriate at this time?

SUGGESTED READINGS

American Heart Association. Recommendations for Human Blood Pressure Determination by Sphygmomanometers. Dallas: Author, 1987.

Baird S, White N, Basinger M. Can you rely on tympanic thermometers? RN August 1992;55:48–51.

Carnevali DL, Patrick M. Nursing Management for the Elderly. 3rd ed. Philadelphia: JB Lippincott, 1993.

Cooper KM. Measuring blood pressure the right way. Nursing April 1992;22:75.

Davis K. The accuracy of tympanic temperature measurement in children. Pediatric Nursing May–June 1993;19:267–272.

Hill MN, Grim CM. How to take a precise blood pressure. American Journal of Nursing February 1991;91:38–42.

Joint National Committee for the Detection, Evaluation, and Treatment of High Blood Pressure. The Fifth Report of the Joint National Committee for the Detection, Evaluation, and Treatment of High Blood Pressure. Bethesda, MD: National Heart, Lung, and Blood Institute, 1993.

Letizia M, Janusek L. The self-defense mechanism of fever. MEDSURG Nursing October 1994;3:373–377.

Mackowiak PA, Wasserman SS, Levine MM. A critical appraisal of 98.6°F, the upper limit of the normal body temperature, and other legacies of Carl Reinhold August Wunderlich. Journal of the American Medical Association September 23/30, 1992;268:1578–1580.

Matteson MA, McConnell ES. Gerontological Nursing. Philadelphia: WB Saunders, 1988.

McConnell EA. Assessing pulse deficit. Nursing November 1993; 23:18.

Nash CA. How do you test a digital sphygmomanometer? American Journal of Nursing January 1992;92:66, 69–70.

Porth CM. Pathophysiology: Concepts of Altered Health States. 4th ed. Philadelphia: JB Lippincott, 1994.

Robinchaud-Ekstrand S, Davis B. Comparison of electronic and glass thermometers: length of time of insertion and type of breathing. Canadian Journal of Nursing Research January 1989; 19:65.

Rousseau P. Management of hypertension in the elderly. Home Healthcare Nurse September–October 1991;9:47–49.

Smeltzer SC, Bare BG. Textbook of Medical–Surgical Nursing. 7th ed. Philadelphia: JB Lippincott, 1992.

Solomon J. Hypertension, new guidelines, new roles. RN December 1993;56:54–58.

Tourangeau A, MacLeod F, Breakwell M. Tap in on ear thermometry. Canadian Nurse September 1993;89:24–28.

Van Buskirk MC, Gradman AH. Monitoring blood pressure in ambulatory patients. American Journal of Nursing June 1993;93: 44–47.

Walczak M. Prevalence of orthostatic hypotension in high-risk ambulatory elders. Journal of Gerontological Nursing November 1991;17:26–29.

Ward L, Kaplan RM, Paris PM. A comparison of tympanic and rectal temperatures in the emergency department. Annals of Emergency Medicine April 1988;17:435.

CHAPTER 12
Physical Assessment

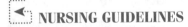

Learning Objectives

An understanding of the content within this chapter will be evidenced by the student's ability to:

- List four purposes for a physical assessment
- Name four assessment techniques
- List at least five items that are needed when performing a basic physical assessment
- Discuss at least three criteria for an appropriate assessment environment
- Identify at least five assessments that can be obtained during the initial survey of patients
- Give two reasons for draping patients
- Explain the difference between a head-to-toe approach to physical assessment and a body systems approach
- List six areas into which the body may be divided for the purpose of organizing data collection
- Identify two self–assessments that nurses should teach adult patients

The first step in the nursing process is assessment, or gathering information. **Physical assessment**, a systematic examination of body structures, is one method for gathering health data.

Timby BK: *Fundamental Skills and Concepts in Patient Care, Sixth Edition* © 1996 Lippincott-Raven Publishers

This chapter describes how to perform a physical assessment from a generalist's or beginning nurse's point of view, and identifies common assessment findings. Advanced physical assessment skills may be learned through additional education and experience or by consulting specialty texts.

PURPOSES FOR PHYSICAL ASSESSMENT

Patients are thoroughly examined on admission and briefly at the beginning of each shift for several reasons:

- To evaluate the patient's current physical condition
- To detect early signs of developing health problems
- To establish a data base for future comparisons
- To evaluate responses to medical and nursing interventions

PHYSICAL ASSESSMENT TECHNIQUES

There are four basic physical assessment techniques: inspection, percussion, palpation, and auscultation.

Inspection

Inspection, the most frequently used assessment technique, involves purposeful observation. More specifically, inspection refers to examining particular parts of the body for specific normal and abnormal characteristics (Fig. 12-1). With advanced instruction, some nurses learn to use special examination instruments.

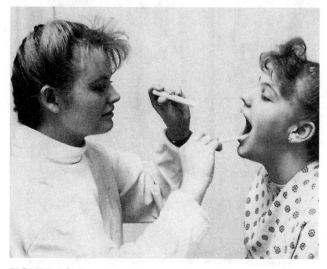

FIGURE 12-1
Inspection of the patient's mouth and throat. (Courtesy of Ken Timby.)

Percussion

Percussion, the assessment technique least used by nurses, involves striking or tapping a particular part of the body (Fig. 12-2). The fingertips are used to produce vibratory sounds. The quality of the sound aids in determining the location, size, and density of underlying structures (Table 12-1). If the sound is different from that which is normally expected, it suggests that there may be some pathologic change in the area being examined.

If percussion is performed correctly, the patient does not experience any discomfort. If pain is experienced, it may indicate the presence of a disease process or tissue injury.

Palpation

Palpation is an assessment technique that includes touch and pressure. *Light palpation* involves the use of the fingertips, the dorsum (back) of the hand, or the palm of the hand (Fig. 12-3). Light palpation is best used when feeling the surface of the skin, structures that lie just beneath the skin, the pulsation from peripheral arteries, and vibrations in the chest. *Deep palpation* is performed by depressing tissue approximately 1 inch (2.5 cm) with the forefingers of one or both hands (Fig. 12-4).

Palpation provides information about:

- The size, shape, consistency, and mobility of normal tissue and unusual masses
- The symmetry or asymmetry of bilateral (both sides of the body) structures, like lobes of the thyroid gland
- The temperature and moisture of the skin
- The presence of tenderness
- Unusual vibrations

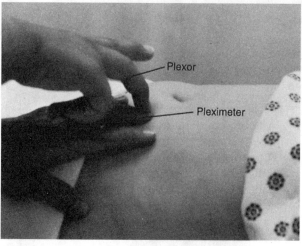

FIGURE 12-2
Percussing the patient's abdomen. (Courtesy of Ken Timby.)

TABLE 12-1. *Percussion Sounds*

Sound	Intensity	Descriptive Term	Common Locations
Muted	Soft	Flat	Muscle, bone
Thud	Soft to moderate	Dull	Liver, full bladder, tumorous mass
Empty	Moderate to loud	Resonant	Normal lung
Cavernous	Loud	Tympanic	Intestine filled with air
Booming	Very loud	Hyperresonant	Barrel-shaped chest overinflated with trapped air due to chronic lung disease

Auscultation

Auscultation is an assessment technique that involves listening to sounds. Loud sounds may be quite audible, but a stethoscope is required for hearing soft sounds (Fig. 12-5). The heart, lungs, and abdomen are the structures that are most often assessed by auscultation.

The technique of auscultation must be practiced repeatedly on a variety of healthy and ill people to gain experience in interpreting data and to become proficient at its use. To ensure obtaining adequate assessment findings, noise within the environment is eliminated or reduced as much as possible.

ASSESSMENT EQUIPMENT

The items that usually are needed for a basic physical assessment are listed in Display 12-1. Additional examination equipment may be used by more advanced practitioners (Fig. 12-6).

ASSESSMENT ENVIRONMENT

Patients may be assessed in a special examination room or at the bedside. Regardless of the assessment location, the area should have:

- Close access to a restroom
- A door or curtain to ensure privacy
- Adequate warmth for patient comfort
- A padded, adjustable table or bed
- Sufficient room for moving to either side of the patient
- Adequate lighting
- Facilities for handwashing
- A clean counter or surface for placing examination equipment
- A lined receptacle for soiled articles

PERFORMING A PHYSICAL ASSESSMENT

The procedure for conducting a physical assessment is described in Skill 12-1. Basic activities involved in a physical assessment include performing an initial survey, gathering general data, draping and positioning, and selecting a systematic approach for collecting data. Specific assessment techniques are described later in the chapter.

Initial Survey

An initial survey actually begins during the nurse's first contact with the patient. At this time the nurse develops an overall appraisal of the patient's general condition.

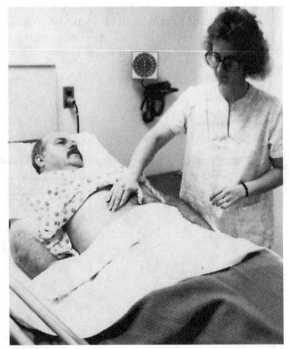

FIGURE 12-3
Light palpation of the patient's abdomen. (Courtesy of Ken Timby.)

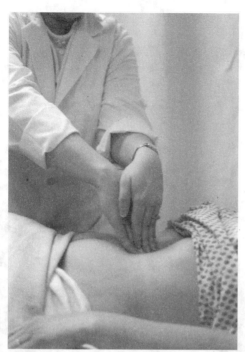

FIGURE 12-4
Deep palation of the patient's abdomen. (Courtesy of Ken

General Data

There is a great deal of general data that can be obtained by observing and interacting with the patient before the actual physical examination begins. For example, the nurse can note (1) the patient's physical appearance in relation to clothing and hygiene, (2) level of consciousness, (3) body size, (4) posture, (5) gait and coordinated movement or lack of it, 6) use of ambulatory aids, and (7) mood and emotional tone.

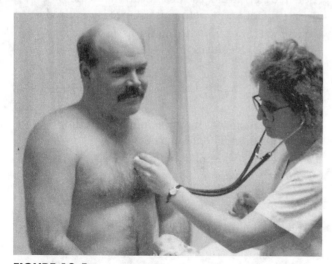

FIGURE 12-5
Auscultation of lung sounds. (Courtesy of Ken Timby.)

> **DISPLAY 12-1. *Physical Assessment Equipment***
>
> For a basic physical assessment, the nurse needs:
> * Gloves
> * Patient gown
> * Cloth or paper drapes
> * Scale
> * Stethoscope
> * Sphygmomanometer
> * Thermometer
> * Penlight or flashlight
> * Tongue blade
> * Assessment form and pen

Preliminary assessments, such as measuring the vital signs and obtaining the patient's height and weight, are documented at this time.

VITAL SIGNS

Because vital signs provide information about many aspects of general health, they are usually obtained during the initial survey (see Chap. 11).

WEIGHT AND HEIGHT

The patient's weight and height are measured and documented because they provide more reliable data than the nurse's subjective assessment of body size. These recorded measurements are extremely important in assessing trends in future weight loss or gain. For hospitalized patients, weight and height may be used to calculate appropriate drug dosages.

In most cases, adult patients and older children can tolerate being weighed and measured with a balanced standing scale (Fig. 12-7). A chair or bed scale is used to weigh critically ill or inactive patients.

NURSING GUIDELINES FOR OBTAINING WEIGHT AND HEIGHT

* Check that the scale is calibrated at zero.
  Rationale: Ensures accuracy
* Ask or assist the patient to remove all but a minimum of clothing, including shoes.
  Rationale: Facilitates measuring actual body weight
* Place a paper towel on the scale before the patient stands on it in bare feet.

(*text continues on page 176*)

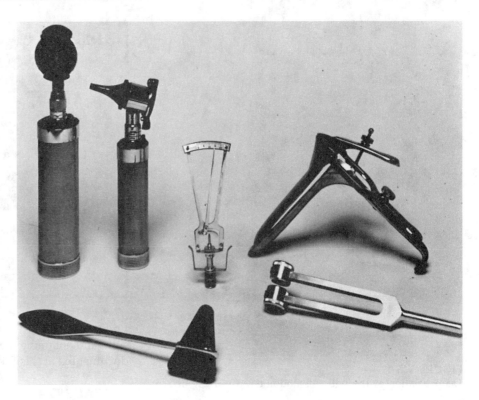

FIGURE 12-6
In a clockwise direction, starting at the top left, additional examination equipment includes an ophthalmoscope, otoscope with speculum attached, tonometer, vaginal speculum, tuning fork, and percussion hammer.

SKILL 12-1
Performing a Physical Assessment

Suggested Action	Reason for Action
Assessment	
Identify the patient.	Ensures that the assessment is performed on the correct person
Determine the age, gender, and race of the patient.	Forms the basis for planning techniques for physical assessment
Note the patient's state of alertness and ability to move about.	Aids in determining the best location for the assessment and whether assistance is required
Ask the patient's opinion about his or her health status and any current or recent signs and symptoms.	Helps focus attention during the assessment on particular structures and their functions
Planning	
Give the patient a specimen container, if a urine sample is needed.	Takes advantage of an opportunity when the patient's bladder contains urine
Have the patient empty his or her bladder before undressing.	Facilitates the examination and reduces discomfort
Ensure privacy and give the patient a drape or grown.	Prepares the patient for proper assessment
Gather assessment equipment and supplies (see Display 12-1 for basic necessities)	Promotes organization and efficient time management

(continued)

SKILL 12-1
Performing a Physical Assessment *(Continued)*

Suggested Action	Reason for Action
Decide on a head-to-toe or body systems approach.	Establishes the plan for assessment and ensures that the data is gathered in a comprehensive manner
Implementation	
Explain the general plan for the assessment procedure.	Informs the patient, which may help reduce anxiety
Explain that all information is kept confidential among those who are involved in the patient's care.	Encourages the patient to be honest and open in identifying health problems
Wash your hands thoroughly and preferably in the presence of the patient.	Provides reassurance that the nurse is clean and conscientious about controlling the spread of microorganisms
Warm your hands before touching the patient.	Demonstrates concern for the patient's comfort.
Obtain the patient's height, weight, and vital signs.	Contributes to the general survey of the patient
Assist the patient to sit at the bottom of an examination table.	Facilitates examination of the upper body without requiring the patient to change positions
Modify the patient's position if the examination is being conducted in locations other than an examination room.	Demonstrates adaptability
Explain each assessment technique before it is performed.	Reduces anxiety
Try to avoid tiring the patient and apologize if the patient experiences discomfort	Demonstrates concern for the patient's comfort
Help the patient to resume sitting after the examination.	Places the patient in the best position for communicating
Wash your hands once again.	Shows responsibility for controlling the spread of microorganisms.
Review pertinent findings, both normal and abnormal, without making medical interpretations.	Demonstrates compliance with the patient's right to information.
Offer the patient an opportunity to ask questions.	Encourages active participation in learning and decision-making
Leave while the patient dresses or dons a bathrobe if safe to do so.	Ensures privacy
Help the patient leave the examination room.	Demonstrates courtesy and concern for the patient's safety
Dispose of soiled equipment, restore cleanliness and order to the examination room, and restock used supplies.	Shows consideration for the next person who uses the examination room

(continued)

SKILL 12-1
Performing a Physical Assessment (Continued)

Suggested Action	Reason for Action

Evaluation

- All aspects of the assessment have been carried out
- A comprehensive amount of data has been collected
- The patient remained safe, warm, and comfortable
- The patient's questions or concerns have been addressed

Document

- Date and time
- All normal and abnormal findings
- Any unexpected outcomes during the procedure and the nursing actions that were taken
- To whom abnormal information was verbally reported, and outcome of the communication

Sample Documentation*

Date and Time   67-year-old male transported from bed to examination room per wheel chair for physical assessment. Able to cooperate without distress. Refer to assessment form for examination findings. _____ **Signature, Title**

*The documentation of an actual assessment is quite lengthy. Students are therefore encouraged to read examples of physical assessment findings documented within the medical records of assigned patients.

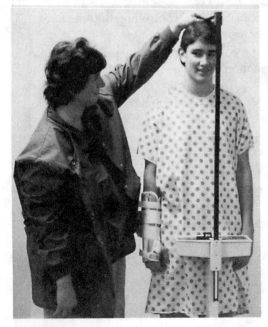

FIGURE 12-7
Assessment of height and weight. (Courtesy of Ken Timby.)

Rationale: Helps reduce contact with microorganisms present on equipment that is used in common with other people
- Assist the patient onto the scale.
  Rationale: Prevents injury should the patient become dizzy or unstable
- Position the heavier weight in a calibrated groove of the scale arm.
  Rationale: Provides a rough approximation of the gross body weight
- Move the lighter weight across the calibrations for individual pounds and ounces until the bar balances in the center of the scale.
  Rationale: Correlates with the actual weight
- Read the weight and write it down.
  Rationale: Ensures accurate documentation
- Raise the measuring bar well above the patient's head.
  Rationale: Provides room for positioning the patient without risk of injury
- Ask the patient to stand straight and look forward.

Rationale: Facilitates measuring actual height
- Lower the measuring bar until it lightly touches the top of the patient's head.
Rationale: Correlates with actual height
- Note the height and write it down.
Rationale: Ensures accurate documentation

Draping and Positioning

Because patients are assessed with very little clothing other than a loose patient gown, they usually appreciate being covered with a drape. A **drape** is a sheet of soft cloth or paper apparel. It provides more for the patient's modesty than it does warmth.

The examination may begin with the patient in a standing or sitting position (Fig. 12-8) and proceed to positions where the patient reclines and turns from side to side. Additional positions for special examinations are described and illustrated in Chapter 13.

Approaches for Data Collection

Once the patient has been draped and positioned, further data collection is facilitated by following some organized pattern. Two common approaches for data collection are the head-to-toe and body systems approaches.

HEAD-TO-TOE APPROACH

A **head-to-toe approach**, as the name suggests, involves gathering data from the top of the body to the feet. This approach has three advantages: (1) it prevents overlooking some aspect of data collection, (2) it reduces the number of position changes required of the patient, and (3) it usually takes the least amount of time because the nurse is not constantly moving about the patient in what may appear to be a haphazard manner.

BODY SYSTEMS APPROACH

A **body systems approach** organizes data collection according to the functional systems of the body, such as the skin or integumentary system, the cardiovascular system, and so on. One advantage of collecting data in this manner is that the assessment findings tend to be clustered, making problems more easily identifiable.

DATA COLLECTION

Regardless of the approach used for data collection, the objective is to obtain essentially the same basic data. Consequently, each nurse may develop his or her own order and sequence for examining patients, or an assessment form may be used as a guide. Whichever the case, nurses strive to conduct the assessment consistently each time to avoid omitting essential information.

When collecting data, the body may be divided into six general areas: (1) the head and neck, (2) the chest, (3) the extremities, (4) the abdomen, (5) the genitalia, and (6) the anus and rectum. The discussion that follows identifies the structures that are commonly assessed, specific assessment techniques, and common assessment findings.

The Head and Neck

The assessments involving the head and neck may involve several body systems.

HEAD

When at the patient's head, the nurse may begin by assessing the patient's mental status, facial structures and their sensory functions, and the condition of the skin, oral and nasal mucous membranes, hair, and scalp.

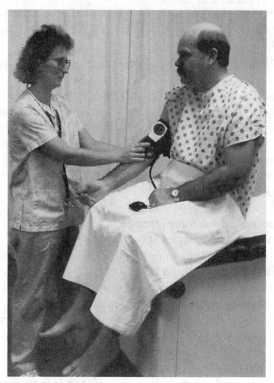

FIGURE 12-8
Patient is prepared for examination. (Courtesy of Ken Timby.)

Mental Status Assessment

A **mental status assessment** is a technique for determining the level of a patient's cognitive functions, such as attention and concentration, memory, and the ability to think abstractly. For most patients, documenting that they are alert and oriented may be all that is necessary. However, more objective assessment data may be important when caring for patients who have:

- Recovered after being unconscious
- Been recently resuscitated
- Had periods of confusion
- Sustained a head injury
- Taken overdoses of drugs
- A history of chronic alcoholism
- Psychiatric diagnoses

◄ NURSING GUIDELINES FOR PERFORMING A MENTAL STATUS EXAMINATION

- Ask the patient to identify the year, season, date, day, and month.
  Rationale: Assesses orientation to time
- Ask the patient to identify the state, county, town, and present location.
  Rationale: Assesses orientation to place
- Ask the patient to explain what kind of work you do or why he or she is in the present location.
  Rationale: Assesses orientation to person
- Name three objects—for example, book, dog, and cup; have the patient repeat the words, and explain that he or she will be asked to give the same list of words in approximately 5 minutes.
  Rationale: Ensures that the patient heard the three words and understands the subsequent task
- Request that the patient add two simple numbers, like 3 plus 5.
  Rationale: Assesses ability to perform simple mathematical computations
- Have the patient count backwards from 100 in a series of three; for example 100, 97, 94, 91, and so on. Stop after five answers.
  Rationale: Assesses attention and concentration
- Ask the patient to spell the word "world" backwards as an alternative to counting backwards by serial threes.
  Rationale: Assesses attention and concentration
- Show the patient a common object, like a watch or pencil, and ask the patient to name the object.
  Rationale: Tests whether the brain can interpret a visual stimulus correctly

- Ask the patient to explain an abstract, but commonly used, figure of speech, such as, "That child is sharp as a tack."
  Rationale: Assesses the patient's ability to think abstractly
- Ask the patient to explain a proverb, such as "Don't cry over spilled milk."
  Rationale: Provides a second method for validating a person's ability to think abstractly
- Have the patient list three large cities in the United States, or the current and last two presidents.
  Rationale: Tests the patient's knowledge and long-term memory
- Hold up a piece of paper and give the following instructions: (1) take the paper in your right hand, (2) fold it in half, and (3) place it on the floor.
  Rationale: Tests the patient's ability to follow instructions
- Ask the patient to recall the names of the three objects listed previously.
  Rationale: Assesses short-term memory

After a mental status assessment, it is important to document the assessment technique and the patient's responses, even if they were correct or normal. The assessment is performed daily to detect an improvement or worsening of mental state.

Facial Structures and Functions

When the head of a patient is examined, the appearance and symmetry of craniofacial structures, like the eyes, ears, nose, and mouth, and their respective functions are included in the physical assessment.

Eyes. Probably one of the most obvious assessments, when examining the head, is the appearance of the eyes. The eyes are usually of similar size and distance from the center of the face. Each iris is the same color, the sclerae (plural for sclera) appear white, the corneas are clear, and eyelashes are present along the margins of each eye. Structures within the eye may be examined by more advanced practitioners with an instrument called an *ophthalmoscope* (see Fig. 12-6).

After gross inspection, functions like visual acuity, pupil size and response, and ocular movement are assessed.

Visual Acuity. Central vision, or the ability to see both far and near, is called **visual acuity**. Although a detailed eye examination is not routinely performed on every patient who is hospitalized, it is always appropriate to inquire whether the patient wears glasses, contact lenses, has a false eye, or considers himself or herself blind.

To grossly assess far vision, the nurse may have the patient cover one eye at a time and from a distance of about 20 feet count the number of fingers being raised. Patients are permitted to wear their corrective lenses during this assessment. For close vision, patients are asked to read newsprint (if they are literate) from approximately 14 inches away.

A more objective method for measuring far vision is the use of a **Snellen eye chart** (Fig. 12-9). Each line on the Snellen eye chart is printed in progressively smaller letters or symbols. Patients are asked to "read" the smallest line that can be seen comfortably from a distance of 20 feet, both with and without their corrective lenses. The patient's vision is then compared with standard norms.

Normal vision is defined as the ability to read printed letters seen by most people without prescription lenses at a distance of 20 feet. Assessment findings are written as a fraction. Normal vision is 20/20. If, for example, at 20 feet from the chart, a person could see only the first line—one that can be seen by people with normal vision from 200 feet away, the patient's visual acuity is written as 20/200. Near vision is tested using a **Jaeger chart**, which has small-sized print (Fig. 12-10).

Pupil Size and Response. The size of each pupil is estimated in millimeters (mm) under normal light conditions (Fig. 12-11). Normal pupils are round and equal in size. They also constrict simultaneously when stimulated with light. That is, *both* pupils get smaller when each respective eye is stimulated with light—a phenomenon referred to as a **consensual response** (Fig. 12-12). Normal pupils also constrict simultaneously when looking at a near object, and dilate when looking at an object in the distance, a process referred to as **accommodation** (Fig. 12-13). Normal findings may be documented using the abbreviation *PERRLA*, meaning: *Pupils Equally Round and React to Light and Accommodation.*

◀ NURSING GUIDELINES FOR ASSESSING PUPILLARY RESPONSE

- Dim the lights in the examination area.
  Rationale: Facilitates pupil dilation
- Instruct the patient to stare straight ahead.
  Rationale: Facilitates pupil dilation
- Bring a narrow beam of light, like that from a penlight or small flashlight, from the temple toward the eye.
  Rationale: Provides a direct stimulus for pupil constriction
- Observe the pupil of the stimulated eye as well as the unstimulated pupil (the response should be the same).
  Rationale: Indicates status of brain function
- Repeat the assessment by directly stimulating the opposite eye.
  Rationale: Provides comparative data
- Ask the patient to look at a finger or object approximately 4 inches (10 cm) from his or her face.
  Rationale: Patient's pupils should get smaller
- Tell the patient to look from the near object to another that is more distant.
  Rationale: Patient's pupils should get larger

Extraocular Movements. Eye movements that can be voluntarily produced are called **extraocular movements** (EOMS). EOMS are controlled by several pairs of eye muscles. To assess EOMS, the patient is asked to focus on and track the nurse's finger or some other object as it is moved in each of six positions (Fig. 12-14). During the assessment, both eyes should move in a coordinated manner. Absence of movement in one or the

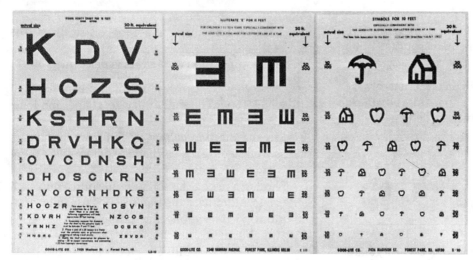

FIGURE 12-9
Snellen eye charts. (Courtesy of Ken Timby.)

Near V. E. %: 5
Jaeger 14

24 Point

Acuity: Approx. 0.12(20/170)
Sight-saving texts.

man oxen   25 37 84 90   OXXO OXXX

Near V. E.%: 10
Jaeger 12

18 Point

Acuity: Approx. 0.15 (20/130)
Books, children 7-8 yrs.

raw see van   90 89 76 60 54   XOXXX OXOOO

Near V. E. %: 15
Jaeger 10

14 Point

Acuity: Approx. 0.2 (20/100)
Books, children 8-9 yrs.

noon even mew   38 72 80 93 54 60 76   XXOX XXXX OOOX

Near V. E. %: 20
Jaeger 8

12 Point

Acuity Approx. 0.25 (20/80)
Books, children 9-12 yrs.

war use worm eve
avenue ransom err

40 53 82 64 79 60 47
809 423 657 980 765

XOOX OOOXO OOXXX
remo romero suma

Near V. E. %: 30
Jaeger 7

10 Point

Acuity: Approx. 0.28 (20/70)
Adult textbooks.

scum crease nervous
cocoon cannon saucer

98 67 45 34 23 50 86 73 98
456 309 582 740 605 482 765

XOOO OXXO OXXX XXXX
saca zarco cascarron

Near V. E. %: 40
Jaeger 6

9 Point

Acuity: Approx. 0.3 (20/65)
Magazines.

arrow scour noose razor
zone reverence sorceress

35 98 20 82 47 30 74 73 42 65 27
740 203 965 423 807 203 460 244

XXXO OOXX OXOOX XOXOX
remanso semana asma

Near V. E. %: 50
Jaeger 5

8 Point

Acuity: Approx. 0.4 (20/50)
Newspaper text.

amaze wares curve scarce
snooze caress sewer wax

82 34 65 90 53 83 67 46 98 65 42 54
426 397 564 782 206 360 375 389 246

OXXO OOOO XOXX XXXX OOOX
remesa   suave   arrancar

Near V. E. %: 90
Jaeger 3

6 Point

Acuity: Approx. 0.5 (20/40)
Telephone directory.

comma worse reason measure vase
census arrears recover crane now

75 23 68 90 44 80 40 93 92 43 79 60 47 35
890 375 204 534 806 867 654 302 246 479 268

XOXX OOXO OXXO OXOO XXOX OOOO
resaca carecer crecer sazonar

Near V. E. %: 95
Jaeger 2

5 Point

Acuity: Approx. 0.6 (20/30)
Want ads.

success numerous assurance consume
cocoa convex morocco uncommon err

56 87 92 30 47 92 45 27 90 80 46 21 45 80
209 354 872 405 625 829 234 350 575 482 981

XOXX OOOX OOXO OOXXX XOXO XXOX OXOO
sesos sucesor vaso zamarra azar

Near V. E. %: 100
Jaeger 1

4 Point

Acuity: Approx. 0.8 (20/25)
Small bibles.

occurrence nevertheless successor romance worm
craze arson crew amorous snow aroma samovar

72 95 40 56 36 55 80 60 30 57 99 46
284 454 306 905 283 400 244 825 350

XXXOX XXOOO OOOO OOXO XXOX XXXO OOOXO
comarcano   rosca   serrano   amanecer

Comparable:
Jaeger 1+

3 Point

Acuity: Approx. 1.0 (20/20)
Mailorder catalogues.

XOXO XXOO OOOO OOXO XXOX XXXO OOOXO
escarcer   mettano   avance   buffo   crasano   calisto

FIGURE 12-10
A Jaeger chart. (Courtesy of Ken Timby.)

other eyes may indicate cranial nerve damage; irregular or uncoordinated movement may suggest other neurologic pathology.

Ears. During a physical assessment, external ears are examined by inspection and palpation. More advanced practitioners may use an instrument called an *otoscope*

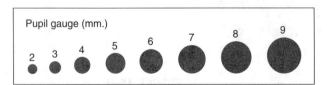

FIGURE 12-11
Pupil sizes can be estimated from printed assessment guides.

to examine the tympanic membrane, or ear drum (see Fig. 12-6).

A gross examination of the ears is performed by:

* Observing the appearance of the ears, both of which should be similar in size, shape, and location.
* Moving the skin behind and in front of the ears as well as the ear's cartilage to determine if there is any tenderness.
* Shining a penlight or other light source into each ear to illuminate the ear canal. To obtain optimum visualization, the curved ear canal is straightened as much as possible. For children, this is done by pulling each ear down and back;

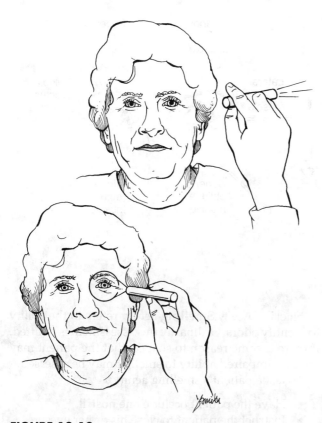

FIGURE 12-12
Testing pupillary response to light.

on an adult, each ear is pulled up and back (Fig. 12-15). **Cerumen**, also known as ear wax, a yellowish-brown, waxy secretion produced by glands within the ear, is a common finding. Any other type of drainage is abnormal, and its characteristics are described and reported.

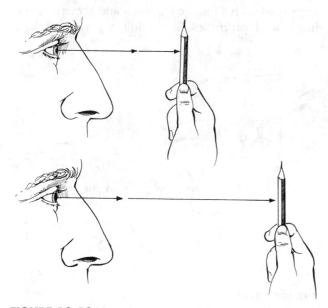

FIGURE 12-13
Testing accommodation.

Gross Hearing Acuity. Gross **hearing acuity**, or the ability to hear and discriminate sound, may be assessed by performing either a **voice test** or **watch-tick test**.

NURSING GUIDELINES FOR PERFORMING A VOICE TEST

- Stand approximately 2 feet behind and to the side of the patient.
  Rationale: Simulates the distance between most people during social interaction and prevents the patient from observing visual cues
- Instruct the patient to cover the ear on the opposite side.
  Rationale: Facilitates sound conduction to only the tested ear
- Whisper a color, number, or name into the uncovered ear.
  Rationale: Delivers a high-pitched sound, the most common type of hearing loss, toward the tested ear
- Instruct the patient to repeat the whispered word.
  Rationale: Reveals the ability to discriminate sound
- Continue the same pattern using several more words; increase the volume from a soft to medium to loud whisper or spoken voice if the patient's response is inaccurate.
  Rationale: Provides more reliable data
- Repeat the test on the opposite ear.
  Rationale: Provides separate assessment findings for each ear

A watch-tick test provides the same data as a voice test but is performed somewhat differently. When the watch-tick test is done:

- The nurse sits beside the patient, but facing the opposite direction
- The patient is told to cover the ear on the side opposite the nurse
- A watch is held an equal distance between the nurse's ear and that of the patient
- The patient is asked to indicate if the ticking can be heard
- The test is repeated for the other ear

Another variation of the watch-tick test consists of moving the watch away from both the nurse and the patient. If the nurse has normal hearing, the patient should be unable to hear the ticking at the same distance as the nurse.

Some nurses may use a tuning fork to determine if patients have impaired hearing due to nerve damage or disorders that interfere with sound conduction. The

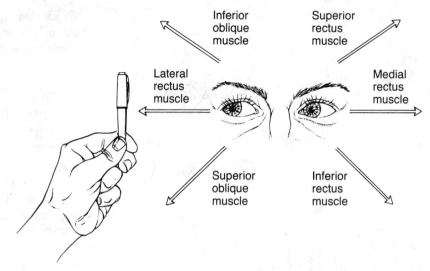

FIGURE 12-14
Assessing extraocular movements.

Weber test (Fig. 12-16) is performed by striking a tuning fork and placing it in the middle of the patient's skull or forehead. This tests aids in determining if sound is heard equally in both ears. If the sound is heard bilaterally, it indicates a normal finding or that the hearing in both ears is equally diminished. Hearing the sound louder in one ear is a sign of unequal hearing loss. The **Rinne test** (Fig. 12-17) is a method for comparing air versus bone conduction of sound. Normally, sound is heard longer by air conduction when the tuning fork is placed beside the ear, rather than pressed behind the ear. If the reverse is true, or if sound is heard for equal periods of time, it indicates a problem with the structures that collect and transmit sound through the ear, or it can indicate nerve damage.

More sophisticated tests may be performed by *audiologists*, professionals who are trained to test hearing with standardized instruments. When audiometric hearing tests are used, exact pitch and volume deficits are measured. Hearing deficits are measured in decibels, the intensity of sound. The greater the intensity of sound before it is perceived, the more impaired the hearing (Table 12-2). Whenever patients rely on a hearing aid for amplifying sound, that information is always noted on the assessment form.

Nose. The nose and nasal passages are inspected by having the patient assume a "sniffing position." The septum, or tissue that divides the nose in half, should be in midline, causing the nasal passages to be equal in size. Deeper inspection may be facilitated by pressing at the tip of the nose. Air should move fairly quietly through the nose during breathing. The mucous membrane within the nose should be pink and moist, but free of obvious drainage. The presence of a deviated septum, lesions or growths of any kind, flaring of the nostrils, and characteristics of unusual drainage are documented in the patient's assessment findings.

Smelling Acuity. **Smelling acuity** refers to the ability to identify odors. Ordinarily this assessment is omitted. If there is some reason to suspect that the patient may have an impaired ability to smell, it may be assessed.

To test a patient's smelling acuity:

* Have the patient occlude one nostril
* Instruct the patient to close his or her eyes
* Place substances with strong odors, like lemon, vanilla extract, coffee, peppermint, or alcohol one at a time, beneath the patent's (open) nostril
* Ask the patient to inhale and identify the substance

Mouth and Oral Mucous Membranes. The mouth is surrounded by the lips and contains the tongue and teeth, which may be inspected by having the patient open his or her mouth widely. The tongue, before it is depressed with a tongue blade, should remain in midline when it protrudes. In an adult, at least 28 of the 32

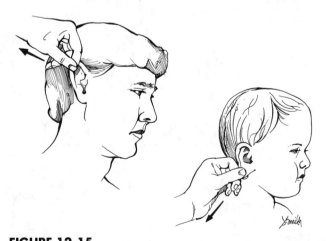

FIGURE 12-15
An adult's ear is pulled up and back; a child's ear is pulled down and back to facilitate inspection.

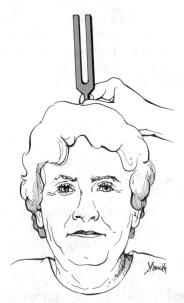

FIGURE 12-16
Performing the Weber test.

TABLE 12-2. *Hearing Acuity Levels*

Hearing Level	Decibel Range
Normal	0–25 dB
Mildly impaired	26–30 dB
Moderately impaired	31–55 dB
Moderately to severely impaired	56–70 dB
Severely impaired	71–90 dB
Profoundly impaired	91 dB or greater

permanent teeth should be present and in good repair. The presence of dentures, missing or malpositioned teeth, or a partial plate is documented. Sometimes there are unusual odors to the breath that may be diagnostic. For example, the odor of alcohol or acetone may suggest health problems.

The oral mucous membranes should appear pink and intact. They are kept moist by salivary glands located below the tongue. When the patient is asked to smile, purse the lips as though preparing to whistle, or show the teeth, the lips should look the same.

Taste. The tongue contains many taste buds that detect particular taste characteristics (Fig. 12-18). Although assessing taste is rarely done, it is facilitated by placing substances on the tongue and asking the patient to identify them. To ensure valid results, the patient is encouraged to sip water between assessments.

Facial Skin. Characteristics of the facial skin may be noted while assessing the head. Although skin assessment may begin in this area, it continues as other areas of the body are examined. Regardless of where the skin

is examined, it should be smooth, unbroken, of uniform color according to the patient's ethnic or racial origin, warm, resilient, and feel neither wet nor unusually dry. Variations in skin color, which may be diagnostic, are listed in Table 12-3.

While examining the skin, the nurse may detect several common changes in its integrity:

- A *wound* is a break in the skin.
- An *ulcer* is an open, crater-like area.
- An *abrasion* is an area that has been rubbed away by friction.
- A *laceration* is a torn, jagged wound.
- A *fissure* is a crack in the skin, especially in or near mucous membranes.
- A *scar* is a mark left by the healing of a wound or lesion.

Other common skin lesions and their characteristics are described in Table 12-4. Additional skin assessments are described in later discussions within this chapter.

Hair

The assessment of the hair includes that which covers the head, including the eyebrows and eyelashes. Usually the color, texture, and distribution—its presence or absence in unusual locations for gender or age—are noted. The hair is also inspected for the presence of unusual debris such as blood in the case of head trauma,

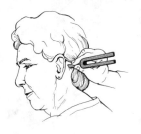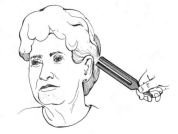

FIGURE 12-17
Performing the Rinne test.

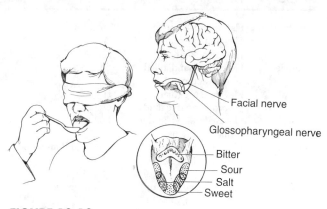

FIGURE 12-18
Assessing taste.

TABLE 12-3. *Common Skin Color Variations*

Color	Term	Possible Causes
Pale, regardless of race (see Chap. 6)	Pallor	Anemia, blood loss
Red	Erythema	Superficial burns, local inflammation, carbon monoxide poisoning
Pink	Flushed	Fever, hypertension
Purple	Ecchymosis	Trauma to soft tissue
Blue	Cyanosis	Low tissue oxygenation
Yellow	Jaundice	Liver or kidney disease, destruction of red blood cells
Brown	Tan	Ethnic variation, sun exposure, pregnancy, Addison's disease

nits (eggs from a louse infestation), or scales from scalp lesions. As the physical assessment progresses, the characteristics of body hair are also observed.

Scalp

The scalp is assessed by separating the hair at random areas and inspecting the skin. Primarily, the nurse looks for signs indicating that the scalp is smooth, intact, and free of lesions. While examining the scalp, the nurse may also palpate the skull for the presence of any unusual contour.

NECK

The neck supports the head in midline. The patient should be able to bend the head forward, backward, and to either side, as well as rotate it in a 180° arc. The trachea, or windpipe, should appear in the center of

TABLE 12-4. *Common Skin Lesions*

Type of Lesion	Description	Examples
Macule	Flat, round, colored	Freckles
Papule	Elevated, obvious raised border, solid	Wart
Vesicle	Elevated, round, filled with serum	Blister
Wheal	Elevated, irregular border, no free fluid	Hives
Pustule	Elevated, raised border, filled with pus	Boil
Nodule	Elevated, solid mass, extends into deeper tissue	Enlarged lymph node
Cyst	Encapsulated, round, fluid-filled, or solid mass beneath the skin	Tissue growth

the neck. The pulsations in the carotid arteries (see Fig. 11-8 in Chap. 11) should be visible and easily palpated.

There should be no unusual bulges or fullness in the neck. Some nurses may palpate the lymph nodes in the neck area (Fig. 12-19) or assess for an enlarged thyroid gland.

The Chest

The chest is a cavity surrounded by the ribs and the spinal vertebrae. It is the area where the heart and lungs are located. When the chest is examined, the nurse observes the shape of the chest and how it moves during breathing, notes the curved appearance of the spine, and assesses skin turgor, the breasts, heart sounds, and lung sounds.

CHEST SHAPE AND MOVEMENT

There may be variations in the appearance of the chest as a result of musculoskeletal abnormalities, cardiac or respiratory diseases, or trauma (Fig. 12-20). When the patient breathes, the chest should rise and fall equally on both sides of the body. To assess if the chest is moving equally in a lateral position:

- Place the thumbs side by side over the posterior vertebrae at about the level of the 10th rib (Fig. 12-21).
- As the patient inhales, note how far the thumbs separate; normally the distance is 1 to 2 inches (3–5 cm).

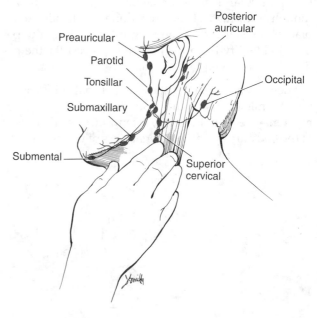

FIGURE 12-19
Light palpation of lymph nodes.

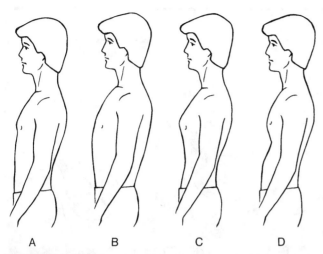

FIGURE 12-20
Common chest variations: (*A*) normal, (*B*) barrel chest, (*C*) pigeon chest, and (*D*) funnel chest.

SPINE

The spine, or column of vertebrae, should appear in midline with gentle concave and convex curves when viewed from the side. The shoulders should appear at equal height. Some common deviations may be noted (Fig. 12-22). For example, *lordosis* is a condition in which the natural lumbar curve of the spine is exaggerated. *Kyphosis* is an increased curve in the thoracic area, and *scoliosis* is a pronounced lateral curvature of the spine.

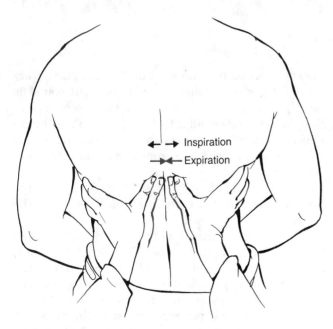

FIGURE 12-21
Checking for equal chest excursion.

SKIN TURGOR

Turgor is a term that refers to the resiliency of the skin. Turgor is a combination of the elastic quality of the skin and the pressure exerted on it by fluid within the tissue. To assess skin turgor, the skin is grasped between the thumb and fingers in an attempt to lift it from the underlying tissue. The area over the chest is a good assessment location because the skin in other areas tends to become loose with aging. When the tissue is released, it should immediately return to its original position. Prolonged tenting may indicate dehydration.

BREASTS

Breasts appear different depending on the gender of the patient. Although abnormalities, such as tumors, may be present in either women or men, they are more common in women. The breast examination may be deferred in certain situations. However, because breast tumors are common and their early diagnosis ensures a better prognosis, nurses have a responsibility for teaching patients about examining their breasts on a routine basis.

Breast self-examination should be combined with additional diagnostic breast examinations to ensure early diagnosis and treatment of cancerous tumors (Table 12-5).

HEART SOUNDS

When assessing the anterior chest, the nurse listens to the heart sounds that are caused by the closing of the atrial and ventricular heart valves.

A beginning nurse may choose to limit the assessment to the apical area (see section on Apical Heart Rate in Chap. 11). With experience, nurses may expand their assessment skills to include auscultation at the aortic, pulmonic, tricuspid, and mitral areas (Fig. 12-23).

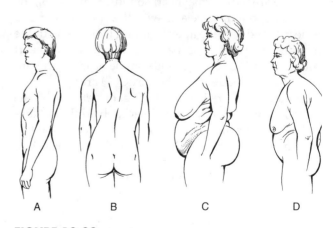

FIGURE 12-22
Variations in spinal curves: (*A*) normal, (*B*) scoliosis, (*C*) lordosis, and (*D*) kyphosis.

PATIENT TEACHING FOR BREAST SELF-EXAMINATION

Teach the patient to do the following:

- Examine the breasts monthly about a week after a menstrual cycle or on a specific date if menstruation has ceased.
- Begin the examination in the shower.
- Use the right hand to examine the left breast and the left hand to examine the right breast.
- Place the hand on the side that will be examined behind the head.
- Glide the flat portion of the fingers over all aspects of each breast in a circular fashion.
- Determine if there are any lumps, hard knots, or thickened areas.
- Next, stand in front of a mirror.
- Look at the appearance of both breasts with the arms relaxed at the side, with the hands pressing on the hips, and elevated above the head.
- Look for dimpling in the skin or retraction of either nipple.
- Lie down for the remainder of the examination.
- Put a pillow or folded towel under the shoulder on the side where the first breast will be examined; reverse the pillow before examining the second breast.
- Again, place the arm behind the head.
- Press the flat surface of the fingers in small circular motions from the outer margin of the breast toward the nipple or as in spokes of a wheel.

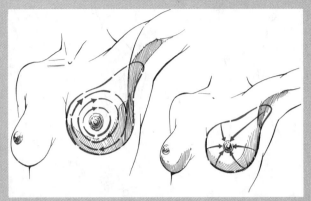

Breast tissue extends well into the axilla; palpation is performed using either of these two techniques.

- Also feel upward toward the axilla of each arm.
- Complete at least three revolutions about the breast.
- Squeeze the nipple gently between the thumb and index finger to determine if there is any clear or bloody discharge.
- Repeat the examination on the opposite breast and axilla.
- Report any unusual findings or changes that become apparent to a physician.

Normal Heart Sounds

There are two normal heart sounds, S_1 and S_2. S_1, the first heart sound, correlates with the "lub" sound and is heard louder at the apex or mitral (M) area with the diaphragm of a stethoscope. Although the second heart sound, S_2 or the "dub" sound, can be heard in the mitral area, it is louder over the aortic (A) area.

Sometimes there is tiny slurring, or *splitting*, of one or both sounds. It may sound like "lubba-dub" or "lub-dubba." Split sounds are usually attributed to the fact that the valves between the atria (or the ventricles) do not always close in exact unison. Splitting, if heard at all, is usually noted with the stethoscope at point "P" or "T" on the chest.

Abnormal Heart Sounds

The nurse may hear two additional sounds, identified as S_3 and S_4, when auscultating the chest. An S_3 may be normal in children, but it is considered abnormal for most adults. When an S_3 heart sound is heard, it appears *after* the S_2 sound in a sequence of S_1-S_2-S_3. It sounds similar to "lub-dub-**dub**" or the cadence of sounds in the syllables of "Ken-tuck-y." A third sound is much more pronounced than a split second sound.

The S_4 sound is heard just *before* the S_1 sound, as in S_4-S_1-S_2. It may sound more like "**lub**-lub-dub" or the syllables in "Ten-nes-see."

Identifying abnormal heart sounds, like S_3 and S_4, and other unique sounds like heart murmurs, clicks, and rubs, is a developed skill that is mastered after becoming proficient at distinguishing between S_1 and S_2. In the meantime, the best advice is to consult with another experienced nurse or the physician if there is any unusual characteristic in the heart sounds.

TABLE 12-5. *Breast Examination Guidelines*

Technique	Age	Frequency
Self-examination	≥20 years	Once per month
Clinical examination by a nurse or physician	20–40 years	Every 3 years
Mammography	≥40 years	Every year
	40 years	First examination
	40–49 years	Every 1–2 years
	≥50 years	Annually

Source: American Cancer Society.

LUNG SOUNDS

Listening to the lungs is a skill that also requires frequent and repeated practice because some sounds are normal and others are abnormal.

Normal Lung Sounds

Normal lung sounds are created by air moving in and out of passageways that vary in their location and size. Therefore, the sounds vary in pitch and duration depending on the area being auscultated (Fig. 12-24). There are four normal lung sounds:

Tracheal sounds are loud and coarse. They are equal in length during inspiration and expiration, and separated by a brief pause in between.
Bronchial sounds, heard over the upper area of the sternum, are harsh and loud, shorter on inspiration than expiration, with a pause between the two.

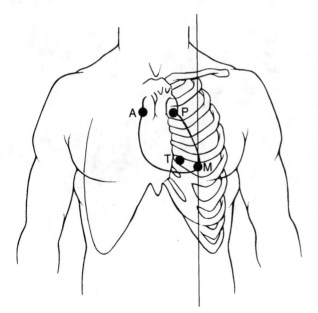

FIGURE 12-23
Locations for assessing heart sounds: M = mitral area, T = tricuspid area, P = pulmonic area, A = aortic area.

Bronchovesicular sounds are heard on either side of the central chest or back. They are medium-range sounds that are equal in length during inspiration and expiration, with no noticeable pause.
Vesicular sounds are located in the periphery of all the lung fields. Their soft, rustling quality is longer on inspiration than expiration, with no pause in between.

Abnormal Lung Sounds

Abnormal lung sounds, known as *adventitious sounds*, are those that are heard *in addition to* normal lung sounds. Most adventitious sounds are created by air moving through secretions or narrowed airways.

Adventitious sounds, named for their descriptive sounds, are divided into four categories:

Crackles, or *rales*, are intermittent, high-pitched, popping sounds heard in distant areas of the lungs primarily during inspiration. They resemble the sound of crisp rice cereal when milk is added. The sound is attributed to the opening of partially collapsed alveoli (terminal air sacs) or the movement of air over minute amounts of fluid in the periphery of the lungs during deep inspiration.
Gurgles, or *rhonchi*, are low-pitched, continuous, bubbling sounds heard in larger airways. They are more prominent during expiration. Some describe gurgles as sounding like "wet snoring." Gurgles may clear with deep breathing or coughing.
Wheezes are whistling or squeaking sounds caused by air moving through a narrowed passage. They can be heard anywhere throughout the chest during inspiration or expiration. Sometimes these sounds are audible without a stethoscope. Coughing and deep breathing do not usually alter a wheeze. In fact, if wheezing suddenly stops, it may mean that the air passage is totally occluded.
Rubs are grating, or leathery, sounds caused by two dry pleural surfaces moving over one another.

Whenever adventitious sounds are heard, the nurse also assesses the characteristics of any cough that may be present and the appearance of sputum that is raised.

NURSING GUIDELINES FOR ASSESSING LUNG SOUNDS

• Wash your hands.
Rationale: Reduces the spread of infection
• Provide privacy.
Rationale: Demonstrates concern for patient modesty
• Raise the bed to a comfortable position for you.

Rationale: Reduces strain on the musculoskeletal system
- Assist the patient to a sitting position, if possible.
Rationale: Facilitates auscultating the anterior, posterior, and lateral aspects of the chest with minimal exertion on the patient's part.
- Remove or loosen the patient's upper clothing.
Rationale: Aids in identifying anatomic landmarks
- Reduce or eliminate sources of environmental noise, such as suction motors and oxygen equipment if possible.
Rationale: Improves the perception of lung sounds
- Ask the patient not to talk.
Rationale: Interferes with concentration and distorts lung sounds
- Warm the diaphragm of the stethoscope in the palm of your hand.
Rationale: Reduces discomfort when applied to the chest
- Instruct the patient to breathe in and out deeply, but slowly, through an open mouth.
Rationale: Reduces noise from air turbulence and prevents hyperventilation
- Apply the chestpiece to the upper back, but avoid placement over the scapulae or ribs.
Rationale: Facilitates hearing sounds and reduces competing sounds from the heart
- Listen for one complete ventilation (inspiration and expiration) at each area that is auscultated.

Rationale: Ensures hearing characteristics during each phase of ventilation.
- Wet body hair that causes noise or press harder with the chestpiece.
Rationale: Reduces sound distortion
- Move the diaphragm from side to side from the apices (top) to the bases (bottom) of the lungs (Fig. 12-25).
Rationale: Aids in comparing the characteristics of sounds
- Auscultate the lateral and anterior chest in a similar fashion (Fig. 12-26).
Rationale: Ensures a comprehensive assessment
- Ask the patient to cough or breathe deeply if crackles or gurgles are heard.
Rationale: Helps to clear the air passages and open the alveoli
- Reapply clothing and lower the patient's bed.
Rationale: Restores comfort and safety
- Wash your hands.
Rationale: Reduces the spread of microorganisms
- Record assessment findings.
Rationale: Documents data that can be used for future comparisons
- Repeat lung sound assessments according to agency policy or condition of the patient.
Rationale: Demonstrates responsibility, accountability, and good clinical judgment

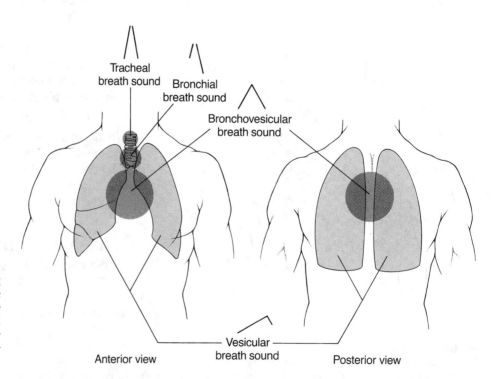

FIGURE 12-24
Locations of normal lung sounds. The symbols indicate the ratio of time they may be heard during inspiration and expiration, as well as the presence or absence of pauses between the two.

Tracheal breath sound
Bronchial breath sound
Bronchovesicular breath sound
Vesicular breath sound
Anterior view
Posterior view

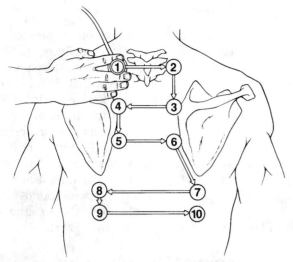

FIGURE 12-25
Systematically comparing posterior lung sounds.

The Extremities

Before examining the abdomen, genitalia, and anus, the nurse may assess the arms and legs. In general, when the extremities are examined, the nurse notes their alignment, mobility, and strength, and compares the size of one with the other.

The nurse also feels the skin temperature, notes the characteristics of the nails and capillary refill time, palpates local peripheral pulses (see Chap. 11), checks for the presence of edema, and may test the perception of skin sensations. Advanced practitioners may assess deep tendon reflexes with a *reflex hammer*.

MUSCLE STRENGTH

All four extremities are assessed separately to determine muscle strength. The patient is asked to grasp, squeeze, and release the nurse's fingers. As the nurse pulls and pushes on the forearm and upper arm, the patient is instructed to resist. To test the strength in the lower extremities, the nurse has the patient push and pull his or her feet against a resisting hand.

FINGER AND TOE NAILS

Changes in the shape and thickness of the finger and toe nails are often signs of chronic cardiopulmonary disease (Fig. 12-27) or fungal infections. Any unusual characteristics of the nails or tissue surrounding it are documented.

Capillary Refill

Capillary refill time is the amount of time it takes blood to resume flowing in the base of compressed nailbeds. Normally, the capillary refill time is less than 3 seconds. To assess capillary refill time, the nurse (1) observes the color in the nailbed, (2) compresses the nailbed, displacing capillary blood, (3) releases the pressure, and (4) notes how many seconds it takes for the preassessment color to reappear. Because watching a clock would interfere with an accurate assessment, the nurse may count "one-one thousand, two-one thousand, three-one thousand" as a gross approximation of the time in seconds.

EDEMA

Edema is fluid that is trapped within the interstitial spaces. Patients with cardiovascular, liver, and kidney dysfunction are prone to development of edema. Subtle indications of edema include weight gain, tight rings, and patterns in the skin after socks or shoes have been removed. To determine the presence and extent of edema, the nurse presses a thumb or finger into the tissue. If an indentation remains—a condition referred to as *pitting edema*, the nurse attempts to quantify its severity (Display 12-2).

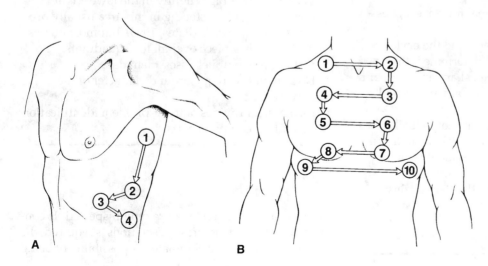

FIGURE 12-26
(*A*) Each side of the chest is auscultated and compared. (*B*) The anterior chest is systematically examined over each lung field.

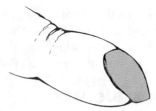

FIGURE 12-27
Clubbing. (Bates B. A Pocket Guide to Physical Examination and History Taking, p 132. Philadelphia: JB Lippincott, 1991)

SKIN SENSATION

During a comprehensive assessment, as opposed to one that is basic, the ability of the patient to differentiate between light touch, warmth, cold, sharp, dull, and vibration may be tested.

◄ NURSING GUIDELINES FOR ASSESSING SENSORY SKIN PERCEPTION

- Gather a cotton ball, safety pin or pointed object, small containers of warmed and iced water, and a tuning fork.
  Rationale: Provides a variety of testing items
- Instruct the patient to keep both eyes closed temporarily.
  Rationale: Reduces the potential for gathering invalid data
- Explain that the skin will be touched at various places and on both sides of the body with test objects and that the patient will be asked to identify the location and the characteristic of the sensation.
  Rationale: Identifies the method of the test and how the patient is expected to respond
- Touch the patient in a random pattern with the test objects.
  Rationale: Avoids the potential for correct guessing
- Use both the pointed, open end and the enclosed, curved end of a safety pin to determine if the patient can discriminate between sharp and dull, but take care that the skin is not actually punctured.
  Rationale: Prevents injury
- Stroke the skin with a wisp of the cotton ball and touch areas with both warm and cold containers.
  Rationale: Assesses the ability to identify fine touch and differences in temperatures
- Strike a tuning fork and place the stem against bony areas like the wrists and along the length of the shin bones.
  Rationale: Tests the ability to sense vibration

The Abdomen

Most of the gastrointestinal and accessory organs for digestion lie within the abdomen. Occasionally the bladder, if distended, may rise into the abdomen and be palpable.

To facilitate describing assessment findings, the abdomen is usually divided into four quadrants (Fig. 12-28). The abdomen is always inspected and then auscultated before using either palpation or percussion techniques. In addition to assessing the condition of the skin, noting the size of the abdomen, and describing palpated masses (Display 12-3), the nurse listens for the presence and characteristics of bowel sounds. Occasionally, the nurse may also detect the sound of blood pulsating through the abdominal aorta.

BOWEL SOUNDS

Bowel sounds are produced by the wave-like contractions of the large and small intestine. They are routinely assessed on admission and once per shift.

Normal bowel sounds resemble clicks or gurgles and occur 5 to 34 times a minute (Bates, 1990). They are more active after food is ingested. Bowel sounds may be described as *hyperactive*, if they are frequent, *hypoactive* if they occur after long intervals of silence, and *absent* if no sound is heard for 2 to 5 minutes (Bates, 1990).

◄ NURSING GUIDELINES FOR ASSESSING BOWEL SOUNDS

- Have the patient recline.
  Rationale: Provides access to the abdomen
- Reduce noise.
  Rationale: Facilitates an accurate assessment
- Warm the diaphragm of the stethoscope.
  Rationale: Promotes comfort
- Place the diaphragm lightly in the lower right quadrant (LRQ). Listening in this area usually provides adequate data (Bates, 1990), but most nurses move the chestpiece over all four quadrants.
  Rationale: Compiles assessment data
- Document the frequency and character of the bowel sounds.
  Rationale: Provides data for problem identification and future comparisons

The Genitalia

In most cases, the genitalia are only inspected. If contact with genital structures or secretions is required, the nurse dons gloves. To eliminate the possibility of being

---

DISPLAY 12-2. *Criteria for Estimating Pitting Edema*

1+	Slight indentation (≤2 mm); returns quickly to previous contour
2+	Deeper indentation (≥2 mm but ≤4 mm); pit remains up to 1 second
3+	Deep pit (up to 6 mm); remains several seconds; surrounding skin appears obviously swollen even after indentation subsides
4+	Pit extends to a depth of 8 mm; remains for minutes; patient may be unable to wear shoes that previously fit
>4	No pitting because of excessive volume; tissue is firm and hard; skin appears shiny, warm, and moist; may be called *brawny edema*

Descriptions adapted from Fuller J, Schaller-Ayers J. Health Assessment: A Nursing Approach. 2nd ed. Philadelphia: JB Lippincott, 1994, p. 133.

---

falsely accused of sexual impropriety, it is a good practice to ask someone who is the patient's gender to be present when the genitalia are touched.

During inspection, the condition of the skin and the distribution and any unusual characteristics of pubic hair are noted (lice may also infest pubic hair). A physician or nurse practitioner may examine women internally with an instrument called a *speculum* (see Chap. 13); the prostate gland of men may be palpated during a rectal examination.

The nurse observes whether men are circumcised and if the scrotum appears of normal size. Whenever possible, men are instructed on self-examination of their testicles (Fig. 12-29).

The Anus and Rectum

Unless the patient describes specific symptoms, only the anus is inspected. If touching is required, gloves are necessary. To examine the anus, the patient is posi-

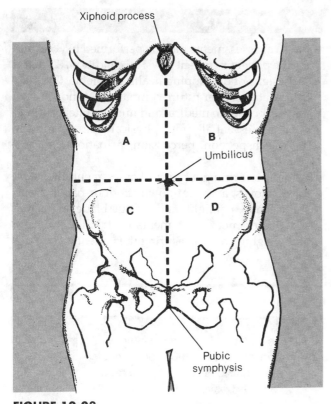

FIGURE 12-28
Four abdominal quadrants. (A) Right upper quadrand (RUQ), (B) Left upper quadrand (LUQ), (C) Right lower quadrant (RLQ), and (D) Left lower quadrant (LLQ).

DISPLAY 12-3. *Characteristics of Palpated Masses*

Characteristic	Description
Mobility	Fixed—Does not move Mobile—Can be moved with palpation
Shape	Round—Resembles a ball Tubular—Is elongated Ovoid—Resembles an egg Irregular—Has no definite shape
Consistency	Edematous—Leaves indentation when palpated Nodular—Feels bumpy to touch Granular—Feels gritty to touch Spongy—Feels soft to touch Hard—Feels firm to touch
Size	Measured in centimeters (1 cm = approximately ½ in)
Tenderness	Amount of discomfort when palpated—none, slight, moderate, or severe

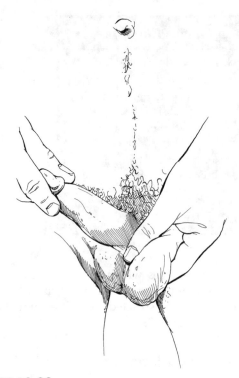

FIGURE 12-29
Testicular self-examination.

tioned on his or her side with the knees bent. The upper buttock is lifted, and the external orifice is inspected. The area should appear intact, moist, and hairless but more pigmented than the adjacent skin. External hemorrhoids, saccular protrusions filled with blood, may extend beyond the external sphincter muscle. There may be fissures present if the patient has a history of chronic constipation. Trauma may also be present due to anal intercourse, forced or otherwise.

NURSING IMPLICATIONS

Assessment findings form the basis for identifying the patient's health problems. Often during the course of a physical assessment, patients reveal situations that

APPLICABLE NURSING DIAGNOSES

- Altered Health Maintenance
- Ineffective Management of Therapeutic Regimen
- Knowledge Deficit
- Noncompliance
- Health Seeking Behaviors

caused their health to fail, or they indicate a desire for more health information. The accompanying Applicable Nursing Diagnoses may be identified after a physical assessment.

The Nursing Care Plan in this chapter is an example of how the nursing process is used whena patient has the nursing diagnosis of Health Seeking Behaviors. Health Seeking Behaviors is defined in the NANDA Taxonomy (1994) as "A state in which an individual is actively seeking ways to alter personal health habits and/or the environment in order to move toward a higher level of health."

KEY CONCEPTS

- Physical assessments may be performed to (1) evaluate the patient's current physical condition, (2) detect early signs of developing health problems, (3) establish a data base for future comparisons, and (4) evaluate responses to medical and nursing interventions.
- There are essentially four physical assessment techniques: inspection, percussion, palpation, and auscultation.
- Before performing a physical assessment, the nurse needs gloves, a patient gown, cloth or paper drape, stethoscope, penlight, and tongue blade, as well as other assessment instruments for taking vital signs and weighing and measuring the patient.

PATIENT TEACHING FOR TESTICULAR SELF-EXAMINATION

Teach the patient to do the following:

- Plan to examine the testicles monthly.
- Use an opportunity when the testicles are warm and positioned loosely within the scrotum, such as when bathing or showering.
- Gently roll each testicle between the thumb and fingers.

- Feel for the presence of an unusual lump; cancerous lumps are more often located on the upper and outer sides of the testes.
- Contact a physician as soon as possible if a lump is detected because an early diagnosis ensures a better prognosis.

NURSING CARE PLAN:
Health-Seeking Behaviors

Assessment

Subjective Data

States, "I've been having sex with a lot of women. None of them have gotten pregnant and I haven't caught any diseases as far as I know. But, I don't want to take chances anymore."

Objective Data

19-year-old man scheduled for inguinal hernia repair as an outpatient in 3 days. Circumcised penis with bilaterally descended testicles. Slight bulge in R. inguinal area. No discharge from penis. Has vaginal sex at least four times a week. Currently has three sexual partners. Requests information on safer sex practices and use of condoms.

Diagnosis

Health Seeking Behaviors: Preventing sexually transmitted diseases and pregnancy.

Plan

Goal

The patient will identify safer sex practices by 10/13 and use them during future sexual activities.

Orders: 10/10

1. Give assorted pamphlets and free condoms from Reproductive Control Clinic.
2. Emphasize the following safer sex practices:
   - Reduce sexual partners to one noninfected, faithful person.
   - Use a latex condom and nonoxynol-9 spermicide either over the tip of the condom or as a vaginal application.
   - Remove the condom-covered penis from the vagina before the penis becomes limp.
   - Do not have sexual contact again unless another condom is applied.
   - In the case that a condom breaks or leaks, urinate immediately and wash the penis with soap and water.

(A) To apply, roll the condom completely over the erect penis while pinching the space at the condom tip. (B) Hold the condom at the base of the penis during its removal from the vagina.

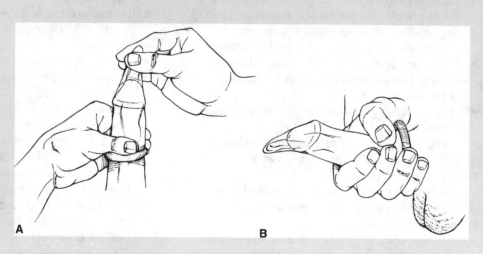

3. Give schedule of Reproductive Control Clinic hours _____ B. Velasquez, RN

(continued)

NURSING CARE PLAN:
Health-Seeking Behaviors *(Continued)*

Implementation 10/10   1300   Given the following pamphlets: "Choices" and "Understanding Safer Sex."
(Documentation)   Identified pages with illustrations for applying condoms. Given sample package of condoms. Clinic hours written on cover of pamphlets. Will discuss reading and use of condoms on return admission._____ B. VELASQUEZ, RN

Evaluation 10/13   0630   Says he has read sex information pamphlets given during preadmission exam.
(Documentation)   Used one sample condom s̄ problems. Asked, "What can my girlfriend do if the condom breaks?" Advised immediate insertion of an applicator filled with foam spermicide. To reduce risks of sexually transmitted diseases, a female sex partner should urinate and also wash well with soap and water. Told to avoid douching as this may push infectious organisms higher into the uterus or Fallopian tubes. Plans to buy more condoms. Says "They're a lot cheaper than babies."_____ B. VELASQUEZ, RN

⚙ FOCUS ON OLDER ADULTS

- The skin of older adults is usually dry, thin, and wrinkled.
- Older adults often have small, brown-pigmented freckles called *lentigines*, or liver spots, on the hands, arms, and face, from a lifetime of exposure to sun and weather.
- Older adults gradually lose height because of a loss of calcium from the skeletal system.
- Kyphosis is a common result of demineralization of bones, especially among older women.
- Older men tend to become thinner, whereas weight gain seems to be the pattern among older women.
- Hair becomes gray with age and may become thin as well.
- Older adults experience a reduction in sweat glands with age, which predisposes them to dry skin.
- The acuity of skin sensation is usually diminished among older adults because of a decrease in sensory receptors.
- The redistribution of subcutaneous fat and the effects of gravity may cause the skin beneath the eyes, chin, and arms to sag.
- All sensory functions tend to diminish with age.
- Older adults often require eyeglasses or eye surgery to maintain their visual acuity.
- High-pitched consonants such as "f," "s," "th," "ch," and "sh" may be more difficult for older

adults to hear (Fuller and Schaller-Ayers, 1994).
- Older adults may have a weaker cough because of the loss of muscle tone in the thorax.
- Menstruation is rare after the age of 50 years; vaginal spotting may indicate uterine pathology.
- Female breasts become flat and pendulous once the levels of estrogen decline after menopause.
- There is an increased incidence in tumors as people age; the risk for breast cancer rises after menopause.
- The mucous membrane that lines the vagina loses its moisture with age, which may lead to discomfort during intercourse.
- Older men usually retain their ability to produce sperm; however, it may take them more time to achieve an erection.
- The prostate gland tends to enlarge as men age, predisposing them to urinary retention and urinary infections.
- Bladder capacity becomes reduced with age, which increases the frequency with which older adults need to urinate.
- Older adults may have more difficulty controlling their urinary and rectal sphincters.
- Muscular strength and joint flexibility decrease with age.

- The best assessment environment is close to a restroom, private, warm, adequately lighted, and contains an adjustable examination table or bed.
- During an initial survey of a patient, the nurse may observe the patient's physical appearance, level of consciousness, body size, posture, gait, movement, use of ambulatory aids, and mood and emotional tone.
- Drapes are used during a physical examination to protect the patient's modesty and provide warmth.
- There are two approaches that may be used for data collection: the head-to-toe approach involves gathering data from the top of the body, working toward the feet; a systems approach organizes data collection according to the functional systems of the body.
- The body may be divided into six general components for the purpose of organizing data collection: (1) the head and neck, (2) the chest, (3) the extremities, (4) the abdomen, (5) the genitalia, and (6) the anus and rectum.
- Whenever an opportunity arises, adult patients are taught how to perform breast and testicular self-examinations.

CRITICAL THINKING EXERCISES

- You have been asked to assess two new patients. One, a preoperative patient, arrived by wheelchair and has been walking about the nursing unit. The other was transported by ambulance, has intravenous fluid infusing, and oxygen is being administered.
  Which patient would you assess first? Why?
  What modifications would you plan when assessing the nonsurgical patient?
- You have assessed a new patient and found that his abdomen is round and tympanic. Bowel sounds are absent, and the patient is breathing rapidly and shallowly. The patient seems anxious and frightened. What actions would be appropriate at this time? Number them in a sequence identifying their priority.
- Make a list of the most important assessments that should be made each shift when caring for stable patients.

SUGGESTED READINGS

Ali NS. Teaching early breast cancer detection strategies. Advancing Clinical Care July–August 1991;6:21–23.

Assessing the lungs. Nursing November 1991;21:32C–32D, 32F.

Bates B. A Guide to Physical Examination and History Taking. 5th ed. Philadelphia: JB Lippincott, 1990.

Coulter JS. ABCD's of assessing skin lesions. Advancing Clinical Care November–December 1991;6:18–19.

Cummings JL. The mental status examination. Hospital Practice May 30, 1993:28:56–58, 60, 65–68.

Finesilver C. Respiratory assessment. RN February 1992;55:22–30.

Fuller J, Schaller-Ayers J. Health Assessment: A Nursing Approach. 2nd ed. Philadelphia: JB Lippincott, 1994.

Gehring PE. Physical assessment begins with a history. RN November 1991;54:26–32.

Holmgren C. Abdominal assessment. RN March 1992;55:28–34.

Irwin MJ. Assessing color changes for dark skinned patients. Advancing Clinical Care November–December 1991;6:8–11.

King PA, Longman AJ, Pergrin JV. Educating nursing home staff in lower extremity assessment and care. Geriatric Nursing November–December 1991;12:297–299.

Lusis SA, Hydo B, Clark L. Nursing assessment of mental status in the elderly. Geriatric Nursing September–October 1993;14:255–259.

McConnell EA. Clinical do's and don'ts: assessing the skin. Nursing April 1992;22:86.

McGovern M, Kuhn JK. Cardiac assessment of the elderly client. Journal of Gerontological Nursing August 1991;18:40–44.

McGovern M, Kuhn JK. Skin assessment of the elderly client. Journal of Gerontological Nursing April 1992;18:39–43.

Performing a rapid assessment of the heart. Nursing February 1992;22:32C–32D.

Sternberger C. Breast self-examination: how nurses can influence performance. MEDSURG Nursing October 1994;3:367–371.

Stiesmeyer JK. A four-step approach to pulmonary assessment. American Journal of Nursing August 1993;93:22–28, 31.

Walbrecker J. Start talking about testicular cancer. RN January 1995;58:34–35.

Examinations and Special Tests

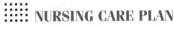
Learning Objectives

An understanding of the content within this chapter will be evidenced by the student's ability to:

- Differentiate between an examination and a test
- List 10 general nursing responsibilities when assisting with special examinations and tests
- Name five positions that are commonly used during tests or examinations
- Explain what is involved in a pelvic examination and Pap smear
- List six categories of tests or examinations that are commonly performed
- Identify four word endings and their meanings that indicate how tests or examinations are performed
- Explain procedures like a sigmoidoscopy, paracentesis, lumbar puncture, throat culture, and measurement of capillary blood glucose
- Discuss at least three factors that are considered when examinations and tests are performed on older adults

In addition to obtaining a health history and performing a physical examination, patients may be further assessed or evaluated by obtaining data from special examinations and tests. An examination is a procedure that involves physical inspection. It may or may not include collecting substances for laboratory or diagnostic testing. A test involves analyzing physical data and comparing the results to normal findings.

This chapter gives an overview of several diagnostic procedures and the nursing responsibilities that are involved in each. In addition, specific nursing activities for assisting with common procedures, like pelvic and sigmoidoscopic examinations, paracentesis, and lumbar puncture are provided. Also, those for which the nurse is primarily responsible, like collecting a throat culture and testing capillary blood glucose, are described. Tests involving the collection of urine and stool specimens are discussed in Chapters 30 and 31, respectively.

GENERAL NURSING RESPONSIBILITIES

When patients undergo examinations and special tests, nurses have specific responsibilities before, during, and after the procedure.

Preprocedural Care

Before a procedure begins, nurses must determine if patients understand the purpose and activities involved in the examination or test and if they agree to proceed with it. Once consent is obtained, the patient is prepared, equipment and supplies are obtained, and the examination area is prepared.

CLARIFYING EXPLANATIONS

In some cases, a signed consent form may be required before examinations or tests may be performed.

According to Corey and colleagues (1988), to be legally sound, consent must contain three elements: *capacity*, *comprehension*, and *voluntariness* (Display 13-1). Although physicians are responsible for explaining proposed examinations and tests, not all patients fully understand the information. Some are too anxious to process details; others feel too insecure to ask questions; and still others express additional concerns after the physician has left. Therefore, it often happens that the nurse must repeat, simplify, clarify, or expand the original explanation.

There are no exact rules for providing information. In general, it is best to find out how much of the physician's explanation each patient understands and use the patient's questions as a guide for further instructions. It may also be beneficial to follow the suggestions for teaching and providing emotional support as discussed in Chapter 8.

PREPARING PATIENTS

Some examinations and tests require special preparation of the patient, like withholding food and fluids or modifying the diet. Because test preparation requirements may vary from one health agency to another, the nurse may refer to written protocols in an agency's manual rather than rely on memory.

Once the specific requirements for a test are known, the nurse provides directions to the patient, nursing staff, and other hospital departments affected by the test. Everyone who is involved must cooperate so that the test is conducted accurately. In the event that the test preparations are not carried out correctly, the information is reported promptly because it may be necessary to cancel and reschedule the procedure.

Because many tests are being done on an outpatient basis, the nurse must be clear as to what the patient's responsibilities include.

DISPLAY 13-1. *Elements of Informed Consent*

Capacity	Indicates that the patient has the ability to make a rational decision; if not, a spouse, parent, or legal guardian must do so
Comprehension	Indicates that the patient understands the physician's explanation of the risks, benefits, and alternatives that are available.*
Voluntariness	Indicates that the patient is acting on his or her own free will without coercion or threat of intimidation.

*Capacity and comprehension may be temporarily affected by sedative drugs or the effects of anesthesia.

PATIENT TEACHING BEFORE SPECIAL EXAMINATIONS OR TESTS

Teach the outpatient or the family to do the following:

- Call (specify the number) if any test preparation instructions are not clearly understood or cannot be followed.
- Refrain from eating or drinking anything for at least 8 to 12 hours before a test or examination that requires a fasting state.
- Follow all dietary specifications for eating or omitting certain foods exactly as directed.
- Check with your physician about taking or readjusting the time schedule for prescribed medications on the day of the test or examination.
- Bathe or shower as usual on the day of the test or examination.

- Dress casually and in layers so that items of clothing can be removed or added to maintain comfort in the test environment.
- Ask a friend or family member for transportation to and from the test or examination if there is a potential for drowsiness, lingering pain, or weakness after the test.
- Come to the test location at least one-half hour before the test is scheduled.
- Identify yourself at the information or appointment desk when you arrive.
- Bring information to verify insurance or Medicare coverage.

Regardless of the type of examination or test, it is always appropriate to help patients change into an examination gown, take vital signs beforehand, and suggest that they empty their bladder. Patients who are experiencing pain may be given prescribed medication.

OBTAINING EQUIPMENT AND SUPPLIES

All the equipment and supplies for a particular examination or test performed at the bedside or on the nursing unit are obtained ahead of time. Nurses are relieved of this responsibility if the examination or test is carried out in other locations, or when a special technician performs the procedure.

Some items the nurse may need are in prepackaged kits kept in a clean utility room (Fig. 13-1) or obtained from a central supply department. If packaged kits are used, the nurse checks the list of contents to determine what, if any, additional items may be needed. A supply of clean gloves, goggles, masks, and gowns is provided for preventing direct contact with blood or body secretions (see Standard Precautions in Chap. 22).

ARRANGING THE EXAMINATION AREA

If the procedure is to be performed at the patient's bedside, the nurse clears the area of unnecessary articles and provides privacy. Many nursing units contain an examination room that is clean, well lighted, and stocked with frequently used equipment (Fig. 13-2). The examination table is covered with sheets of paper dispensed from a roll. A lined receptacle is nearby for disposing of soiled items.

Necessary equipment and supplies are arranged for easy access by the examiner. Sterile items remain wrapped or covered until just before their use. Instruments that require electric power, batteries, or lights are checked before the examiner arrives, so as to replace nonfunctioning equipment before the examination begins.

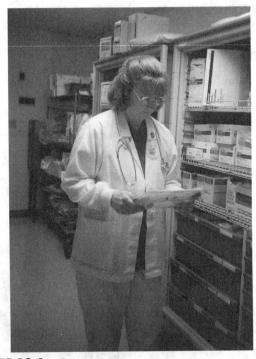

FIGURE 13-1
Obtaining equipment from the supply room. (Courtesy of Ken Timby.)

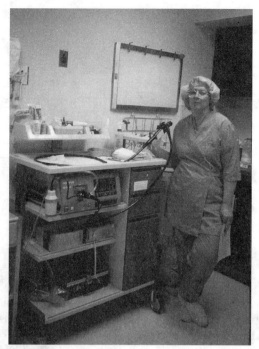

FIGURE 13-2
An examination room. (Courtesy of Ken Timby.)

TABLE 13-1. *Indications for Common Examination Positions*	
Position	Uses
Dorsal recumbent	• External genitalia inspection • Vaginal examination • Rectal examination • Urinary catheter insertion
Lithotomy	• Internal pelvic examination (female) • Obstetric delivery • Cystoscopic (bladder) examination • Rectal examination
Sims'	• Rectal examination • Vaginal examination • Rectal temperature assessment • Suppository insertion • Enema administration
Knee–chest	• Rectal and lower intestinal examinations • Prostate gland examination
Modified standing	• Prostate gland examination

Procedural Responsibilities

Before the examination or test, the patient is positioned and draped, the examiner is provided with technical assistance, and the patient is supported physically and emotionally.

POSITIONING AND DRAPING

There are five positions that are commonly used, depending on the type of examination, condition of the patient, and preference of the examiner. They include the dorsal recumbent position, Sims' or left lateral position, lithotomy position, knee–chest or genupectoral position, and a modified standing position (Table 13-1).

Dorsal Recumbent Position
The **dorsal recumbent position** (Fig. 13-3) is achieved by having the patient recline, bend the knees, rotate the hips outward, and keep the feet flat. A bath blanket is used to drape the patient. A disposable pad may be placed under the patient's buttocks to absorb drainage.

Lithotomy Position
The **lithotomy position** (Fig. 13-4) is similar to the dorsal recumbent position except that the feet are placed in metal supports called *stirrups*. To facilitate an internal examination, the buttocks are brought to the very end of the examination table. A drape is used to cover the exposed perineum and legs.

Sims' Position
Sims' position (Fig. 13-5) is essentially a left lateral side-lying position with the chest leaning slightly forward. When this position is used, the patient's right knee is sharply bent toward the head. The right arm is forward and the left arm is extended behind the body.

Knee–Chest Position
A **knee–chest position** (Fig. 13-6) is one in which the patient rests on the knees and chest. The head is turned to one side and may be supported on a small pillow. A pillow may also be placed under the chest for added comfort. The arms may be above the head or bent at the elbows so as to rest alongside the patient's head. A drape is placed so that the patient's back, buttocks, and thighs are covered.

This is a very difficult position for most patients—especially the elderly—to assume for any length of time. Therefore, conscientious nurses wait to position patients in this manner until just before the examination. However, there are examination tables with movable sections that facilitate maintaining this position without much patient effort.

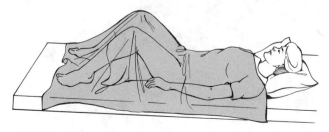

FIGURE 13-3
Dorsal recumbent position.

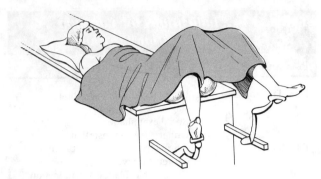

FIGURE 13-4
Lithotomy position.

Modified Standing Position

A **modified standing position** (Fig. 13-7) is used primarily when the prostate gland is examined. To assume this position, the patient stands in front of the examination table and leans forward from the waist.

ASSISTING THE EXAMINER

Technical assistance involves being familiar with the examination equipment and the order in which it will be used. To facilitate the examination, instruments and equipment are placed on the side of the examiner's dominant hand, if that is possible. If not, the nurse anticipates what may be needed during the procedure and hands one item at a time to the examiner.

If the skin and underlying tissue require local anesthesia, the nurse may be required to hold a glass container of the medication as the physician withdraws some of its contents (Fig. 13-8). The nurse always checks the drug name and concentration on the label carefully. A second method for ensuring that the correct drug is being used is to hold the container in such a manner that the physician can read the label.

If the nurse is responsible for performing the test or examination, all equipment and supplies are obtained so that the patient is not left alone. If assistance or additional equipment is required, a telephone or call light may be used to summon help.

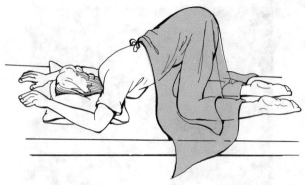

FIGURE 13-6
Knee-chest position.

PROVIDING PHYSICAL AND EMOTIONAL SUPPORT

Throughout any examination or testing procedure, the nurse constantly surveys the patient's physical and emotional reactions. For example, comfort measures may be in order if the patient is cold or in pain. Holding the patient's hand and offering words of encouragement may help the patient endure temporary discomfort. The nurse's assessments often alert the physician to shorten or modify the examination in some manner.

Postprocedural Care

After examinations and tests are completed, the nurse attends to the patient's comfort and safety, cares for specimens, and records and reports pertinent data.

ATTENDING TO THE PATIENT

First, the patient is helped to a position of comfort. Vital signs are rechecked to verify that the patient's condition is stable. Then the patient is cleaned of any substances that caused soiling. Hospitalized patients may be offered a clean gown; outpatients are directed to dress in their own clothing. When it is safe to do so,

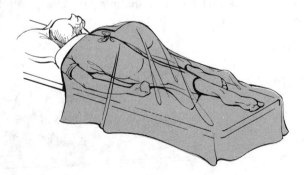

FIGURE 13-5
Sims' position.

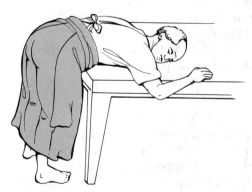

FIGURE 13-7
Modified standing position.

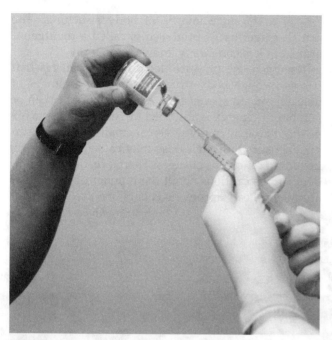

FIGURE 13-8
Withdrawing local anesthetic. (Courtesy of Ken Timby.)

patients are escorted to their rooms or to the discharge area, and instructions for follow-up care are provided.

CARING FOR SPECIMENS

Specimens are samples of tissue or body fluids. If specimens are collected during an examination or test, they must be cared for in such a way as to ensure their accurate analysis. Therefore, the nurse:

1. Collects the specimen in an appropriate container
2. Labels the specimen container with correct information
3. Attaches the proper laboratory request form
4. Ensures that the specimen does not rapidly decompose before it can be examined
5. Delivers the specimen to the laboratory as soon as possible

Refer to Display 13-2 for factors that often interfere with accurate examinations or invalidate test results.

RECORDING AND REPORTING DATA

Certain information requires documentation whenever a patient undergoes a special examination or test. General information includes (1) the date and time, (2) pertinent preexamination assessments and preparation, (3) the type of the examination or test, (4) who performed the test or where it was performed, (5) the response of the patient during the examination and afterward, and (6) type of specimen, if any was col-

---

> **DISPLAY 13-2.** *Common Factors That Invalidate Examination or Test Results*
>
> - Incorrect diet preparation
> - Failure to remain fasting
> - Insufficient bowel cleansing
> - Drug interactions
> - Inadequate specimen volume
> - Failure to deliver specimen in a timely manner
> - Incorrect or missing test requisition

lected; its appearance, size, or volume; and where the specimen was taken.

In addition to the written account of the examination, the nurse reports significant information to other nursing team members. When the nursing team is kept aware of current events and changes in the patient's condition, the plan of care can be revised and kept up to date.

ASSISTING WITH A PELVIC EXAMINATION

Skill 13-1 incorporates the nursing responsibilities that have been previously described when assisting a physician with a pelvic examination. A **pelvic examination** is a physical assessment in which the vagina and adjacent organs are inspected and palpated.

The suggested actions in Skill 13-1 also include how to assist with collecting a specimen of cervical secretions for a Pap (Papanicolaou) smear. A **Pap smear** is a test to determine whether cancer cells are present, the status of reproductive hormone activity, or the presence of normal or infectious microorganisms within the uterus or vagina (Table 13-2). The American College of Obstetricians and Gynecologists (1989) and the American Cancer Society (1980) recommend Pap smear screening for all adult women every 1 to 3 years.

COMMON DIAGNOSTIC EXAMINATIONS AND TESTS

Besides pelvic examinations and Pap smears, there are many other types of diagnostic examinations that are commonly performed to assess and evaluate patients. By learning root words and suffixes or word endings, which come primarily from Latin or Greek origins, it is possible to decipher many unfamiliar names of diagnostic tests or examinations (Table 13-3).

Some common diagnostic tests and examinations include those that involve the use of x-rays, recordings of electrical impulses, absorption and detection of radioactive substances, detection of sound waves, use of endoscopes, and examinations of body fluids. More specific information may be obtained by referring to laboratory and test manuals, courses where specific diseases are studied, or through experience in clinical settings.

Radiography

Radiography, or **roentgenography**, is a general term referring to all procedures that use roentgen rays, or x-rays, to produce images of body structures. The actual image that is produced is called a **roentgenogram,** but it is commonly known as an **x-ray**.

Roentgen rays produce electromagnetic energy that passes through body structures, leaving an image of dense tissue on special film. X-rays cannot be seen or felt, but the energy is absorbed by cells. Long-term exposure to roentgen rays, even at small doses, or a single exposure to a high dose may cause cell damage, including cancerous changes. Therefore, there is a tendency to be cautious about the number of x-rays that are taken. Lead aprons or collars are used to shield

(text continues on page 206)

SKILL 13-1
Assisting With a Pelvic Examination

Suggested Action	Reason for Action
Assessment	
Determine the identity of the patient on whom the examination will be performed.	Prevents errors
Determine if a Pap smear will be collected.	Indicates the need for additional equipment and supplies
Find out if the patient has ever had a pelvic examination before.	Provides a basis for teaching
Ask if the patient is currently menstruating or had intercourse within the last 24–48 hours.	Interferes with microscopic examination of collected specimens; the examiner may wish to delay obtaining a Pap smear
Inquire if the patient has douched in the last 24 hours.	Suggests a need to reschedule the Pap smear because an adequate sample of cells and secretions may not be available
Ask the patient's age, the date of the last menstrual cycle, the number of pregnancies and live births, and a description of symptoms such as bleeding or drainage, itching, or pain characteristics.	Provides data with which to determine the possibility of pregnancy, to compare cellular specimens with hormonal activity, and to provide clues as to possible pathology and the need for additional tests
Determine if and what type of birth control is being used if the patient is premenopausal. For oral contraceptives, identify the name of the drug and dosage.	Correlates the influence of presribed hormones on cellular specimens
Ask menopausal patients if they are taking estrogen replacements, the brand name, and dosage.	Correlates the influence of prescribed hormones on cellular specimens
Observe for impaired strength or joint limitation.	Suggests the need to modify the examination position
Planning	
Explain the procedure and give the patient an opportunity to ask questions.	Tends to reduce anxiety
Provide an examination gown and direct the patient to empty her bladder.	Facilitates palpation of the uterus and ovaries

(continued)

SKILL 13-1
Assisting With a Pelvic Examination (Continued)

Suggested Action	Reason for Action
Place a **speculum**, an instrument for widening the vagina, gloves, examination light, lubricant, and the following materials for the Pap smear: long, soft applicators and spatula and at least three glass slides, chemical fixative, and a container for holding the slides, on the counter or on a tray in the examination room.	Promotes efficient time management; specula (plural of speculum) may be made of disposable plastic or metal; the latter are reused after sterilization; it is best to select an appropriate size according to the individual patient

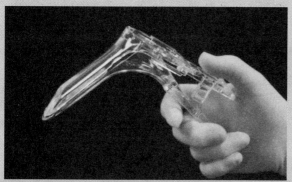

Vaginal speculum. (Courtesy of Ken Timby.)

Suggested Action	Reason for Action
Mark one slide with an "E" for endocervical, another with "C" for cervical, and the last with a "V" for vaginal.	Identifies the location from which the specimens are taken; *endocervical* means "inside the cervix"; the cervix is the lower portion of the uterus, or womb

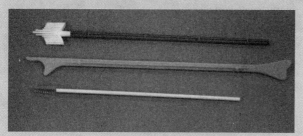

Applicators and spatula for obtaining cervical and vaginal specimens. (Courtesy of Ken Timby.)

Suggested Action	Reason for Action
Arrange to be with the patient during the examination, especially if the examiner is a man.	Reduces the potential for claims of sexual impropriety
Plan to assist with the collection of the vaginal and cervical secretions for the Pap smear before the examiner proceeds to palpate the internal organs.	Lubricant interferes with microscopic examination of the specimens

Implementation

Suggested Action	Reason for Action
Place the patient in a lithotomy position or use an alternate position, like Sims' or dorsal recumbent positions, if the patient is disabled.	Provides access to the vagina
Cover the patient with a cotton or paper drape.	Maintains modesty

(continued)

SKILL 13-1
Assisting With a Pelvic Examination (Continued)

Suggested Action	Reason for Action
Introduce the examiner to the patient if the two are strangers.	Tends to reduce anxiety by extending common courtesies
Fold back the drape just before the examination begins.	Exposes the genitalia
Direct the examination light from behind the examiner's shoulder toward the vaginal opening.	Illuminates the area, facilitating inspection
Wet the speculum with warm water, or if a Pap smear will not be obtained, apply water-soluble lubricant to the speculum blades.	Provides comfort during insertion
Prepare the patient to expect the momentary insertion of the speculum and explain that a loud click may be heard as it is locked in place.	Tends to reduce anxiety and aids in relaxation
Hand the examiner a soft-tipped applicator, the spatula, and another applicator, in that order.	Facilitates collection of secretions for the Pap smear
Hold the slide marked "E" so the examiner can roll the specimen across the slide; follow a similar pattern as the second and third samples are collected from the cervix and vagina.	Deposits intact cells and secretions according to their source

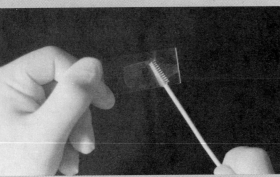

Transferring secretions to a glass slide. (Courtesy of Ken Timby.)

Suggested Action	Reason for Action
Position the lined receptacle so the examiner may dispose of each collection device and the speculum after they are used.	Controls the spread of microorganisms

(continued)

SKILL 13-1
Assisting With a Pelvic Examination (Continued)

Suggested Action	Reason for Action
Place each slide in a chemical fixative solution, or spray it with a similar chemical.	Preserves the integrity of the specimens

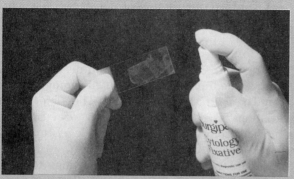

Preserving specimen. (Courtesy of Ken Timby.)

Suggested Action	Reason for Action
Lubricate the gloved fingers of the examiner's dominant hand and prepare the patient for an internal examination of the vagina (and in some cases the rectum as well).	Reduces friction and keeps the patient informed of continuing aspects of the examination
Don gloves and clean the skin of lubricant when the examination is completed; then remove the gloves.	Prevents the transmission of microorganisms; promotes comfort and hygiene
Lower both feet simultaneously from the stirrups and assist the patient to sit up.	Reduces strain on abdominal and back muscles
Assist the patient from the room after she has dressed.	Maintains patient safety
Wash hands.	Reduces the number of microorganisms on the hands

Evaluation
- Understood the purpose for the examination
- Assumed and maintained a satisfactory position for examination
- Comfort and safety were maintained
- Specimens have been collected, identified, and preserved

Document
- Date and time
- Pertinent preassessment data, if any
- Type of examination
- Examiner and location
- Condition of the patient afterwards
- Disposition of specimens

Sample Documentation

Date and Time Taken to examination room by wheelchair for pelvic examination by Dr. Wood. Able to assume lithotomy position without difficulty. Smears of endocervical, cervical, and vaginal specimens obtained and sent to lab. Returned to room by wheelchair and assisted into bed. _____ **Signature, Title**

TABLE 13-2. *Pap Smear Results*

Test Component	Interpretation
Cellular Examination	
Class I	Negative; no abnormal cells
Class II	Unusual, but not cancerous
Class III	Suggestive of cancer, but not definite
Class IV	Strongly suggestive of cancer
Class V	Definitely cancerous
Hormonal Effects *(on a 6-point scale)*	
1	Marked estrogen effect
2	Moderate estrogen effect
3	Slight estrogen effect
4	Absent estrogen effect
5	Compatible with pregnancy
6	Too bloody, inflamed, or scanty to analyze
Identifiable Microorganisms *(on a 5-point scale)*	
1	Normal microorganisms
2	Scanty or absent microorganisms
3	*Trichomonas vaginalis* (protozoan organism)
4	*Monilia* (yeast-like fungus)
5	Other or mixed collection of microorganisms

Adapted from Fischbach F. A Manual of Laboratory and Diagnostic Tests. 4th ed. Philadelphia: JB Lippincott, 1992.

parts of the body during x-rays (Fig. 13-9). Because a developing fetus is at greater risk for cellular damage from x-rays, radiography is contraindicated during pregnancy if at all possible.

Magnetic resonance imaging (MRI) is one alternative for producing an image without exposing patients to radiation from x-rays. Instead, the body is scanned while the magnetic forces are disturbed with radiofrequency signals (Fig. 13-10). However, because metal devices on or within the body can be affected, patients with metal implants, pacemakers, or staples are excluded from this type of diagnostic imaging.

USING CONTRAST MEDIUM

A **contrast medium** is a substance, like barium sulfate or iodine, that fills a body organ or cavity, making it appear more dense. This serves to make the shape of the structure more distinct when imaged on x-ray film. One of the newest forms of x-ray to use contrast medium is the **computed tomography** (CT) scan. The contrast medium makes it possible to identify variations in tissue density when x-ray images are obtained from various angles and levels in the body (Fig. 13-11).

Some patients have allergic reactions to contrast media (plural for "medium"). An **allergy** is an unfavorable reaction to a substance to which the body is sensitive. Allergic reactions to contrast media that contain iodine are relatively common. The reactions may be mild, causing nausea and vomiting, a skin rash, or itching. Others may experience severe reactions involving shock and death. Therefore, it is essential to identify the patient's allergy history before a test in which a contrast medium is used. If a patient is allergic to iodine or shellfish, which correlates with an iodine allergy, the information is reported immediately.

Whenever contrast media are used, it is important to promote their excretion and elimination. This may be done by increasing fluid intake in the case of intravenously administered contrast medium, or by administering a laxative if the contrast medium is given by the oral or rectal route.

TABLE 13-3. *Deciphering Diagnostic Terms*

Suffix	Meaning	Examples	Description
-graphy	To record	Angiography	Test that records an image of blood vessels
-gram	An image	Angiogram	The actual image recorded during angiography
-scopy	To see	Sigmoidoscopy	Test in which the lower intestine is inspected
-scope	Examination instrument	Sigmoidoscope	A tube with a light and lens for looking within the lower intestine
-centesis	To puncture	Thoracentesis	Procedure in which a needle is used to puncture the thorax and withdraw fluid
-metry	To measure	Pelvimetry	Procedure in which the pelvis is measured
-meter	Instrument for obtaining measurements	Glucometer	Instrument for measuring glucose

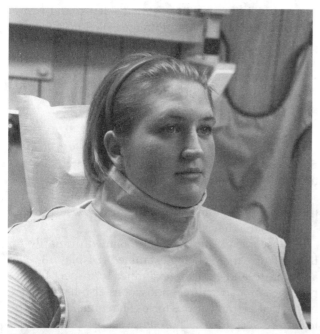

FIGURE 13-9
Lead thyroid collar and apron. (Courtesy of Ken Timby.)

Electrical Impulse Recordings

Diagnostic information can be obtained by using machines that record electrical impulses from structures like the heart, brain, and skeletal muscles. These tests are identified by the prefix "electro," as in **electrocardiography** (ECG or EKG), **electroencephalography** (EEG), and **electromyography** (EMG).

To detect the electrical impulses, wires, called *electrodes*, are attached to the skin. They in turn transmit the electrical activity to a machine that converts it to a series of waveforms (Fig. 13-12). Except for an awareness of the presence of electrodes, the patient usually does not experience any other sensations during the test.

Radionuclide Studies

Radionuclides are elements whose atomic structures are altered so as to produce radiation. They may be identified by a number followed by their chemical symbol, such as ^{131}I (radioactive iodine) and ^{99}Tc (radioactive technetium).

When radionuclides are instilled within the body, usually by the intravenous route, they are absorbed by particular tissues or organs. With the use of a scanning device that detects radiation, the size, shape, and function of the radiated structure can be assessed. The term **hotspot** indicates an area where the radionuclide is concentrated and the radiation is intense, whereas a **coldspot** is an area with diminished absorption. **Positron emission tomography** (PET) combines the technology of radionuclide scanning with the layered analysis of tomography.

Tests using radionuclides are contraindicated for pregnant women and nursing mothers. The energy that is released can be harmful to the rapidly growing cells of an infant or fetus.

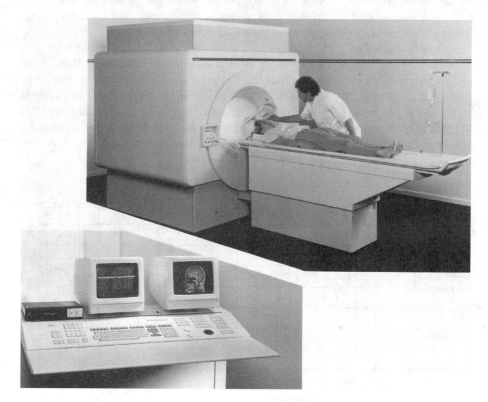

FIGURE 13-10
Magnetic resonance imaging. (Courtesy of Kalamazoo Neuro-Imaging Center, Inc., Kalamazoo, MI.)

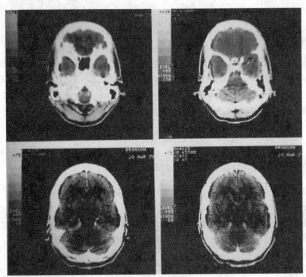

FIGURE 13-11
Cross-sections of cranial CT scan. (Courtesy of Ken Timby.)

Ultrasonography

Ultrasonography, also known as **echography**, is an examination that uses sound waves in ranges beyond human hearing to produce an image of internal organs. Ultrasound examinations do not involve radiation or contrast media, which makes them an extremely safe diagnostic tool.

Ultrasonography is used to study the position and size of various stationary or moving structures such as the lens of the eye, the heart, placenta, or fetus. Air-filled structures, like the lung or intestine, and extremely dense tissue, like bones, do not image well. When examining the abdomen, patients are often required to drink a quart of water to promote distention of the bladder.

During ultrasonography, which is similar in principle to the echo location used by bats and dolphins or the sonar devices on submarines, sound is projected through the body's surface from a hand-held probe. The sound waves cause vibrations within body tissues and images are produced as the waves are reflected back toward the machine. The reflected sound waves are converted into a visual image called an *ultrasonogram*, *sonogram*, or *echogram*, which can be viewed on a television-like monitor and recorded for future analysis. Doppler ultrasound, discussed in Chapter 11, is a variation of this type of technology.

Endoscopy

Endoscopy is a visual examination of an internal structure with an instrument called an *endoscope*. Endoscopes have a lighted mirror–lens system attached to a tube and are flexible enough to be advanced through structures that have anatomic curves.

Endoscopic examinations are named primarily for the structure that is being examined (Display 13-3). In addition to allowing the examiner to inspect the appearance of a structure, endoscopes also have attachments that permit various forms of treatment or the collection of specimens. Those endoscopic examinations that produce discomfort or anxiety may be performed under light, short-acting anesthesia.

Endoscopic examinations are being performed more and more on an outpatient basis, making them an economic alternative to invasive tests and procedures that previously required surgery.

ASSISTING WITH A SIGMOIDOSCOPY

A **sigmoidoscopy**, an examination that involves inspection of the rectum and sigmoid section of the lower intestine, is a common screening tool used to detect cancer of the rectum and colon.

Cancer of the colon and rectum is the second highest cause of deaths from cancer among both men and women in the United States. Consequently, the American Cancer Society (1985) advocates that everyone older than 50 years of age have a sigmoidoscopic examination, and that the examination be repeated at 3- to 5-year intervals after two negative examinations performed 1 year apart.

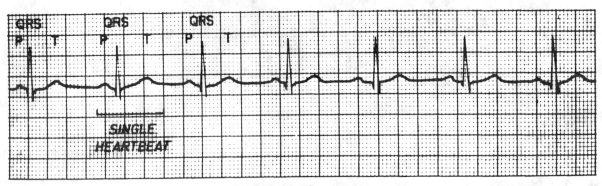

FIGURE 13-12
Normal electrocardiogram.

DISPLAY 13-3. *Examples of Endoscopic Examinations*

- *Bronchoscopy*—inspection of the bronchi
- *Gastroscopy*—inspection of the stomach
- *Colonoscopy*—inspection of the colon
- *Esophagogastroduodenoscopy* (EGD)—inspection of the esophagus, stomach, and duodenum
- *Laparoscopy*—inspection of the abdominal cavity
- *Cystoscopy*—inspection of the urinary bladder

Considering the growing population of older adults, it is highly probable that nurses will be called on to assist at some time or another with a sigmoidoscopic examination. Skill 13-2 provides suggestions for the nurse's responsibilities.

Patients usually are instructed to eat a light or liquid diet the evening before the examination. Good bowel cleansing is essential for visualizing the tissue. Therefore, a suppository or small-volume enema is usually required the night before unless the patient has a previously existing bowel disorder or diarrhea. About an hour before the examination, another enema or two may be administered (see Chap. 31).

With the patient in bed or on an examination table, the sigmoidoscope is inserted through the anus and advanced up to 24 inches (60 cm) if the scope is flexible, or 10 inches (25 cm) if a rigid scope is used. Because no anesthesia is used, passage of the scope and the instillation of air to distend the walls of the intestine may be accompanied by a feeling of pressure and the urge to have a bowel movement. The sensation is brief and passes after the scope is removed. Ordinarily the examination lasts 10 to 20 minutes, unless the bowel is suctioned to remove debris that obstructs the examiner's view, or a **biopsy**, a sample of tissue, is taken.

(text continues on page 212)

SKILL 13-2
Assisting With a Sigmoidoscopy

Suggested Action	Reason for Action
Assessment	
Identify the patient on whom the examination will be performed.	Prevents errors
Check for a signed consent form.	Provides legal protection
Ask the patient to describe the sigmoidoscopic procedure.	Indicates the accuracy of the patient's understanding and provides an opportunity for clarifying the explanation
Inquire about the patient's current symptoms and family history of significant diseases.	Provides information about the purpose for performing the procedure and an opportunity for reinforcing the need for future sigmoidoscopic examinations
Ask for a description of the patient's dietary and fluid restrictions and bowel-cleansing results.	Indicates if the patient complied with proper preparation for the procedure
Assess the patient's vital signs and obtain other physical assessments according to agency policy, such as weight or characteristics of bowel sounds.	Provides a baseline for future comparisons
Ask for an allergy history and a list of any current medications that are being taken.	Influences drugs that may be prescribed and alerts staff to other medical problems
Planning	
Direct the patient to undress, don an examination gown, and use the restroom.	Facilitates the examination and gives the patient an opportunity to empty the bowel and bladder again

(continued)

SKILL 13-2
Assisting With a Sigmoidoscopy (Continued)

Suggested Action	Reason for Action
Prepare for the examination by placing a sigmoidoscope, gloves, gown, mask, goggles, lubricant, suction machine, and containers for biopsied tissue in the examination room.	Promotes efficient time management

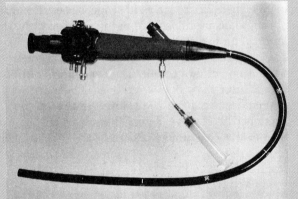

Flexible sigmoidoscope. (Courtesy of Ken Timby.)

Suggested Action	Reason for Action
Check that the light at the end of the sigmoidoscope and the suction equipment are operational.	Avoids delay, inconvenience, and discomfort once the examination is in progress
Implementation	
Help the patient to assume a Sims' position, if a flexible sigmoidoscope will be used, or a knee–chest position, if a rigid sigmoidoscope is used.	Facilitates passage of the scope; an endoscopic table may be used in lieu of a self-maintained knee–chest position
Cover the patient with a cloth or paper drape.	Maintains modesty
Introduce the examiner to the patient if the two are strangers.	Tends to reduce anxiety by extending common courtesies
Lubricate the examiner's gloved fingers.	Reduces discomfort when the fingers are used to dilate the anal and rectal sphincters
Prepare the patient for the introduction of the examiner's fingers followed by the insertion of the sigmoidoscope.	Tends to reduce anxiety by keeping the patient informed of each step and the progress that is being made
Acknowledge any discomfort that the patient may be experiencing and explain that the discomfort should be short-lived.	Indicates that the nurse empathizes with the patient's distress
Inform the patient if, and before, suction is used, air is introduced, or a sample of tissue is obtained.	Prepares the patient for unexpected sensations or temporary increase in discomfort
Open the specimen container, cover the specimen with preservative, and recap the container.	Prevents loss and decomposition of the specimen
Inform the patient when the scope will be withdrawn.	Keeps the patient informed of progress
Don gloves and clean the skin of lubricant and stool after the examination is completed; then remove the gloves.	Prevents the transmission of microorganisms; promotes comfort and hygiene

(continued)

SKILL 13-2
Assisting With a Sigmoidoscopy *(Continued)*

Suggested Action	Reason for Action
Assist the patient from the room to an area where his or her personal clothing is located, or provide a clean gown in exchange for a soiled one.	Maintains patient safety and dignity
Wash hands.	Reduces the number of microorganisms
Explain that there may be slight abdominal discomfort until the instilled air has been expelled, and that some rectal bleeding may be observed if a biopsy was taken.	Provides anticipatory health teaching
Stress that if severe pain occurs or the bleeding is excessive, the physician is to be notified.	Identifies significant reportable data
Advise that food and fluids may be consumed whenever the patient desires.	Clarifies dietary guidelines
Clean the sigmoidoscope and any other soiled equipment according to infection control guidelines.	Prevents the transmission of microorganisms
Restore order and cleanliness to the examination room; restock supplies.	Prepares the room for future use
Complete laboratory requisition form, label specimen, and take both to the lab for analysis.	Facilitates microscopic examination

Evaluation

- Understood the purpose for the examination
- Carried out the appropriate dietary and bowel preparation
- Assumed required position
- Comfort and safety were maintained
- Postprocedural instructions were given
- Specimen was preserved, identified, and delivered appropriately

Document

- Date and time
- Pertinent preassessment data, if any
- Type of examination
- Examiner and location
- Condition of the patient afterwards
- Instructions provided
- Disposition of specimen

Sample Documentation

Date and Time   Arrived ambulatory for routine sigmoidoscopic examination. No current symptoms, no known allergies. Takes Tenormin for hypertension. Last dose was @0700. BP 142/90 in right arm while sitting. T—98.2 P—90 R—22. Bowel sounds are active in all four quadrants. Has eaten lightly this morning and self-administered two enemas last night with good results, and one this morning with very little stool expelled. Placed in Sims' position for examination. Biopsy omitted. Instructed to resume eating and taking fluid as desired. Explained that gas pains are possible and that walking about will help, but to notify Dr. Ross if the discomfort is prolonged. Discharged ambulatory accompanied by wife. _____ **Signature, Title**

Tests Involving Body Fluids

Body fluids may include blood, urine, stool, sputum, intestinal secretions, spinal fluid, and drainage from wounds or infected tissue. Specimens for body fluid examinations and tests may be collected by laboratory personnel, physicians, or nurses, and the tests may be repeated at intervals to monitor the progress of patients. Beginning students are encouraged to refer to laboratory manuals for the purposes of specific tests and the nursing responsibilities that are involved in each.

Several examples of specimen collection are discussed in later chapters, where they are more pertinent. Nursing responsibilities for assisting with a paracentesis and lumbar puncture, collecting a throat culture, and measuring capillary blood glucose follow.

ASSISTING WITH A PARACENTESIS

A *paracentesis* is a procedure that involves puncturing the skin and subsequently the abdominal cavity so that body fluid may be withdrawn. This procedure is always performed by a physician with the assistance of a nurse.

A paracentesis is most commonly done to relieve abdominal pressure and improve breathing, which generally becomes labored as fluid crowds the lungs. Sometimes up to 1 quart (liter) or more of fluid is removed. In some cases, a fluid specimen is sent to the laboratory for microscopic examination.

◄····: NURSING GUIDELINES FOR
⋮····⋮   ASSISTING WITH A PARACENTESIS

- Explain the procedure or clarify the physician's explanation to the patient.
  Rationale: Prepares the patient for an unfamiliar experience and promotes a clearer understanding
- Check to see if a signed consent form is required.
  Rationale: Provides legal protection
- Take the patient's weight, blood pressure, respiratory rate, and measure the abdominal girth at its widest point with a tape measure.
  Rationale: Serves as a basis for postprocedural comparisons
- Obtain a prepackaged paracentesis kit along with a glass vial of local anesthetic.
  Rationale: Promotes efficient time management
- Make sure that extra gloves, gown, mask, and goggles are available.
  Rationale: Offers protection from contact with microorganisms, like the AIDS virus, that may be present in blood or other body fluids
- Encourage the patient to empty his or her bladder just before the paracentesis is performed.

Rationale: Prevents accidental puncturing of the bladder
- Place the patient in a sitting position (Fig. 13-13).
  Rationale: Pools abdominal fluid in the lower areas of the abdomen and displaces the intestines posteriorly
- Hold the container of local anesthetic so the physician can withdraw a sufficient amount.
  Rationale: Prevents contaminating the physician's sterile gloves
- Offer patient support as an area of the abdomen is anesthetized and then pierced with an instrument called a *trocar*, and a hollow sheath, called a *cannula*, is inserted.
  Rationale: Relieves anxiety through empathetic concern
- Reassess the patient periodically; expect that the blood pressure and respiratory rate may decrease.
  Rationale: Monitors the patient's response
- Place a bandaid or small dressing over the puncture site after the cannula is withdrawn.
  Rationale: Acts as a barrier to microorganisms and absorbs drainage
- Assist the patient to a position of comfort
  Rationale: Demonstrates concern for the patient's welfare
- Measure the volume of fluid withdrawn.
  Rationale: Contributes to accurate assessment of fluid volume
- Label the specimen, if so ordered, and send it to the lab with the appropriate requisition form.
  Rationale: Facilitates appropriate analysis

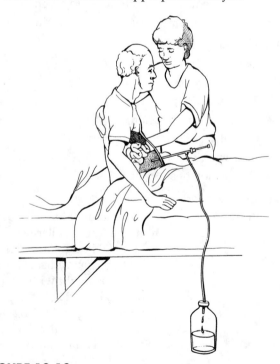

FIGURE 13-13
Positioning for an abdominal paracentesis.

- Document pertinent information such as the appearance and volume of the fluid, patient assessments, and disposition of the specimen.
Rationale: Adds essential data to the patient's medical record

ASSISTING WITH A LUMBAR PUNCTURE

A **lumbar puncture** or **spinal tap** is a procedure in which a needle is inserted between lumbar vertebrae at a level below the spinal cord itself. The tip of the needle is advanced until it is located beneath the middle layer of the meningeal membrane. Spinal fluid pressure is measured and then a small amount of fluid is withdrawn.

This test is performed for various reasons. It may be used to diagnose conditions that raise the pressure within the brain, such as brain or spinal cord tumors, or infections like meningitis. Spinal fluid may also be withdrawn to instill contrast medium for x-rays of the spinal column. Finally, some conditions are treated by instilling drugs directly into the spinal fluid after an equivalent amount has been withdrawn.

NURSING GUIDELINES FOR ASSISTING WITH A LUMBAR PUNCTURE

- Explain the procedure or clarify the physician's explanation to the patient.
Rationale: Prepares the patient for an unfamiliar experience, or promotes a clearer understanding
- Check to see if a signed consent form is required.
Rationale: Provides legal protection
- Perform a basic neurologic examination including pupil size and response and muscle strength and sensation in all four extremities.
Rationale: Provides a baseline for future comparisons
- Encourage the patient to empty his or her bladder.
Rationale: Promotes comfort during the procedure
- Administer a prescribed sedative drug if it has been ordered.
Rationale: Reduces anxiety
- Obtain a prepackaged lumbar puncture kit along with a glass vial of local anesthetic.
Rationale: Promotes efficient time management
- Make sure that extra gloves, gown, mask, and goggles are available.
Rationale: Offers protection from contact with microorganisms, like the AIDS virus, that may be present in blood or other body fluids

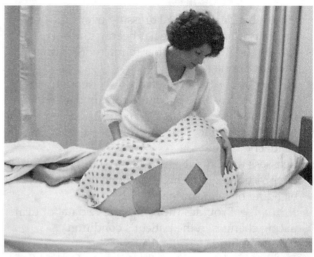

FIGURE 13-14
Positioning for lumbar puncture. (Courtesy of Ken Timby.)

- Place the patient on his or her side with the knees and neck acutely flexed (Fig. 13-14), or in a sitting position in which the patient bends from the hips.
Rationale: Separates the bony vertebrae
- Instruct the patient that once the needle has been inserted, movement must be avoided.
Rationale: Prevents injury
- Hold the container of local anesthetic so the physician can withdraw a sufficient amount.
Rationale: Prevents contamination of the physician's sterile gloves
- Stabilize the patient's position at the neck and knees.
Rationale: Reinforces the need to remain motionless
- Support the patient emotionally as the skin is injected with local anesthesia and the needle is inserted.
Rationale: Relieves anxiety through empathetic concern
- Tell the patient that it is not unusual to feel pressure or a shooting pain down the leg.
Rationale: Prepares the patient for expected sensations
- Perform *Queckenstedt's test*, if asked, by compressing each jugular vein separately for approximately 10 seconds while the pressure is being measured.
Rationale: Indicates that an obstruction in spinal fluid flow is present if the pressure remains unchanged, rises slightly, or takes longer than 20 seconds to return to baseline
- Observe that the physician fills three separate, numbered containers with 5 to 10 mL in their appropriate sequence if laboratory analysis is desired.
Rationale: Suggests that if blood is present, but in decreasing amounts in the third container, its source is most likely the trauma of the procedure rather than central nervous system pathology

- Place a bandaid or small dressing over the puncture site after the needle has been withdrawn.
  Rationale: Acts as a barrier to microorganisms and absorbs drainage
- Position the patient flat on his or her back or abdomen; instruct the patient to remain flat and roll from side to side for the next 6 to 12 hours.
  Rationale: Reduces the potential for a severe headache
- Reassess the patient's neurologic status, as before the procedure, and check the puncture site for bleeding or clear drainage.
  Rationale: Provides the comparative data for evaluating changes in the patient's condition
- Offer oral fluids frequently.
  Rationale: Helps restore the volume of spinal fluid
- Label the specimens, if so ordered, and send them to the lab with the appropriate requisition form.
  Rationale: Facilitates appropriate analysis
- Document pertinent information such as the appearance of the fluid, patient assessments, and disposition of the specimen.
  Rationale: Adds essential data to the patient's medical record

COLLECTING A THROAT CULTURE

A **culture** is a test in which cells or body fluids suspected of containing infectious microorganisms are collected, placed in other living tissue or a nonliving nutritive substance, and examined for growth of microorganisms. Bacteria, a common cause of throat infections, are one type of microorganism that will grow in a nonliving medium. Conclusive results of a bacterial culture usually require a minimum of 24 hours and as long as 72 hours for sufficient growth to take place. However, an abbreviated test that takes approximately 10 minutes can be performed on a throat swab to rapidly determine a preliminary diagnosis.

Once the specimen is obtained, bacteria, if they are present, can be identified microscopically by their shape and by the color they acquire when stained with special dyes. Treating the specimen with dye, a process known as **Gram staining** for the Danish physician who developed the technique, helps determine whether a bacteria is gram positive or gram negative. *Gram-positive bacteria* appear violet after staining. Those that repel the violet dye but appear red, the color of a counterstain, are called *gram-negative bacteria* (Fischbach, 1992). Streptococci, bacteria that frequently infect the throat, are gram positive.

Determining if and exactly what microorganism is present helps in choosing the most appropriate treatment. A throat culture is most often performed on young children, who are susceptible to complications from upper respiratory infections and infection of the tonsils. However, adults who tend chronically to harbor infectious microorganisms in their pharynx, the passageway for air and food, may also be tested from time to time.

NURSING GUIDELINES FOR COLLECTING A THROAT CULTURE

- Check with the physician about proceeding with the throat culture if the patient is taking any antibiotic drugs.
  Rationale: Affects the diagnostic value of the test
- Delay collecting a specimen if an antiseptic gargle has recently been used.
  Rationale: Affects the diagnostic value of the test
- Explain the purpose and technique for obtaining the culture.
  Rationale: Reduces anxiety and promotes cooperation
- Collect supplies, which include a sterile culture swab, glass slide, tongue blade, gloves, mask if the patient is coughing, paper tissues, and an emesis basin in case the patient gags.
  Rationale: Facilitates organization and efficient time management
- Have the patient sit where there is optimum light.
  Rationale: Enhances inspection of the throat
- Don gloves and a mask, if necessary.
  Rationale: Reduces the potential for transferring microorganisms
- Loosen the cap on the tube in which the swab is located.
  Rationale: Facilitates hand dexterity
- Tell the patient to open his or her mouth widely, stick out the tongue, and tilt the head back.
  Rationale: Promotes access to the back of the throat
- Depress the middle of the tongue with a tongue blade in your nondominant hand (Fig. 13-15).
  Rationale: Opens the pathway for the swab
- Rub and twist the tip of the swab about the tonsil areas and the back of the throat without touching the lips, teeth, or tongue (Fig. 13-16).
  Rationale: Transfers microorganisms from the inflamed tissue to the swab
- Be prepared for gagging.
  Rationale: Stroking back of throat stimulates gag reflex
- Remove the swab and discard the tongue blade in a lined receptacle.
  Rationale: Controls the spread of microorganisms
- Spread the secretions on the swab across the glass slide.
  Rationale: Prepares the specimen for quick staining

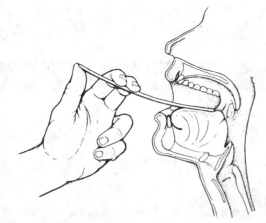

FIGURE 13-15
Depressing the tongue. (Smeltzer SC, Bare BG: Brunner and Suddarth's Textbook of Medical-Surgical Nursing, 7th ed, p 484. Philadelphia: JB Lippincott, 1992)

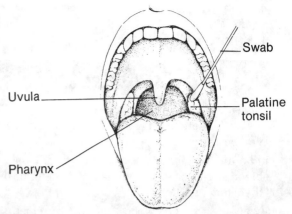

FIGURE 13-16
Obtaining a specimen for a throat culture. (Smeltzer SC, Bare BG: Brunner and Suddarth's Textbook of Medical-Surgical Nursing, 7th ed, p 484. Philadelphia: JB Lippincott, 1992)

- Replace the swab securely within the tube, taking care not to touch the outside of the container.
  Rationale: Avoids collecting unrelated microorganisms and provides containment for the collected specimen
- Crush the packet in the bottom of the tube.
  Rationale: Releases nourishing fluid to promote growth of bacteria
- Remove your gloves, discard them in a lined receptacle, and wash your hands.
  Rationale: Reduces the transmission of microorganisms
- Label the culture tube with the patient's name, date, time, and the source of the specimen.
  Rationale: Provides laboratory personnel with essential information
- Attend to staining and examining the prepared glass slide.
  Rationale: Provides tentative identification of streptococci bacteria
- Deliver the sealed culture tube to the laboratory or refrigerate it if there will be a delay longer than 1 hour.
  Rationale: Ensures that the microorganisms will grow when transferred to other culture media

MEASURING CAPILLARY BLOOD GLUCOSE

Glucose is the type of sugar present in blood as a result of eating carbohydrates. A certain amount is always present to keep cells supplied with a source of instant energy. The amount of blood sugar in a nonfasting state is generally between 80 to 120 mg/dl (milligrams per deciliter). Normal blood levels are maintained by the body's production of glucagon and insulin, hormones that regulate glucose metabolism.

Diabetics, who have an impaired ability to produce insulin, have difficulty regulating their blood sugar levels. They must attend to their diet, exercise, and use medications to do what the body ordinarily does naturally.

Diabetics may experience low or high blood sugar levels—each of which can have life-threatening consequences. Therefore, many diabetics measure their own capillary blood sugar levels rather than having venous blood drawn for laboratory analysis, which is more expensive and inconvenient.

A **glucometer** is an instrument that measures the amount of glucose present in capillary blood by assessing the amount of light that is reflected through a chemical test strip. Based on the amount of measured sugar in the blood, diabetics may adjust their intake of food or medication.

Because diabetes is such a common disorder, nurses are frequently called on to teach newly diagnosed diabetic patients how to test their own blood sugar. In addition, nurses measure capillary blood sugar levels for diabetics who are hospitalized or being cared for in long-term institutions. Therefore, Skill 13-3 is offered here to introduce this skill as early as possible, even though the specifics of the disease may be learned much later.

There are several important points to remember about measuring blood glucose. First, there are several types of glucometers that are available, and the manufacturer's instructions must be followed for accurate use. Skill 13-3 describes the actions to follow for using an Ames' glucometer. Second, the blood sugar is usually measured about a half hour before eating a meal and before bedtime to determine what are likely the lowest levels of glucose. This allows time for increasing or decreasing the consumption of food or administer

(text continued on page 220)

SKILL 13-3
Using a Glucometer

Suggested Action	Reason for Action
Assessment	
Identify the patient on whom the examination will be performed.	Prevents errors
Find out if the patient has ever had his or her blood sugar measured with a glucometer or if there any questions.	Provides a basis for teaching
Review the previous blood sugar measurements and the trends.	Helps evaluate the reliability of the assessed measurement when it is obtained
Check to see if insulin coverage has been ordered if the glucose levels are higher than normal.	Aids in quickly reducing high levels of blood glucose
Check that the glucometer has been calibrated at least once within the last 24 hours.	Confirms that the machine is operating correctly
Check the date on the container of test strips.	Determines if the test strips are still appropriate for use
Observe the code number on the container of test strips and compare it with the code number that is programmed into the glucometer.	Ensures accuracy

Comparing code number on test strip bottle to glucometer code number. (Courtesy of Ken Timby.)

Suggested Action	Reason for Action
Inspect the patient's fingers and thumb for a non-traumatized area; the earlobes may be used as an acceptable alternate.	Avoids secondary trauma
Planning	
Test the machine's calibration with a control strip or solution supplied by the manufacturer if it has not been done in 24 hours.	Verifies the machine's accuracy
Arrange the plan of care so that the test will be performed about one-half hour before a meal and at bedtime.	Ensures consistency in obtaining data and facilitates the detection of trends
Collect the necessary equipment and supplies, which include the glucometer, lancets, lancet holder, test strips, gloves, and a paper tissue.	Promotes efficient time management

(continued)

SKILL 13-3
Using a Glucometer (Continued)

Suggested Action	Reason for Action
Open the container of test strips, lay one on a clean surface, and fold a paper tissue in quarters.	Organizes supplies needed during the test
Implementation Have the patient wash his or her hands with soap and warm water and towel dry.	Reduces the number of microorganisms on the skin; warmth dilates the capillaries and increases blood flow
Turn on the machine.	Prepares the machine for testing the blood sample
Assemble the lancet within the spring-loaded holder.	Conceals the sharp tip while preparing it for a rapid thrust into the skin
Avoid wiping the skin with alcohol.	Alters the test results if it has not totally evaporated
Don clean gloves after washing your hands.	Provides a barrier against contact with blood
Apply the lancet to the margin around a nontraumatized fingertip, avoiding the central pad area.	Avoids puncturing an area where there are sensitive nerve endings.

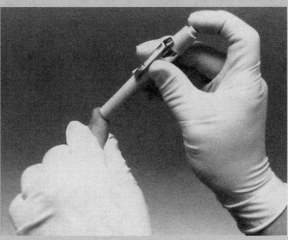

Punture made with lancet holder. (Courtesy of Ken Timby.)

Release the spring, causing the lancet to pierce the skin.	Opens a path for blood

(continued)

SKILL 13-3
Using a Glucometer (Continued)

Suggested Action	Reason for Action
Hold the finger or thumb so that a large hanging drop of blood forms.	Uses gravity to aid in collecting blood

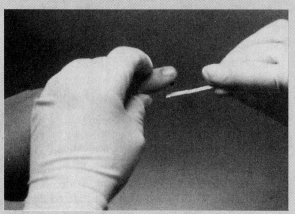

One large drop of blood is necessary for test. (Courtesy of Ken Timby.)

Suggested Action	Reason for Action
Touch the hanging drop of blood to the pad on the test strip, making sure that the test area is completely covered.	Saturates the test area to ensure accurate test results
Press the start button on the glucometer.	Activates the timing mechanism
Offer the patient a bandaid or paper tissue.	Absorbs blood and controls bleeding
Place the test strip on the folded tissue; blot and reblot for 1 to 2 seconds when the machine beeps audibly.	Removes excess blood
Insert the blotted test strip into the window of the glucometer immediately after blotting and before the timer reaches zero.	Ensures accurate test results

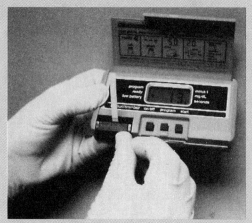

Inserting the test strip. (Courtesy of Ken Timby.)

Suggested Action	Reason for Action
Shut the door of the test window.	Secures the test strip and prevents light from entering, which may alter the test results

(continued)

SKILL 13-3
Using a Glucometer (Continued)

Suggested Action	Reason for Action
Observe the number displayed on the screen at the end of the test.	Indicates the current level of blood sugar
Remove the test strip and compare the color change with the color code on the test strip container.	Provides a second method for checking the accuracy of the displayed glucose measurement
Turn off the machine.	Extends the life of the battery
Press the sharp tip of the lancet into its plastic protector.	Prevents accidentally puncturing oneself

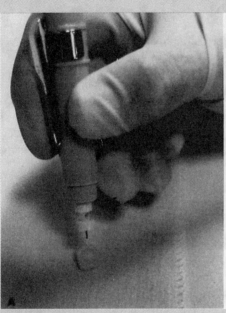 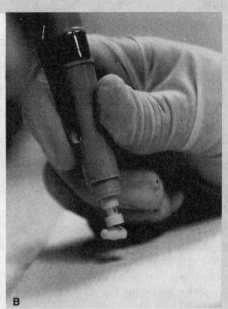

(*A*) Position used lancet above the protective cap. (*B*) Pierce the cap with the sharp point. (Courtesy of Ken Timby.)

Dispose of the lancet into a puncture-resistant container.	Prevents injury and the possible transmission of blood-borne infectious microorganisms
Clean the light window with a clean, dry, lint-free cloth.	Keeps the window free of debris that may impair light detection
Remove gloves and immediately wash your hands.	Reduces the number of microorganisms
Remove the equipment from the bedside if it does not belong to the patient.	Facilitates the use of equipment that may be needed for other patients
Store the test strips in a cool dry place between 37°F to 85°F (1.7°–30°C).	Prevents decomposition due to heat and humidity
Record the glucose measurement on the patient's record.	Documents essential data
Report the blood sugar level to the nurse in charge.	Communicates information for making treatment decisions

(continued)

SKILL 13-3
Using a Glucometer (Continued)

Suggested Action	Reason for Action

Evaluation
- Understood the purpose for the examination
- Adequate amount of blood obtained for testing glucose
- Results were consistent with the patient's present condition, previous trends, and concurrent treatment
- Additional treatment provided depending on glucose measurement

Document
- Date and time
- Pertinent preassessment data, if any
- Results obtained when using the glucometer (*Note*: In most health agencies, the test data may be recorded on a flow sheet specific for glucometer results, rather than being charted in narrative nursing notes)
- Treatment provided based on abnormal test results

Sample Documentation

Date and Time   Blood sugar 210 mg per glucometer. 5 Units of Humulin R given subcutaneously as
coverage. _____ **Signature, Title**

---

ing additional prescribed insulin (see Chap. 34), referred to as *coverage*. Third, measuring blood glucose involves a potential risk for contact with blood. Because blood may contain infectious viruses, gloves are *always* worn when performing this test.

NURSING IMPLICATIONS

Most patients who undergo special examinations and tests have emotional needs related to the stress of a potential diagnosis or the anxiety created by undergoing something that is unfamiliar to them. The accompanying list of Applicable Nursing Diagnoses indicate some nursing diagnoses that may be identified during the preprocedural and postprocedural stages of nursing care.

The Nursing Care Plan in this chapter is an example of the nursing process as it relates to the nursing diagnosis of Decisional Conflict. Decisional Conflict is defined in the NANDA taxonomy (1994) as "The state of uncertainty about the course of action to be taken when choice among competing actions involves risk, loss, or challenge to personal life values."

⬥ APPLICABLE NURSING DIAGNOSIS

- Knowledge Deficit
- Anxiety
- Fear
- Impaired Adjustment
- Decisional Conflict
- Health Seeking Behaviors
- Powerlessness
- Spiritual Distress

KEY CONCEPTS

- An examination is a procedure that involves physical inspection. A test involves analyzing physical data to determine how the results compare to normal findings.
- Whenever patients undergo special examinations and tests, the nurse is usually responsible for (1) determining the patient's understanding of the procedure, (2) checking on a signed consent form, (3) following test preparation requirements or teaching outpatients how to prepare themselves, (4) obtaining equipment and supplies, 5) arranging the examination area, (6) positioning and draping patients, (7) assisting the examiner, (8) providing patients with

NURSING CARE PLAN:
Decisional Conflict

Assessment	**Subjective Data**
	States, "I don't know what to do now that the amniocentesis shows that my baby will have cystic fibrosis. I know I can have an abortion, but I'm not sure I want to do that. I remember what it was like when my brother was always sick and then died. Why did this have to happen to me? I don't feel that any decision is possible right now."
	Objective Data
	28-year-old married woman who is 20 weeks pregnant. Date of last menstrual period: 7/2. Fetal heart rate is 140 in left lower quadrant. Says she has felt fetal movement. Had a younger brother who died at age 5 from cystic fibrosis. Sits with rigid posture almost immobile except wringing hands. Very little eye contact during interaction.
Diagnosis	Decisional Conflict related to birthing options of fetus with genetic disorder detected by amniocentesis.
Plan	**Goal**
	The patient will make an informed choice concerning the outcome of the current pregnancy by the return office visit on 11/10.

Orders: 11/5

1. Ask to compose a written list of advantages and disadvantages to possible choices before return appointment on 11/10.
2. Encourage to discuss options with husband and other significant persons.
3. Offer referrals to the Cystic Fibrosis Foundation, pro-choice or right-to-life groups.
4. Support patient's decision even if it is contrary to one's personal choice.

———————————————————————————————— F. BROWN, RN

Implementation 11/5 1415 Shared that this decision is difficult—other women dealing with these same
(Documentation) circumstances have felt similarly. Reinforced that the choice is hers to make and also confident that she can make the one that is best for her. Asked to list any and all advantages and disadvantages in writing to help clarify options. Offered referral to supportive agencies. Asked for and was given the phone number of the Cystic Fibrosis Foundation. Encouraged to come with husband for sharing questions and concerns. ———————————— F. BROWN, RN

Evaluation 11/10 1300 Returned for office conference with husband. Contacted Cystic Fibrosis
(Documentation) Foundation and attended a support group of parents. List of advantages and disadvantages completed by both patient and husband. Stated "The treatment of cystic fibrosis seems to have improved in the 20 years since my brother died. We talked it over and even if we had a normal baby, there's the risk it would die while we are alive. The people at the CF meeting made us feel like we're not alone." Scheduled next prenatal visit for 12/15. ———————— F. BROWN, RN

physical and emotional support, (9) caring for specimens, and (10) recording and reporting significant information.

- There are five common examination positions: the dorsal recumbent position, Sims' position, lithotomy position, knee–chest position, and modified standing position.

- During a physical examination, the nurse may be called on to assist with a pelvic examination, which involves an inspection and palpation of the vagina and adjacent organs. This examination often includes the collection of secretions for a Pap smear, a test used to identify the presence of cancerous cells, levels of hormone activity, or the identity of infectious microorganisms.

FOCUS ON OLDER ADULTS

- Reference values for test results are often determined using averaged statistics from younger adult age groups. Consequently, unless separate age-specific norms are available, test findings acquired from older adults may be misinterpreted.
- Prescription medications prescribed for older adults may affect test results.
- Older adults often take medications on a daily basis for multiple chronic conditions. Therefore, the physician is consulted about administering medications with a small amount of water when older adults must fast before a test or examination.
- Older adults, especially those who are ill, may not be able to tolerate having food and fluids withheld for long periods of time before examinations. Assessing urinary output, blood pressure, and state of alertness may provide data on how well an older adult is tolerating a fasting state.
- Dehydration, a common problem among older ill adults, may cause blood values in test results to seem elevated because of their concentration in a reduced volume of plasma.
- The frequent and urgent need to defecate (eliminate stool) in response to bowel preparations involving laxatives and enemas may exhaust some older adults.
- It may be helpful to provide a bedside commode and to anticipate the need for assistance when older adults are given laxatives or enemas before diagnostic tests or examinations.
- A bed alarm that sounds when a patient gets out of bed may be considered as a safety measure for older adults who require assistance in toileting after being given harsh laxatives or enemas.
- Because some older adults may fatigue easily, it is helpful to coordinate the timing of tests or examinations that take place in other departments so that older adults are not required to wait long periods of time before or after examinations.
- Older adults often have compromised circulation and may become cold in drafty hallways or air-conditioned testing areas. Therefore, many appreciate a bathrobe, slippers, and access to one or more blankets that may be warmed before being applied.
- After an examination, it may be best to offer fluids and food and then allow a period during which an older adult can rest before resuming physically taxing nursing activities.

- There are six common categories of tests and examinations. They include those that involve the use of x-rays, recordings of electrical activity, absorption and detection of radioactive substances, detection of sound waves, use of endoscopes, and tests involving body fluids.
- To aid in determining how particular tests are performed, it is helpful to understand four word endings: *graphy* (as in angiography) means to record an image; *scopy* (as in bronchoscopy) means to look through a lensed instrument; *centesis* (as in amniocentesis) means to puncture; and *metry* (as in pelvimetry) means to measure with an instrument.
- Nurses are often called on to assist with a sigmoidoscopy, paracentesis, and lumbar puncture, or to collect a throat culture and measure capillary blood glucose levels.
- A sigmoidoscopy involves inspecting the rectum and sigmoid section of the lower intestine with an endoscope. A paracentesis involves puncturing the skin and withdrawing fluid from the abdominal cavity. A lumbar puncture requires the insertion of a needle between lumbar vertebrae in the spine, but below the spinal cord itself. When a throat culture is obtained, microorganisms are collected and examined. Capillary blood glucose is measured with an instrument called a glucometer.
- Older adults undergoing special examinations and tests present certain challenges to the nurse, such as avoiding fatigue and dehydration, maintaining or adjusting current drug therapy, and avoiding misinterpretation of laboratory test results that may be based on norms of younger adults.

CRITICAL THINKING EXERCISES

- Discuss how a test or examination like a sigmoidoscopy may differ if it is performed on an outpatient basis rather than on an inpatient in a health agency.
- Explain how diminished mentation (capacity to understand), reduced strength and stamina, and pain may affect a diagnostic examination like a pelvic examination.
- Propose how a pelvic examination may be modified if the patient had diminished mentation, reduced strength and stamina, or pain.

SUGGESTED READINGS

American College of Obstetricians and Gynecologists. Report of Task Force on Routine Cancer Screening. Washington, DC: Author, 1989.

American Cancer Society. Guidelines for the cancer-related checkup: recommendations and rationale. CA: A Cancer Journal for Clinicians 1980;30:195–230.

American Cancer Society. Taking Control (Publication No. 2019.05). New York: Author, 1985.

Buffington S. How much do you know about laboratory studies? Nursing December 1991;21:46–49.

Carnevali DL, Patrick M. Nursing Management for the Elderly. 3rd ed. Philadelphia: JB Lippincott, 1993.

Corey G, Corey MS, Callahan P. Issues and Ethics in the Helping Professions. Pacific Grove, CA: Brooks/Cole Publishing Company, 1988.

Fischbach F. A Manual of Laboratory and Diagnostic Tests. 4th ed. Philadelphia: JB Lippincott, 1992.

Lewis K, Joyce-Nagata B, Fite EG. The effect of time and temperature on blood glucose measurements. Home Healthcare Nurse May–June 1992;10:56–61.

Murray S, Preuss M, Schultz F. How do you prep the bowel without enemas? American Journal of Nursing August 1992;92:66–67.

Renkes J. GI endoscopy: managing the full scope of care. Nursing June 1993;23:50–55.

UNIT V

Assisting With Basic Needs

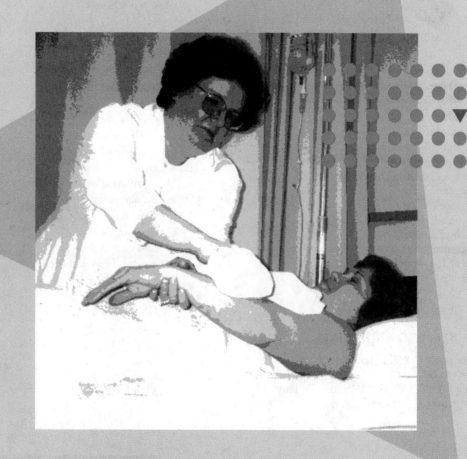

CHAPTER 14

Nutrition

Learning Objectives

An understanding of the content within this chapter will be evidenced by the student's ability to:

- Define the terms "nutrition" and "malnutrition"
- List six components of basic nutrition
- List at least five factors that influence nutritional needs
- Discuss the purpose and components of the food pyramid
- Describe three facts that may be obtained from a current nutritional label
- Explain protein complementation

- Identify four objective assessments for determining a person's nutritional status
- Discuss the purpose of a diet history
- List five common problems that may be identified after a nutritional assessment
- Plan nursing interventions for resolving problems affecting nutrition
- List seven common hospital diets
- Discuss four nursing responsibilities for meeting the nutritional needs of patients
- Identify three facts the nurse must know about a patient's diet
- Satisfactorily demonstrate how to feed patients
- Discuss at least three unique aspects of nutrition that apply to older adults

Nutrition is the process by which the body uses food. **Malnutrition** is a condition resulting from a lack of proper nutrients in the diet. Malnutrition is a common problem among people in poor, developing countries. However, there are groups of people within the United States who tend to be undernourished or marginally nourished. They include the socially isolated elderly living on fixed incomes, children of economically deprived parents, pregnant teenagers, and people with substance abuse problems like alcoholism.

More and more data support the fact that the quality of one's nutrition influences health and well-being. Therapeutic diets have been a standard technique in the treatment of diseases. Now, there is an emphasis on improving nutrition to prevent diseases. Healthy people in general are becoming selective about the quantity and quality of their daily food consumption. Consequently, nurses are prepared to advise others about what and how much to eat, discourage food fads and unsafe dieting, and manage the care of patients whose ability to eat, digest, absorb, or eliminate food is impaired.

EATING HABITS

Eating is a basic human need. Most eating habits are learned early in life. The kind of food that is consumed and eating patterns are affected by cultural (Fig. 14-1), economic, emotional, and social variables. Some factors include:

- Food preferences acquired during childhood
- Established patterns for meals
- Attitudes about nutrition
- Knowledge of nutrition
- Level of income
- Time, or lack of it, for food preparation
- Number of individuals within a household
- Access to food markets
- Use of food for comfort, celebration, or symbolic reward
- Satisfaction or dissatisfaction with body weight

HUMAN NUTRITIONAL NEEDS

Despite variations in food preferences and eating customs, all humans have the same basic nutritional needs for health. Through the scientific study of nutrition,

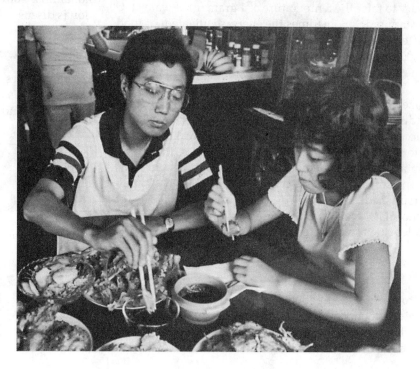

FIGURE 14-1
Cultural influences affect eating habits. (Ellis JR, Nowlis EA: Nursing: A Human Needs Approach, 5th ed, p 469. Philadelphia, JB Lippincott, 1994)

standards have been determined for the recommended daily amounts of the following:

- Calories
- **Nutrients**, which are those food sources like proteins, carbohydrates, and fats that provide the calories and chemicals for energy, growth, and repair of body structures, and
- Vitamins and minerals, which are essential for regulating and maintaining physiologic processes necessary for health, but do not supply calories.

Water, which is also necessary for life, is discussed in Chapter 15.

Although standards have been established for the types and amounts of dietary components needed to sustain health, individual nutritional needs are influenced by and may require adjustment according to:

- Age
- Weight and height
- Growth periods
- Activity
- Health status

Calories

Food is the source of energy for humans. Some nutrients produce more energy than others. Using a calorimeter, a device for measuring heat, the nutrients in food are burned in a laboratory and then analyzed to quantify their energy-producing value.

The energy, or heat equivalent, of food is measured in calories. A **calorie** (cal) is the amount of heat necessary to raise the temperature of 1 gram (g) of water 1°C (centigrade). Sometimes the energy equivalent of food is expressed in **kilocalories** (kcal), the equivalent of 1,000 calories, or the amount of heat necessary to raise the temperature of 1 kilogram (kg) of water 1°C.

When proteins, carbohydrates, and fats are metabolized, they produce energy (Display 14-1). Average adults need between 2,000 and 3,000 calories per day according to the National Research Council of the National Academy of Science. However, unless the caloric intake includes adequate sources of all three nutrients, a person may still be marginally nourished or malnourished. In other words, consuming 3,000 calories of chocolate, exclusive of any other food, would not be adequate to sustain a healthy state.

Proteins

Protein is a component of food that contains **amino acids**, chemical compounds made up of nitrogen, carbon, hydrogen, and oxygen. Twenty-two amino acids have been identified. Nine of the 22 are referred to

---

DISPLAY 14-1. *Energy Value of Nutrients**

Proteins	4 kcal/g
Carbohydrates	4 kcal/g
Fats	9 kcal/g

*Alcohol yields 7 kcal/g, but because it is not considered an essential nutrient, its value is not emphasized in this display.

---

as **essential amino acids** because they must be obtained from food. The body is able to manufacture the remaining or **nonessential amino acids**. The term "nonessential" is somewhat misleading; it refers to the fact that the body does not depend on dietary intake for these amino acids–not that they are unnecessary for health.

Besides the potential for providing energy, proteins are used primarily to build, maintain, and repair body tissue. The body spares protein for energy use as long as calories are available from carbohydrates and fats.

Proteins come from animal and plant food sources. Foods that are good sources of protein include milk, meat, fish, poultry, eggs, legumes (peas, beans, peanuts), nuts, and components of grains. Animal sources are referred to as **complete proteins** because they contain all the essential amino acids, whereas plant sources are called **incomplete proteins** because they contain some, but not all, of the essential amino acids. However, by combining certain plant sources, a practice referred to as **protein complementation**, it is possible to acquire all the essential amino acids from nonanimal sources (Fig. 14-2). Protein complementation is discussed later in relation to vegetarian diets.

Carbohydrates

Carbohydrates, abbreviated CHO because they contain molecules of carbon, hydrogen, and oxygen, are generally found in plant food sources. They are classi-

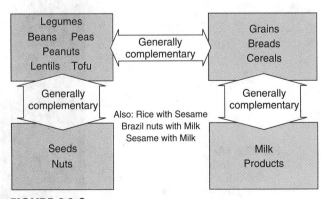

FIGURE 14-2
Complementary protein guide for meatless meals.

fied according to the number of sugar, or saccharide, units they contain. Carbohydrates are subdivided into sugars like **monosaccharides** and **disaccharides**, and starches called **polysaccharides**. Good sources of carbohydrates include cereals and grains, such as rice, wheat and wheat germ, oats, barley, and corn and corn meal; fruits and vegetables; molasses, maple, and corn syrups, honey, and common table sugar.

Carbohydrates, which make up the chief component of most diets, are used primarily as a quick energy source. In addition to providing calories, the undigestible fiber, called **cellulose**, found in the stems, skins, and leaves of many fruits and vegetables provides intestinal bulk that promotes bowel elimination.

Fats

Fats, known collectively as **lipids**, are combinations of molecules composed of glycerol and fatty acids called **glycerides**. Depending on the number of fatty acids that make up the fat molecule, fats may be referred to as mono-, di-, or triglycerides.

Saturated fats are those that contain as much hydrogen as their molecular structure can hold. As a result, saturated fats are usually solid. Most saturated fats come from animal sources. **Unsaturated fats**, found in plant sources like corn, are missing some hydrogen, and therefore assume the composition of a liquid oil. The following foods are rich in fat: red meat, such as beef and pork; butter, margarine, and vegetable oils; egg yolk; whole milk and cheese; peanut butter; salad dressings; avocados; chocolate; and nuts.

Because fats are insoluble in water, they are carried throughout the bloodstream within molecules of protein. The combination of the two is referred to as **lipoproteins**. Lipoproteins vary in the proportion of protein to fat (Table 14-1). The more protein the molecule contains, the higher its density. The ratio of low-density lipoprotein, which contains substantial amounts of cholesterol, to high-density lipoprotein is significant in predicting the risk for cardiovascular disease.

Fats are a concentrated source of energy, supplying more than twice the calories per gram than either proteins or carbohydrates. Although fats are high in calories, they should not be totally eliminated from the diet. Fats provide energy and are necessary for many chemical reactions in the body. Fat is necessary for the absorption of some vitamins. They also add flavor to food, and because they leave the stomach slowly, they promote a feeling of having satisfied appetite and hunger.

In general, Americans eat more fats than people in most countries. The influence of fat consumption and obesity on disorders like heart disease, hypertension, diabetes, and some types of cancer is becoming well documented. In an effort to improve the health of the nation, the United States Department of Health and Human Resources (1992), in *Healthy People 2000: National Health Promotion and Disease Prevention Objectives*, has set a goal that Americans will reduce their present fat intake to no more than 30% of their daily calories, which is 17% less than the average currently consumed.

Minerals

Minerals, like calcium, are noncaloric substances in food that are essential to all cells. Minerals play a role in the regulation of many of the body's chemical processes, such as blood clotting and the conduction of nerve impulses. Table 14-2 lists some of the major and trace minerals of the body, their chief functions, and common dietary sources.

Vitamins

Vitamins are chemical substances that are necessary in minute amounts for normal growth, maintenance of health, and functioning of the body (Table 14-3). When

TABLE 14-1. *Classification of Lipoproteins*

Type of Lipoprotein	Function	Recommended Blood Level*
Very low density (VLDL)	Delivers triglycerides to cells; becomes a major source of LDL	Not usually reported
Low density (LDL)	Transports cholesterol to cells and tissues	<130 mg/dl
High density (HDL)	Mobilizes cholesterol from tissues; transfers cholesterol to the liver for eventual excretion	30–85 mg/dl

*Values must be adjusted for age and gender.

TABLE 14-2. *Common Dietary Minerals*

Mineral	Chief Functions	Common Dietary Sources
Sodium	Maintenance of water and electrolyte balance	Table salt Processed meat
Potassium	Maintenance of electrolyte balance Neuromuscular activity Enzyme reactions	Bananas Oranges Potatoes
Chloride	Maintenance of fluid and electrolyte balance	Table salt Processed meat
Calcium	Formation of teeth and bones Neuromuscular activity Blood coagulation Cell wall permeability	Milk Milk products
Phosphorus	Buffering action Formation of bones and teeth	Eggs Meat Milk
Iodine	Regulation of body metabolism Promotion of normal growth	Seafoods Iodized salt
Iron	Component of hemoglobin Assistance in cellular oxidation	Liver Egg yolk Meat
Magnesium	Neuromuscular activity Activation of enzymes Formation of teeth and bones	Whole grains Milk Meat
Zinc	Constituent of enzymes and insulin	Seafoods Liver

they were first discovered, vitamins were named according to the sequence of letters in the alphabet. Numbers were subsequently added to some letters as more were identified. Chemical names are now replacing the letter–number system of identification. **Water-soluble vitamins**, the complex of B vitamins and vitamin C, are eliminated with body fluid and thus require daily replacement. **Fat-soluble vitamins**, which are vitamins A, D, E, and K, can be stored as a reserve for future needs.

With the exceptions of vitamin K (menadione) and biotin, vitamins cannot be manufactured by the body. Vitamin requirements, however, are easily met by eating a variety of foods. Cooking, processing, and lack of refrigeration can deplete the content of some vitamins in food. Various commercially packaged foods like margarine, milk, and flour have been vitamin enriched or fortified to promote health among consumers of those products.

Vitamin and mineral supplements usually are not necessary as long as people eat a well balanced diet. On the other hand, consuming megadoses, amounts exceeding those considered adequate for health, can be dangerous. Unfortunately, some people with terminal diseases follow unconventional diets and take large doses of nutritional supplements in a desperate attempt to be cured. Although various deficiency diseases develop from inadequate nutrition, there is no conclusive evidence at this time that consuming excessive amounts of vitamins or minerals is a reliable substitute for established medical treatment.

NUTRITIONAL STANDARDS

Several recent national efforts have aimed at educating the public about nutrition and promoting healthy or informed choices when purchasing food. Examples include the United States Department of Agriculture's (USDA) food pyramid, requiring simpler, yet informative, nutritional labeling on processed and packaged foods, and establishing standard definitions for terms used on food labels.

The Food Pyramid

The **food pyramid** is a guide for promoting a healthy dietary intake of food (Fig. 14-3). With a simple design like a pyramid, average citizens can easily learn what foods and how much of them to consume on a daily basis. To ensure easy recall and use of the information it contains, the number of servings from each category is sequenced from greater to lesser amounts. The top of the food pyramid includes the oils, fats, and sweets that should be consumed sparingly. On a daily basis, adults should eat 2 to 3 servings from both the animal and plant protein group and dairy group; 3 to 5 servings of vegetables, 2 to 4 servings of fruit; and 6 to 11 servings

TABLE 14-3. *Vitamins*

Vitamin	Chief Functions	Common Dietary Sources
A (Retinol) Not destroyed by ordinary cooking temperatures	Growth of body cells Promotion of vision, healthy hair and skin, and integrity of epithelial membranes Prevention of xerophthalmia, a condition characterized by chronic conjunctivitis	Animal fats: butter, cheese, cream, egg yolk, whole milk Fish liver oil and liver Green leafy and yellow fruits and vegetables
B_1 (Thiamine) Not readily destroyed by ordinary cooking temperatures	Carbohydrate metabolism Functioning of nervous system Normal digestion Prevention of beriberi, a condition characterized by neuritis	Fish Lean meat and poultry Glandular organs Milk Whole gain cereals Peas, beans, and peanuts
B_2 (Riboflavin) Not destroyed by heat except in presence of alkali	Formation of certain enzymes Normal growth Light adaptation in the eyes	Eggs Green leafy vegetables Lean meat Milk Whole grains Dried yeast
B_3 (Niacin)	Carbohydrate, fat, and protein metabolism Enzyme component Prevention of appetite loss Prevention of pellagra, a condition characterized by cutaneous, gastrointestinal, neurologic, and mental symptoms	Lean meat and liver Fish Peas, beans Whole grain cereals Peanuts Yeast Eggs Liver
B_6 (Pyridoxine) Destroyed by heat, sunlight, and air	Healthy gums and teeth Red blood cell formation Carbohydrate, fat, and protein metabolism	Whole grain cereals and wheat germ Vegetables Yeast Meat Bananas Black strap molasses
B_9 (Folic acid)	Protein metabolism Red blood cell formation Normal intestinal tract functioning	Green leafy vegetables Glandular organs Yeast
B_{12} (Cyanocobalamin)	Protein metabolism Red blood cell formation Healthy nervous system tissues Prevention of pernicious anemia, a condition characterized by decreased red blood cells	Liver and kidney Dairy products Lean meat Milk Saltwater fish and oysters
C (Ascorbic acid) Readily destroyed by cooking temperatures	Healthy bones, teeth, and gums Formation of blood vessels and capillary walls Proper tissue and bone healing Facilitation of iron and folic acid absorption Prevention of scurvy, a condition characterized by bleeding and abnormal bone and teeth formation	Citrus fruits and juices Tomatoes Berries Cabbage Green vegetables Potatoes
D (Calciferol) Relatively stable with refrigeration	Absorption of calcium and phosphorus Prevention of rickets, a condition characterized by weak bones	Fish liver oils, salmon, tuna Milk Egg yolk Butter Liver Oysters Formed in the skin by exposure to sunlight
E (Alpha-tocopherol) Heat stable in absence of oxygen	Red blood cell formation Protection of essential fatty acids Important for normal reproduction in experimental animals (i.e., rats)	Green leafy vegetables Wheat germ oil Margarine Brown rice

(continued)

TABLE 14-3. *Vitamins (Continued)*

Vitamin	Chief Functions	Common Dietary Sources
Pantothenic acid	Metabolism	Liver Egg yolk Milk
H (Biotin) 　Heat sensitive	Enzyme activity Metabolism of carbohydrates, fats, and proteins	Egg yolk Green vegetables Milk Liver and kidney Yeast
K (Menadione)	Production of prothrombin	Liver Eggs Green leafy vegetables Synthesized in the gastrointestinal 　tract by bacteria

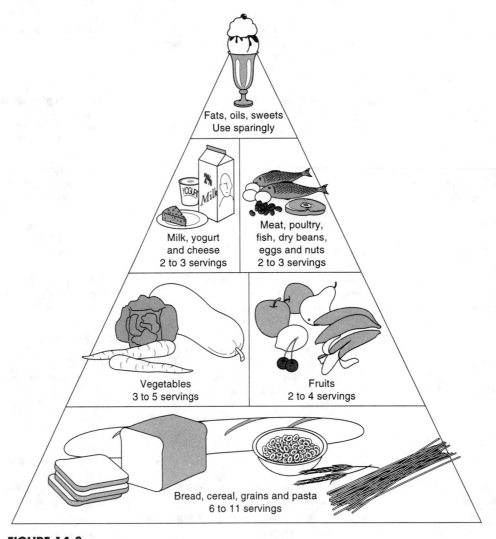

FIGURE 14-3
The food pyramid. (Scherer JC, Timby BK: Introductory Medical–Surgical Nursing, 6th ed, p 113. Philadelphia, JB Lippincott, 1995)

from the cereal, bread, and grain group. By following the pyramid's guidelines, Americans can achieve the dietary recommendations set by the United States Department of Health and Human Services and USDA for promoting health and preventing chronic disease (Display 14-2).

Modifications in the number of servings still need to be made in certain circumstances. Children, adolescents, pregnant women, and breast-feeding mothers require more servings per day of certain food groups, particularly the milk group.

Nutritional Labeling

Nutritional information has appeared on food labels since 1974, but until 1994, there were no new labeling requirements. Now, however, all packages of fresh meat and poultry must provide printed disease prevention guidelines. In addition, there are some major changes in the way nutritional information is provided on approximately 90% of processed and packaged food labels (Fig. 14-4).

The labels continue to identify the amounts of nutrients per serving size, as had been done in the past, but the serving sizes are identified in household measurements rather than in metric amounts, which was the case before. However, to interpret the labeled information accurately, consumers must become familiar with some new or revised terms. For example, daily value (DV) is a term that replaces the previously used standard, recommended daily allowance (RDA).

All DVs are calculated in percentages based on standards set for total fat, saturated fat, cholesterol, sodium, carbohydrate, and fiber within a 2,000-calorie diet. Those standards are:

- Total fat, 65 g
- Saturated fat, ≤ 20 g
- Cholesterol, 300 mg
- Sodium, < 2,400 mg
- Total carbohydrate, 300 g
- Dietary fiber, 25 g

People who are limited to less or require more than 2,000 calories must mathematically adjust the percentage of DVs according to their individual needs, which may prove difficult for the average consumer.

An expanded table showing the DV equivalents for both a 2,000- and 2,500-calorie diet may appear on some, but not all, commercial food labels. Because requirements for vitamins and minerals do not depend on calories, those amounts apply universally to all consumers.

Universal Labeling Terms

The federal Nutrition Labeling and Education Act now requires that food companies comply with standard

definitions if they choose to use health-related claims, like "low-fat," on their labels (Display 14-3).

VEGETARIANISM

People who for religious or personal reasons restrict their consumption of animal food sources are called **vegetarians**. Vegetarianism may be practiced in various forms, from **vegans**, who rely exclusively on plant sources for protein, to semivegetarians, who exclude only red meat.

Vegetarians, as a whole, have a lower incidence of colorectal cancer and fewer problems with obesity and diseases that are associated with a high-fat diet. However, a vegan diet has the potential, unless skillfully planned, for being inadequate in complete protein, calcium, riboflavin, vitamins B_{12} and D, and iron. Refer to the display on patient teaching for information to provide to persons interested in vegetarianism.

ASSESSING NUTRITIONAL STATUS

Because eating is a basic need, it is important for the nurse to identify any current or potential problems associated with nutrition. One place to begin is by gathering objective data using physical assessment techniques, and obtaining subjective information by asking focused questions in a diet history.

Objective Data
ANTHROPOMETRIC DATA

Anthropometric data are measurements that pertain to body size and composition. These data are usually obtained by measuring the patient's height, weight, triceps skin fold thickness, and mid-arm circumference. More sophisticated tests, like bioelectrical

---

DISPLAY 14-2. *Dietary Guidelines for Americans*

- Eat a variety of foods
- Maintain a healthy weight
- Choose foods low in fat (particularly saturated fat) and cholesterol
- Consume plenty of vegetables, fruits, and grain products
- Use sugars, salt, sodium, and alcohol only in moderation

Source: United States Department of Agriculture and United States Department of Health and Human Services, 1990.

Nutrition Facts
Serving Size 1/2 of package (21g)
Servings Per Container 2

Amount Per Serving	
Calories 70	Calories from Fat 20

	% Daily Value*
Total Fat 2.5g	4%
Saturated Fat 1.5g	6%
Cholesterol Less than 5mg	1%
Sodium 940mg	39%
Total Carbohydrate 12g	4%
Dietary Fiber 1g	6%
Sugars 4g	
Protein 2g	
Vitamin A 0% •	Vitamin C 0%
Calcium 6% •	Iron 2%

* Percent Daily Values are based on 2,000
calorie diet. Your daily values may be higher
or lower depending on your calorie needs:

	Calories:	2,000	2,500
Total Fat	Less than	65g	80g
Sat Fat	Less than	20g	25g
Cholesterol	Less than	300mg	300mg
Sodium	Less than	2,400mg	2,400mg
Total carbohydrate		300g	375g
Dietary Fiber		25g	30g

Calories per gram:
Fat 9 • Carbohydrate 4 • Protein 4

FIGURE 14-4
Sample label with nutritional information.

impedance analysis, which calculates lean body mass, body fat, and total body water based on changes in conduction of an applied electrical current, may be used by staff at eating disorder clinics or fitness centers.

Height and Weight

In general, the patient's height and weight are sufficient anthropometric data unless a severe nutritional problem is suspected or long-term therapy is anticipated. When measuring the patient's height, it is preferable to do so without shoes. An actual weight, rather than the patient's estimation, is essential. A standing, chair, or bed scale is used depending on the patient's condition. The date, time, type of scale, and the clothing worn by the patient are recorded. It is important to duplicate the same conditions when taking subsequent weights for comparison.

The patient's height and weight may then be graphed using a **nomogram**, a scale for determining numeric relationships. One such nomogram aids in determining a patient's **body mass index** (BMI), a numeric figure that is used to identify whether the patient's weight is within acceptable limits (Fig. 14-5). To calculate BMI, draw a line from the patient's weight in the column on the left to the patient's height in the column on the right. The BMI is the number where the line crosses the center scale. A BMI between 19 and 27 is considered within the normal range for adults through middle age (Eschleman, 1996). In the absence of a nomogram, another quick technique for determining a patient's ideal weight is to use the following formulas:

For women: 100 pounds for the first 5 feet + 5 pounds
for each additional inch

For men: 106 pounds for the first 5 feet + 6 pounds
for each additional inch (Hamwi, 1964)

Mid-Arm Circumference

When measuring the mid-arm circumference:

- Use the nondominant arm
- Find the midpoint of the upper arm between the shoulder and elbow
- Mark the mid-arm location
- Position the arm loosely at the patient's side
- Encircle the arm with a tape measure at the marked position
- Record the circumference in centimeters

DISPLAY 14-3. *Regulations for Labeling Terms*

Calorie free: <5 calories*
Low calorie: ≤40 calories
Reduced calorie: at least 25% fewer calories than standard product
Light or lite: 1/3 fewer calories or 50% less fat than regular product
Fat free: <0.5 g fat
Low fat: ≤3 g of fat
Reduced fat: at least 25% less fat than regular product
Cholesterol free: <2 mg cholesterol and ≤2 g saturated fat
Low cholesterol: <20 mg cholesterol and ≤2 g saturated fat
Sugar free: <0.5 g sugar

Per serving for all figures.

NOMOGRAM FOR BODY MASS INDEX

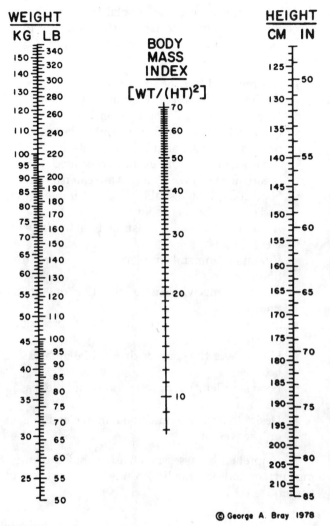

© George A. Bray 1978

FIGURE 14-5
Nomogram for calculating body mass index (BMI). (George A. Bray, M.D., copyright 1978.)

To calculate how much of the mid-arm circumference is actual muscle, multiply the triceps skin fold measurement, described next, by 0.314.

Skin Fold Thickness
The thickness of the skin fold at the triceps or subscapular areas is usually obtained (Fig. 14-6). To measure the triceps skin-fold thickness:

- Use the same arm as measured for mid-arm circumference.
- Grasp and pull the skin away from the muscle at the previously marked location.
- Place the calipers about the skin fold.
- Record the measurement in millimeters.

To interpret the significance of the mid-arm circumference measurement and the triceps skin fold thick-

---

<table>
<tr><td colspan="2">⬥⬥ PATIENT TEACHING FOR VEGETARIANS</td></tr>
</table>

Teach the patient or the family to do the following:

- Pre-plan menus a day or week at a time.
- Eat a wide variety of foods.
- Use complementary plant proteins.
- Include dried fruit, molasses, and dried peas for iron.
- Enhance the absorption of iron by including a good source of vitamin C, like orange juice, at each meal.
- Use whole grains and enriched flour, rather than refined, to obtain riboflavin.
- Add brewer's yeast, a dietary source of B vitamins, to the dough of baked goods.
- Take a calcium supplement that supplies at least 800 mg, and preferably 1,200 mg per day.
- Use soybean milk fortified with vitamin B_{12}, or consult with a physician concerning replacement therapy of at least 2 μg/day.
- Broccoli, collard and mustard greens, kale, and tofu are good sources of calcium.
- Breast-feed infants, if at all possible.
- Consider taking cod liver oil as a source of vitamin D.
- Purchase meat analogs, products that mimic the taste and appearance of meat, poultry, or fish, but are made from textured vegetable protein, in health food stores.
- Contact a Seventh Day Adventist church, whose members practice vegetarianism, for information on market sources for meatless products and food preparation classes.

ness, the measurements are compared with averages provided in standardized charts (Table 14-4). Skin fold thickness norms do not exist for adults older than 75 years of age. Matteson and McConnell (1988) indicate that abdominal circumference may be a more accurate anthropometric measurement for older adults, but standardized norms have not been established.

PHYSICAL ASSESSMENT

In addition to the anthropometric data, the nurse assesses the following:

- General appearance
- Integrity of the mouth
- Condition of the teeth
- Ability to chew and swallow

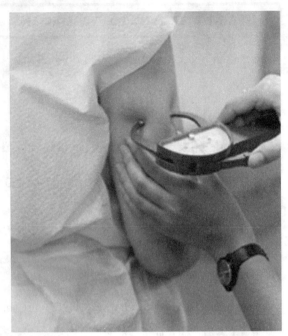

FIGURE 14-6
Measuring triceps skin-fold thickness with calipers. (Courtesy of Ken Timby.)

- Gag reflex
- Characteristics of skin and hair
- Joint flexibility
- Hand strength
- Attention and concentration

LABORATORY DATA

Laboratory tests that may support other physical evidence that a patient is overnourished or undernourished include a complete blood count, especially the hemoglobin, hematocrit, and number of lymphocytes; serum albumin and transferrin levels, which indicate protein status; and cholesterol, triglycerides, and lipoprotein levels, which may reflect a need to adjust the amount of fat in the patient's diet.

Subjective Data
THE DIET HISTORY

A diet history is a method of obtaining facts about a person's eating habits and factors that may affect nutrition. Common information acquired in a diet history includes:

- Self-reported level of appetite
- Weight loss or gain of 10 lbs in the past 6 months
- Number of meals consumed per day
- List of food eaten in the previous 24 hours in approximate household measurements
- Time when meals are usually consumed
- Frequency with which meals are eaten alone
- Food likes, dislikes, allergies, and intolerances, and cultural beliefs about food
- Amount of alcohol consumed on a daily or weekly basis
- Vitamin or mineral supplements taken on a routine basis
- Any problems with eating, digestion, or elimination
- Special diets that have been medically prescribed or self-imposed
- Use of over-the-counter drugs, like antacids or laxatives
- Food supplements or restrictions and the reason for them
- Desire to improve nutritional intake and to gain or lose weight

A comprehensive assessment also includes identifying current and past medical conditions, and types of surgery.

MANAGING NUTRITIONAL PROBLEMS

Based on the assessment data, the nurse may identify any one or more of the nursing diagnoses listed in the accompanying Applicable Nursing Diagnoses.

TABLE 14-4. *Anthropometric Measurements for Adults*		
Measurement	Gender	Normal Range*
Mid-arm circumference (MAC)	Male	29.3–17.6 cm
	Female	28.5–17.1 cm
Mid-arm muscle circumference (MAMC)	Male	25.3–15.2 cm
	Female	23.2–13.9 cm
Triceps skin fold (TSF)	Male	12.5–7.3 mm
	Female	16.5–9.9 mm

*If measurements are below the lowest range for normal, nutritional support may be indicated.
Adapted from Jelliffe DB. The assessment of the nutritional status of the community. World Health Organization Monograph No. 53. Geneva: World Health Organization, 1986.

If a nutritional problem is beyond the scope of independent nursing practice, the nurse consults with the physician. If the problem can be resolved through independent nursing measures, the nurse may proceed by collaborating with the dietitian, selecting appropriate nursing interventions, and continuing to monitor the patient to evaluate the effectiveness of the nursing plan for care. Refer to the Focus on Older Adults at the end of the chapter for unique nutritional aspects among the older population of patients.

The accompanying Nursing Care Plan for Impaired Swallowing illustrates how the nurse might manage the care of a patient who has a nursing diagnosis of Impaired Swallowing. This diagnostic category is defined in the NANDA Taxonomy (1994) as, "The state in which an individual has decreased ability to voluntarily pass fluids and/or solids from the mouth to the stomach." Nursing guidelines follow with measures for managing the care of patients with other problems associated with nutrition and eating.

Obesity

It is important to confirm that people who are dissatisfied with their appearance actually have a need to lose weight. A desire to lose weight may be based solely on a wish to resemble an unrealistic cultural ideal. **Obesity** is a condition in which there is an excessive amount of body fat, usually over 20% of the ideal weight, or a triceps skin fold measurement greater than 15 mm in men and 17 mm in women, or a BMI greater than 27. People who are extremely overweight are medically evaluated to determine if there are any physical etiologies for the disorder or health risks associated with a weight loss program.

To lose one pound of weight, a person must reduce caloric intake by 3,500 calories. The nurse explains that decreasing the current daily intake of food by 500 calories would have a net effect of a 1 pound weight loss per week. By omitting 1,000 calories per day, 2 pounds could be lost over a week's time. In general, a sustained weight loss of 2 pounds per week is a healthy goal. Obese people are advised against the hazards of unsupervised weight loss techniques like fasting, fad diets, or diet drugs.

Emaciation

Progressive or prolonged weight loss resulting in a weight that is 20% or less than ideal or a BMI of less than 19 can have serious consequences. **Emaciation** is excessive leanness. **Cachexia** is a general wasting away of body tissue. Severe malnourishment is confirmed by a 20% to 25% loss in previously stable body weight. States of severe malnourishment require treatment in collaboration with a physician. The physician may prescribe measures that ensure adequate nourishment, such as gastric or enteral tube feedings and parenteral nutrition, which are discussed in Chapter 29.

Independent nursing interventions are appropriate for thin people who need to increase their weight by approximately 10 pounds to achieve ideal body weight. To gain one pound, a person must consume 3,500 calories more than his or her metabolic needs. This is best done gradually over a period of a time.

Anorexia

Anorexia is a loss of appetite or a lack of desire for food. There are many factors that may produce anorexia, including illness, altered taste and smell, oral problems, and feeling tense and depressed. Simple anorexia is usually a short-lived symptom that requires no medical or nursing intervention. However, the nurse never ignores the fact that a patient is not eating. If food is uneaten, the nurse assesses for physiologic, emotional, cultural, or social etiologies that may be contributing factors.

NURSING GUIDELINES FOR OVERCOMING SIMPLE ANOREXIA

- Cater to the patient's food preferences.
  Rationale: Promotes food consumption
- Serve nutrient-dense foods, that is, foods that are calorie loaded.
  Rationale: May compensate for a low intake of food
- Offer small servings of food at frequent intervals.
  Rationale: May result in a cumulative intake that is within acceptable nutritional levels
- Ensure that the patient is rested before meal time.
  Rationale: Conserves energy for eating
- Provide an opportunity for oral hygiene before meals.
  Rationale: Stimulates salivation and potentiates the pleasure from eating
- Help the patient to a sitting position.
  Rationale: Stimulates the appetite center and promotes access to the food
- Arrange for the patient to eat with others, such as at a group table.
  Rationale: May encourage the patient to eat more food

- Serve food attractively.
  Rationale: Stimulates the appetite center
- Suggest adding spices and herbs to foods.
  Rationale: May stimulate a desire to eat, but may have the opposite effect as well; when experimenting, add new seasonings to small amounts of food

- Serve foods at their appropriate temperature.
  Rationale: Promotes food consumption
- Serve cool, bland foods to patients with mouth irritation.
  Rationale: Minimizes irritation of oral structures

NURSING CARE PLAN:
Impaired Swallowing

Assessment

Subjective Data
States "I'm losing weight. I've almost given up trying to eat. I get more on me than in me since my stroke."

Objective Data
67-year-old woman recovering from a cerebral vascular accident (CVA). Gag reflex is present on stimulating the throat with a cotton-tipped swab. Produces an audible cough on request. Food lodges in pockets of left cheek. Drools from left side of mouth when attempting to swallow.

Diagnosis

Impaired Swallowing related to neuromuscular impairment.

Plan

Goal
The patient will demonstrate swallowing techniques that result in an empty mouth and maintenance of present weight of 110 lb. by 2/5.

Orders: 2/1
1. Weigh every day on standing scale at 0730 wearing slippers, patient gown, and cotton robe.
2. Maintain suction machine, suction catheter, and oxygen per mask at the bedside in case of choking.
3. Seat in a high-backed chair for meals.
4. Cover chest with towel.
5. Open sealed food containers.
6. Sit with patient and remain throughout meals.
7. Remind to place food on the unaffected (right) side of the mouth and chew well.
8. Repeat the following instructions for swallowing:
   - Work the food to the back of mouth
   - Lift tongue up to the roof of mouth
   - Close lips tightly
   - Lower chin toward chest
   - Swallow once and repeat
9. Give patient a hand mirror for inspecting the mouth.
10. Have patient use a finger to clear food from the cheek and repeat instructions for swallowing. _____ T. BERENSON, RN

Implementation
(Documentation) 2/2

0745 Weighed 109 lbs. using standing scale. Up in chair for breakfast. Places food on R. side of mouth with spoon. Given instructions for swallowing as identified in care plan. _____ V. HILL, RN

Evaluation
(Documentation)

0830 Mouth suctioned twice. Food still under tongue after several swallowing attempts. States, "I can't feel were the food's at." Used a mirror to visualize retained food. Able to swallow food after finger sweep. Ate half of breakfast. States, "I'm so discouraged. I don't think I'll ever be able to eat in public again." _____ V. HILL, RN

Nausea

Nausea is a feeling of sickness with a desire to vomit. The feeling of nausea is produced when gastrointestinal sensations, sensory data, and drug effects stimulate a portion of the medulla that contains the vomiting center.

Nausea may be associated with feeling faint or weak. Often, dizziness, perspiration, skin pallor, a rapid pulse rate, and a headache are present. The physician is consulted when nursing measures like the ones that follow are unsuccessful for overcoming nausea. Prescribed medications may be necessary.

NURSING GUIDELINES FOR RELIEVING NAUSEA

- Check to see if something as simple as an annoying odor or sight is contributing to nausea.
  Rationale: Removes offensive sensory data, which can stimulate the vomiting center in the brain
- Have the patient take deep breaths.
  Rationale: Redirects conscious attention away from the unpleasant sensation
- Avoid abrupt movements and limit activities.
  Rationale: Prevents shifting of gastrointestinal structures and their contents, which may intensify stimulation of the vomiting center
- Limit the intake of food and fluid temporarily until signs of nausea subside.
  Rationale: Prevents distention of the stomach, a common trigger of the vomiting center
- Avoid making negative comments about food.
  Rationale: Prevents creation of visual images that may stimulate the vomiting center

Once nausea has been relieved, resuming fluid intake and nourishment becomes a priority. This process is always begun gradually. Sips of clear fluids are offered first. Soft, bland food can be added in small amounts when fluids are tolerated.

Vomiting

Vomiting results when the contents of the stomach are expelled through the mouth. The vomited content is called **emesis** or **vomitus**. **Retching**, which is the act of vomiting without producing vomitus, may also occur. Nausea is usually present before vomiting occurs. Bringing stomach contents to the throat and mouth without the effort of vomiting is called **regurgitation**; it is quite common among infants after eating.

Projectile vomiting is that which occurs with great force. Nausea may be present, but often is not. Projectile vomiting is associated with certain disease conditions, such as increased pressure in the brain.

NURSING GUIDELINES FOR MANAGING THE CARE OF A VOMITING PATIENT

- Temporarily limit the intake of food.
  Rationale: Shortens episodes of vomiting
- Lean the vomiting patient's head forward over a container or the toilet.
  Rationale: Reduces the possibility that vomitus will enter the lungs
- Adjust the light, sound, ventilation, and temperature to a comfortable level.
  Rationale: May reduce the urge to vomit by decreasing sensory stimulation
- Apply a cool washcloth to the forehead or back of the neck.
  Rationale: Alleviates the increase in perspiration and the clammy feeling to the skin that often accompany vomiting
- Rinse the mouth, offer mouthwash, or provide mouth care as soon as possible after vomiting.
  Rationale: Protects tooth enamel from the harmful effects of gastric acid, and removes the unpleasant aftertaste of emesis
- Turn an unconscious or weak patient onto the abdomen or side.
  Rationale: Helps emesis drain from the mouth rather than remain in the throat, where it may be aspirated into the lungs
- Use a suction machine to clear vomitus from the mouth and throat of a weak or unconscious patient.
  Rationale: Removes fluid from the oral cavity and airway, thus preventing choking and aspiration (see Chap. 36)
- Provide firm support with the hands or a pillow to an abdominal incision of a vomiting surgical patient. An abdominal binder may also provide incisional support (see Chap. 28).
  Rationale: Decreases pain and discomfort caused by strong muscle contractions pulling on stitches
- Remove the container of emesis from the patient's bedside as soon as possible. Provide ventilation to remove any lingering odors.
  Rationale: Removes the sight and odor of vomitus, which may stimulate more vomiting

The characteristics of the emesis are described in the patient's medical record. If it is possible, the amount of emesis is measured and the volume is recorded. Documentation includes the amount, color, appearance, and any unusual odor, such as the odor of fecal material or alcohol. If the characteristics of the emesis are unusual, a specimen is saved in case the physician may want to examine it. If there are any doubts about whether to discard or save the emesis, it is best to check with a more experienced nurse. The physician is always consulted when vomiting is prolonged. It may be necessary to administer prescribed medications to relieve it.

Stomach Gas

Stomach gas primarily results from swallowing air. It only becomes a problem when it accumulates. **Eructation**, or belching, is a discharge of stomach gas from the stomach through the mouth. **Flatus** is gas that is formed in the intestine and released from the rectum. Nursing measures for relieving intestinal gas are discussed in Chapter 31.

NURSING GUIDELINES FOR PREVENTING AND RELIEVING STOMACH GAS

- Suggest that patients chew food with their mouth closed.
  Rationale: Decreases amount of air swallowed
- Eliminate the use of straws.
  Rationale: Prevents swallowing the air within the straw
- Advise against chewing gum and smoking cigarettes.
  Rationale: Reduces factors that contribute to swallowing air
- Limit or restrict foods that contain large volumes of air such as soufflés, yeast breads, and carbonated beverages.
  Rationale: Prevents swallowing air trapped within food and drinking beverages that contain dissolved gas
- Recommend that when under tension, avoid eating.
  Rationale: Avoids delayed gastric emptying with concomitant trapping of gas in the stomach
- Propose walking about if uncomfortable.
  Rationale: Helps gas rise to its highest point, making it easier to be belched through the mouth
- Consult with the physician about the use of medications that relieve accumulating gas. Instruct patients who purchase over-the-counter drugs to follow label directions for their use.

Rationale: Promotes the elimination of air by reducing the surface tension of gas bubbles, using a chemical such as simethicone, an ingredient in several nonprescription antacid products

COMMON HOSPITAL DIETS

Some common hospital diets include regular, light, soft, mechanical soft, full liquid, clear liquid, and various therapeutic modifications for which components are adjusted to treat the symptoms of a patient's medical disorder (Table 14-5). Most hospitals have a dietitian who plans the meals that are served to patients and a centralized food service that prepares patient meals.

Nurses are usually responsible for ordering and canceling diets for patients, serving and collecting dietary trays, helping patients eat, and recording how well or how much food has been eaten. It is important that the nurse know the type of diet prescribed for each patient, the purpose of the diet, and its characteristics. Care is taken that patients receive the correct diet and restricted foods are withheld.

SERVING AND REMOVING DIETARY TRAYS

Patients are usually served food at their bedside. Some hospitals have cafeterias for patients who are ambulatory. Nursing homes usually have a large dining room

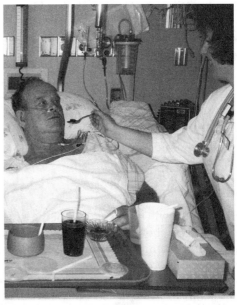

FIGURE 14-7
Feeding a patient. (Courtesy of Ken Timby.)

PATIENT TEACHING FOR PROMOTING WEIGHT LOSS

Teach the patient or the family to do the following:

- Comply with the numbers of servings recommended by the food pyramid to meet the requirements for 2,000 calories.
- Limit servings from the food pyramid to their suggested amounts as follows:
  Grains: one slice of bread, one ounce of cereal, or one-half cup of cooked pasta, rice, or cereal
  Vegetables: one cup of raw or one-half cup cooked, or three-fourths cup of vegetable juice
  Fruits: one medium fresh or one-half cup chopped, or three-fourths cup of fruit juice
  Dairy: one cup of milk or yogurt, or one-half ounce of natural cheese, or two ounces of processed cheese
  Meat: two to three ounces of cooked lean meat, poultry, or fish, or one-half cup cooked dry beans, or one egg, or two tablespoons of peanut butter

- Use fats, oils, and sugar sparingly.
- Eliminate junk food, which contributes calories but not much nutrition, and alcoholic beverages.
- Eat small meals, but more frequently, rather than three large meals per day; any nutrients not used from large meals are stored as fat
- Sit at the table to eat, and do not do other things, such as reading, while eating; distraction often fools the brain into thinking that food has not been consumed.
- Increase fiber in the diet from fresh fruits, vegetables, and whole grains; fiber is not digested and may provide a full feeling without large numbers of calories.
- Participate in some regular, active form of exercise. Exercise raises the **metabolic rate**, the rate at which calories are used, while actually suppressing the appetite. Information on activity and exercise can be found in Chapter 24.

---

where patients eat together in small groups. Nurses and dietary personnel work cooperatively in making sure that patients receive food at mealtimes and the trays are collected afterward. The nursing responsibilities for serving and removing trays are identified in Skill 14-1.

FEEDING PATIENTS

Some patients need help with eating. Skill 14-2 provides suggested actions for feeding patients who can bite, sip, chew, and swallow, but for some reason lack the ability to cut food and use utensils for eating (Fig. 14-7). Nursing suggestions follow for helping patients with **dysphagia** (difficulty swallowing), those who are blind or have both eyes patched, and those who suffer from dementia (impairment of intellectual functioning).

Feeding the Dysphagic Patient

The following techniques can be used when caring for patients who have difficulty chewing and swallowing food:

- Always have equipment for oral and pharyngeal suctioning at the bedside (see Chap. 36).
- If the patient has a tracheostomy tube or endotracheal tube, make sure that the cuff is inflated (see Chap. 36).

(text continues on page 243)

PATIENT TEACHING FOR PROMOTING WEIGHT GAIN

Teach the patient or the family to do the following:

- Eat a variety of foods from the food pyramid, but increase the number of servings or serving sizes.
- Eat small amounts frequently.
- Eat with others.

- Snack on high-calorie but nutritious foods such as hard cheese, milk shakes, and nuts.
- Disguise extra calories by fortifying foods with powdered milk, gravies, or sauces.
- Garnish food with the addition of cubed or grated cheese, diced meat, nuts, or raisins.
- Rest after consuming food.

TABLE 14-5. *Common Types and Characteristics of Prescribed Diets*

Type of Diet	Characteristics
Regular or general	Allows unrestricted selections of food
Light or convalescent	Differs from a regular diet primarily in the method of preparing food. Fried foods, rich pastries, fat-rich foods, gas-forming foods, and raw foods are typically omitted.
Soft	Contains foods that are soft in texture. The diet is low in residue, is readily digested, contains few or no spices or condiments, and has fewer fruits, vegetables, and meats than a light diet.
Mechanical soft	Resembles a light diet but is used for people who have problems chewing food. Vegetables and fruits are cooked and meats are ground.
Full liquid	Contains fruit and vegetables juices, creamed or blended soups, milk, ices, ice cream, gelatin, junket, custards, and cooked cereals.
Clear liquid	Consists of water, clear broth, clear fruit juices, plain gelatin, tea, and coffee. Carbonated beverages may or may not be permitted.
Special therapeutic	Consists of foods that are prepared to meet special needs. A few examples include: caloric, sodium, fat, and fiber restricted diets.

SKILL 14-1
Serving and Removing Dietary Trays

Suggested Action	Reason for Action
Assessment	
Check on the usual time for meals.	Facilitates planning nursing care
Determine which patients are undergoing tests, or for some other reason require that food be withheld.	Ensures that therapeutic outcomes are not affected by eating
Note the type of diet that is currently prescribed for each patient.	Follows the patient's therapeutic management plan
Review the Kardex for information concerning patients' food allergies or food intolerances.	Reduces the potential for adverse reactions.
Planning	
Prepare patients so that they are ready to eat at the designated time.	Ensures that the food is served at its appropriate temperature
Meet patients' needs for comfort, hygiene, and elimination before dietary trays arrive.	Promotes appetite and eating
Help patients to a sitting position.	Assists ambulatory patients to a comfortable position
Implementation	
Wash hands before serving trays.	Prevents transmission of microorganisms
Deliver dietary trays, one by one, as soon as possible.	Facilitates the enjoyment of eating through prompt delivery of food at its intended temperature
Compare the name on the tray with the name on the patient's identification bracelet, or ask the patient to identify himself or herself by name.	Avoids dietary errors
Place the tray so that it is facing the patient.	Provides ease of access to the food
Uncover the food and check its appearance.	Ensures that the tray is complete, orderly, and tidy

(continued)

SKILL 14-1
Serving and Removing Dietary Trays *(Continued)*

Suggested Action	Reason for Action
Assist the patient as necessary with opening cartons and preparing food.	Demonstrates consideration and facilitates independence
Replace food that is objectionable or request special additional items from the dietary department.	Demonstrates respect for unique needs
Check if the patient has any further requests, like adjustment of the pillows or donning eyeglasses, before leaving the room.	Reduces inconveniences during meal time
Make sure the signal cord is handy in case a need arises later.	Provides a means for summoning assistance
Check on the patient's progress from time to time.	Indicates a willingness to provide assistance
Remove the food tray when the patient is finished eating.	Restores order and cleanliness to the environment
Record the amount of fluid consumed from the dietary tray on the bedside flow sheet, if the patient's fluid intake is being monitored (see Chap. 15).	Ensures accurate fluid assessment
Note the percentage of food that the patient has eaten.	Ensures that dietary intake is documented according to JCAHO on precise current standards rather than using vague terms like *good*, *fair*, and *poor*
Assist the patient to brush and floss his or her teeth, if desired.	Removes food residue that may support microbial growth
Place the patient in a position of comfort.	Demonstrates care and concern

Evaluation
- Feels hunger is satisfied
- Majority of food is consumed

Document
- Type of diet and percentage of food consumed

*Sample Documentation**

Date and Time   Ate 100% of mechanical soft diet with need for assistance. _____ **Signature, Title**

* In many agencies the percentage of consumed food is recorded on a flow sheet or checklist. Other pertinent data are recorded within the medical record.

- Place the patient in a sitting position.
- Provide oral hygiene to moisten the mouth.
- Initially avoid dry foods, like crackers, and sticky foods, like bananas.
- Request semisolid foods with some texture, like oatmeal, poached eggs, and mashed potatoes, which are easier to swallow than liquids and watery, pureed food.
- Offer quarter- to half-teaspoon size amounts.
- Observe the patient's swallowing.

- Ask the patient to speak; if the patient's voice sounds normal, not wet and gurgly, the food is most likely in the esophagus. If not, have the patient swallow several more times, cough to clear the airway, or you may need to suction the pharynx.
- Check the mouth for pockets of food that remain unswallowed before offering more.
- Keep the patient in a sitting position for at least a half hour after eating to avoid pulmonary complications should regurgitation or vomiting occur.

(text continues on page 246)

SKILL 14-2
Feeding a Patient

Suggested Action	Reason for Action
Assessment	
Compare the dietary information on the Kardex with the medical record.	Ensures accuracy in providing current therapeutic management
Verify that food or fluids are not temporarily being withheld.	Prevents delaying or having to cancel diagnostic tests
Determine if the patient's fluid intake is being measured.	Ensures accurate documentation of data
Assess the patient to determine what or how much assistance is necessary.	Aids in identifying specific problems and selecting nursing interventions
Review the medical record for how well and how much the patient has eaten during previous meals, and weight trends.	Helps in establishing realistic goals and evaluating progress
Review the characteristics of the diet order.	Helps in determining if the correct food is served
Analyze the purpose for the prescribed diet.	Assists in evaluating therapeutic responses
Assess the patient's current needs for elimination or relief from pain, nausea, fatigue.	Identifies current unmet physiologic needs
Check the medication record for drugs that must be administered before or with meals.	Facilitates optimum drug absorption and reduces drug side effects
Planning	
Set realistic goals for how much food the patient will eat, and how much the patient will participate in self-feeding.	Establishes criteria for evaluating patient responses
Select appropriate nursing measures for promoting the patient's comfort, such as administering an analgesic.	Helps resolve problems that, if ignored, may interfere with eating
Complete priority responsibilities for assigned patients.	Allows a period during which feeding is uninterrupted
Provide for oral hygiene and handwashing before the tray is served.	Controls the transmission of microorganisms; promotes appetite and aesthetics
Prepare medications that must be given before or with meals, or delegate that responsibility.	Coordinates drug and nutritional therapy
Clear clutter and soiled articles from the eating area.	Promotes orderliness and a sanitary environment
Implementation	
Wash hands before preparing food.	Prevents transmission of microorganisms
Obtain or clean special utensils or containers that have been adapted for use by a patient with a physical disability, such as a fork to which a hand grip has been attached.	Promotes independence and self-reliance
Raise the head of the bed to a sitting position or assist to a chair.	Promotes safety by facilitating swallowing
Check that the correct diet and tray are served to the correct patient.	Indicates responsibility and accountability for therapeutic management

(continued)

SKILL 14-2
Feeding a Patient *(Continued)*

Suggested Action	Reason for Action
Cover the patient's upper chest and lap with a napkin or towel.	Protects bedclothes and linen
Sit beside or across from the patient.	Promotes socialization and communication
Uncover the food, open cartons, season food.	Stimulates gastric secretions and motility
Encourage the patient to assist to the limit of his or her abilities.	Maintains or supports independence and self-care
Avoid rushing.	Communicates a relaxed atmosphere while eating
Collaborate with the patient on which foods are desired before loading a fork or spoon.	Accommodates for the individual's preferences
Provide manageable amounts of food with each bite.	Prevents choking or airway obstruction
For a stroke patient, direct the food toward the unparalyzed side of the mouth.	Places food in an area where there is feeling and muscle control for chewing and swallowing
Give the patient time to chew thoroughly and swallow.	Aids digestion by grinding the food and mixing it with saliva and enzymes
Let the patient indicate when ready for more food or a sip of beverage.	Promotes an independent locus of control
Talk with the patient about pleasant subjects.	Combines eating with socialization
Record fluid intake if the patient's intake is being measured.	Documents essential assessment data
Remove the tray and make the patient comfortable (it is best for patients to remain in a sitting or semisitting position for at least 30 minutes after eating unless there is a medical reason for doing otherwise).	Prevents the reflux of stomach contents into the esophagus and reduces the potential for aspiration
Offer the patient an opportunity for oral hygiene.	Removes sugar and starches that support microbial growth and tooth decay
Estimate the percent of food that has been eaten.	Provides data for determining current and future nutritional needs

Evaluation

- Eats approximately 75% of meal
- Maintains body weight
- Participates at maximum capacity

Document

- Type of diet
- Percentage of food consumed
- Tolerance of food
- Patient's ability to participate
- Problems encountered with chewing or swallowing.
- Approaches taken to resolve problems.

Sample Documentation

Date and Time   Stated "I'm full" after consuming 75% of full liquid diet. Unable to hold spoon or glass, but could direct straw into mouth. _____ **Signature, Title**

Feeding the Visually Impaired Patient

When caring for patients who are temporarily or permanently sightless, do the following:

- Place a thick towel across the patient's chest and over the lap.
- If the patient is able to eat independently, consider using dishes with rims or bowls to prevent spilling.
- Arrange as much as possible to have finger foods (foods that may be eaten with the hands) prepared for the patient.
- Describe the food and indicate where it is located on the tray.
- Use the analogy of a clock when describing where food may be found on the plate. For example, "the potatoes are at 3 o'clock."
- Guide the patient's hand to reinforce the location of food and utensils.
- Prepare the food by opening cartons, cutting bite-size pieces, adding salt and pepper, buttering bread, pouring coffee, and so on.
- If the patient needs to be fed, tell him or her what kind of food is being offered with each mouthful.
- Devise a system whereby the patient can indicate when he or she is ready for more food or beverage, such as asking or raising a finger.
- Do not rush the patient; eating should take place at a leisurely pace.

Assisting the Patient With Dementia

Dementia refers to the deterioration of previous intellectual capacity. It is a common problem among patients with neurologic conditions like Alzheimer's disease. Demented patients often can be helped to retain their ability to carry out activities of daily living, like self-feeding, by ensuring their attention and concentration and repeating actions over and over. Therefore, it may be helpful for the nurse to do the following:

- Have the same staff person help the patient, if at all possible, so as to develop a rapport with the patient and promote continuity of care.
- Be consistent with the time and place for eating.
- Reduce or eliminate distractions within the eating environment to promote concentration on the task at hand.
- Place the food tray close to the patient, not the staff person, to communicate visually and spatially that the food is to be eaten by the patient.
- Remove unnecessary wrappers, containers, and food covers to reduce confusion.

- Pour milk from a carton into a glass so it is easily recognizable.
- Encourage the patient's participation by offering finger foods and utensils to stimulate awareness and memory.
- Ensure that the patient can see at least one other individual who is also eating; self-feeding may occur by watching another person model the desired behavior.
- Guide the hand with food to the patient's mouth.
- Positively reinforce a desired response by praising, touching, and smiling at the patient.
- Remain with the patient; do not begin feeding, leave, and then return because this interrupts the patient's attention and concentration.

KEY CONCEPTS

- Nutrition is the process by which the body uses food. Malnutrition results from inadequate consumption of nutrients.
- The components of basic nutrition include adequate amounts of calories, proteins, carbohydrates, fats, vitamins, and minerals.
- Some factors that affect nutritional needs include age, height and weight, growth, activity, and health status.
- The food pyramid is a guide for promoting a healthy dietary intake of food. It provides recommended servings and sizes of servings for meat or its substitute, dairy products, fruits, vegetables, and grain products to acquire 2,000 calories per day.
- Nutritional labels now indicate the serving size in household measurements and the daily value for specific nutrients per serving, and must meet established criteria for using health-related claims.
- Protein complementation is the practice of combining two plant food sources for protein to obtain all the essential amino acids required for healthy nutrition.
- Data that provide objective information about a person's nutritional status include anthropometric measurements, physical examination data, and results from laboratory tests.
- A diet history is the information obtained by asking a person to describe his or her eating habits and factors that may affect nutrition.
- Common problems that may be identified after performing a nutritional assessment include weight problems, anorexia, nausea, vomiting, and stomach gas.

FOCUS ON OLDER ADULTS

When caring for older adults, it is common to find that :

- A decline in smell and taste may affect appetite and food intake.
- As a whole, the diet of older adults tends to be high in carbohydrates, which are more affordable on a fixed income.
- To compensate for a decrease in appetite, it may be helpful for older adults to consume more nutrient-dense foods, like meat and milk, rather than taking in nutrient-deficient calories from sweets like cake or cookies.
- As adults get older, there is progressive loosening and loss of teeth. Oral and dental problems interfere with adequate nutrition.
- Approximately 20% of the population older than 65 years of age suffer from **xerostomia**, a dry mouth caused by decreased salivation (Matteson & McConnell, 1988). Xerostomia may be caused by medication side effects, but whatever the cause, it affects the ability to mix food with saliva and swallow it.
- Chronic health conditions, like arthritis, paralysis due to stroke and dementia, and visual impairments affect the ability of older adults to remain independent and self-reliant in accomplishing their activities of daily living.
- Older adults in general take more than four medications on a regular basis to treat various chronic diseases (William & DiPalma, 1992).

This factor increases the incidence of medication–nutrient interactions.
- Nutrition may be affected by a painful or burning tongue due to oral infections, poorly fitting dentures, or vitamin deficiencies.
- In older adults, dysphagia may be the result either of a dilated or constricted esophagus, dilated pouches in the esophagus known as diverticula, or pressure from abdominal disorders.
- It may be difficult for older adults to obtain food because of an inability to find transportation for shopping.
- Social isolation and accompanying depression may affect the quality and amount of food that is consumed by older adults.
- Environmental barriers, such as high cupboards, may prevent older adults from storing or preparing a variety of foods.
- Older adults may benefit from being referred to community services that provide group meals at centralized meal sites or home delivery such as the Meals on Wheels program, and those funded by the National Nutrition Program for the Elderly, established under the Older Americans Act.
- Some commercial vendors, even hospital food services, may provide special meals for minimal fees to discharged patients.
- Older adults may be referred to the state's Commission on Aging, which may assist with obtaining food stamps or other social welfare services based on income.

- Some common hospital diets include regular, light, soft, mechanical soft, full liquid, clear liquid, and various therapeutic modifications of these diets.
- Nurses are usually responsible for ordering and canceling diets for patients, serving and collecting dietary trays, helping patients eat, and recording how much food has been eaten.
- Nurses must know the type of diet prescribed for each patient, the purpose for the diet, and its characteristics.
- The nutrition of older adults may be affected by oral problems, like the loss of teeth and reduced saliva; side effects caused by medications or their interaction with nutrients; physical disabilities; social isolation; and living on a fixed income.

CRITICAL THINKING EXERCISES

- Design a dinner menu for a young, middle-aged, and older adult that meets the daily requirements in the food pyramid, but also reflects their unique age-related differences.
- Take your own anthropometric measurements, or those of some other person, and analyze the information according to the norms provided in this chapter. Based on your analysis, what recommendations are appropriate?
- A patient tells the nurse that she eats the following on a daily basis: cereal, milk, and banana for breakfast; a sandwich made with processed meat, mayonnaise, and a soft drink for lunch; a candy bar in the late af-

ternoon; and meat, potatoes, vegetable, and glass of milk for supper. In the late evening, she snacks on potato chips. Using the food pyramid, what would be appropriate recommendations to improve this patient's nutrition?

SUGGESTED READINGS

Cerrato PL. Becoming a vegetarian: the risks and the benefits. RN March 1991;54:73–77.

Earnest VV. Clinical Skills in Nursing Practice. 2nd ed. Philadelphia: JB Lippincott, 1993.

Eschleman MM. Introductory Nutrition and Nutrition Therapy. 3rd ed. Philadelphia: Lippincott-Raven, 1996.

Fishbach F. A Manual of Laboratory and Diagnostic Tests. 4th ed. Philadelphia: JB Lippincott, 1992.

Gray GE, Gray LK. Anthropometric measurements and their interpretation: principles, practices and problems. Journal of the American Dietetic Association 1980;77:534.

Hamwi GJ. Therapy: changing dietary concepts. In: Diabetes Mellitus: Diagnosis and Treatment. New York: American Diabetes Association, 1964.

Keithley JK, Kohn CL. Advances in nutritional care of medical–surgical patients. MEDSURG Nursing September 1992;1:13–20.

Matteson MA, McConnell ES. Gerontological Nursing: Concepts and Practice. Philadelphia: WB Saunders, 1988.

Meehan M. Nursing Dx: potential for aspiration. RN January 1992;55:30–35.

Miller CA. Nursing Care of Older Adults: Theory and Practice. Glenview, IL: Scott, Foresman/Little, Brown, 1990.

NANDA Nursing Diagnoses: Definitions and Classification 1994–1995. Philadelphia: North American Nursing Diagnosis Association, 1994.

National Center for Nutrition and Dietetics. Labeling Logic: Healthful Eating With the New Food Label. Chicago: American Dietetic Association, 1994.

Osborn CL, Marshall M. Promoting mealtime independence. Geriatric Nursing September–October 1992;13:254–256.

The new food labels. American Health May 1994;4:101.

United States Department of Agriculture and United States Department of Health and Human Services. Dietary Guidelines for Americans. Washington, DC: U.S. Government Printing Office, 1990.

United States Department of Health and Human Services. Healthy People 2000: National Health Promotion and Disease Prevention Objectives. Boston: Jones and Bartlett, 1992.

Van Ort S, Phillips L. Feeding nursing home residents with Alzheimer's disease. Geriatric Nursing September–October 1992;13:249–253.

Williams SG, DiPalma JA. Medication-induced digestive system injury in the elderly. Geriatric Nursing January–February 1992;13:39–42.

Yen PK. Nutrition: a vital sign. Geriatric Nursing January–February 1992;13:52–53.

CHAPTER 15

Fluid and Chemical Balance

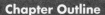 NURSING GUIDELINES

 SKILLS

 NURSING CARE PLAN

Fluid Volume Deficit

Key Terms

Active Transport	Intake and Output
Air Embolism	Interstitial Fluid
Anions	Intracellular Fluid
Cations	Intravascular Fluid
Circulatory Overload	Intravenous Fluids
Colloidal Osmotic Pressure	Ions
Colloids	Isotonic Solution
Colloid Solutions	Medication Lock
Crystalloid Solutions	Nonelectrolytes
Drop Factor	Osmosis
Electrolytes	Parenteral Nutrition
Emulsion	Passive Diffusion
Extracellular Fluid	Peripheral Parenteral Nutrition
Facilitated Diffusion	
Filtration	Phlebitis
Fluid Imbalance	Pulmonary Embolus
Hypertonic Solution	Third-spacing
Hypotonic Solution	Thrombus Formation
Hypovolemia	Total Parenteral Nutrition
Infiltration	Venipuncture
Infusion Pump	Volumetric Controller

Learning Objectives

An understanding of the content within this chapter will be evidenced by the student's ability to:

- Name four components of body fluid
- List five physiologic processes by which fluid and its constituents are distributed

- Name ten assessments that provide data about a patient's fluid status
- Describe three methods for maintaining or restoring fluid volume
- Describe four methods for reducing fluid volume
- List six reasons for administering intravenous fluids
- Differentiate between crystalloid and colloid solutions and give examples of each
- Explain the terms "isotonic," "hypotonic," and "hypertonic" in reference to intravenous solutions
- List four factors that affect the choice of tubing used to administer intravenous solutions
- Name three techniques for infusing intravenous solutions
- Discuss at least five criteria for selecting a vein through which to administer intravenous fluid
- List seven complications associated with administering intravenous fluid
- Discuss two purposes for inserting a medication lock
- Identify three differences between administering blood and crystalloid solutions
- Name at least five types of transfusion reactions
- Explain the concept of parenteral nutrition

Body fluid is a mixture of water, chemicals called electrolytes and nonelectrolytes, and blood cells. Because water is the vehicle for transporting these substances, it is the very essence of life. And, because water is not stored in any great reserve, daily replacement is the key to maintaining survival.

In this chapter, the mechanisms for maintaining fluid balance and restoring fluid volume and the components that are present in body fluid are discussed.

WATER

The human body is composed of approximately 45% to 75% water depending on age and gender (Table 15-1). Body water is normally supplied and replenished from three sources:

- Drinking liquids
- Consuming food
- Oxidizing nutrients during metabolism

Once the water is absorbed, it is distributed among various locations, called compartments, within the body.

Fluid Compartments

Body fluid is located in two general compartments: inside and outside cells (Fig. 15-1). The fluid inside cells is referred to as **intracellular fluid**, and that which is outside the cells is called **extracellular fluid**. Extracellular fluid is further subdivided into **interstitial fluid**, or that located in the tissue space between and around cells, and **intravascular fluid**, which refers to the watery plasma, or serum, portion of blood.

ELECTROLYTES

Electrolytes (Table 15-2) are chemical compounds such as sodium and chloride, and others present in food, that become dissolved in body fluid. Once dissolved, they enable the body to perform chemical activities like facilitating muscle contraction and forming enzymes, acids, and bases.

Electrolytes, also known as **ions**, carry either a positive or negative electrical charge. A **cation** is an electrolyte with a positive charge; an **anion** is an electrolyte with a negative charge. Overall, the amounts of cations and anions, measured in *milliequivalents* (mEq), are similar, although they may be distributed differently in each of the fluid compartments. For example, there are more potassium ions inside cells than outside. When the overall ratio changes or any individual component becomes excessive or deficient, there is said to be an electrolyte imbalance. Any imbalance in electrolytes can lead to dangerous physiologic problems. Changes in fluid volumes very often are accompanied by electrolyte imbalances as well.

NONELECTROLYTES

Nonelectrolytes are chemical compounds that remain bound together when dissolved in a solution, and therefore cannot conduct electricity. The chemical end-products of carbohydrate, protein, and fat metabolism—glucose, amino acids, and fatty acids,

TABLE 15-1. *Percentages of Body Fluid According to Age and Gender*				
Fluid Compartment	Infants	Adult Men	Adult Women	Elderly
Intravascular	4%	4%	5%	5%
Interstitial	25%	11%	10%	15%
Intracellular	48%	45%	35%	25%
Total	77%	60%	50%	45%

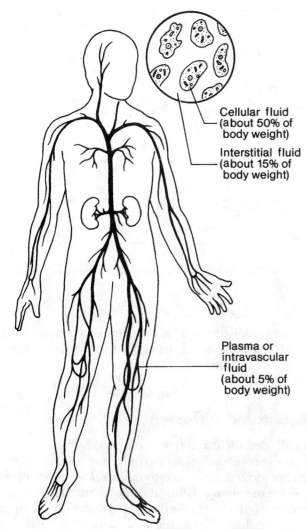

FIGURE 15-1
Normal distribution of body fluid.

respectively—provide a continuous supply of non-electrolytes.

In the absence of metabolic diseases, as long as people consume adequate amounts of these nutrients, there ought to be stable amounts of nonelectrolytes circulating in body fluid. Deficiency states may occur when body fluid is lost or when the ability to eat is compromised.

BLOOD

Blood consists of 3 liters of plasma, or fluid, and 2 liters of blood cells, making a total of 5 liters of circulating volume. Blood cells include erythrocytes, or red blood cells; leukocytes, or white blood cells; and platelets, also known as thrombocytes. For every 500 red blood cells, there are approximately 30 platelets and 1 white blood cell (Fischbach, 1992).

Any disorder that alters the volume of body fluid, whether it be fluid retention or loss, also affects the plasma volume of blood. Blood cell volume may be affected by chronic bleeding or hemorrhage, infection, disease conditions that destroy the blood cells, and disorders that affect the bone marrow's production of blood cells. Deficits in either fluid or cell volume may be treated by administering fluid, whole blood or packed cells, or individual blood components.

FLUID AND ELECTROLYTE DISTRIBUTION

Although fluid compartments are identified separately, water and the substances dissolved therein continuously circulate throughout all areas of the body. The movement and relocation of water and substances within body fluid are governed by physiologic processes such as *osmosis, filtration, passive diffusion, facilitated diffusion,* and *active transport.*

Osmosis

Osmosis is a process that regulates the distribution of water from one compartment to another. Under the influence of osmosis, water moves through semipermeable membranes, like those surrounding body cells, from an area where the fluid is more dilute to an area where the fluid is more concentrated (Fig. 15-2). Once the fluid is of equal concentration on both sides of the membrane, the balance of fluid between compartments does not change appreciably—fluid

TABLE 15-2. *Major Serum Electrolytes*			
Electrolyte	**Chemical Symbol**	**Cation/Anion**	**Normal Serum Level**
Sodium	NA	Cation	135–148 mEq/L
Potassium	K	Cation	3.5–5.0 mEq/L
Chloride	Cl	Anion	90–110 mEq/L
Phosphate	PO$_4$	Anion	1.7–2.6 mEq/L
Calcium	Ca	Cation	2.1–2.6 mEq/L
Magnesium	Mg	Cation	1.3–2.1 mEq/L
Bicarbonate	HCO$_3$	Anion	22–26 mEq/L

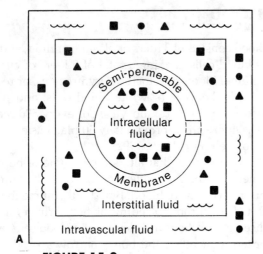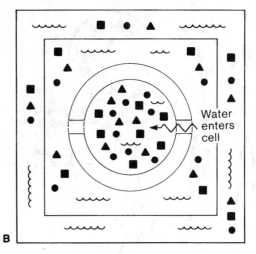

FIGURE 15-2
(*A*) Equal concentration of fluid in all fluid compartments. (*B*) Fluid moves by osmosis to areas of greater concentration.

may continue to be transferred, but equal volumes are exchanged between compartments.

Osmosis is influenced by the presence and quantity of colloids on either side of the semipermeable membrane. **Colloids** are undissolved substances like albumin and blood cells that are within body fluids and do not readily pass through a membrane wall. Their very presence contributes to fluid concentration, and therefore acts as a force for attracting water, a property referred to as **colloidal osmotic pressure**.

Filtration

Filtration, on the other hand, is a process that promotes the movement of fluid and some dissolved substances through a semipermeable membrane according to pressure differences. Filtration regulates the movement of water and substances from a compartment where the pressure is higher to one where the pressure is lower. Thus, at the arterial end of a capillary, where the fluid is under higher pressure than at the venous end, fluid and some dissolved substances like oxygen are forced into the interstitial compartment. Water is then reabsorbed from the interstitial fluid in comparable amounts at the venous end of the capillary as a result of colloidal osmotic pressure (Fig. 15-3).

Filtration also affects the manner in which the kidney excretes fluid and wastes and then selectively reabsorbs water and substances that need to be conserved.

Passive Diffusion

Passive diffusion refers to a physiologic process in which dissolved substances, like electrolytes, move from an area of high concentration to an area of lower

concentration through a semipermeable membrane. Passive diffusion, like osmosis, remains fairly static once equilibrium is achieved.

Facilitated Diffusion

Facilitated diffusion refers to a process in which certain dissolved substances require the assistance of a carrier molecule to pass through one side of a semipermeable membrane to the other. For example, the distribution of glucose molecules is facilitated by a carrier substance known as insulin.

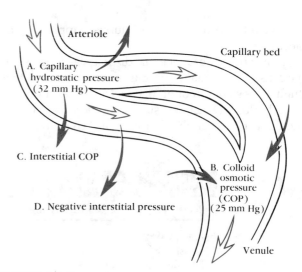

FIGURE 15-3
Dynamics of capillary fluid filtration. (Bullock BL, Rosendahl PP: Pathophysiology: Adaptations and Alterations in Function, 3rd ed, p 184. Philadelphia, JB Lippincott, 1992)

Active Transport

Active transport requires an energy source, a substance called *adenosine triphosphate* (ATP), to drive dissolved chemicals from an area of low concentration to one that is higher—just the opposite of passive diffusion.

An example of active transport is the *sodium–potassium pump system* on cellular membranes that moves potassium from lower concentrations in the extracellular fluid into cells where it is highly concentrated. It also moves sodium, which is in lower amounts within the cells, to extracellular fluid, where it is more abundant.

Metabolic disorders that diminish the supply of ATP seriously affect normal cellular functions by impairing the distribution of chemicals within intracellular and extracellular fluid.

FLUID LOSS

Normal mechanisms for fluid loss are urination, bowel elimination, perspiration, and breathing. Losses from the skin in areas other than where sweat glands are located and from the vapor in exhaled air are referred to as *insensible losses* because they are, for practical purposes, unnoticeable and unmeasurable.

FLUID REGULATION

In healthy adults, fluid intake generally averages approximately 2,500 mL per day, but it can range between 1,800 to 3,000 mL per day with a similar volume of fluid loss (Table 15-3).

Under normal conditions, several mechanisms maintain a match between fluid intake and output. For example, as body fluid becomes concentrated, the brain triggers the sensation of thirst, which then stimulates a person to drink fluid. And, as fluid volume expands, the kidneys excrete a proportionate volume of water to maintain or restore proper balance.

However, there are circumstances in which oral intake or fluid losses may be altered. Therefore, nurses assess patients for signs of fluid deficit or excess, particularly among those who are prone to fluid imbalances (Display 15-1).

FLUID VOLUME ASSESSMENT

Fluid status may be assessed through a combination of physical assessment techniques (Table 15-4) and measuring intake and output volumes.

Intake and Output

Intake and output (I & O) refers to measuring a patient's fluid intake and fluid loss over a 24-hour period. Agencies often specify which types of patients are automatically placed on I & O. In general, they include:

- All postoperative patients, until they are eating, drinking, and voiding in sufficient quantities
- All patients who are receiving intravenous (IV) fluids
- All patients who are receiving tube feedings
- All patients who have some type of wound drainage or suction equipment
- All patients with urinary catheters, until it can be determined that they have an adequate output or are voiding well after the catheter has been removed

In addition to the previous list, many agencies allow nurses independently to order I & O assessment for those patients who have an actual or potential fluid imbalance problem. The nurse may also discontinue the nursing order when the assessment is no longer indicated.

Each agency has a specific I & O form that is kept at the bedside so that the type of fluid and amounts can be conveniently recorded throughout the day (Fig. 15-4). The amounts are subtotaled at the end of each shift or more frequently in critical care areas. The grand

TABLE 15-3. *Daily Fluid Intake and Losses*			
Sources of Fluid		**Mechanisms of Fluid Loss**	
Oral liquids	1,200–1,500 mL/day	Urine	1,200–1,700 mL/day
Food	700–1,000 mL/day	Feces	100–250 mL/day
Metabolism	200–400 mL/day	Perspiration	100–150 mL/day
		Insensible losses	
		Skin	350–400 mL/day
		Lungs	350–400 mL/day
Total	2,100–2,900 mL/day	**Total**	2,100–2,900 mL/day
Median amount	2,500 mL/day	**Median amount**	2,500 mL/day

DISPLAY 15-1. *Conditions that Predispose to Fluid Imbalances*

Fluid Deficit	Fluid Excess
• Starvation • Impaired swallowing • Vomiting • Gastric suction • Diarrhea • Laxative abuse • Potent diuretics • Hemorrhage • Major burns • Draining wounds • Fever and sweating • Exercise and sweating • Environmental heat and humidity	• Kidney failure • Heart failure • Rapid administration of intravenous fluid or blood • Administration of albumin • Corticosteroid drug therapy • Excessive intake of sodium • Pregnancy • Premenstrual fluid retention

---

total may be documented in a designated area within the patient's medical record, such as on the graphics sheet with other vital sign information.

FLUID INTAKE

Fluid intake is the sum of all fluid consumed by a patient or instilled into the body. It includes:

- All the liquids a patient drinks
- The liquid equivalent of ice chips, which is half of the frozen volume
- Some foods that are considered as liquids by the time they are swallowed, such as gelatin, ice cream, and thin cooked cereal
- Fluid infusions, like IV solutions
- Fluid instillations, such as those administered through feeding tubes or tube irrigations

Fluid volumes are usually recorded in milliliters (mL), a metric measurement. The approximate equivalent for 1 ounce is 30 mL; a teaspoon is 5 mL, and a tablespoon is 15 mL. Packaged beverage containers like milk cartons often indicate their specific fluid volume somewhere on

TABLE 15-4. *Signs of Fluid Imbalance*

Assessment	Fluid Deficit	Fluid Excess
Weight	Weight loss $\geq$ 2 lbs/24 hr	Weight gain $\geq$ 2 lbs/24 hr
Blood pressure	Low	High
Temperature	Elevated	Normal
Pulse	Rapid, weak, thready	Full, bounding
Respirations	Rapid, shallow	Moist, labored
Urine	Scant, dark yellow	Light yellow
Stool	Dry, small volume	Bulky
Skin	Warm, flushed, dry	Cool, pale, moist
	Poor skin turgor	Pitting edema
Mucous membranes	Dry, sticky	Moist
Eyes	Sunken	Swollen
Lungs	Clear	Crackles, gurgles
Breathing	Effortless	Dyspnea, orthopnea
Energy	Weak	Fatigues easily
Jugular neck veins	Flat	Distended
Cognition	Reduced	Reduced
Consciousness	Sleepy	Anxious

24 HOUR INTAKE/OUTPUT RECORD

DATE 2-17		WEIGHT 137#		TIME 0700		TYPE OF WEIGHT ☒ STANDING ☐ CHAIR ☐ BED						
CVP READING: TIME READING		TIME READING		TIME READING								

INTAKE 7-3 SHIFT						OUTPUT 7-3 SHIFT								
Time	Oral	IV	Piggyback	Blood	Tube/Feed	Time	Irrig.	Urine	NG	Emesis	Other	Tube	Tube	BM
0730	100	600				0700		250						
0900			50			0800				100				
1130	240					1200		300						
1300			50			1400		400						
8 HR TOTAL	340	600	100					950		100				
			8° GRAND TOTAL	1040							8° GRAND TOTAL			1050

INTAKE 3-11 SHIFT						OUTPUT 3-11 SHIFT								
Time	Oral	IV	Piggyback	Blood	Tube/Feed	Time	Irrig.	Urine	NG	Emesis	Other	Tube	Tube	BM
1600	30					1530				50				
1700		6.00	50											
1730	30					1800		200						
2000	100					2200		300						
8 HR TOTAL	160	600	50					500		50				
			8° GRAND TOTAL	810							8° GRAND TOTAL			550

INTAKE 11-7 SHIFT						OUTPUT 11-7 SHIFT								
Time	Oral	IV	Piggyback	Blood	Tube/Feed	Time	Irrig.	Urine	NG	Emesis	Other	Tube	Tube	BM
0030	30	600				0100		300						
						0400		200						
						0600		100						
8 HR TOTAL	30	600						600						
			8° GRAND TOTAL	630							8° GRAND TOTAL			600
			24° GRAND TOTAL	2480							24° GRAND TOTAL			2200

FORM 96 (9/92)   CIRRUS 3025

24 HOUR INTAKE / OUTPUT RECORD

FIGURE 15-4

Intake and output volumes are recorded throughout a 24-hour period and subtotaled at the end of each 8-hour shift.

the label. Hospitals may identify the volume equivalents that are contained within the cups, glasses, and bowls used to serve food and beverages from the dietary department (Display 15-2). If an equivalency chart is not available, nurses may use a calibrated container (Fig. 15-5) for measuring specific amounts because, more often than not, estimated volumes are inaccurate.

FLUID OUTPUT

Fluid output is the sum of all liquid eliminated from the body. This includes all of the following:

- Urine
- Emesis (vomitus)
- Blood loss

DISPLAY 15-2. Volume Equivalents for Common Containers

Container	Volume (mL)
Teaspoon	5
Tablespoon	15
Juice glass	120
Drinking glass	240
Coffee cup	210
Milk carton	240
Water pitcher	900
Paper cup	180
Soup bowl	200
Cereal bowl	120
Ice cream cup	120
Gelatin dish	90

- Diarrhea
- Wound or tube drainage
- Aspirated irrigations

In some cases where accurate assessment is critical to a patient's treatment, the nurse may weigh wet linen, pads, diapers, or dressings and subtract the weight of a similar dry item. An estimate of fluid loss is based on the equivalency: *1 pound (0.47 kg) = one pint (475 mL).*

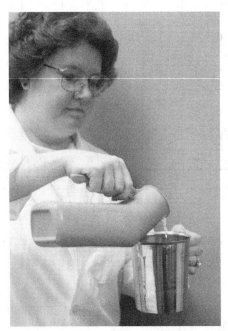

FIGURE 15-5
Calibrated containers used to measure liquid volumes. (Courtesy of Ken Timby.)

Patient cooperation often ensures accurate I & O assessment records. Therefore, those patients whose intake and output volumes are being recorded are given instructions on the purpose and goals for fluid replacement or restrictions and the ways that they may assist in the procedure.

Suggested actions for maintaining an I & O record are provided in Skill 15-1.

COMMON FLUID IMBALANCES

Fluid imbalance is a general term describing any of several conditions in which the body's water is not in the proper volume or location within the body. Common fluid imbalances include hypovolemia, hypervolemia, and third-spacing.

Hypovolemia

Hypovolemia is a term that refers to a low volume of extracellular fluid. **Dehydration** (Fig. 15-6) results when the volume of fluid is reduced in both extracellular and intracellular compartments. Causes for fluid volume deficits include:

- Inadequate fluid intake
- Fluid loss in excess of fluid intake
- Translocation of large volumes of intravascular fluid to the interstitial compartment (see later discussion of third-spacing) or to areas with only potential spaces, like the peritoneal cavity, pericardium, and pleural space

Fluid balance is restored by treating the disorder causing hypovolemia, increasing oral intake, administering IV fluid replacements, controlling fluid losses, or a combination of all of these measures.

(text continues on page 260)

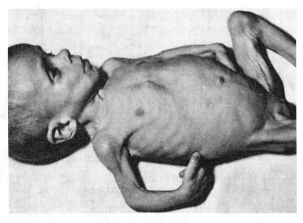

FIGURE 15-6
A severe case of dehydration.

PATIENT TEACHING REGARDING INTAKE AND OUTPUT

Teach the patient or the family to do the following:

- Write down the amount or notify the nurse whenever oral fluid is consumed.
- Use a common household measurement, like one glass or cup to describe the volume that was consumed, or refer to an equivalency chart.
- Do not let a staff person remove a dietary tray until the fluid amounts have been recorded.
- Do not empty a urinal or void (urinate) directly into the toilet bowl.

- Make sure that a measuring device is within the toilet bowl if the bathroom is used for voiding.
- If a urinal needs to be emptied, call the nurse or empty its contents into a calibrated container.
- Use a container like a bedpan or bedside commode if diarrhea occurs so the stool can be measured.
- If vomiting occurs, use an emesis basin rather than the toilet.

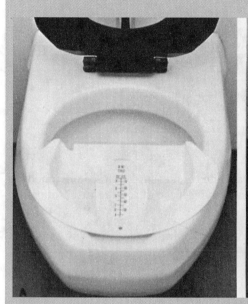
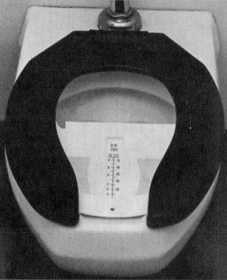

(*A*) The toilet seat is raised to insert a calibrated container. (*B*) The urine is collected in the container. (Courtesy of Ken Timby.)

 SKILL 15-1
Recording Intake and Output

Suggested Action	Reason for Action
Assessment	
Check the Kardex or listen in report to determine if an assigned patient is on intake and output (I & O).	Ensures compliance with the plan for care
Verify during report how much intravenous fluid has been accounted for from any currently infusing solution.	Indicates the credited volume for calculating fluid intake at the end of the shift
Review the nursing care plan for any previously identified fluid problem and nursing orders for specific interventions.	Promotes continuity of care

(*continued*)

SKILL 15-1
Recording Intake and Output

Suggested Action	Reason for Action
Review the patient's medical record and analyze the trends in I & O, vital sign measurements, laboratory findings, and weight records.	Aids in analyzing trends in fluid status
Perform a physical assessment to obtain data that reflect the patient's fluid status (see Table 15-1).	Provides current data
Inspect all tubings and drains to determine that they are patent (open).	Ensures that methods for instilling or removing fluids are functional
Notice if all suction containers or drainage containers have been emptied at the end of the previous shift.	Ensures accurate record keeping
Determine how much the patient understands about I & O measurements, fluid intake goals, or fluid restrictions.	Verifies if additional teaching is needed
Look for a calibrated container and bedside I & O record.	Facilitates keeping accurate data
Obtain a collection device for inside the toilet if the patient has none and uses the toilet for urinary elimination.	Facilitates measuring voided urine
Measure the amount of water in the patient's bedside carafe at the beginning of the shift.	Provides a baseline for measuring fluid consumed in addition to that served at regular meal times
Planning	
Place the patient on I & O or plan to measure I & O if the patient is at high risk for fluid imbalance or the assessment data suggest that there may be a problem.	Demonstrates safe and appropriate nursing care
Identify the goal for fluid intake or restriction; a minimum of 1,000 mL in 8 hours is not unrealistic for a patient who may be in fluid deficit, whereas an amount prescribed by the physician or an intake equal to the patient's previous hourly output may be used as a guideline for fluid restrictions.	Provides a target for patient care
Implementation	
Explain or reinforce the purpose and procedures that will be followed for measuring I & O.	Facilitates patient cooperation
Record the volume for all fluids consumed from the dietary tray and other sources of oral liquids.	Contributes to accurate assessment records
Make sure that all infusions of intravenous fluids or tube feedings are instilling at the prescribed rate.	Ensures compliance with medical therapy
Check that the nurse who adds additional intravenous fluid containers also records the instilled volume when the infusion is complete or replaced.	Ensures accurate record keeping

(continued)

SKILL 15-1
Recording Intake and Output *(Continued)*

Suggested Action	Reason for Action
Keep track of the fluid volumes used to irrigate drainage tubes or flush feeding tubes (see Chap. 29).	Ensures accurate record keeping
Measure and record the volume of voided urine; although urine is not considered a vehicle for the transmission of blood-borne microorganisms unless it contains blood, gloves may be worn as a standard precaution (see Chap. 22).	Ensures accurate record keeping and reduces the transmission of microorganisms
Measure and record the volume of urine collected in a catheter drainage bag near the end of the shift.	Ensures accurate record keeping

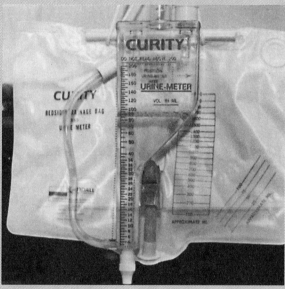

Urine drainage bag. (Courtesy of Ken Timby.)

Wear gloves to measure liquid stool or other body fluids and record their measured amounts.	Prevents the transmission of microorganisms and provides assessment data
Wash your hands thoroughly after removing and disposing of the gloves.	Reduces the presence and potential transmission of microorganisms
Check the volume remaining in currently infusing intravenous fluids; subtract the remaining volume from the credit provided at the beginning of the shift.	Ensures accurate assessment data
Total all fluid intake volumes and all fluid output volumes for the current 8-hour shift and record the amounts.	Ensures accurate record keeping

(continued)

SKILL 15-1
Recording Intake and Output *(Continued)*

Suggested Action	Reason for Action
Compare the data to determine if the intake and output are approximately the same and if the goals for fluid intake or restrictions have been met.	Demonstrates concern for safe and appropriate patient care
Report major differences in I & O to the nurse in charge or the patient's physician.	Demonstrates concern for safe and appropriate care
Review the plan of care and make revisions if the goals have not been met or if additional nursing interventions seem appropriate.	Demonstrates responsibility and accountability
Report the I & O volumes, intravenous fluid credit amount, and any other pertinent data to the nurse who will be assuming responsibility for the patient's care.	Demonstrates responsibility and accountability

Evaluation
- Intake approximates output
- Goals for fluid intake or restriction have been met
- Significant data have been reported
- The patient's fluid status justifies continuing the care as planned or the care plan has been revised

Document
- Date and time
- I & O volumes for the previous 8 hours

*Sample Documentation**
Date and Time   Fluid intake for the previous 8 hours is 1,200 mL and output is 1,000 mL.
_____ **Signature, Title**

* These data are usually recorded on a graphic flow sheet rather than in the narrative nursing notes; however, for teaching purposes, this example has been provided.

◀ **NURSING GUIDELINES FOR INCREASING ORAL INTAKE**

- Explain to the patient the reasons for increasing consumption of oral fluids.
  Rationale: Facilitates patient cooperation
- Obtain a list of beverages the patient enjoys drinking.
  Rationale: Promotes patient compliance
- Develop a schedule for providing small portions of the total fluid volume over a 24-hour period.

  Rationale: Ensures that the final goal is reached by meeting short-term goals
- Plan to provide the bulk of the projected fluid intake during times when the patient is awake.
  Rationale: Avoids disturbing sleep
- Offer verbal recognition, frequent feedback, or design a method for demonstrating the patient's progress such as coloring a bar graph or pie chart.
  Rationale: Motivates compliance and maintains goal-directed efforts through positive reinforcement
- Keep fluids handy at the bedside and place them in containers that the patient can handle.

Rationale: Availability and convenience promote compliance

- Vary the types of fluid, serving glass, or container frequently.
  Rationale: Reduces boredom and maintains interest in working toward the goal
- Serve fluids in small containers and in small amounts.
  Rationale: Avoids overwhelming the patient
- Ensure that the fluids are at an appropriate temperature.
  Rationale: Promotes pleasure and enjoyment
- Include gelatin, popsicles, ice cream, and sherbert as alternatives to liquid beverages, if they are allowed.
  Rationale: Provides texture as an alternative to items that are sipped or consumed from a glass

Hypervolemia

Hypervolemia means there is a high volume of water in the intravascular fluid compartment. As the excess volume of fluid is distributed to the interstitial space, edema may be noted. Edema (Fig. 15-7) does not usually occur unless there is a 3-liter excess in body fluid (Monahan et al., 1994). Hypervolemia can lead to **circulatory overload**, or severely compromised heart function, if it remains unresolved.

Fluid balance is restored by treating the disorder contributing to the increased fluid volume, by restricting or limiting oral fluids, reducing salt consumption (Display 15-3), discontinuing IV fluid infusions or reducing the infusing volume, administering drugs that promote urine elimination, or a combination of these interventions.

NURSING GUIDELINES FOR RESTRICTING ORAL FLUIDS

- Explain the purpose for the restrictions.
  Rationale: Facilitates patient cooperation
- Identify the total amount of fluid the patient may consume using measurements with which the patient is familiar.
  Rationale: Helps the patient understand the extent of the restrictions
- Work out a plan with the patient for distributing the allotted volume over a 24-hour period.
  Rationale: Promotes cooperation by including the patient in decision-making
- Ration the fluid so that the patient will have an opportunity to consume beverages at times other than just with meals.
  Rationale: Ensures that the patient's thirst will be relieved

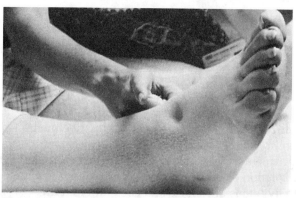

FIGURE 15-7
Evidence of pitting edema.

- Avoid sweet drinks and foods that are dry or salty.
  Rationale: Reduces thirst and the desire for fluid
- Serve liquids at their proper temperature.
  Rationale: Demonstrates concern for the patient's pleasure and enjoyment
- Offer ice chips as an occasional substitute for liquids.
  Rationale: Appears to be greater than its actual volume and prolongs the time over which the fluid may be consumed
- Provide water or other fluid in a plastic squeeze bottle or spray atomizer.
  Rationale: Decreases thirst while using only a small volume of fluid
- Help the patient with frequent oral hygiene.
  Rationale: Relieves thirst, moistens oral mucous membranes, and prevents drying and chapping of lips

---

DISPLAY 15-3. *Foods High in Salt (Sodium)*

- Processed meats like frankfurters and cold cuts
- Smoked fish
- Frozen egg substitutes
- Peanut butter
- Dairy products, especially hard cheese
- Powdered cocoa or hot chocolate mixes
- Canned vegetables, especially sauerkraut
- Pickles
- Tomato and tomato–vegetable juice
- Canned soup and bouillon
- Boxed casserole mixes
- Baking mixes
- Salted snack foods
- Seasonings like catsup, gravy mixes, soy sauce, monosodium glutamate (MSG), pickle relish, tartar sauce

- Allow the patient to rinse his or her mouth with water yet avoid swallowing it.
  Rationale: Reduces thirst and keeps the mouth moist

Third-Spacing

Third-spacing is a term used to describe the transmigration of intravascular fluid to nonvascular fluid compartments, where it becomes trapped and useless. The depletion of fluid in the intravascular space may lead to hypotension, shock, and circulatory failure.

Third-spacing is associated with disorders in which albumin levels are low, like liver failure and chronic kidney disease, and disorders in which capillary and cellular permeability is altered, such as burns and severe allergic reactions.

Fluid therapy becomes quite a challenge during third-spacing. The priority is to restore the circulatory volume. This may be accomplished by providing IV fluids—sometimes in large volumes at rapid rates. Blood transfusions or the administration of albumin by IV infusion may also be used to restore colloidal osmotic pressure and pull the trapped fluid back into the intravascular space. When this occurs, patients who were previously hypovolemic can suddenly become hypervolemic. Consequently, they must be monitored closely for signs of circulatory overload.

Policies and practices vary concerning how much responsibility practical/vocational nurses may assume with regard to IV fluid therapy. The discussion that follows is provided to meet the needs of those nurses who are expected to administer IV fluids.

ADMINISTERING INTRAVENOUS FLUIDS

Intravenous fluids are solutions that are infused through a patient's vein. They may be used for the following purposes:

- To maintain or restore fluid balance when oral replacement is inadequate or impossible
- To maintain or replace electrolytes
- To administer water-soluble vitamins
- To provide a source of calories
- To administer drugs (see Chap. 35)
- To replace blood and blood products

Types of Solutions

There are two types of IV solutions: crystalloid and colloid solutions. **Crystalloid solutions** consist of water and other uniformly dissolved crystals such as salt and sugar. **Colloid solutions** consist of water and molecules of suspended substances like blood cells and blood products like albumin.

CRYSTALLOID SOLUTIONS

Crystalloid solutions are subdivided into isotonic, hypotonic, and hypertonic solutions (Table 15-5), referring to the concentration of dissolved substances in relation to plasma. When administered to patients, the concentration of the solution influences the osmotic distribution of body fluid (Fig. 15-8).

Isotonic Solutions

An **isotonic solution** is one that contains the same concentration of dissolved substances as is normally found in plasma. Isotonic solutions are usually administered to maintain fluid balance among patients who may not be able to eat or drink for a short period of time. Because of its equal concentration, an isotonic solution does not cause any appreciable redistribution of body fluid.

Hypotonic Solutions

A **hypotonic solution** contains fewer dissolved substances than normally found in plasma. Hypotonic solutions are administered to patients who are experiencing fluid losses in excess of their fluid intake, such as those who have diarrhea or vomiting.

Because hypotonic solutions are dilute, the water in the solution passes through the semipermeable membrane of blood cells, causing them to swell. This can temporarily increase blood pressure because it expands the circulating volume. The water may also pass through capillary walls and become distributed within other body cells and the interstitial spaces. Hypotonic solutions, therefore, are an effective mechanism for rehydrating patients experiencing fluid deficits.

Hypertonic Solutions

A **hypertonic solution** is more concentrated than body fluid. Consequently, it draws fluid into the intravascular compartment from the more dilute areas within the interstitial spaces and cells, causing them to shrink. Hypertonic solutions are not used very frequently except for extreme cases in which it is necessary to reduce cerebral edema or expand the circulatory volume rapidly.

COLLOID SOLUTIONS

Colloid solutions are used to replace circulating blood volume because the suspended molecules pull fluid from other compartments. Examples of colloid solutions include blood, blood products, and solutions known as plasma expanders.

TABLE 15-5. *Types of Intravenous Solutions*

Solution	Components	Special Comments
Isotonic Solutions		
0.9% saline, also called normal saline	0.9 g of sodium chloride/100 mL of water	Contains amounts of sodium and chloride in physiologically equal amounts to that found in plasma
5% dextrose and water, also called D_5W	5 g of dextrose (glucose/sugar)/100 mL of water	Isotonic when infused but the glucose is metabolized quickly, leaving a solution of dilute water
Ringer's Solution or Lactated Ringer's	Water and a mixture of sodium, chloride, calcium, potassium, bicarbonate, and in some cases, lactate	Replaces electrolytes in amounts similarly found in plasma. The lactate, when present, helps maintain acid–base balance
Hypotonic Solutions		
0.45% sodium chloride, or also called half-strength saline	0.45 g of sodium chloride/100 mL of water	A smaller ratio of sodium and chloride than found in plasma causing it to be less concentrated in comparison
5% dextrose in 0.45% saline	5 g of dextrose and 0.45 sodium chloride/100 mL of water	The sugar provides a quick source of energy, leaving a hypotonic salt solution
Hypertonic Solutions		
10% dextrose in water, also called $D_{10}W$	10 g of dextrose/100 mL of water	Twice the concentration of glucose than present in plasma
3% saline	3 g of sodium chloride/100 mL of water	The high concentration of salt in the plasma will dehydrate cells and tissue
20% dextrose in water	20 g of dextrose/100 mL water	Rapidly increases the concentration of sugar in the blood, causing a fluid shift to the intravascular compartment

Blood

Whole blood or packed cells are probably the most common types of colloid solutions that are administered to patients. One unit of whole blood contains approximately 475 mL of blood cells and plasma with 60 to 70 mL of preservative and anticoagulant added (Smeltzer & Bare, 1992), whereas packed cells have most of the plasma removed. Packed cells are preferred for patients who need cellular replacements but do not need, or may be harmed by, the administration of additional fluid.

Most of the blood that is administered to patients comes from public donors. In some cases, the patient's own blood may be infused (see Chap. 27, section on Autologous Blood Donation).

Blood Collection and Storage. Blood donors are screened to ensure that the person giving the blood is healthy and will not be endangered by the temporary loss in blood volume. Blood can be stored for 21 to 35 days, after which it must be discarded.

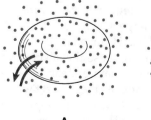
A

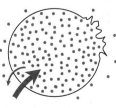
B

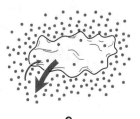
C

FIGURE 15-8
(*A*) Isotonic solutions. (*B*) Hypotonic solutions. (*C*) Hypertonic solutions. (Scherer J, Timby BK: Introductory Medical–Surgical Nursing, 6th ed, p 188. Philadelphia, JB Lippincott, 1994)

Blood Safety. Once collected, the donated blood is tested for syphilis, hepatitis, and human immunodeficiency virus (HIV) antibodies to exclude administering blood that may transmit these blood-borne diseases. Blood that tests positive is automatically discarded. Unfortunately, disease-causing viruses may be present in donated blood and go undetected if the antibodies have not reached a high enough level to be measured.

Blood Compatibility. There may be several hundred differences among the proteins present in the blood of a donor and recipient, any one of which can cause minor or major transfusion reactions. However, one of the most dangerous differences involves the antigens, or protein structures, on membranes of red blood cells. Antigens determine the characteristic blood group—A, B, AB, and O, and Rh factor. Rh positive means the protein is present; Rh negative means the protein is absent.

Before donated blood is administered, the blood of the potential recipient is typed and mixed, or crossmatched with a sample of the stored blood to determine that the two are compatible. To avoid an incompatibility reaction, it is best to administer the same blood group and Rh factor. There are some exceptions (Table 15-6).

Type O blood is considered the *universal donor* because it lacks both A and B blood group markers on its cell membrane. Therefore, type O blood can be given to anyone because it will not trigger a reaction when given to recipients with other blood types. Persons with type AB are referred to as *universal recipients* because their red blood cells have proteins that are compatible with either type A or B blood, and O as well. Rh-positive people may receive Rh-positive or Rh-negative blood because the latter does not contain the sensitizing protein. The reverse, however, is not true: *Rh-negative people must never receive Rh-positive blood.*

Blood Substitutes. In response to the needs of patients who object to receiving blood for religious reasons, like Jehovah's Witnesses, and because of the potential risks for blood-borne diseases, like AIDS, scientists have been working on perfecting blood substitutes. Cur-

rently, a chemical group called *perfluorocarbons* appears promising (Ingbar, 1990).

Perfluorocarbons, in general, and Fluosol DA, in particular, have been tested and used on a limited basis as artificial substitutes for blood in humans. When administered to patients, Fluosol DA carries 20 times the oxygen found in plasma; however, the serum must be highly oxygenated first. In addition, the administration is not entirely without risk.

Other applications for perfluorocarbons are being explored based on the fact that they have a smaller molecular size than red blood cells. This unique characteristic permits oxygen-carrying molecules to pass through blood vessels that have been narrowed because of blood clots. Therefore, Fluosol DA seems to have a potential use in restoring oxygen to tissues experiencing impaired circulation, such as the brain after a stroke or the heart after a heart attack. Scientists theorize that the same effect could be used in the treatment of patients experiencing a sickle cell crisis. Furthermore, this same chemical could prolong the preservation of organs for transplantation and improve the oxygenation of cancer cells, making them more vulnerable to the standard medical treatments now in use.

Besides perfluorocarbons, other substances are being tested to discover a safe, effective substitute for whole blood. For example, solutions containing just hemoglobin have been used successfully in animals. Also, attempts are being made to recycle outdated red blood cells in donated blood by sealing them within a lipid capsule. This product is referred to as *microencapsulated hemoglobin*. With continued research, these substances and others may improve the treatment of disorders previously dependent on blood transfusions. Finding a blood substitute may eventually reduce the need to rely on human blood donors.

Blood Products

There are several types of blood products that may be administered to patients who need specific substances yet do not need all the fluid or cellular components in whole blood (Table 15-7).

Plasma Expanders

Various types of nonblood solutions may be used to pull fluid into the vascular space. Two examples are dextran 40 (Rheomacrodex; Pharmacia Laboratories, Piscataway, NJ) and hetastarch (Hespan; American Critical Care, McGraw Park, IL). Each of these two substances are polysaccharides (eg, complex carbohydrates). Polysaccharides are large-sized, insoluble molecules. Therefore, when either is mixed with water, they form colloidal solutions. Because the suspended particles cannot move through semipermeable membranes when instilled intravenously, they attract water from other fluid compartments. Consequently, plasma expanders are used as an economic and virus-free sub-

TABLE 15-6. *Blood Groups and Compatible Types*

Blood Groups	Percentage of Population	Compatible Blood Types
A	41%	A and O
B	9%	B and O
O	47%	O
AB	3%	AB, A, B, and O
Rh+	85% Whites 95% African Americans	Rh+ and Rh−
Rh−	15% Whites 5% African Americans	Rh− only

TABLE 15-7. *Types of Blood Products*

Blood Product	Description	Purpose for Administration
Platelets	Disk-shaped cellular fragments that promote coagulation of blood	Restores or improves the ability to control bleeding
Granulocytes	Types of white blood cells	Improves the ability to overcome an infection
Plasma	Serum minus blood cells	Replaces clotting factors or increases intravascular fluid volume by increasing colloidal osmotic pressure
Albumin	Plasma protein	Pulls third-spaced fluid by increasing colloidal osmotic pressure
Cryoprecipitate	Mixture of clotting factors	Treats blood clotting disorders like hemophilia

stitute for blood and blood products when treating hypovolemic shock.

Regardless of the prescribed solution, the nurse prepares the solution for administration, performs a venipuncture, regulates the rate of administration, monitors the infusion, and discontinues its administration when the patient's fluid balance is restored.

Preparing Intravenous Solutions

Intravenous solutions are most commonly stored in plastic bags containing 1,000, 500, 250, 100, and 50 mL of solution. A few solutions may be stocked in glass containers. The physician specifies the type of solution, additional additives, and the volume in milliliters per hour for infusing the solution. To reduce the potential for infection, it is a standard of practice to replace IV solutions every 24 hours even if the total volume has not been instilled.

Before preparing the solution, the nurse inspects the container and determines that:

- The type of solution is the same as that prescribed by the physician
- The solution is clear and transparent
- The expiration date has not elapsed
- No leaks are apparent
- A separate label is attached identifying the type and amount of other drugs added to the commercial solution

SELECTING TUBING

All IV tubing consists of a spike for accessing the solution, a drip chamber for holding a small amount of fluid, a length of plastic tubing with one or more ports for instilling IV medications (see Chap. 35), and a roller or slide clamp for regulating the rate of the infusion (Fig. 15-9).

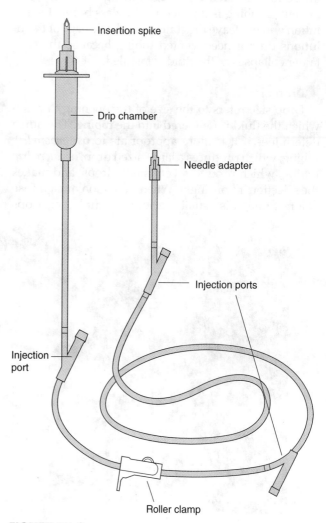

FIGURE 15-9
Basic intravenous tubing.

Despite the common components on tubings, the nurse may select from various options in their basic design. The choice depends on five considerations: (1) whether to use primary or secondary tubing, (2) whether to use vented or unvented tubing, (3) the drop size most convenient for administering the prescribed volume, and (4) whether a filter is needed.

Primary Versus Secondary Tubing

Primary tubing is longer than secondary tubing. Primary tubing is used when the tubing must span the distance from a solution that hangs several feet above the infusion site. Secondary tubing, which is shorter, is used for administering smaller volumes of solution into a port within the primary tubing.

Vented Versus Unvented Tubing

Vented tubing draws air into the container, whereas unvented tubing does not (Fig. 15-10). The choice depends on the type of container in which the solution is packaged. Vented tubing is necessary for administering solutions that are packaged in rigid containers. If unvented tubing is inserted into a glass bottle, the solution will not leave the container. Plastic bags of IV solutions do not need vented tubing because the container collapses as the fluid is instilled.

Drop Size

Drop size refers to the size of the opening through which the fluid is delivered into the tubing. The nurse determines if it is more appropriate to use *macrodrip* tubing, which produces a large-sized drop, or *microdrip* tubing, which produces very small drops, and makes the selection accordingly. When a solution must infuse at a fast rate, it is usually easier to count larger drops than smaller ones. When the rate must be infused very precisely or at a slow rate, smaller drops are preferred.

Microdrip tubing, regardless of the tubing manufacturer, delivers a standard volume of 60 drops per mL. Macrodrip tubing manufacturers, on the other hand, have not been consistent in designing the size of the opening. Therefore, the nurse must read the package label to determine the **drop factor**, or number of drops per milliliter. Some common drop factors are 10, 15, and 20 drops/mL. Knowing the drop factor also becomes important in calculating the infusion rate, which is discussed later in this chapter.

Filters

An in-line filter (Fig. 15-11) removes air bubbles as well as undissolved drugs, bacteria, and large-sized substances. Filtered tubing is usually used when:

- Administering parenteral nutrition
- Patients are at high risk for infections
- Infusing IV solutions to pediatric patients
- Administering blood and packed cells

Another factor that may affect the type of tubing selected is the technique that will be used to administer the IV solution.

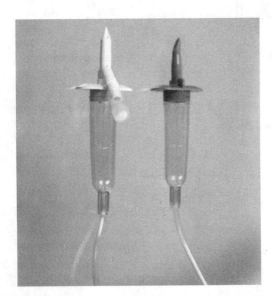

FIGURE 15-10
Vented and unvented tubing. (Courtesy of Ken Timby.)

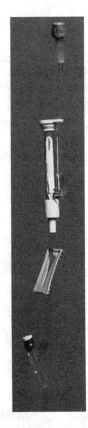

FIGURE 15-11
An in-line filter removes air bubbles as well as undissolved debris that is 0.22 microns in diameter or larger. (Courtesy of Ken Timby.)

Infusion Techniques

Intravenous infusions are instilled by gravity or with an infusion device, an electric or battery-operated machine that regulates and monitors the administration of IV solutions. If the infusion is administered with an infusion device, it may affect the type of tubing that is used.

GRAVITY INFUSION

Most of the basic types of tubing can be used for infusing a solution by gravity. The height of the IV solution, rather than the tubing, is the most important factor affecting gravity infusions.

To overcome the pressure in the patient's vein, which is higher than atmospheric pressure, the solution is elevated at least 18 to 24 inches (45–60 cm) above the site of the infusion. The height of the solution affects the rate of flow. The higher the solution, the faster it infuses, and vice versa.

ELECTRONIC INFUSION DEVICES

There are two general types of infusion devices: infusion pumps and volumetric controllers. Both infusion pumps and volumetric controllers are programmed to deliver a preset volume per hour. They may sound audible and visual alarms if the infusion is not progressing at the rate intended. They may also produce an audible sound when the infusion container is nearly empty, contains air within the tubing, or senses an obstruction or resistance to delivering the fluid.

Infusion Pumps

An **infusion pump** (Fig. 15-12) is a device that uses pressure to infuse solutions. Infusion pumps usually require special tubing that contains a cassette for creating sufficient pressure to push fluid into the vein. The machine adjusts the pressure according to the resistance it meets. This feature explains one of the major disadvantages in using a pump: if the catheter or needle within the vein becomes displaced, a pump may continue to infuse fluid into the tissue for a period of time.

Volumetric Controllers

A **volumetric controller** (Fig. 15-13) is an infusion device that infuses IV solutions by gravity, but mechanically compresses the tubing at a certain frequency to infuse the solution at a precise preset rate. Volumetric controllers may or may not require special tubing.

Newer models allow the nurse to program the infusion of more than one solution. And, in some cases, when one container of fluid finishes infusing, the controller automatically resumes the infusion of the other solution.

The suggestions provided in Skill 15-2 may be used when preparing to administer an IV solution.

(text continues on page 271)

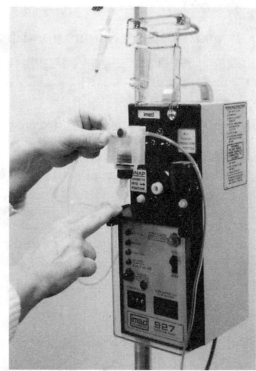

FIGURE 15-12
Special tubing with a cassette is inserted into this electronic infusion pump. (Courtesy of Ken Timby.)

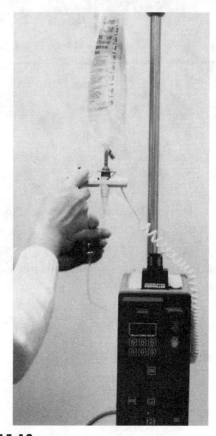

FIGURE 15-13
A volumetric controller monitors and regulates the infusion of intravenous solutions. (Courtesy of Ken Timby.)

SKILL 15-2
Preparing Intravenous Solutions

Suggested Action	Reason for Action
Assessment	
Check the medical order for the type, volume, and projected length of fluid therapy.	Ensures accuracy and guides the selection of equipment
Determine if the solution is in a bag or bottle and if the infusion will be administered by gravity or infusion device.	Affects the selection of tubing
Review the patient's medical record for information on the risk for infection.	Determines if there is a need for filtered tubing
Read the label on the solution at least three times.	Helps to prevent errors
Planning	
Mark a time strip and attach it to the side of the container.	Facilitates future monitoring

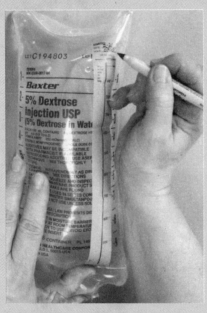

Marking a time strip. (Courtesy of Ken Timby.)

Suggested Action	Reason for Action
Implementation	
Wash your hands.	Reduces the transmission of microorganisms
Select the appropriate tubing and stretch it once it has been removed from the package.	Straightens the tubing by removing bends and kinks

(continued)

SKILL 15-2
Preparing Intravenous Solutions *(Continued)*

Suggested Action	Reason for Action
Tighten the roller clamp.	Aids in filling the drip chamber

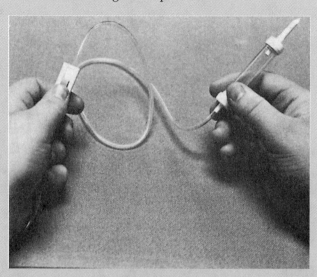

Tightening the roller clamp. (Courtesy of Ken Timby.)

Suggested Action	Reason for Action
Remove the cover from the access port.	Exposes the spike
Insert the spike by puncturing the seal on the container.	Provides an exit route for fluid

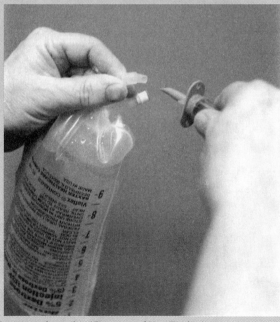

Inserting the spike. (Courtesy of Ken Timby.)

Suggested Action	Reason for Action
Hang the solution container from an IV pole or suspended hook.	Inverts the container and facilitates proceeding

(continued)

SKILL 15-2
Preparing Intravenous Solutions (Continued)

Suggested Action	Reason for Action
Squeeze the drip chamber, filling it no more than half full.	Leaves space to count the drops when regulating the rate of infusion

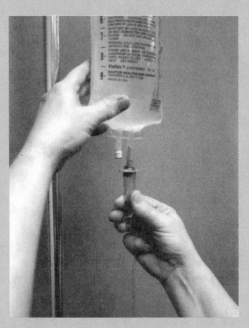

Squeezing the drip chamber. (Courtesy of Ken Timby.)

Suggested Action	Reason for Action
Release the roller clamp.	Flushes air from the tubing
Invert ports within the tubing as the solution approaches.	Displaces air that may be trapped in the junction

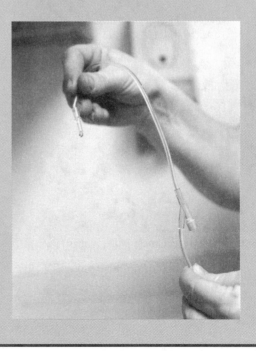

Inverting all the ports. (Courtesy of Ken Timby.)

(continued)

SKILL 15-2
Preparing Intravenous Solutions (Continued)

Suggested Action	Reason for Action
Tighten the roller clamp when all the air has been removed.	Prevents loss of fluid
Attach a piece of tape or a label on the tubing identifying the date, time, and your initials.	Provides a quick reference for determining when the tubing needs to be changed
Take the solution and tubing to the patient's room.	Facilitates administration

Evaluation
- Solution and tubing are properly labeled
- Tubing has been purged of air

Document
- Date and time
- Type and volume of solution
- Rate of infusion once venipuncture has been performed
- Location of venipuncture site

Sample Documentation

Date and Time   1,000 mL of 5% D/W infusing at 125 mL/hr through IV in L. forearm.
_____ **Signature, Title**

Performing a Venipuncture

Venipuncture, as the name implies, means gaining access to the venous system by piercing a vein with a needle. Venipunctures on peripheral veins are usually performed by nurses. When performing a venipuncture, the nurse assembles needed equipment, inspects and selects a vein, and inserts the venipuncture device.

VENIPUNCTURE DEVICES

There are several devices that may be used for accessing a vein. The nurse may use a butterfly needle, an over-the-needle catheter, or a through-the-needle catheter (Fig. 15-14). Over-the-needle catheters are most commonly used.

Regardless of the design, venipuncture devices come in various diameters or gauges; the larger the gauge number, the smaller the diameter. The diameter of the venipuncture device should always be smaller than the vein into which it will be inserted. This reduces the potential for occluding blood flow. An 18, 20, or 22 gauge are the sizes most used for adults.

Besides a device for puncturing the vein, the following items are usually necessary when performing a venipuncture: gloves; tourniquet; antiseptic swabs to cleanse the skin; antiseptic ointment; a bandaid, sterile gauze, or transparent dressing for covering the puncture site; and adhesive tape for securing the needle, dressing, and tubing. An armboard may be needed to prevent dislodging the venipuncture device when a patient may not be relied on to be cautious when moving about.

SELECTING A VEIN

The veins in the hand and forearm are most commonly used for inserting a venipuncture device (Fig. 15-15). Scalp veins are used for infants and small children. Several additional criteria are used when selecting a venipuncture site.

NURSING GUIDELINES FOR SELECTING A VENIPUNCTURE SITE

- Use veins in the nondominant hand or arm.
  Rationale: Reduces the potential for dislodging the device due to movement and use
- Refrain from using foot and leg veins.
  Rationale: Avoids restricting mobility and reduces the potential for forming blood clots where circulation is naturally reduced
- Exclude veins on the side where a breast has been removed.

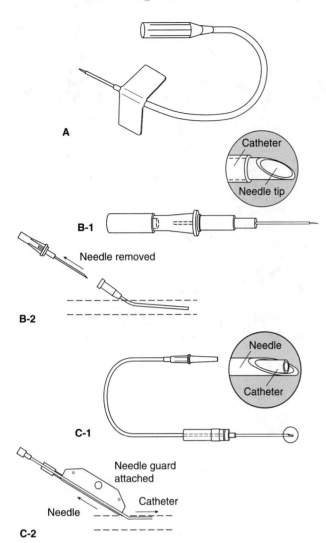

FIGURE 15-14
Venipuncture devices. (*A*) Butterfly needle. (*B-1*) Over-the-needle catheter. (*B-2*) Needle removed. (*C-1*) Through-the-needle catheter. (*C-2*) A needle guard covers the tip of the needle, which remains outside the skin.

Rationale: Reduces the potential for complications due to compromised circulation
- Choose a vein in a location that will be unaffected by joint movement.
  Rationale: Prevents the potential for displacement
- Look for a vein that is larger than the needle or catheter.
  Rationale: Prevents circulatory impairment
- Avoid veins on the inner surface of the wrist.
  Rationale: Prevents pain and discomfort
- Always look for a vein proximal to the previous site.
  Rationale: Promotes healing
- Feel and look for a vein that is fairly straight.
  Rationale: Promotes the ability to cannulate (thread) the device within the vein

- Exclude the use of any vein that appears inflamed or looks impaired in any way.
  Rationale: Prevents additional trauma

Once the general site is selected, the nurse applies a tourniquet to select a specific vein (Fig. 15-16). Display 15-4 identifies several techniques for promoting vein distention.

A blood pressure cuff may be substituted for a rubber tourniquet. Whichever technique is used, the radial pulse should be palpable to indicate that arterial blood flow is being maintained.

INSERTING A VENIPUNCTURE DEVICE

The suggestions in Skill 15-3 may be used when inserting an over-the-needle catheter within a vein.

Monitoring and Maintaining the Infusion

Once the venipuncture has been performed and the solution is infusing, the nurse regulates the rate of infusion, assesses for complications, cares for the venipuncture site, and replaces equipment as needed.

REGULATING THE INFUSION RATE

The nurse is responsible for calculating, regulating, and maintaining the rate of infusion according to the physician's order. If an infusion device is being used, the electronic equipment is programmed according to milliliters per hour. If the solution is being infused by gravity, the rate is calculated in drops (gtt) per minute. Formulas for calculating infusion rates are provided in Display 15-5.

For gravity infusions, the nurse counts the number of drops falling into the drip chamber per minute. By adjusting the roller clamp, the number of drops can be increased or decreased until the infusion rate matches the calculated rate. Thereafter, the nurse monitors the time strip on the the side of the container at hourly intervals to ensure that the infusion is being administered at the prescribed rate.

ASSESSING FOR COMPLICATIONS

There are several complications associated with the infusion of IV solutions (Table 15-8). They include circulatory overload, in which the intravascular volume becomes excessive; **infiltration**, the infusion of IV fluid into the tissue; **phlebitis**, inflammation of a vein; **thrombus formation**, a stationary blood clot; **pulmonary embolus**, a blood clot that travels to the lung; infection, growth of microorganisms at the site or within the bloodstream;

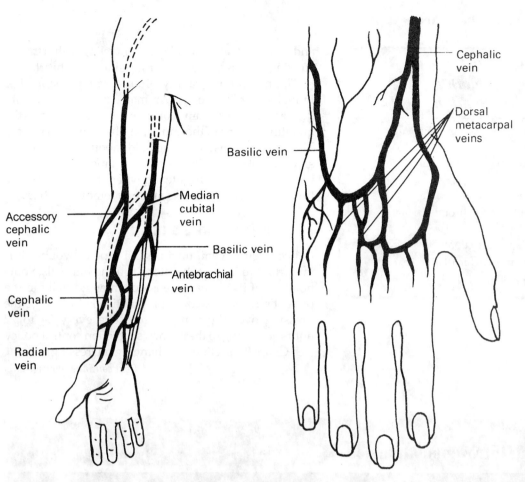

Accessory
cephalic
vein

Median
cubital
vein

Basilic vein

Antebrachial
vein

Cephalic
vein

Radial
vein

Cephalic
vein

Basilic vein

Dorsal
metacarpal
veins

FIGURE 15-15
Potential venipuncture
sites.

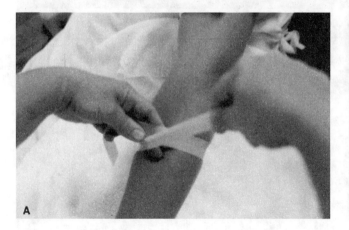

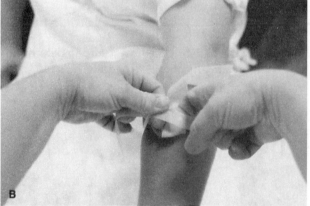

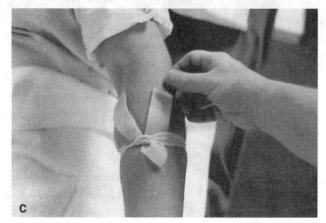

FIGURE 15-16
To apply a tourniquet, the ends are (*A*) pulled tightly in
opposite directions. Then one end is (*B*) tucked beneath
the other so that it can be (*C*) easily released by pulling
one of the free ends. (Courtesy of Ken Timby.)

DISPLAY 15-4. *Techniques for Promoting Vein Distention*

- Apply a tourniquet or blood pressure cuff tightly about the arm
- Have the patient make a fist and pump the fist intermittently
- Tap the skin over the vein several times
- Lower the patient's arm to promote distal pooling of blood
- Stroke the skin in the direction of the fingers
- Apply warm compresses for 10 minutes to dilate veins and then reapply the tourniquet

and **air embolism**, a bubble of air traveling within the circulating venous blood to the right side of the heart.

The minimum quantity of air that may be fatal to humans is not known. Animal experimentation indicates that fatal volumes of air are much larger than the quantity present in the entire length of infusion tubing. The average infusion tubing holds about 5 mL of air, an amount not ordinarily considered dangerous. Patients, however, are often frightened when they see air in the tubing, and every effort is made to remove bubbles.

CARING FOR THE SITE

Because the venipuncture is a type of wound, it is important to inspect the site at routine intervals. Some notation of its appearance is documented daily in the patient's record. A common practice is to change the dressing over the venipuncture site every 24 to 72 hours according to the agency's infection control policy (see Chap. 28, section on Changing a Dressing).

(text continues on page 281)

SKILL 15-3
Starting an Intravenous Infusion

Suggested Action	Reason for Action
Assessment	
Check the identity of the patient.	Prevents errors
Review the patient's medical record to determine if there are any allergies to iodine or tape.	Influences supplies that will be used and modifications in the procedure
Inspect and palpate several potential venipuncture sites.	Provides an alternative if the first attempt is unsuccessful

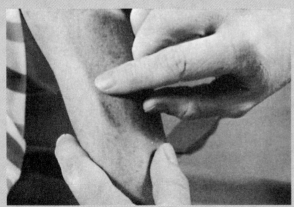
Palpating veins.

Planning	
Bring all the necessary equipment to the bedside.	Promotes organization and efficient time management

SKILL 15-3
Starting an Intravenous Infusion *(Continued)*

Suggested Action	Reason for Action
Position the patient on his or her back or in a sitting position.	Promotes comfort and facilitates inspection of the arm
Place an absorbent pad beneath the hand or arm.	Saves having to change bed linen if the site bleeds
Select a site that will most likely facilitate the purpose for the infusion and comply with the criteria for vein selection.	Facilitates continuous fluid administration and minimizes potential complications
Clip body hair at the site if it is excessive.	Facilitates visualization and reduces future discomfort when adhesive tape is removed
Tear strips of tape, open the package with the venipuncture device, and place antiseptic ointment on an opened bandaid or gauze square.	Saves time and ensures that the venipuncture device is not displaced once it is inserted

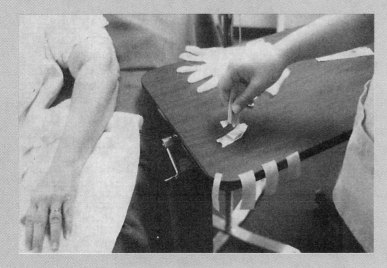

Preparing supplies. (Courtesy of Ken Timby.)

Implementation

Wash your hands.	Reduces the number of microorganisms
Apply a tourniquet or a blood pressure cuff 2 to 4 inches (5–10 cm) above the vein that will be used.	Distends the vein

(continued)

SKILL 15-3
Starting an Intravenous Infusion (Continued)

Suggested Action	Reason for Action
Use Betadine and/or alcohol to cleanse the skin, starting at the center of the site outward 2 to 4 inches.	Reduces the potential for infection

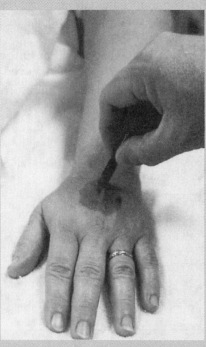

Cleaning the site. (Courtesy of Ken Timby.)

Suggested Action	Reason for Action
Allow the antiseptic to dry.	Potentiates the effectiveness of antispetic and prevents burning when the needle is inserted
Don clean gloves.	Provides a barrier against blood-borne viruses

(continued)

Suggested Action	Reason for Action
Use the thumb to stretch and stabilize the vein and soft tissues about 2 inches (5 cm) below the intended site of entry.	Helps straighten the vein and prevents it from moving about underneath the skin

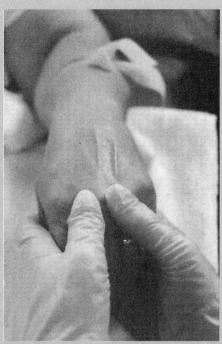

Stabilizing the vein. (Courtesy of Ken Timby.)

Suggested Action	Reason for Action
Position the venipuncture device with the bevel up and at approximately a 45° angle above or to the side of the vein.	Facilitates piercing the vein

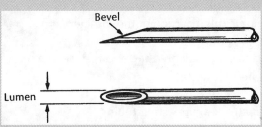

Placing the bevel up.

Suggested Action	Reason for Action
Warn the patient just before inserting the needle.	Prepares the patient for experiencing discomfort
Feel for a change in resistance and look for blood to appear behind the needle.	Indicates the vein has been pierced

(continued)

SKILL 15-3
Starting an Intravenous Infusion (Continued)

Suggested Action	Reason for Action
Once blood is observed, advance the needle about 1/8 to 1/4 inch.	Positions the catheter tip within the inner wall of the vein

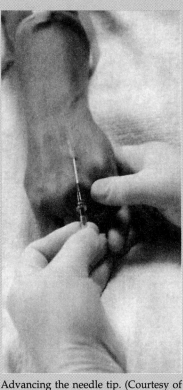

Advancing the needle tip. (Courtesy of Ken Timby.)

Suggested Action	Reason for Action
Withdraw the needle slightly so that the tip is within the catheter.	Prevents puncturing through the outside of the vein wall
Slide the catheter into the vein until only the end of the infusion device can be seen.	Ensures full insertion of the catheter
Release the tourniquet.	Reduces venous pressure and restores circulation
Apply pressure over the internal tip of the catheter.	Limits blood loss
Remove needle from catheter.	Prepares for connecting tubing
Remove the protective cap covering the end of the IV tubing and insert it into the end of the venipuncture device.	Facilitates infusing the solution
Release the roller clamp and begin instilling solution slowly.	Clears blood from the venipuncture device before it can clot
Remove gloves when there is no longer a potential for direct contact with blood.	Facilitates handling tape

(continued)

SKILL 15-3
Starting an Intravenous Infusion *(Continued)*

Suggested Action	Reason for Action
Place a small amount of antiseptic ointment onto the site or dressing.	Reduces the potential for infection

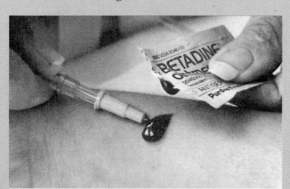

Applying antiseptic ointment. (Courtesy of Ken Timby.)

Suggested Action	Reason for Action
Secure the catheter by criss-crossing a piece of tape from beneath the tubing.	Prevents catheter displacement

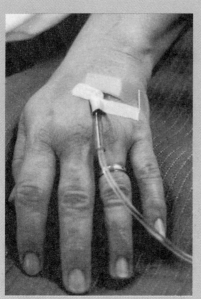

Stabilizing catheter. (Courtesy of Ken Timby.)

(continued)

SKILL 15-3
Starting an Intravenous Infusion (Continued)

Suggested Action	Reason for Action
Cover the entire site with additional strips of tape, taking care to loop and secure the tubing.	Prevents tension on the tubing, which may cause its displacement

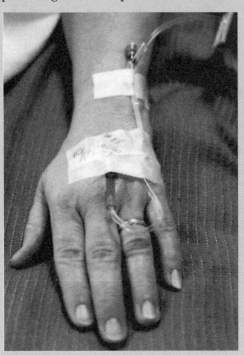

Securing the tubing.

Write the date, time, gauge of the catheter, and your initials on the outer piece of tape.	Provides a quick reference for determining when the site must be changed
Tighten or release the roller clamp to regulate the rate of fluid infusion.	Facilitates compliance with the medical order

Evaluation
- A flashback of blood was observed before advancing the catheter
- Minimal discomfort and blood loss occurred
- Fluid is infusing according to the prescribed rate

Document
- Date and time
- Gauge and type of venipuncture device
- Site of venipuncture
- Type and volume of solution
- Rate of infusion

Sample Documentation

Date and Time   #20 gauge over-the-needle catheter inserted into vein in L. forearm. 1,000 mL 0.9% saline infusing at 42 gtt/min._____**Signature, Title**

DISPLAY 15-5. *Formulas for Calculating Infusion Rates*

When using an infusion device:

$$\frac{\text{Total volume in mL}}{\text{Total hours}} = \text{mL/hr}$$

Example:

$$\frac{1,000 \text{ mL}}{8 \text{ hr}} = 125 \text{ mL/hr}$$

When infusing by gravity:

$$\frac{\text{Total volume in mL}}{\text{Total time in minutes}} \times \text{drop factor*} = \text{gtt/min}$$

$$\frac{1,000 \text{ mL}}{480 \text{ min}} \times 20 = 42 \text{ gtt/min}$$

* *The macrodrip drop factor varies among manufacturers.*

◄ NURSING GUIDELINES FOR REMOVING AIR BUBBLES FROM INTRAVENOUS TUBING

- Flush the tubing with IV solution before inserting the adapter into the venipuncture device.
Rationale: Purges air from the tubing
- Tighten the roller clamp if small bubbles are observed.

Rationale: Prevents continued forward movement of the air
- Tap the tubing below the air bubbles (Fig. 15-17).
Rationale: Promotes movement of the air in an upward direction above the fluid in the drip chamber
- Milk the air in the direction of the drip chamber or filter, if one is incorporated within the tubing.
Rationale: Pushes the air physically to an area where it can be trapped or released
- Wrap the tubing around a circular object, like a

TABLE 15-8. *Complications of Intravenous (IV) Therapy*

Complication	Signs and Symptoms	Cause(s)	Action
Infection	Swelling Discomfort Redness at site Drainage from site	Growth of microorganisms	Change site. Apply antiseptic and dressing to previous site. Report findings.
Circulatory overload	Elevated blood pressure Shortness of breath Bounding pulse Anxiety	Rapid infusion Reduced kidney function Impaired heart contraction	Slow the IV rate. Contact the physician. Elevate the patient's head. Give oxygen.
Infiltration	Swelling at the site Discomfort Decrease in infusion rate Cool skin temperature at the site	Displacement of the venipuncture device	Restart the IV. Elevate the arm.
Phlebitis	Redness, warmth, and discomfort along the vein	Administration of irritating fluid Prolonged use of the same vein	Restart the IV. Report the findings. Apply warm compresses.
Thrombus formation	Swelling Discomfort Slowed infusion	Stasis of blood at the catheter, needle tip, or vein	Restart the IV. Report the findings. Apply warm compresses.
Pulmonary embolus	Sudden chest pain Shortness of breath Anxiety Rapid heart rate Drop in blood pressure	Movement of previously stationary blood clot	Stay with the patient. Call for help. Administer oxygen.
Air embolism	Same as pulmonary embolus	Failure to purge air from the tubing	Same as for pulmonary embolus, but also: Place the patient's head lower than the feet. Position the patient on left side.

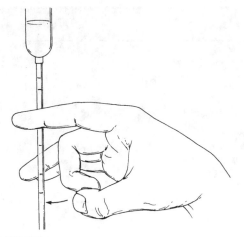

FIGURE 15-17
Tapping the tubing may help air bubbles rise into the drip chamber.

pencil, starting below the trapped air (Fig. 15-18). *Rationale:* Moves the air toward the drip chamber where it can escape from the liquid into the empty air space
- Insert a syringe within a port below the air and open the roller clamp. *Rationale:* Siphons the air from the tubing as it passes by the bevel of the needle

REPLACING EQUIPMENT

Solutions are replaced when they finish infusing or every 24 hours, depending on which occurs first (Skill 15-4).

Intravenous tubing is changed every 72 hours depending on agency policy, with some exceptions. Tubing used to instill parenteral nutrition is replaced daily. Tubing used to administer whole blood can be reused for a second unit, if one unit immediately follows the

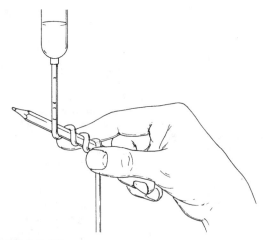

FIGURE 15-18
Twisting the tubing around a pencil or other object may displace air bubbles toward the drip chamber.

other. Whenever equipment is changed, it is more convenient to replace both the solution and the tubing at the same time. However, Skill 15-5 describes how to replace just the tubing.

Discontinuing an Intravenous Infusion

Intravenous infusions are discontinued when the solution has infused and no more is scheduled to follow. Alternatively, the venipuncture device may be temporarily capped, and kept patent with the use of a medication lock.

NURSING GUIDELINES FOR DISCONTINUING AN INTRAVENOUS INFUSION

- Wash your hands.
  Rationale: Reduces the spread of microorganisms
- Clamp the tubing and remove the tape that held the dressing and venipuncture device in place. *Rationale:* Facilitates removal without leaking fluid
- Don gloves.
  Rationale: Prevents contact with blood
- Gently press a gauze square over the site of entry. *Rationale:* Absorbs blood
- Remove the catheter or needle by pulling it out without hesitation, following the course of the vein. *Rationale:* Prevents discomfort and injury to the vein
- Apply pressure to the injection site for 30 to 45 seconds while elevating the forearm (Fig. 15-19). *Rationale:* Controls bleeding
- Cover the site with a dressing or bandaid. *Rationale:* Reduces the potential for infection
- Remove your gloves when the bleeding has been controlled and wash your hands again. *Rationale:* Removes microorganisms from the hands
- Flex and extend the arm or hand several times. *Rationale:* Helps the patient regain sensation and mobility in the area where the venipuncture device was located
- Record the amount of fluid infused during the current shift on the I & O sheet. *Rationale:* Demonstrates responsibility for documenting fluid intake volumes
- Document and sign a notation on the patient's record indicating the time the infusion was discontinued and the condition of the venipuncture site. *Rationale:* Demonstrates responsibility and accountability for patient care

(text continues on page 286)

SKILL 15-4
Changing Intravenous Solution Containers

Suggested Action	Reason for Action
Assessment	
Assess the volume that remains in the infusing container and the rate at which it is infusing.	Helps to establish a time frame for replacing the solution
Check the medication record or physician's orders to determine what solution is to follow.	Ensures compliance with the medical treatment
Planning	
Obtain the replacement solution well in advance.	Ensures that the infusion will be uninterrupted
Attach a time strip to the new container indicating the date, your initials, and the hourly infusion volumes.	Avoids having to complete this responsibility later
Organize patient care so as to be ready to change the container as the current infusion becomes low.	Demonstrates efficient time management
Implementation	
Check the identity of the patient.	Prevents errors in nursing care
Wash your hands.	Reduces the transmission of microorganisms
Tighten the roller clamp slightly or slow the rate of infusion on an infusion device.	Ensures that the drip chamber remains filled with solution
Remove the almost empty solution container from the suspension hook with the tubing still attached.	Facilitates separating the tubing from the container
Invert the empty solution container and pull the spike free.	Prevents minor loss of remaining solution
Deposit the empty bag within a lined waste receptacle.	Keeps the environment clean and orderly
Remove the seal from the replacement solution container.	Provides access to the port
Insert the spike into the port of the new container.	Provides a route for infusing fluid
Hang the new container from the suspension hook on the IV standard or infusion device.	Restores height to overcome venous pressure
Inspect for the presence of air within the tubing and proceed to remove it if present.	Reduces the potential for air embolism or an alarm from an infusion device detecting air
Readjust the regulator clamp or reprogram the infusion device to restore the prescribed rate of infusion.	Demonstrates compliance in carrying out the medical order
Evaluation	
• Solution container is replaced	
• Infusion continues	

(continued)

SKILL 15-4
Changing Intravenous Solution Containers (Continued)

Suggested Action	Reason for Action
Document	
• Volume infused from previous container on intake and output record	
• Time, volume, type of solution, and signature on the medication record or wherever the agency specifies documenting the administration of intravenous solutions	
• Condition of the patient	

Sample Documentation

Date and Time   1,000 mL lactated Ringer's instilling at 42 gtt/min. Dressing over venipuncture is dry and intact. No swelling or discomfort in the area of the infusing fluid.

_____ **Signature, Title**

SKILL 15-5
Changing Intravenous Tubing

Suggested Action	Reason for Action
Assessment	
Determine the agency's policy for changing IV tubing.	Demonstrates responsibility for complying with infection control policies
Check the date and time on the label attached to the tubing.	Determines the approximate time when the tubing must be changed
Determine if the solution container will need replacing before the time expires on the tubing.	Facilitates changing both the container and tubing at the same time
Planning	
Obtain appropriate replacement tubing and supplies for changing the dressing.	Ensures that equipment will be available and ready when needed
Attach a new label to the tubing indicating the date and time the tubing is changed, and your initials.	Provides a quick reference for determining when the tubing must be changed again
Implementation	
Wash your hands.	Reduces the transmission of microorganisms
Prepare adhesive tape and dressing materials and place them in a convenient location.	Facilitates dexterity later in the procedure
Open the new package of tubing, stretch the tubing, and tighten the roller clamp.	Prepares the tubing for insertion into the solution container
Remove the solution container from the suspension hook with the tubing still attached.	Facilitates separating the tubing from the container

(continued)

SKILL 15-5
Changing Intravenous Tubing *(Continued)*

Suggested Action	Reason for Action
Invert the solution container and pull the spike free.	Prevents minor loss of remaining solution
Secure the spike to the IV pole with a strip of previously torn tape.	Facilitates continued infusion
Insert the spike from the new tubing into the container of solution.	Provides a route for the fluid
Squeeze the drip chamber to fill it half full, open the roller clamp, and purge the air from the tubing.	Prepares the tubing for use
Remove the tape and dressing from the venipuncture site.	Provides access to the venipuncture device
Don gloves.	Provides a barrier against contact with blood
Tighten the roller clamp on the expired tubing.	Temporarily interrupts the infusion
Stabilize the hub of the venipuncture device and separate the tubing from it.	Prevents accidental removal of the catheter or needle from the vein
Remove the cap from the end of the new tubing and attach it to the end of the venipuncture device.	Connects the venipuncture device to the tubing without contaminating the tip of the tubing
Continue to hold the venipuncture device with one hand while releasing the roller clamp on the new tubing.	Reestablishes the infusion.
Proceed to replace the dressing on the venipuncture site and secure the tubing	Covers the site and keeps the tubing and venipuncture device from being pulled out
Readjust the rate of infusion.	Complies with the medical order
Write the date, time, and your initials on the new dressing, and include the gauge of the venipuncture device and original date of insertion.	Provides a quick reference for determining future nursing responsibilities for infection control
Dispose of the expired tubing in a lined receptacle.	Maintains a clean and orderly environment

Evaluation
• Tubing is replaced
• Solution continues to infuse at the prescribed rate

Document
• Date and time
• Assessment findings of venipuncture site
• Dressing change

Sample Documentation

Date and Time   No redness, swelling, or tenderness at venipuncture site in L. forearm. Dressing changed after replacement of IV tubing. _____ **Signature, Title**

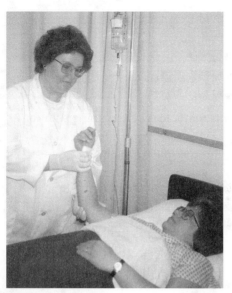

FIGURE 15-19
Applying pressure. (Courtesy of Ken Timby.)

INSERTING A MEDICATION LOCK

A **medication lock** is a sealed chamber that is inserted into a venipuncture device (Skill 15-6 and Fig. 15-20). A medication lock may also be known as a *saline lock* or *heparin lock* because the chamber is filled with either of these two solutions and periodically flushed with one or the other to prevent blood from clotting at the tip of the catheter or needle.

Medication locks are used when patients:

- No longer need continuous infusions of fluid
- Need intermittent administrations of IV medications
- May need emergency IV fluid or medications if their condition deteriorates

Medication locks are replaced if and when the venipuncture site is changed. The use of a medication lock when administering IV drugs is discussed further in Chapter 35.

(text continues on page 289)

SKILL 15-6
Inserting a Medication Lock

Suggested Action	Reason for Action
Assessment	
Confirm that the physician has written an order to discontinue the continuous infusion of intravenous fluid and insert a medication lock.	Demonstrates responsibility and accountability for carrying out medical orders
Check the patient's identity.	Prevents errors
Inspect the site for signs of redness, swelling, or drainage.	Provides data indicating if the site can be maintained or if a new venipuncture should be performed
Observe if the infusion is instilling at the predetermined rate.	Indicates whether the vein and catheter are currently patent (open)
Determine if the patient understands the purpose and technique for inserting a medication lock.	Indicates the need for patient teaching
Planning	
Assemble necessary equipment, which includes the medication lock, syringe containing 2 mL of sterile normal saline (0.9% sodium chloride) or heparinized saline (10 U/mL or 100 U/mL), depending on the agency's policy, alcohol swabs, gloves, and supplies for changing or reinforcing the dressing over the site.	Promotes organization and efficient time management
Implementation	
Wash your hands.	Reduces the spread of microorganisms
Prefill the chamber of the medication lock with saline or heparin solution.	Displaces air from within the empty chamber

(continued)

SKILL 15-6
Inserting a Medication Lock *(Continued)*

Suggested Action	Reason for Action
Loosen the tape over the dressing to expose the connection between the hub of the catheter or needle and the tubing adapter; also remove the tape that is stabilizing the tubing to the patient's arm.	Facilitates removing the tubing from the patient
Loosen the protective cap from the end of the medication lock.	Maintains sterility while preparing for the insertion of the lock
Don clean gloves.	Provides a barrier against contact with blood
Tighten the roller clamp on the tubing and stop the infusion pump or controller if one is being used.	Prevents fluid from leaking during removal of the tubing

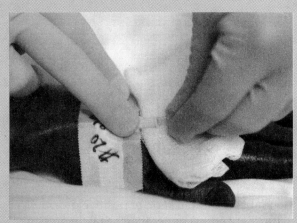

Applying pressure over the catheter tip. (Courtesy of Ken Timby.)

Apply pressure over the tip of the catheter or needle.	Controls or prevents blood loss
Remove the tip of the tubing from the venipuncture device and insert the medication lock.	Seals the opening in the catheter or needle

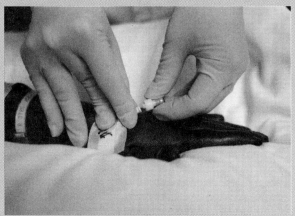

Inserting the lock. (Courtesy of Ken Timby.)

(continued)

SKILL 15-6
Inserting a Medication Lock (Continued)

Suggested Action	Reason for Action
Screw the lock onto the end of the catheter or needle.	Stabilizes the connection
Swab the rubber port on the medication lock with alcohol.	Cleans the port
Pierce the port with the needle or blunt needleless adapter on the syringe and gradually instill 1 mL of saline or heparin until the syringe is almost empty.	Clears blood from the venipuncture device and lock before it can clot

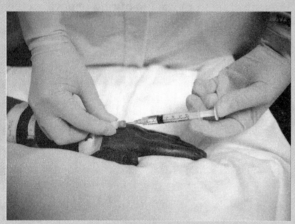

Instilling saline or heparin solution. (Courtesy of Ken Timby.)

Suggested Action	Reason for Action
Begin to remove the needle from the port as the last volume of solution is instilled.	Continues the application of positive pressure (pushing effect) rather than negative pressure (pulling effect) during the time the needle is removed; negative pressure may pull blood into the catheter or needle tip and cause it to become obstructed.
Retape or secure the dressing.	Reduces the possibility that the lock and catheter may be accidentally dislodged
Plan to flush the lock at least every 8 hours with 1 or 2 mL of flush solution (either saline or heparin solution) when it is not used, or after each use.	Ensures continued patency

Evaluation
• Site appears free of inflammation
• Patency is maintained
• Flush solution instills easily
• Device is stabilized

Document
• Date and time
• Discontinuation of infusing solution
• Volume of infused intravenous solution

(continued)

SKILL 15-6
Inserting a Medication Lock (Continued)

Suggested Action	Reason for Action

- Insertion of medication lock
- Volume and type of flush solution
- Assessment findings

Sample Documentation

Date and Time   Infusion of 5% D/W discontinued. 700 mL of IV solution infused. Medication lock inserted into IV catheter in R. hand and flushed with 1 mL of normal saline. No redness, swelling, or discomfort at site. _____ **Signature, Title**

ADMINISTERING BLOOD

The nursing responsibilities for administering blood are similar to those already discussed for administering crystalloid solutions. However, before blood is administered, vital signs are obtained and documented. They provide a baseline for comparison in case the patient experiences a transfusion reaction. Also, the numbers on the patient's color-coded bracelet are checked to make sure they correlate with the unit of blood that will be administered. Furthermore, IV medications are *never* infused through tubing that is administering blood.

There are also some differences in regard to equipment and potential complications.

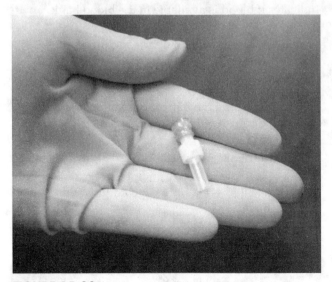

FIGURE 15-20
Medication lock. (Courtesy of Ken Timby.)

Blood Administration Equipment

When blood is administered, there are certain standards for the gauge of catheter or needle and tubing that are used.

CATHETER OR NEEDLE GAUGE

Because blood contains cells in addition to water, it is usually infused through at least a 20-gauge, but preferably an 18-gauge catheter or needle. Any smaller gauge may prolong the infusion beyond 4 hours, the maximum safe period for administering blood.

BLOOD ADMINISTRATION TUBING

Blood is administered through tubing referred to as a *Y-set* (Fig. 15-21). As the name implies, there are two branches at the top of the tubing. One is used for administering normal saline solution and the other is used for administering blood. Normal saline (0.9% sodium chloride) is the *only* solution that is used when administering blood. Other types of solutions cause destruction of red blood cells.

The two branches of the Y-set join together above a filter that removes clotted blood and debris. The normal saline is always administered before the blood is hung and follows after the blood has been infused. It may also be used during the infusion, if patients experience a transfusion reaction.

Skill 15-7 describes how blood is administered.

Transfusion Reactions

Serious, life-threatening transfusion reactions generally occur within the first 5 to 15 minutes of the infusion. For this reason, nurses usually remain with patients during this critical time. The fact that the potential for grave consequences diminishes as the transfusion progresses uneventfully, however, is no absolute guarantee that

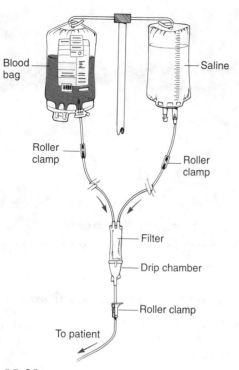

FIGURE 15-21
Blood administration set.

adverse reactions will not occur. Therefore, patients are monitored frequently during a transfusion. They are instructed to call for assistance if they experience any unusual sensations because various types of reactions may occur at any time (Table 15-9).

PROVIDING PARENTERAL NUTRITION

The term *parenteral* literally means "a route other than enteral or intestinal." Therefore, **parenteral nutrition** refers to a technique for providing nutrients, such as protein, carbohydrate, fat, vitamins, minerals, and trace elements, intravenously rather than orally.

Depending on the concentration of these substances, parenteral nutrition may be administered through an IV catheter in a peripheral vein or through a catheter that terminates in a central vein near the heart.

Peripheral Parenteral Nutrition

Peripheral parenteral nutrition (PPN) is an isotonic or hypotonic nutrient solution that provides temporary nutritional support, promotes nitrogen balance, and fa-

(text continues on page 293)

SKILL 15-7
Administering Blood

Suggested Action	Reason for Action
Assessment	
Check the patient's identity.	Prevents errors
Determine if a special signed consent is required.	Complies with legal responsibilities
Check the size of the current venipuncture device if an IV is presently infusing.	Indicates if another venipuncture must be performed
Review the medical record for results of the type and cross-match.	Indicates if blood is available in the blood bank
Take temperature, pulse, respirations, and blood pressure within 30 minutes of obtaining blood.	Provides a baseline for comparison during the transfusion
Planning	
Complete major nursing activities before starting the infusion of saline unless the blood must be given immediately.	Avoids disturbing the patient once the blood is being administered
Plan to perform a venipuncture or start the infusion of saline just before obtaining the blood.	Prevents administering fluid unnecessarily
Obtain necessary equipment, which includes a 250 mL container of normal saline (0.9% NaCl) and a Y-set.	Complies with the standards of care for administering blood
Tighten the roller clamp on one branch of the Y-tubing and the roller clamp below the filter.	Prepares the tubing for purging with saline

(continued)

SKILL 15-7
Administering Blood (Continued)

Suggested Action	Reason for Action
Insert the unclampled branch of the Y-set into the container of saline and squeeze the drip chamber until it and the filter are half-full.	Moistens the filter and fills the upper portion of the tubing with saline
Release the lower clamp and flush air from the remaining section of tubing.	Reduces the potential for infusing a bolus of air

Implementation

Suggested Action	Reason for Action
Perform the venipuncture or connect the Y-set to the present venipuncture device if it is at least an 18-gauge.	Provides access to the venous circulation and ensures that the blood will move freely through the catheter or needle
Begin the infusion of saline.	Ensures that the site is patent and that there will be no delay once the unit of blood is obtained
Go to the blood bank to pick up the unit of blood, making sure to take a form identifying the patient.	Prevents mistaken identity when releasing the matched blood
Cross-check the information on the blood bag and the lab slip with the blood bank personnel.	Prevents releasing the wrong unit of blood or blood that is not a compatible blood group and Rh factor
Check that the blood has not passed the expiration date.	Ensures maximum benefit from the transfusion
Inspect the container of blood and reject the blood if it appears black or has obvious gas bubbles inside.	Indicates deteriorated or tainted blood
Plan to give the blood as soon as it is brought to the unit.	Demonstrates an understanding that blood must be infused within 4 hours after being released from the blood bank
Rotate the blood, but do not shake or squeeze the container, if the serum has separated from the cells.	Avoids damaging intact cells
At the bedside, check the label on the blood bag with the numbers on the patient's wristband with a second nurse; sign in the designated areas on the transfusion record.	Reduces the potential for administering incompatible blood
Spike the container of blood.	Provides a route for administering the blood
Tighten the roller clamp on the saline branch of the tubing and release the roller clamp on the blood branch.	Fills the tubing and filter with blood
Regulate the rate of infusion at 2 mL/minute for the first 15 minutes (check the drop factor to determine the rate in gtt/minute).	Establishes a slow rate of infusion so as to be able to monitor and respond to signs of a transfusion reaction
Increase the rate to 7 to 9 mL/minute after the first 15 minutes if no signs of a reaction have occurred.	Increases the rate of administration so as to infuse the unit within 4 hours or less.
Assess the patient at 15- to 30-minute intervals during the transfusion.	Ensures the patient's safety

(continued)

SKILL 15-7
Administering Blood (Continued)

Suggested Action	Reason for Action
Clamp the tubing from the blood and release the clamp on the saline when the blood has infused.	Flushes blood cells from the tubing
Take vital signs one more time.	Documents the condition of the patient at the completion of the blood administration
Tighten the roller clamp below the filter when the tubing looks reasonably clear of blood.	Prevents leaking when the IV is discontinued
Don gloves.	Provides a barrier against contact with blood
Loosen the tape covering the venipuncture site and remove the catheter, or remove the blood tubing and reconnect the previously infusing solution.	Discontinues the infusion or restores previous fluid therapy
Apply a dressing or bandaid over the venipuncture site if the IV is discontinued.	Prevents infection
Dispose of the blood container and tubing according to agency policy.	Blood is a biohazard and requires special bagging to ensure that others will not accidentally come in direct contact with the blood

Evaluation

- Entire unit of blood is administered within 4 hours
- No evidence of transfusion reaction, or
- Reactions have been minimized by appropriate interventions
- Infusion has been discontinued or previous orders have been resumed

Document

- Venipuncture procedure if initiated for the administration of blood
- Preinfusion vital signs
- Names of nurses who checked armband and blood bag container
- Time blood administration began
- Rate of infusion during first 15 minutes and remaining period of time
- Signs of reaction, if any, and nursing actions
- Periodic vital sign assessments
- Time blood infusion was completed
- Volume of blood and saline that infused

Sample Documentation

Date and Time   #18 gauge over-the-needle catheter inserted into L. forearm and connected to 250 mL of 0.9% saline infusing at 21 mL/hr. T—98^2 (tympanic), P—90, R—22, BP 116/64 in R. arm while lying flat. One unit of type O+ whole blood #684381 obtained from the blood bank and checked by E. Rogers, RN and D. Baker, RN. Blood bag and wrist band information found to be compatible. Blood infusing at 2 mL/min (20 gtt/min) for 15 min. Rate increased to 7 mL/min (70 gtt/min) during remainder of infusion. Blood transfusion completed at 1600. No evidence of transfusion reaction. T—98^2 (tympanic), P—86, R—20, BP 122/70 in R. arm at end of transfusion. Total of 100 mL of saline and 500 mL of blood infused before IV discontinued.

_____ **Signature, Title**

TABLE 15-9. Transfusion Reactions

Type of Reaction	Signs and Symptoms	Cause(s)	Action
Incompatibility	Hypotension, rapid pulse rate, difficulty breathing, back pain, flushing	Mismatch between donor and recipient blood groups	Stop the infusion of blood. Infuse the saline at a rapid rate. Call for assistance. Administer oxygen. Raise the feet higher than the head. Be prepared to administer emergency drugs. Send first urine specimen to laboratory. Save the blood and tubing.
Febrile	Fever, shaking chills, headache, rapid pulse, muscle aches	Allergy to foreign proteins in the donated blood	Stop the blood infusion. Start the saline. Check vital signs. Report findings.
Septic	Fever, chills, hypotension	Infusion of blood that contains microorganisms	Stop the infusion of blood. Start the saline. Report findings. Save the blood and tubing.
Allergic	Rash, itching, flushing, stable vital signs.	Minor sensitivity to substances in the donor blood	Slow the rate of infusion. Assess the patient. Report findings. Be prepared to give an antihistamine.
Moderate chilling	No fever or other symptoms	Infusion of cold blood	Continue the infusion. Cover and make the patient comfortable.
Overload	Hypertension, difficulty breathing, moist breath sounds, bounding pulse	Large volume or rapid rate of infusion; inadequate cardiac or kidney function	Reduce the rate. Elevate the head. Give oxygen. Report findings. Be prepared to give a diuretic.
Hypocalcemia (low calcium)	Tingling of fingers, hypotension, muscle cramps, convulsions	Multiple blood transfusions containing anticalcium agents	Stop the blood infusion. Start saline. Report findings. Be prepared to give antidote, calcium chloride.

cilitates weight gain when oral intake is inadequate or contraindicated (Dudek, 1993). It may also be used for a transitional period of time as a patient begins to resume eating.

Peripheral parenteral nutrition solutions usually provide between 2,000 to 2,500 calories. This form of nutrition may be provided when oral intake is expected to resume within 7 to 10 days. Because these solutions are not extremely concentrated, they may be infused through peripheral veins.

Total Parenteral Nutrition

Total parenteral nutrition (TPN) is a hypertonic solution of nutrients designed to meet nearly all the caloric and nutritional needs of patients who are severely malnourished or who may not be able to consume food or liquids for a long period of time. Display 15-6 provides a profile of patients who may benefit from TPN.

DISPLAY 15-6. *Candidates for Total Parenteral Nutrition*

- Patients who have not eaten for 5 days and are not likely to eat during the next week
- Patients who have had a 10% or more loss of body weight
- Patients exhibiting self-imposed starvation (anorexia nervosa)
- Patients with cancer of the esophagus or stomach
- Patients with postoperative gastrointestinal complications
- Patients with inflammatory bowel disease in an acute stage
- Patients with major trauma or burns
- Patients with liver and renal failure

Because TPN solutions are extremely concentrated, they are delivered to an area where they may be diluted in a fairly large volume of blood. This excludes peripheral veins. Consequently, TPN solutions are infused through a catheter inserted into the subclavian or jugular vein but which terminates in the superior vena cava. This type of a catheter is referred to as a *central venous catheter* (Fig. 15-22). Sometimes a *peripherally inserted central catheter* (PICC) may be used. A PICC is a long catheter that is inserted in a peripheral arm vein but terminates in the superior vena cava as well (Fig. 15-23).

NURSING GUIDELINES FOR ADMINISTERING TOTAL PARENTERAL NUTRITION

- Weigh the patient daily.
  Rationale: Aids in monitoring the patient's response to treatment
- Use tubing that contains a filter.
  Rationale: Absorbs air and bacteria, two potential complications among patients with central venous catheters

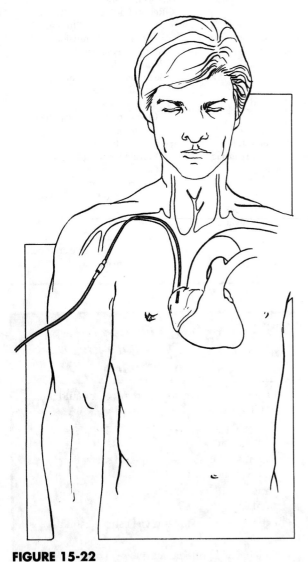

FIGURE 15-22
Central venous catheter inserted into the subclavian vein and threaded into the heart. (Ellis JR, Nowlis EA, Bentz PM: Modules for Basic Nursing Skills, 5th ed, p 467. Philadelphia, JB Lippincott, 1992)

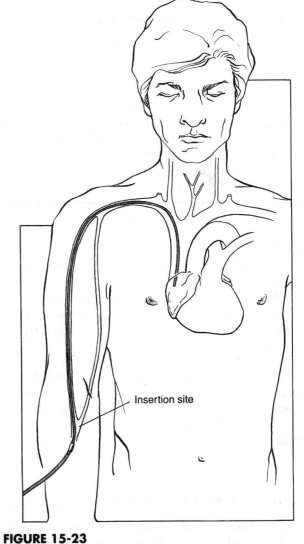

FIGURE 15-23
Peripherally inserted central catheter with distal tip in the heart. (Ellis JR, Nowlis EA, Bentz PM: Modules for Basic Nursing Skills, 5th ed, p 475. Philadelphia, JB Lippincott, 1992)

- Change TPN tubings daily.
  Rationale: Reduces the potential for infection
- Tape all connections in the tubing and central catheter.
  Rationale: Prevents accidental separation and the potential for an air embolism
- Clamp the central catheter and have the patient bear down whenever separating the tubing from its catheter connection.
  Rationale: Prevents an air embolism
- Use an infusion pump to administer TPN solution.
  Rationale: Monitors and regulates precise fluid volumes
- Infuse initial TPN solutions gradually (eg, 25–50 mL/hour).
  Rationale: Allows time for physiologic adaptation
- Never increase the rate of infusion to make up for an uninfused volume unless the physician has been consulted.
  Rationale: Tends to create a potential for high blood sugar levels
- Monitor intake and especially urine output.
  Rationale: Monitors for diuresis (increased urine excretion), which can be triggered by high blood glucose levels, resulting in outputs greater than intake
- Monitor capillary blood glucose levels (see Chap. 13).
  Rationale: Determines the ability to metabolize glucose and the potential need for insulin
- Wean from TPN gradually.
  Rationale: Prevents sudden drop in blood sugar level

Lipid Emulsions

An **emulsion** is a mixture of two liquids, one of which is insoluble in the other, but when combined is distributed throughout as small droplets within the other. A lipid emulsion is a mixture of water and fats in the form of soybean or safflower oil, egg yolk phospholipids, and glycerin (Dudek, 1993).

Lipid solutions, which look milky white (Fig. 15-24), are often given intermittently with TPN solutions. They provide additional calories and promote adequate blood levels of fatty acids. Lipid solutions may be administered peripherally or in a port in the central catheter below the filter and close to the vein. If the lipid solution is squeezed or mixed with TPN solutions in larger volumes than those moving through the catheter, the lipid molecules tend to "break" and separate in the solution.

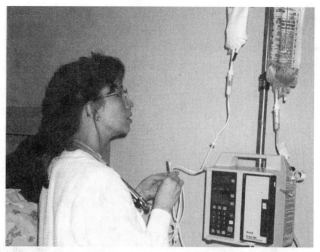

FIGURE 15-24
Administration of lipid emulsion. (Courtesy of Ken Timby.

When lipids are administered, patients may experience adverse reactions within 2 to 5 hours of the infusion (Dudek, 1993). Some common manifestations include fever, flushing, sweating, dizziness, nausea, vomiting, headache, chest and back pain, dyspnea, and cyanosis. Delayed reactions, which may be manifested up to 10 days later, are characterized by enlargement of the liver and spleen accompanied by jaundice, reduced white blood cell and platelet counts, elevated blood lipid levels, seizures, and shock.

NURSING IMPLICATIONS

Patients who have fluid, electrolyte, blood, and nutritional imbalances are likely to have one or more of the nursing diagnoses listed in the accompanying Applicable Nursing Diagnoses.

The Nursing Care Plan in this chapter illustrates the nursing process as it applies to a patient with Fluid Volume Deficit. This diagnostic category is defined by the North American Nursing Diagnosis Association (1994) as, "The state in which an individual experiences vascular, cellular, or intracellular dehydration."

APPLICABLE NURSING DIAGNOSES

- Feeding Self-Care Deficit
- Fluid Volume Deficit
- Fluid Volume Excess
- Altered Oral Mucous Membrane
- Risk for Impaired Skin Integrity
- Knowledge Deficit

NURSING CARE PLAN:
Fluid Volume Deficit

Assessment

Subjective Data
States, "I've been living on the streets. I don't have a job. I haven't eaten in several days."

Objective Data
56-year-old homeless man brought to the Emergency Department after being found by police wandering and confused near Main St. Outdoor daytime temperatures have been in the 90° ranges. Height 5'10", weight 137 lbs. States usual weight is around 160 lbs. T—100° orally, P—100 and weak, R—28. Oral mucous membranes are dry. Able to void 50 mL of dark, amber urine. BP 100/68 in R. arm while sitting up. Skin is dry and tents for >5 seconds when compressed.

Diagnosis

Fluid Volume Deficit related to inadequate oral intake and increased insensible fluid loss.

Plan

Goal
The patient's oral fluid intake will be between 1,500 to 3,000 mL in the next 24 hours. (8/15).

Orders: 8/14
1. Compile a list of food and fluid likes and dislikes.
2. Provide a minimum of 100 to 200 mL/hour of preferred liquids/hour over the next 16 hours. Avoid disturbing hours of sleep.
3. Request dietary department to send foods that are good sources of sodium, such as milk, cheese, bouillon, ham.
4. Refer to Salvation Army shelter for the homeless before discharge
———————————————————————————————— R. ARMSTRONG, RN

Implementation 8/14 1000
(Documentation)

States "I like just about anything. I'm so thirsty. A big, cool glass of lemonade sounds wonderful right now." Also lists ginger ale and orange juice as favorite beverages. Dietary department notified to send sodium-rich foods for next 24 hours. Discharge planner notified for referral to Salvation Army.
———————————————————————————————— L. O'CONNELL, LPN

Evaluation
(Documentation)

1030   200 mL of orange juice provided and consumed. Weakness and tremors of the hand noted. Able to use a straw with glass. ——————————— L. O'CONNELL, LPN

1230   Ate macaroni and cheese, sausage, stewed tomatoes, and whole milk for lunch.
———————————————————————————————— L. O'CONNELL, LPN

1430   Total oral fluid intake since 1000 has been 1,000 mL. Urine is lighter in color. Voided a total of 600 mL since admission. Vital signs improving; see graphic sheet for specifics. Discharge planner will visit in A.M. 8/15. ———————————
———————————————————————————————— L. O'CONNELL, LPN

FOCUS ON OLDER ADULTS

- Older adults are more likely to have chronic diseases affecting the heart and kidneys, which places them at risk for fluid and electrolyte imbalances.
- Diuretics, drugs prescribed for older adults with cardiovascular disorders, place them at greater risk for fluid and electrolyte imbalances.
- Compromised mobility and self-care may lead to fluid deficits in older adults who cannot eat or drink independently.
- When caring for older adults, nurses must frequently offer and assist with oral fluids rather than assume that they will be consumed independently.
- More fluid may be consumed when it is offered, rather than inquiring as to whether the older adult would like a drink.
- The potential for dehydration is greater among older adults because they tend to have a reduced sensation of thirst (Matteson and McConnell 1988).
- To maintain an adequate consumption of nutrients, it is best to offer fluids at times other than meals. Distending the stomach with liquids may reduce dietary intake because it creates a sensation of satiety (fullness).

- Older adults may restrict their own fluid intake as a self-prescribed intervention for preventing incontinence. This practice may lead to postural hypotension, falls, and injury if fluid volumes fall to dangerous limits.
- Assess for possible fluid volume or electrolyte deficits among older adults who become confused.
- When providing instructions for older adults who must fast before certain procedures, advise them to increase their oral fluid intake in the hours before beginning fluid restrictions to prevent dehydration.
- Because the skin of older adults tends to lose elasticity, assessing skin turgor is often inadequate in determining the status of hydration. Instead, the nurse may assess for a dry, furrowed tongue, dark color to the urine, and low urine volume as more useful indicators of fluid volume deficit.
- The response of older adults to intravenous infusions must be monitored closely. They may not be able to tolerate comparable volumes that can safely be administered to younger adults.

KEY CONCEPTS

- Body fluid is a mixture of water, chemicals called electrolytes and nonelectrolytes, and blood cells.
- Body fluid is distributed inside cells, called the intracellular compartment, and outside the cells, in the extracellular compartment. The extracellular compartment is further subdivided into the interstitial compartment and the intravascular compartment.
- Fluid and the components within it are distributed by osmosis, filtration, passive diffusion, facilitated diffusion, and active transport.
- Fluid volume status is assessed by measuring a patient's intake and output, obtaining daily weights, obtaining vital signs, monitoring bowel elimination patterns and stool characteristics, observing the color of urine, and assessing skin turgor, the condition of the oral mucous membranes, lung sounds, and level of consciousness.

- A fluid volume deficit can be corrected by treating the underlying disorder, increasing oral intake, administering IV fluid replacements, controlling fluid losses, or a combination of all of these measures.
- Fluid volume excess is reduced or eliminated by treating the underlying disorder, restricting or limiting oral fluids, reducing salt consumption, discontinuing IV fluid infusions or reducing the infusing volume, administering drugs that promote urine elimination, or a combination of these interventions.
- Intravenous fluids are administered to (1) maintain or restore fluid balance, (2) maintain or replace electrolytes, (3) administer water-soluble vitamins, (4) provide calories, (5) administer drugs, and (6) replace blood and blood products.
- Crystalloid solutions are mixtures of water and substances like salt and sugar that totally dissolve. Col-

loid solutions are mixtures of water and suspended, undissolved substances like blood cells.

- The term "isotonic" refers to a solution that has the same concentration of dissolved substances as plasma; "hypotonic" refers to one that has fewer dissolved substances; and "hypertonic" is a term that describes a solution that is more concentrated than plasma.
- When selecting tubing for administering IV solutions, the nurse must consider whether to use primary or secondary tubing, vented or unvented tubing, which drop size is most appropriate, and if a filter is needed.
- Intravenous fluids may be infused by gravity or with the assistance of an infusion device such as a pump or volumetric controller.
- When selecting a vein before venipuncture, the nurse gives priority to one in the nondominant hand or arm that is fairly straight, larger than the needle or catheter gauge, likely to be undisturbed by joint movement, and unimpaired by previous trauma or use.
- Complications of IV fluid therapy include infiltration, phlebitis, infection, circulatory overload, thrombus formation, pulmonary embolus, and air embolism.
- A medication lock may be used for patients who require intermittent IV fluid or medication administration, or for emergency access to the vascular system should their condition rapidly deteriorate.
- When administering blood, the nurse (1) assesses vital signs before and during the administration; (2) uses no smaller than a 20-gauge needle or catheter, normal saline solution, and Y-set tubing; and (3) infuses the blood within 4 hours or less.
- During blood administration, the nurse monitors patients closely for incompatibility and febrile, septic, and allergic reactions, as well as chilling, circulatory overload, and signs of hypocalcemia.
- Parenteral nutrition refers to a technique for providing nutrients, such as protein, carbohydrate, fat, vitamins, minerals, and trace elements, intravenously rather than orally.

CRITICAL THINKING EXERCISES

- When calculating a patient's I & O, you find that the patient has had a total intake of 1,000 mL and output of 750 mL. What other assessment findings are you likely to observe?
- What nursing interventions would you plan to restore the patient's fluid imbalance in the previous sit-

uation? What criteria would indicate that the patient's fluid imbalance has been corrected?

- Several people involved in a serious motor vehicle accident are brought to an Emergency Department. All of the victims have lost a great deal of blood. Identify methods for restoring their fluid volume and the substances, including possible blood products and blood groups that may be used for people who have types A, B, O, AB, and Rh-positive antigens.
- A patient you are caring for is scheduled to receive a blood transfusion shortly. What are your plans for assessing the patient before, during, and following the transfusion? What is the basis for your assessment concerns?
- If the patient receiving a blood transfusion suddenly develops hypotension tachycardia, and you observe flushing and dyspnea, what action should you take? Rank interventions in order of priority.

SUGGESTED READINGS

Alford DM. Tips on promoting food and fluid intake in the elderly. Journal of Gerontological Nursing November 1991;17:44–46.

Angelucci D, Todaro A. Reversing acute dehydration. Nursing June 1993;23:33.

Bove LA. How fluids and electrolytes shift after surgery. Nursing August 1994;24:34–39.

Carnevali DL, Patrick M. Nursing Management for the Elderly. 3rd ed. Philadelphia: JB Lippincott, 1993.

Cullen L. Interventions related to fluid and electrolyte balance. Nursing Clinics of North America June 1992;27:569–597.

Dennison RD, Blevins BN. Myth and facts . . . about acid–base imbalance. Nursing March 1992;22:69.

Dennison RD, Blevins BN. Myth and facts . . . about fluid imbalance part 1. Nursing January 1992;22:22.

Dennison RD, Blevins BN. Myth and facts . . . about fluid imbalance part 2. Nursing February 1992;22:26.

Dudek SG. Nutritional Handbook for Nursing Practice. 2nd ed. Philadelphia: JB Lippincott, 1993.

Ingbar DH. The quest for a red blood cell substitute. Respiratory Care 35(3):260–272, 1990.

Fischbach F. A Manual of Laboratory & Diagnostic Tests. 4th ed. Philadelphia: JB Lippincott, 1992.

Masiak MJ, Naylor MD, Hayman LL. Fluids and Electrolytes Through the Life Cycle. Norwalk, CT: Appleton-Century-Crofts, 1985.

Matteson MA, McConnell ES. Gerontological Nursing: Concepts and Practice. Philadelphia: WB Saunders, 1988.

Monahan FD, Drake T, Neighbors M. Nursing Care of Adults. Philadelphia: WB Saunders, 1994.

NANDA Nursing Diagnoses: Definitions and Classifications 1994–1995. Philadelphia: North American Nursing Diagnosis Associat, 1994.

Newbern VB. Failure to thrive: a growing concern in the elderly. Journal of Gerontological Nursing August 1992;18:21–25, 38–39.

Osato EE, Stone JT, Phillips SL. Clinical manifestations: failure to thrive in the elderly. Journal of Gerontological Nursing August 1993;19:28–34.

Smeltzer SC, Bare BG. Medical-Surgical Nursing. 7th ed. Philadelphia: JB Lippincott, 1992.

Thompson J. Parenteral nutrition. Nursing Times January 8–14, 1992; 88:62, 64.

Weinstein SM. Administering P.P.N. Nursing January 1992;22:32H, 32J.

Yen PK. Liquid nutrition boosters. Geriatric Nursing September-October 1991;12:262.

CHAPTER 16

Hygiene

Chapter Outline

The Integumentary System
Hygiene Practices
Visual and Hearing Devices
Nursing Implications
Key Concepts
Critical Thinking Exercises
Suggested Readings

 NURSING GUIDELINES

Bathing Patients
Shaving Patients

 SKILLS

Providing a Tub Bath or Shower
Administering Perineal Care
Giving a Bed Bath
Giving Oral Care to Unconscious Patients
Shampooing Hair

 NURSING CARE PLAN

Bathing/Hygiene Self-Care Deficit

Key Terms

Bag Bath	Oral Hygiene
Bed Bath	Partial Bath
Caries	Perineal Care
Dentures	Periodontal Disease
Feedback	Plaque

Gingivitis	Podiatrist
Hygiene	Pruritus
Integument	Sordes
Ophthalmologist	Tartar
Optometrist	Towel Bath

Learning Objectives

An understanding of the content within this chapter will be evidenced by the student's ability to:

• Explain what the term "hygiene" means
• Name five hygiene practices that most people perform regularly
• Give two reasons why a partial bath may be more appropriate for older adults than daily bathing
• List at least three advantages for towel or bag baths
• Name two situations in which shaving with a safety razor may be contraindicated
• Name three items that are recommended for oral hygiene
• Identify the chief hazard in providing oral hygiene for unconscious patients and two methods for preventing its occurrence
• Describe two techniques for preventing damage to dentures during cleaning
• Describe two methods for removing hair tangles
• Name two types of patients for whom nail care must be provided with extreme caution
• Name four types of visual and hearing devices
• List two alternatives for patients who are unable to insert or care for their own contact lenses
• Discuss four reasons for sound disturbances experienced by people who wear hearing aids
• Describe an infrared listening device

Timby BK: *Fundamental Skills and Concepts in Patient Care, Sixth Edition* © 1996 Lippincott-Raven Publishers

ygiene refers to practices that promote health through personal cleanliness. Hygiene is fostered through activities like bathing, tooth brushing, cleaning and maintaining fingernails and toenails, and shampooing and grooming hair. It may also apply to the care and maintenance of devices like eyeglasses and hearing aids so that they continue to function properly.

Hygiene practices and needs may differ according to age, inherited characteristics of the skin and hair, cultural values, and health problems. This chapter offers suggestions for carrying out hygiene practices when providing patient care.

Most hygiene practices are based on maintaining or restoring healthy qualities of the integumentary system.

THE INTEGUMENTARY SYSTEM

The word **integument** actually means *covering*. The integumentary system includes the skin, mucous membranes, hair, and nails. Because the mouth, or oral cav-ity (which is lined with mucous membrane) also contains teeth, a discussion of this accessory structure is also included.

Skin

The skin consists of the epidermis, dermis, and subcutaneous layers (Fig. 16-1). The *epidermis*, or outermost layer, contains dead skin cells that form a tough protein called *keratin* that protects the underlying layers and structures within the skin. The cells in the epidermis are continuously shed and replaced from the *dermis*, or true skin, which contains most of the secretory glands (Table 16-1). The *subcutaneous layer* separates the skin from skeletal muscles, and contains fat cells, blood vessels, nerves, and the roots of hair follicles and glands.

The structures that make up the skin carry out such functions as:

* Protecting inner structures of the body from injury and infection
* Regulating body temperature

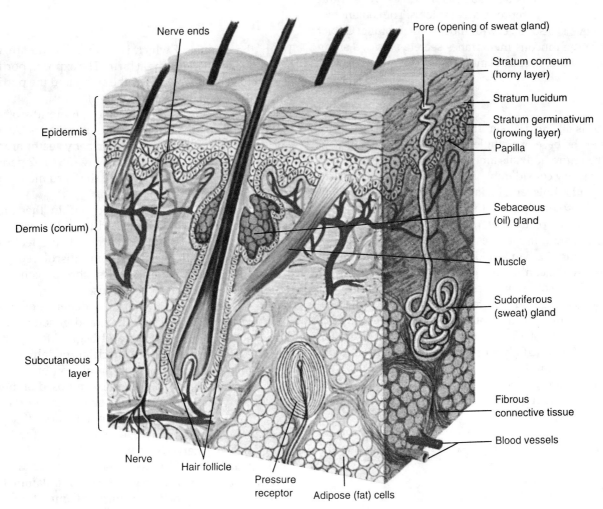

FIGURE 16-1
Cross-section of the skin. (Memmler RL, Cohen BJ, Wood DL: The Human Body in Health and Disease, 7th ed, p 69. Philadelphia, JB Lippincott, 1992)

TABLE 16-1. *Types of Skin Glands*

Gland	Location	Secretion	Purpose
Sudoriferous	Throughout the dermis and subcutaneous layers, especially in the axillae and groin	Sweat	Regulates body temperature
Ceruminous	Ear canals	Cerumen	Has antimicrobial properties
Sebaceous	Throughout the dermis	Sebum	Lubricates skin and hair
Ciliary	Eyelids	Sweat and sebum	Protects lid margin and lubricates eyelash follicles

- Maintaining fluid and chemical balance
- Providing sensory information such as pain, temperature, touch, and pressure
- Converting preforms of vitamin D when exposed to sunlight

Mucous Membranes

The mucous membranes are continuous with the skin. They line body passages such as the digestive, respiratory, urinary, and reproductive systems. The conjunctiva of the eye is also lined with mucous membrane. Goblet cells in the mucous membranes secrete *mucus*, a slimy substance that keeps the membranes soft and moist.

Hair

A hair is a thread of keratin. Each hair is formed from cells at the base of a single follicle. Although hair covers the entire body, its amount, distribution, color, and texture vary considerably among men and women, infants and adults, and racial groups.

Besides contributing to a person's unique appearance, hair helps to prevent heat loss. As heat escapes from the skin, it becomes trapped in the air between and among the hairs. Body heat can be further maintained by the contraction of small muscles around the hair follicle, commonly described as "goose bumps."

Sebaceous glands located within the hair follicle release sebum, which is oily. The oily secretion adds weight to the shafts of hair, causing them to flatten against the skull. Oily hair further attracts dust and debris as it accumulates.

The texture, elasticity, and porosity of hair are inherited characteristics that are influenced by the amount of keratin and sebum that is produced. To alter the basic structure that has been genetically inherited, some people use chemicals to curl, relax, or lubricate their hair.

Nails

Fingernails and toenails are also made of keratin, which, in concentrated amounts, gives them their tough texture. Fingernails and toenails obviously provide some measure of protection to the tips of fingers and toes.

Normal nails are thin, pink, and smooth. The free margin ordinarily extends from the end of each finger or toe, and the skin around the nails is intact. Changes in the shape, color, texture, thickness, and integrity of the nails provide evidence of local injury or infection and even systemic diseases (see Chap. 12, section on Fingernails and Toenails).

Teeth

Teeth, the enamel of which is a keratin structure, are present beneath the gums at birth. The exposed portion of each tooth is referred to as the *crown* and the portion within the gum is the *root* (Fig. 16-2).

The teeth begin to erupt at about 6 months of age and continue to do so for 2 or 2½ more years. As the jaw grows, the *deciduous teeth*, or baby teeth, are replaced by *permanent teeth*. Adults have 28 to 32 permanent teeth, depending on whether the third molars, so-called "wisdom teeth," are present.

Healthy teeth are firmly fixed within the gums. Their alignment, which is related to jaw structure, is usually a result of heredity. Although the teeth are white originally, they may become discolored from drugs like tetracycline antibiotics, chronic consumption of coffee or tea, and tobacco use.

The integrity of the teeth largely depends on a person's oral hygiene practices, diet, and general health. Saliva, which moistens food and begins its digestive processes, tends to keep the teeth clean and inhibits bacterial growth. However the accumulation of food debris, especially sugar, and **plaque**, composed of mucin and other gritty substances in saliva, supports the growth of mouth bacteria. The combination of sugar, plaque, and bacteria may eventually erode the tooth enamel, causing **caries**, or dental cavities (Fig. 16-3).

Hardened plaque, known as **tartar**, is more difficult to remove and may lead to **gingivitis**, or inflammation of the gums. The pockets of gum inflammation may promote bacterial growth well into the tooth-supporting structures and jaw bone, resulting in **periodontal disease**.

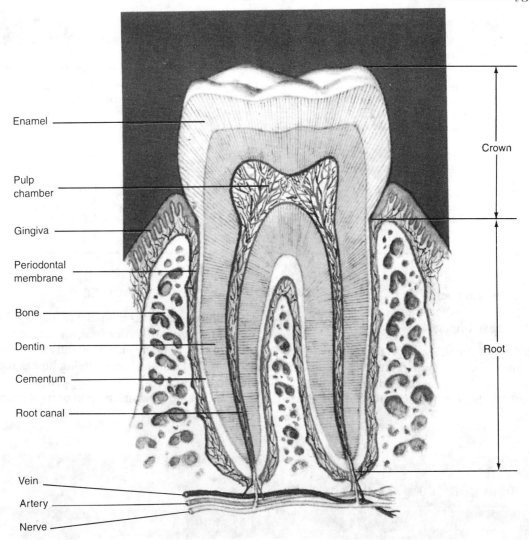

FIGURE 16-2
Cross-section of a tooth. (Cohen B: Medical Terminology: An Illustrated Guide, p 165. Philadelphia, JB Lippincott)

Because the teeth are prone to decay and because the integument contains many types of secretory glands that produce odors and attract debris, hygiene measures are beneficial for maintaining personal cleanliness and healthy structures of the integument.

FIGURE 16-3
Good oral hygiene breaks the chain of factors that contribute to cavity formation.

HYGIENE PRACTICES

Although there may be wide variations, most Americans include bathing, shaving, toothbrushing, shampooing, and nail care among their hygiene practices.

Bathing

Bathing is a hygiene practice in which soap and water are used to remove sweat, oil, dirt, and microorganisms from the skin. Although restoring cleanliness is the primary objective for bathing, there are several other benefits, such as the following:

*   Eliminating body odor
*   Reducing the potential for infection

TABLE 16-2. *Therapeutic Baths*

Type	Description	Purpose
Sitz bath	Immersion of the buttocks and perineum in a small basin of continuously circulating water	Removes blood, serum, stool or urine Reduces local swelling Relieves discomfort (see Chap. 28)
Sponge bath	Applications of tepid water or water and alcohol to the skin	Reduces a fever (see Chap. 11)
Medicated bath	Soaking or immersing in a mixture of water and another substance like baking soda (sodium bicarbonate), oatmeal, or cornstarch	Relieves itching or a rash
Whirlpool bath	Warm water that is continuously agitated within a tub or tank	Improves circulation Increases joint mobility Relieves discomfort Removes dead tissue

- Stimulating circulation
- Providing a refreshed and relaxed feeling
- Improving self-image

In addition to bathing for hygiene purposes, there are other types of therapeutic baths that may be administered (Table 16-2). In general, most bathing is done in a tub or shower, at a sink, or administered at the bedside.

TUB BATH OR SHOWER

As long as the risks to safety are negligible and there are no other contraindications, the nurse may encourage patients to bathe independently in a tub or shower (Skill 16-1). Hospitals and nursing homes usually have bathing facilities that are equipped with a variety of rails and handles, which help to promote patient safety (Fig. 16-4).

SKILL 16-1
Providing a Tub Bath or Shower

Suggested Action	Reason for Action
Assessment	
Check the Kardex or nursing care plan for hygiene directives.	Ensures continuity of care
Assess the patient's level of consciousness, orientation, strength, and mobility.	Provides data for evaluating the patient's ability to carry out hygiene practices independently
Check for gauze dressings, plaster cast, or electrical or battery-operated equipment.	Contraindicates taking a tub bath or shower
Determine if and when any laboratory or diagnostic procedures are scheduled.	Aids in time management
Check the occupancy and cleanliness of the tub or shower.	Helps in organizing the plan for care
Planning	
Clean the tub or shower if it appears to need it.	Reduces the potential for spreading micro-organisms
Consult with the patient about a convenient time for tending to hygiene needs.	Promotes cooperation between the patient and nurse
Assemble supplies: floor mat, towels, face cloth, soap, clean pajamas or gown.	Demonstrates organization and efficient time management

(continued)

SKILL 16-1
Providing a Tub Bath or Shower (Continued)

Suggested Action	Reason for Action
Implementation	
Escort the patient to the shower or bathing room.	Shows concern for the patient's safety
Demonstrate how to operate the water faucet and drain.	Ensures the patient's safety and comfort
If the patient cannot operate the water faucet, fill the tub approximately half-full with water between 105°F to 110°F (40°C–43°C), or adjust the shower to a similar temperature.	Demonstrates concern for the patient's safety and comfort
Place a DO NOT DISTURB or IN USE sign on the outer door.	Ensures privacy
Help the patient into the tub or shower if assistance is needed; this may be done by: • Placing a chair next to the tub • Having the patient swing his or her feet over the edge of the tub • Leaning forward, grabbing a support bar, and raising the buttocks and body until they can be lowered within the tub	Reduces the risk of falling
Have the patient sit on a stool or seat within the tub or shower, if the patient will have difficulty exiting from the tub or may become weak while bathing.	Ensures safety
Show the patient how to summon help.	Promotes safety
Stay close at hand.	Ensures proximity in case there is a need to assist the patient
Check on the patient at frequent intervals by knocking at the door and waiting for a response.	Shows respect for privacy yet concern for safety
Escort the patient back to his or her room after the bath or shower is finished.	Demonstrates concern for safety and welfare
Clean the tub or shower with an antibacterial agent and dispose of the soiled linen in its designated location.	Reduces the spread of microorganisms and demonstrates a conscientious concern for the next person who will use the tub or shower
Remove the IN USE sign from the door.	Indicates that the bathing room is unoccupied

Evaluation
• Patient is clean
• Patient remains uninjured

Document
• Date and time
• Tub bath or shower

*Sample Documentation**

Date and Time   Tub bath taken independently. _____ **Signature, Title**

* Routine hygiene measures usually are documented on a checklist, but for teaching purposes an example of narrative charting has been provided.

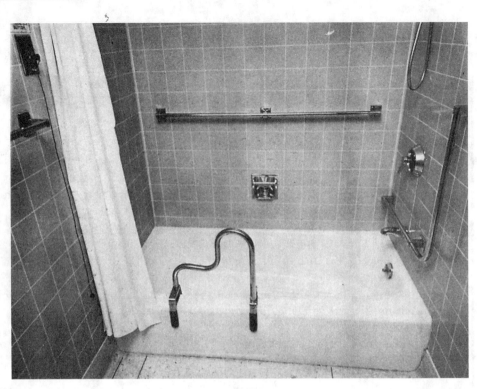

FIGURE 16-4
Tub and shower equipped for patient safety.

PARTIAL BATH

A daily bath or shower is not always necessary. In fact, for older adults who do not perspire as much as younger adults and who are prone to dry skin, frequent washing with soap may further deplete the oil from their skin. Therefore, there may be certain instances when partial bathing may be appropriate.

A **partial bath** consists of washing those areas of the body that are subject to the greatest soiling or sources of body odor, such as the face, hands, and axillae. Partial bathing may be done at a sink or with a basin at the bedside.

There may be situations in which just the *perineum*, the area around the genitals and rectum are bathed.

Perineal Care

Perineal care, or peri-care, refers to techniques used for cleansing the perineum (Skill 16-2). Perineal care (text continues on page 310)

SKILL 16-2
Administering Perineal Care

Suggested Action	Reason for Action
Assessment Inspect the genital and rectal areas of the patient.	Provides data for determining if perineal care is necessary
Planning Wash your hands.	Reduces the spread of microorganisms
Gather gloves, soap, water, and clean cloths or antiseptic wipes or a container of cleansing solution in a squeeze bottle, and several towels or absorptive pads.	Provides a means of removing debris and micro-organisms
Explain the procedure to the patient.	Reduces anxiety and promotes cooperation
Pull the privacy curtain.	Demonstrates respect for modesty

(continued)

SKILL 16-2
Administering Perineal Care (Continued)

Suggested Action	Reason for Action
Place the patient in a dorsal recumbent position (see Chap. 13) and cover with a bath blanket.	Provides access to the perineum

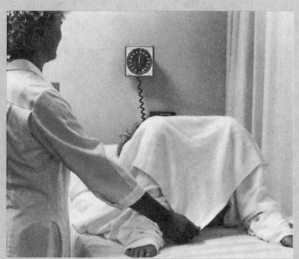

Positioning and draping the patient. (Courtesy of Ken Timby.)

Suggested Action	Reason for Action
Fanfold the top linen to the foot of the bed.	Keeps upper linen clean and dry
For a female patient, place a towel beneath the buttocks or place the patient on a bedpan; for a male patient, place a towel under the penis in addition to the towel beneath the buttocks.	Aids absorption of liquid that may drip downward during cleansing

Implementation

Suggested Action	Reason for Action
Bend the female patient's knees and spread the legs.	Exposes area for cleansing
Put on gloves.	Prevents contact with blood, secretions, or excretions

(continued)

SKILL 16-2
Administering Perineal Care (Continued)

Suggested Action	Reason for Action
Separate the folds of the labia on a female patient and wash from the pubic area toward the anus.	Cleans toward more soiled areas of the body
Never go back over an area that has already been cleansed.	Prevents reintroducing sources of microorganisms into previously cleaned areas

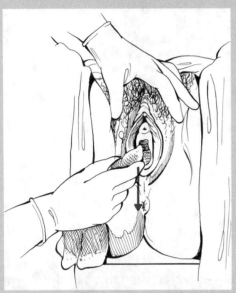

Cleansing the labia.

| Use a clean area of the cloth or a separate antiseptic wipe for each stroke. | Avoids resoiling areas that have already been cleaned |
| Squeeze the solution container starting at the upper areas of the labia downward toward the anus. | Ensures that solution will drain toward more soiled areas of the body; prevents reintroducing sources of microorganisms into previously cleaned areas |

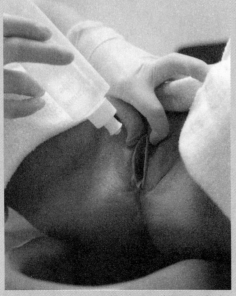

Rinsing the perineum. (Courtesy of Ken Timby.)

(continued)

SKILL 16-2
Administering Perineal Care (Continued)

Suggested Action	Reason for Action
For male patients, grasp the penis and retract the foreskin if the patient is uncircumcised.	Facilitates removing debris and secretions that may be trapped beneath the skin fold
Clean the tip of the penis using circular motions.	Keeps the urethral opening clean
Never go back over an area that has already been cleansed.	

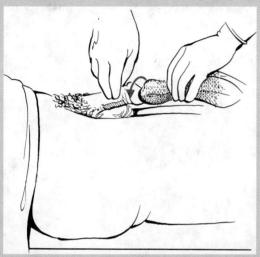

Cleansing the glans penis.

Replace the foreskin.	Prevents trauma
Wash the shaft of the penis toward the scrotum.	Keeps the urethral opening clean

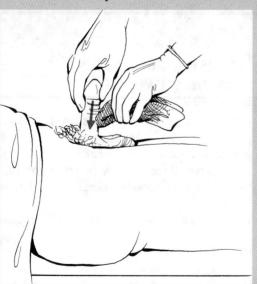

Cleansing the shaft of the penis.

Spread the male patient's legs and wash the scrotum.	Removes debris where it may be trapped and harbor microorganisms
Pat the skin dry with a towel.	Removes excess moisture

(continued)

SKILL 16-2
Administering Perineal Care (Continued)

Suggested Action	Reason for Action
Turn the patient to the side and wash from the perineum toward the anus.	Cleans more soiled areas of the body
Rinse and pat the skin dry.	Prevents skin irritation from soap residue and retained moisture
Remove towels and recover with bed linen.	Ensures comfort and maintains dignity
Deposit wet cloths, soiled wipes, and towels in an appropriate container.	Controls the spread of microorganisms
Empty and rinse the bedpan.	Controls the spread of microorganisms
Remove gloves and wash your hands again.	Reduces the spread of microorganisms
Attend to the comfort and safety of the patient.	Demonstrates concern for the patient's welfare

Evaluation
- Genital, perineum, and rectal areas are clean and dry
- Cleansing has been from lesser to more soiled areas of the body.
- There has been no direct contact with drainage, secretions, or excretions
- Soiled articles have been properly disposed

Document
- Date and time
- Care provided
- Description of drainage and tissue

Sample Documentation

Date and Time	Peri-care provided to remove moderate amount of bloody drainage coming from vagina. Perineal tissue is intact. _____**Signature, Title**

may be necessary after a vaginal delivery or gynecologic or rectal surgery so that the impaired skin is kept as clean as possible. It may also be appropriate whenever male or female patients have bloody drainage, urine, or stool that collects in this area of the body.

Two principles guide the provision of perineal care: (1) preventing direct contact between the nurse and the secretions or excretions that may be present, and (2) cleansing in such a manner as to remove secretions and excretions from less soiled to more soiled areas. Following these principles helps prevent the transfer of infectious microorganisms to the nurse and uncontaminated areas within the patient.

BED BATH

Patients who cannot take a tub bath or shower independently may be given a bed bath. A **bed bath** consists of washing the patient from a basin of water at the bedside. The patient may actively assist with some aspects of the bed bath or the nurse may wash the patient completely (Skill 16-3).

NURSING GUIDELINES FOR BATHING PATIENTS

- Ask each patient if he or she uses special soap, lotion, or other hygiene products.
  Rationale: Individualizes care
- Wear gloves if there is any potential for direct contact with blood, bloody drainage, or other body fluid.
  Rationale: Reduces the potential for acquiring an infection
- Keep the patient covered during the bath.
  Rationale: Demonstrates respect for modesty
- Wash cleaner areas of the body first and dirtier areas last.
  Rationale: Reduces the spread of microorganisms
- Encourage the patient to participate at whatever level is appropriate.
  Rationale: Promotes independence and self-esteem

- Monitor the patient's tolerance of activity.
  Rationale: Indicates if the activity is too strenuous and needs to be terminated and continued later
- Inspect the body as it is being washed.
  Rationale: Provides an excellent opportunity for physical assessment
- Communicate with the patient and use the opportunity to do informal health teaching.
  Rationale: Demonstrates respect for the patient as a person rather than an object being washed; promotes health
- Wash one part of the body at a time.
  Rationale: Prevents chilling

- Place a towel under the part of the body being washed.
  Rationale: Absorbs moisture
- Use firm but gentle strokes.
  Rationale: Avoids friction that may damage the skin
- Wash and dry well between folds of skin.
  Rationale: Removes debris and microorganisms where they are apt to breed
- Keep the washcloth wet, but not so wet that it drips.
  Rationale: Demonstrates concern for the patient's comfort

(text continues on page 315)

SKILL 16-3
Giving a Bed Bath

Suggested Action	Reason for Action
Assessment	
Check the Kardex or nursing care plan for hygiene directives.	Ensures continuity of care
Inspect the skin for signs of dryness and presence of drainage or secretions.	Provides data for determining if a complete or partial bath is appropriate
Planning	
Consult with the patient as to a convenient time for tending to hygiene needs.	Promotes cooperation between the patient and nurse
Assemble supplies: bath blanket, towels, face cloths, soap, wash basin, clean pajamas or gown, clean bed linen, other hygiene articles such as deodorant or antiperspirant, and a razor for men.	Demonstrates organization and efficient time management
Implementation	
Wash your hands.	Reduces the spread of microorganisms.
Pull the privacy curtain.	Demonstrates respect for modesty
Raise the bed to an appropriate height.	Reduces muscle strain on the back when providing care
Remove extra pillows or positioning devices and place the patient on his or her back.	Prepares the patient for washing the anterior body surface
Cover the patient with a bath blanket.	Shows respect for the patient's modesty and provides warmth
Remove the patient's gown.	Facilitates washing the patient
Fanfold the top linen to the bottom of the bed or fold it and lay it on a chair.	Keeps linen, which may be reused, clean
If linen is too soiled to be reused, place it in a laundry hamper.	Reduces the spread of microorganisms
Prevent the linen from contacting your uniform.	Reduces the spread of microorganisms
Fill a basin with 105°F–110°F (40°C–43°C) water and place the basin on the overbed table.	Provides comfortably warm water for bathing in easy access

(continued)

SKILL 16-3
Giving a Bed Bath *(Continued)*

Suggested Action	Reason for Action
Wet the wash cloth and fold it to fashion a mitt.	Keeps water from dripping from the margins of the cloth

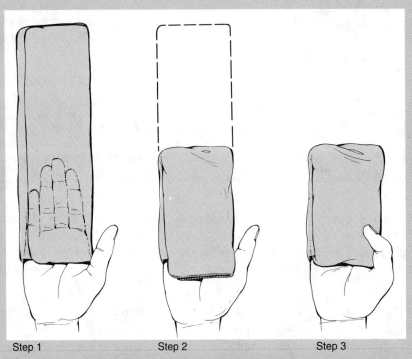

Making a mitt. Step 1   Step 2   Step 3

Suggested Action	Reason for Action
Wipe each eye from the nose toward the ear with a separate corner of the mitt.	Prevents getting soap in the patient's eyes

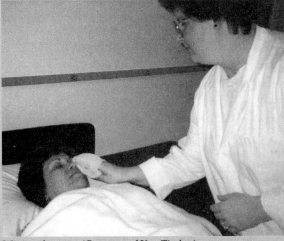

Wiping the eyes. (Courtesy of Ken Timby.)

Suggested Action	Reason for Action
Lather the wet washcloth with soap and finish washing the face.	Soap removes oil, sweat, and microorganisms

(continued)

Suggested Action	Reason for Action
Rinse the washcloth and remove soapy residue, then dry well.	Prevents drying the skin
Bathe each of the patient's arms separately; the axillae may be included now or when the chest is washed.	Cleanses soiled material and keeps the patient from becoming too chilled

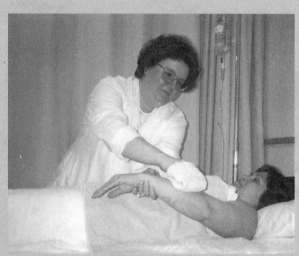

Washing the arm. (Courtesy of Ken Timby.)

Offer to apply deodorant or an antiperspirant after the axillae have been washed.	Demonstrates respect for the patient's usual hygiene practices; reduces perspiration and body odor
Place each hand in the basin of water as it is washed.	Facilitates more thorough washing than just using the washcloth

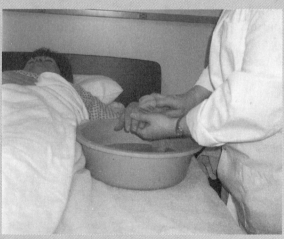

Washing a hand. (Courtesy of Ken Timby.)

Discard and replace the water in the wash basin; rinse the washcloth well or replace it with a clean one.	Eliminates debris, microorganisms, and soap residue, and increases the warmth of the water in preparation for washing cleaner areas of the body

(continued)

Suggested Action	Reason for Action
Wash the chest, abdomen, each leg, and the feet, following the steps described for the upper body.	Follows the principle of washing from cleaner to more soiled areas

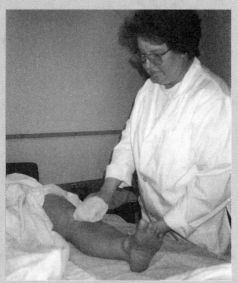

Washing a leg. (Courtesy of Ken Timby.)

Suggested Action	Reason for Action
Help the patient onto his or her side.	Repositions the patient so the posterior of the body can be bathed
Change the water and bathe the patient's back.	Washing begins at cleaner area on the posterior aspect of the body
Offer to apply lotion and provide a back rub (see Chap. 18).	Improves circulation and relaxes the patient
Don gloves and wash the buttocks, genitals, and anus last.	Reduces the potential for contact with lesions or drainage that may contain infectious microorganisms
Discard the water and wipe the basin dry.	Controls the growth and spread of microorganisms
Remove your gloves and assist the patient with donning a fresh gown.	Restores comfort and modesty

Evaluation
- Patient is completely bathed
- No discomfort or intolerance of activity has been noted

Document
- Date and time
- Type and extent of hygiene
- Response of the patient
- Assessment findings observed during bath

*Sample Documentation**

Date and Time   Complete bed bath given. Able to wash face and genitals independently. Skin is intact. No dyspnea noted during bath. _____**Signature, Title**

* Routine hygiene measures usually are documented on a checklist, but for teaching purposes an example of narrative charting has been used.

- Wash areas that are more soiled, like the anus, last.
  Rationale: Prevents transferring microorganisms to cleaner areas of the body
- Remove all soapy residue.
  Rationale: Prevents drying the skin and itching
- Dry the skin after it has been rinsed.
  Rationale: Prevents chilling
- Replace the water as it cools.
  Rationale: Shows concern for the patient's comfort
- Apply an emollient lotion to the skin after bathing.
  Rationale: Restores lubrication to the skin

There are two variations of the bed bath that may be implemented in some health agencies: the towel bath or bag bath.

Towel Bath

A **towel bath** is one in which a single large towel measuring 3 feet × 7½ feet or a bath sheet is used to cover and wash a patient. No basin or soap is used. The towel is prefolded and moistened with approximately ½ gallon (2 L) of 115°F to 120°F (46.1°C–48.8°C) water and 1 ounce (30 mL) of nonrinsable liquid cleanser such as Septi-Soft or Sproam.

After covering the patient (Fig. 16-5), a separate section is used to wipe each part of the body, beginning at the feet and moving upward toward the face. The soiled areas of the towel are folded to the inside as each area is bathed and the skin is allowed to air dry for 2 to 3 seconds. A dry bath blanket or sheet is pulled up to cover the bathed areas.

Once the front of the body has been washed, the patient is positioned on his or her side and the procedure is repeated. The towel is unfolded in such a manner that the clean surface covers the patient. The back is bathed followed by the buttocks. When the towel bath is complete the bed linen is changed.

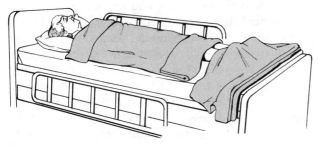

FIGURE 16-5
Giving a towel bath.

DISPLAY 16-1. *Advantages of Towel or Bag Baths*

- Reduces the potential for skin impairment because the nonrinsable cleanser lubricates rather than dries the skin
- Prevents the transmission of microorganisms that may be growing in wash basins
- Reduces the spread of microorganisms from one part of the body to another because separate cloths or regions of the towel are used
- Preserves the integrity of the skin because friction is not used while drying the skin
- Promotes self-care among patients who may lack the strength or dexterity to wet, wring, and lather a washcloth
- Saves time compared to conventional bathing
- Promotes comfort because the moist towel or cloths are used so quickly they are warmer when applied

Bag Bath

A **bag bath** gets its name from the fact that 8 to 10 face cloths are placed in a large plastic bag. The face cloths are moistened with 1 gallon (4 L) of water and 2 to 4 ounces (60–120 mL) of nonrinsable cleanser. The entire bag is microwaved just before being used or the bag is microwaved and then placed in an insulated container to maintain its heat. At the bedside a separate face cloth is used to wash each part of the body. Air drying circumvents the need for a towel.

Display 16-1 lists some of the advantages of towel and bag baths.

Shaving

Shaving involves removing unwanted body hair. In the United States, it is common for men to shave their face daily and for women to shave their axillae and legs on a regular basis. There may be personal or cultural differences, however, that must be respected. Therefore, it is always appropriate to ask each patient about their preferences before assuming otherwise.

Shaving is accomplished by using an electric or safety razor; there may be some contraindications to using a safety razor (Display 16-2). If contraindications exist, use of an electric or battery-operated razor may be an appropriate substitute. When patients are too ill or unable to shave, the nurse may assume responsibility for this hygiene practice.

DISPLAY 16-2. *Contraindications to Using a Safety Razor*

Use of a safety razor may be contraindicated for those patients:

- Receiving anticoagulants (drugs that interfere with clotting)
- Receiving thrombolytic agents (drugs that dissolve blood clots)
- Taking high doses of aspirin
- With blood disorders like hemophilia
- With liver disease who have impaired clotting
- With rashes or elevated or inflamed skin lesions about the face
- Who are suicidal

NURSING GUIDELINES FOR SHAVING PATIENTS

- Prepare a basin of warm water, soap, face cloth, and towel.
  Rationale: Aids in wetting, rinsing, and lathering the face
- Wash the skin with warm, soapy water.
  Rationale: Removes oil, which helps to raise the shafts of hair
- Lather the skin with soap or shaving cream.

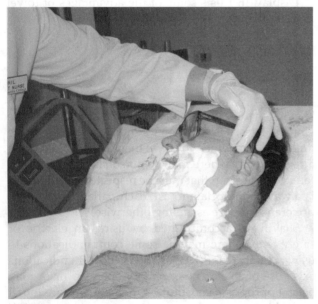

FIGURE 16-6
Face shaving. (Courtesy of Ken Timby.)

Rationale: Reduces the surface tension as the razor is pulled across the skin
- Start at the upper areas of the face or other area of the body that requires shaving and work downward (Fig. 16-6).
  Rationale: Provides more control of the razor
- Pull the skin taut in the area about to be shaved.
  Rationale: Evens the level of the skin
- Pull the razor in the direction of hair growth.
  Rationale: Reduces the potential for irritating the skin
- Use short strokes.
  Rationale: Provides more control of the razor
- Rinse the razor after each stroke or as hair accumulates.
  Rationale: Keeps the cutting edge of the razor clean
- Rinse the soap lather from the skin.
  Rationale: Reduces the potential for drying the skin
- Apply direct pressure to areas that seem to bleed or apply alum sulfate (styptic pencil) at the site of bleeding.
  Rationale: Helps to promote clotting
- Apply after-shave lotion, cologne, or cream to the shaved area if the patient desires it.
  Rationale: Reduces and retards microbial growth within the tiny microabrasions caused by the razor (alcohol in lotions and cologne); restores oil to the skin (creams)

Oral Hygiene

Oral hygiene refers to those practices used to clean the mouth, especially the teeth. Oral hygiene usually includes brushing and flossing the teeth or caring for dentures or bridges.

TOOTHBRUSHING AND FLOSSING

Patients who are alert and physically capable can usually attend to their own oral hygiene at a bathroom sink. For patients who are confined to bed, the nurse assembles the items that are needed such as a toothbrush, toothpaste, a glass of water, emesis basin, and floss.

Most dentists recommend using a soft-bristled toothbrush and toothpaste. Flossing removes plaque and food debris from the surfaces of teeth that the brush may not reach. The choice of unwaxed or waxed floss is a personal one. Waxed floss is thicker than unwaxed and may be difficult to insert between teeth that are very close together. Unwaxed floss frays somewhat more quickly.

Although conscientious oral hygiene does not totally prevent dental problems, it reduces their potential. Therefore, it is appropriate to teach patients measures for maintaining the structure and integrity of their natural teeth.

ORAL CARE FOR UNCONSCIOUS PATIENTS

Oral hygiene is not neglected just because a patient is unconscious. In fact, because unconscious patients are not salivating in response to seeing, smelling, and eating food, they need oral care even more frequently than conscious patients. **Sordes**, which are dried crusts containing mucus, microorganisms, and epithelial cells shed from the mucous membrane, are common on the lips and teeth of unconscious patients.

Toothbrushing is the preferred technique for providing oral hygiene for unconscious patients (Skill 16-4). However, patients who are not alert are at risk for

SKILL 16-4
Giving Oral Care to Unconscious Patients

Suggested Action	Reason for Action
Assessment	
Check the nursing care plan for the frequency for providing oral hygiene.	Maintains continuity of care
Inspect the patient's mouth.	Helps determine equipment and supplies that will be used
Look for oral hygiene supplies that may already be at the patient's bedside.	Controls costs
Planning	
Arrange to brush the patient's teeth once per shift and provide additional oral care at least every 2 hours.	Promotes a schedule for removing plaque and microorganisms, moistening, and refreshing the mouth
Assemble the following equipment: toothbrush, toothpaste, suction catheter, water, bulb syringe, padded tongue blade, emesis basin, towel or absorbent pad, and gloves. Some agencies may stock a toothbrushing device that is connected directly to a suction catheter.	Promotes organization and efficient time management

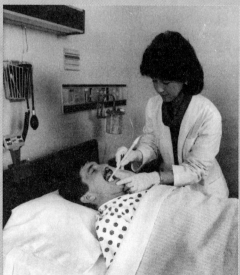

Special toothbrush with suction attachment (Courtesy of Trademark Medical, Fenton, MO.)

(continued)

SKILL 16-4
Giving Oral Care to Unconscious Patients (Continued)

Suggested Action	Reason for Action
Implementation	
Explain what you are about to do to the patient.	Reduces anxiety in the event that the patient has the cognitive capacity to understand
Position the patient on his or her side with the head slightly lowered.	Prevents liquids from draining into the airway
Place a towel beneath the head.	Absorbs liquids
Connect a Yankeur suction tip or suction catheter to a portable or wall-mounted suction source.	Promotes safety
Spread toothpaste over a moistened toothbrush.	Prepares the toothbrush for use
Don gloves.	Prevents direct contact with blood or micro-organisms in the mouth
Use a tongue blade to open the mouth and separate the teeth.	Serves as a safe substitute for the nurse's fingers

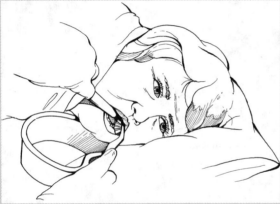

Brushing with tongue blade separating teeth.

Brush all the surfaces of the teeth with the toothbrush.	Removes plaque and microorganisms
Instill water and suction the mouth.	Removes debris and reduces the potential for aspiration

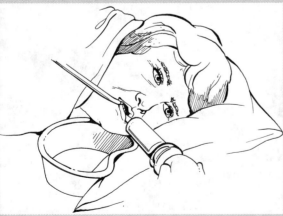

Rinsing and suctioning.

(continued)

SKILL 16-4
Giving Oral Care to Unconscious Patients *(Continued)*

Suggested Action	Reason for Action
Clean and store oral hygiene supplies.	Restores cleanliness and order to the patient environment
Remove wet towel and gloves; restore patient to a position of comfort and safety.	Demonstrates concern for the patient's dignity and welfare

Evaluation
- The teeth are clean
- The oral mucosa is smooth, pink, moist, and intact
- Safety has been maintained

Document
- Date and time
- Assessment findings, if significant
- Type of oral care
- Unusual events, like choking, if they occurred and nursing action that was taken
- Outcome of any nursing action

*Sample Documentation**

Date and Time   Teeth brushed and mouth rinsed. Liquid suctioned from the mouth using a Yankeur suction catheter. No choking during oral care. Lung sounds are clear bilaterally. _____**Signature, Title**

* Routine hygiene measures usually are documented on a checklist, but for teaching purposes an example of narrative charting has been used.

aspirating (inhaling) saliva and liquid oral hygiene products into their lungs. Aspirated liquids predisposes patients to pneumonia. Therefore, the nurse uses special precautions to avoid getting fluid in the patient's airway.

In addition to toothbrushing, the mouth may be moistened and refreshed with oral swabs. Various substances also may be used for oral hygiene depending on the circumstances and assessment findings of each patient (Table 16-3).

DENTURE CARE

Dentures are artificial teeth that substitute for a person's lower or upper set of teeth, or both. A **bridge** is a dental appliance that replaces one or several teeth.

TABLE 16-3. *Optional Substances for Oral Care*

Substance	Use
Antiseptic mouthwash diluted with water	Reduces bacterial growth within the mouth; freshens breath
Equal parts of baking soda and table salt in warm water, or baking soda mixed with normal saline	Removes accumulated secretions
One part hydrogen peroxide to 10 parts of water	Releases oxygen and loosens dry sticky particles; prolonged use may damage tooth enamel
Milk of magnesia	Reduces oral acidity; dissolves plaque, increases flow of saliva, and soothes oral lesions
Lemon and glycerin swabs	Increases salivation and refreshes the mouth; glycerin may absorb water from the lips and cause them to become dry and cracked if used for more than several days
Petroleum jelly	Lubricates lips

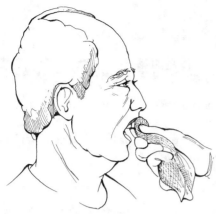

FIGURE 16-7
Removing an upper denture.

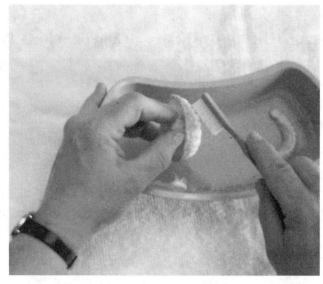

FIGURE 16-8
Cleaning dentures. (Courtesy of Ken Timby.)

A bridge may be fixed permanently to other natural teeth so that it cannot be removed, or it may be fastened with a clasp that allows it to be detached from the mouth.

For patients who are unable to remove their own dentures, the nurse dons gloves and uses a dry gauze square or clean face cloth to grasp and free the denture from the mouth (Fig. 16-7). Dentures and removable bridges are cleaned with a toothbrush, toothpaste, and cold or tepid water (Fig. 16-8). Care is taken to hold dentures over a plastic basin or towel so that they do not break if dropped.

Dentists recommend that dentures and bridges re-main in place except while they are being cleaned. Keeping dentures and bridges out for long periods of time permits the gum lines to change, affecting the fit. If the dentures or bridge are removed during the night, they are stored in a disposable, covered cup. Plain water is most often used to cover dentures when they are not in the mouth, but some may wish to add mouth-wash or denture cleaner to the water.

 PATIENT TEACHING FOR REDUCING DENTAL DISEASE AND INJURIES

Teach the patient or family to do the following:

- Brush and floss the teeth as soon as possi-ble after each meal using the following techniques:

  Moisten the toothbrush and apply tooth-paste.
  Hold the toothbrush at a 45° angle to the teeth.
  Brush the front and back of all the teeth from the gum line toward the crown of the teeth using circular motions.

Wrap floss around the middle fingers of each hand.

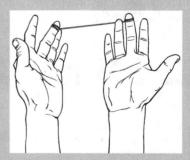

Wrapping floss. (Adapted from How to Brush and Floss. Chicago, American Academy of Periodontology, 1989)

Slide the floss between two teeth until it is next to the gum.
Move the floss back and forth.

(continued)

⬡ **PATIENT TEACHING FOR REDUCING DENTAL DISEASE AND INJURIES** *(Continued)*

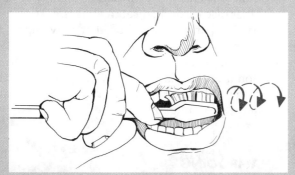

Brushing toward the crown of the teeth. (Adapted from How to Brush and Floss. Chicago, American Academy of Periodontology, 1989)

Brush back and forth over the chewing surfaces of the molars.

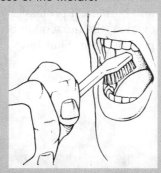

Brushing chewing surfaces. (Adapted from How to Brush and Floss. Chicago, American Academy of Periodontology, 1989)

Rinse the mouth periodically to flush loosened debris.

- Use a battery-operated oral irrigating device that uses pulsating jets of water to flush debris from teeth, bridges, or braces.
- Reduce consumption of sweets, such as soft drinks containing sugar, candy, gum that contains fructose or another form of sugar, pastries, and sweet desserts.
- Increase consumption of raw fruit, like apples, and vegetables, like carrots, that naturally remove plaque and other food as they are chewed.
- Consume three servings of dairy products per day as a dietary source for calcium.

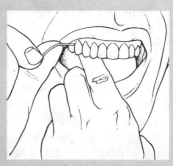

About 1/2 inch of approximately 18 inches of wrapped floss is used at any one time. (Adapted from How to Brush and Floss. Chicago, American Academy of Periodontology, 1989)

Repeat flossing with unwrapped sections of the floss until all the teeth have been flossed, including the outer surface of the last molar.

- Use a tartar control toothpaste or rinse containing fluoride.
- If brushing is impossible rinse the mouth with water after eating.
- If antacids are used, select those with added calcium.
- Select frozen orange juice concentrate that has been fortified with calcium.
- Do not use the teeth to open packages or containers.
- Use scissors rather than the teeth to cut thread.
- Do not chew ice cubes or crushed ice.
- Avoid chewing unpopped or partially popped kernels of popcorn.
- Have dental check-ups at least every 6 months.

Hair Care

Sometimes patients need assistance with grooming or shampooing their hair.

HAIR GROOMING

The following are recommendations for grooming patients' hair:

- Try to use the hairstyle a patient prefers.
- Brush the hair slowly and carefully to avoid damaging the hair.
- Brush the hair to increase circulation and distribution of sebum.
- Use a wide-toothed comb and start at the ends of the hair rather than from the crown downward if the hair is matted or tangled.
- Apply a conditioner or alcohol to loosen tangles.
- Use oil on the hair if it is dry. There are many preparations on the market, but pure castor oil, olive oil, and mineral oil are satisfactory.

- Braid the hair to prevent tangles.
- Provide the patient with a turban or baseball hat, if there is hair loss from cancer therapy or some other disease or medical treatment.
- Avoid hair pins or clips that may injure the scalp.
- Always obtain the patient's or family's permission if the hair is hopelessly tangled and cutting seems to be the best solution for providing adequate grooming.

SHAMPOOING

Hair is washed as often as necessary to keep it clean. A weekly shampoo is sufficient for most people, but shampooing more or less often will not damage the hair.

Long-term health facilities often employ the services of beauticians and barbers. If professional services are unavailable, however, the nurse may be the one who shampoos the patient's hair (Skill 16-5).

SKILL 16-5
Shampooing Hair

Suggested Action	Reason for Action
Assessment	
Inspect the patient for oily and limp hair, or signs of accumulating secretions or lesions on the scalp.	Provides data for determining if shampooing is necessary and what supplies may be appropriate to use
Assess for respiratory symptoms, pain, or other conditions that may increase or contribute to activity intolerance.	Aids in establishing priorities for care
Determine if and when medical treatments or tests are scheduled.	Ensures that hygiene measures will not interrupt therapeutic or diagnostic procedures
Discuss the types of products that are used when shampooing is performed and if they are currently available.	Facilitates individualized care
Planning	
Collaborate with the patient on the time of day that is best for shampooing.	Involves the patient in the decision-making process
Assemble equipment, which may include: shampoo, conditioner, hair oil treatment, towels, water pitcher, shampoo basin or trough.	Promotes organization and efficient time management

(continued)

Suggested Action	Reason for Action

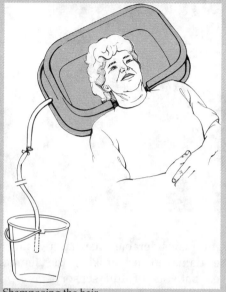
Shampooing the hair.

Implementation

Close the door and pull the privacy curtain.

Remove the pillow and protect the upper area of the bed with towels; cover the patient's chest and shoulders with a towel.

Don gloves if there are any open lesions.

Wet the hair thoroughly and apply shampoo.

Work the shampoo into a lather.

Rinse the hair with water.

Apply conditioner if requested.

Wrap the head and fluff the hair with a dry towel.

Remove and discard gloves when there is no threat of direct contact with blood or secretions.

Comb, braid, or style the hair according to the patient's preference.

Clean and store shampooing supplies.

Reduces the potential for chilling	
Absorbs moisture	
Prevents direct contact with blood or secretions	
Dilutes and distributes the shampoo	
Facilitates cleansing throughout the hair	
Removes oil and shampoo from the hair	
Relaxes the hair and reduces tangles	
Absorbs water and shortens the drying time	
Facilitates hair care	
Promotes patient's self-esteem	
Restores cleanliness and order to the patient environment	

Evaluation

• The hair is clean and dry

Document

• Date and time
• Assessment findings
• Type of care
• Response of the patient

Sample Documentation

Date and Time   Scalp and hair appear oily. Skin is intact. Bed shampoo provided. Hair dried, combed, and styled in braids. Scalp is clean and intact. No evidence of chilling, fatigue, or discomfort during shampoo. States, "I feel so much better."

                                                                      Signature, Title

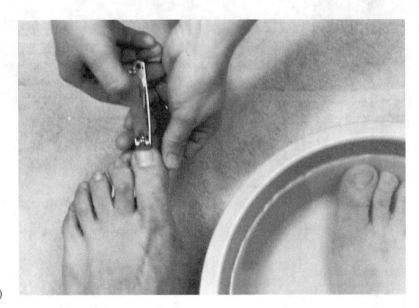

FIGURE 16-9
Foot care. (Courtesy of Ken Timby.)

Nail Care

Nail care involves keeping the fingernails and toenails clean and trimmed. Patients who have diabetes, impaired circulation, or thick nails may need the services of a **podiatrist**, a person with special training in caring for feet. Therefore, it is best to check with the patient's physician before cutting fingernails or toenails.

If there are no contraindications, nails may be cared for in the following manner:

- Soak the hands or feet in warm water to soften the keratin and loosen trapped debris.
- Clean under the nails with a wooden orange stick or other sturdy, but blunt instrument.
- Push *cuticles*, the thin edge of skin at the base of the nail, downward with a soft towel.
- Use a file, emery board, metal clippers, or manicure scissors to shorten long fingernails.
- Trim toenails straight across so as to avoid sharp or jagged points, which may injure the adjacent skin (Fig. 16-9).

To keep the skin and nails soft and supple, lotion or an emollient cream may be applied after bathing and nail care. If foot perspiration is a problem, an antifungal, deodorant powder may be used. Because impaired skin, especially about the feet, is often slow to heal and susceptible to infection, any abnormal assessments are reported immediately. To avoid injuring the feet, it is best to encourage patients to wear sturdy slippers or clean socks and supportive shoes.

VISUAL AND HEARING DEVICES

Visual and hearing devices like eyeglasses and hearing aids improve communication and socialization. Both represent a considerable financial investment. If they become damaged or broken, the temporary loss deprives patients of full sensory perception. It is extremely important, then, to make sure that they are well maintained and safely stored when they are not used.

Although eyeglasses and hearing aids are not body structures, they are worn in close contact to the body for long periods of time. Consequently, they tend to collect secretions, dirt, and debris, which may interfere with their function and use. Therefore, the nurse cares for these devices at the same time that other hygiene measures are provided.

Eyeglasses

Eyeglasses are prescription lenses that are worn within a frame. They enable the wearer to see more clearly. Optical lenses are either glass or plastic. Plastic lenses are considerably lighter in weight, but they are more easily scratched. Glass lenses are more apt to break if dropped. When not being worn, eyeglasses are best placed in a soft case or rested on the frame.

Glass and plastic lenses are cleaned by:

- Holding the eyeglasses at the nose or ear braces
- Running tepid water over both sides of the lenses; hot water may damage plastic lenses
- Washing the lenses with soap or detergent
- Rinsing them with running tap water, and
- Drying them with a clean, soft cloth like a handkerchief

Some people prefer to use commercial glass cleaners, although they are not necessary. However, paper tissues should never be used as a substitute for a soft cloth. Some paper tissues contain wood fibers and pulp that can scratch the lenses.

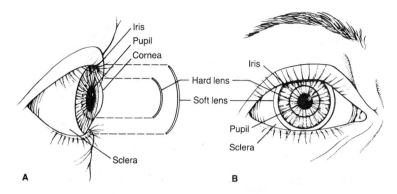

A
B

FIGURE 16-10
Location and size of contact lenses. (*A*) Side view, (*B*) Front view.

Contact Lenses

A contact lens is a small plastic disk that is placed directly on the cornea (Fig. 16-10) for the purpose of improving vision. Some people prefer contact lenses to eyeglasses.

Contact lenses are usually worn in each eye, but some patients who have had cataract surgery on one eye may wear a single contact lens or a single contact lens and eyeglasses. For this reason, the nurse should not assume that a patient who wears eyeglasses does not use a contact lens, and vice versa.

There are several types of contact lenses available. Contact lenses are hard, soft, or gas permeable. All contact lenses, except disposable types that are worn for approximately 1 week and then discarded, require removal for cleaning and eye rest, periodic disinfection, and proper storage. Patients who are not dedicated to following a routine for the care of their contact lenses risk infection, eye abrasion, and permanent damage to the cornea.

When caring for patients who wear contact lenses, it is best to have the patient remove and insert the lens or lenses and care for them according to their established routine. For patients who are no longer able to do so, the nurse consults with the patient's **ophthalmologist**, a medical doctor who treats eye disorders, or **optometrist**, a person who prescribes corrective lenses, about alternatives for promoting adequate vision and safety. Some patients may wish to resume wearing eyeglasses temporarily, use a magnifying glass, or totally do without any visual aid.

Artificial Eyes

An artificial eye is simply a plastic shell that acts as a cosmetic replacement for the natural eye (Fig. 16-11). There is no way to restore vision once the eye has been removed.

The artificial eye needs to be removed and cleaned from time to time. Patients who have an artificial eye usually assume responsibility for its care. If that is not the case, the nurse removes the shell by depressing the lower eyelid until the lid margin is wide enough to allow the artificial eye to slide free. The eye socket is irrigated with water or saline before reinserting the artificial eye.

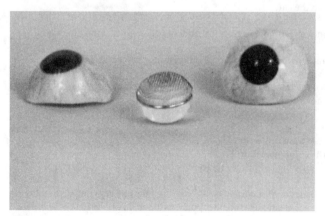

FIGURE 16-11
Front and side views of an artificial eye. The round implant in the center is positioned permanently within the bony orbit from which the natural eye has been removed. Only the cosmetic shell is removed for cleaning. (Courtesy of Ken Timby.)

Hearing Aids

Hearing aids, which are usually worn in or about one or both ears, amplify sound. There are three types of hearing aids: (1) *in-the-ear* devices, which are small, self-contained hearing aids that fit entirely within the patient's ear; (2) *behind-the-ear* devices, consisting of a microphone and amplifier worn behind the ear that delivers sound to a receiver within the ear; and (3) *body aid* devices whose electrical components, enclosed within a case carried somewhere on the body, deliver the sound via a wire connected to an ear mold receiver

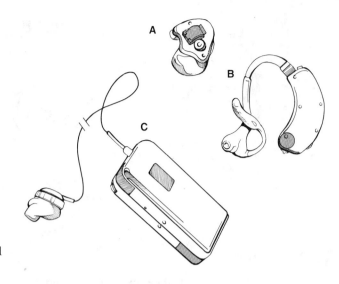

FIGURE 16-12
Types of hearing aids. (*A*) In-the-ear, (*B*) Behind-the-ear, and (*C*) Body aid.

(Fig. 16-12). In-the-ear and behind-the-ear models are most common. Behind-the-ear models can be attached to a person's eyeglass frame. Body aids are used primarily by people who have a severe hearing loss or who are unable to care for a small device (Brinkmann, 1991). All hearing aids are powered by small mercury or zinc batteries that require replacement after 100 to 200 hours of use.

Most patients insert and remove their own hearing aids. However, the nurse may need to assess and troubleshoot problems that develop (Table 16-4). In addition, the following is taught to nursing personnel as well as patients and their families:

- Keep a supply of extra batteries at all times
- Avoid exposing the electrical components to ex-

TABLE 16-4. *Troubleshooting Hearing Aid Problems*

Problem	Possible Causes	Action
Reduced or absent sound	Weak or dead battery	Test and replace battery.
	Incorrect battery position	Match the positive pole of the battery to the positive symbol in the case.
	Cracked tubing leading to the receiver	Repair tubing.
	Broken wire between body aid and receiver	Repair wire.
	Accumulation of cerumen within the ear	Clean the ear.
	Cerumen plugging the receiver	Remove cerumen with an instrument called a wax loop, tip of a pin, or needle on a syringe.
	Ear congestion due to an upper respiratory infection	Consult with the physician about administering a decongestant.
	Damaged electrical components	Have the device inspected by a person who services hearing aids.
Shrill noise, called **feedback**, caused by conditions that return sound to the microphone	Malposition or failure to fully insert the receiver within the ear	Remove and reinsert.
	Kinked receiver tubing	Remove and untwist.
	Excessive volume	Reduce volume control.
	Hearing aid left on while removed from the ear	Turn hearing aid off or replace it in the ear.
Garbled sound	Poor battery contact	Check battery for correct size; make sure the battery compartment is closed; clean metal contact points with an emery board.
	Dirty components	Clean with a soft cloth.
	Debris in the on/off switch	Move the switch back and forth several times.
	Corroded battery	Remove and replace.
	Cracked case	Repair or replace.

treme heat, water, cleaning chemicals, or hair spray

- Wipe the outer surface of a body aid or behind-the-ear case occasionally
- Turn the hearing aid off when not being worn to prolong the life of the battery
- Store the hearing aid in a safe place where it will not fall or become lost

Infrared Listening Devices

Infrared listening devices (IRLDs), which resemble earphones attached to a hand-held receiver, are an alternative to conventional hearing aids. According to Walczak and colleagues (1993), an IRLD converts sound into infrared light and sends it via a wall- or ceiling-mounted receiver to people who are wearing the listening device. The light is then converted back into sound. An advantage of an IRLD, compared to a conventional hearing aid, is that it reduces background noise. Hearing background noise is a common reason people give for not wearing their hearing aids. The disadvantage of IRLDs is that they cannot be used outdoors, in rooms that contain many windows, or rooms that are brightly lit because environmental infrared light jams the signal, causing audio interference. However, IRLDs are being successfully used by hearing-impaired adults who need help in hearing lectures,

television, or live performances. Some geriatric centers are also installing IRLDs in rooms used for social and recreational activities.

NURSING IMPLICATIONS

Patients who require assistance with personal hygiene may have one or more of the nursing diagnoses listed in the accompanying Applicable Nursing Diagnoses.

The accompanying Nursing Care Plan is an example of the care developed for a patient with a nursing diagnosis of Bathing/Hygiene Self-Care Deficit. This diagnosis is defined in the NANDA Taxonomy (1994) as "A state in which the individual experiences an impaired ability to perform or complete bathing/hygiene activities for oneself."

 APPLICABLE NURSING DIAGNOSES

- Bathing/Hygiene Self-Care Deficit
- Dressing/Grooming Self-Care Deficit
- Activity Intolerance
- Risk for Impaired Skin Integrity

NURSING CARE PLAN:
Bathing/Hygiene Self-Care Deficit

Assessment	**Subjective Data** States, "I can't bathe myself and I need help brushing my teeth."
	Objective Data 52-year-old woman admitted for the repair of fractures sustained as a result of falling down the basement stairs of home. Arm cast on right. Right hand is dominant. Uses exposed right thumb and fingers for grasping objects. Right elbow not enclosed within cast and has full range of motion. Left arm in traction and suspension.
Diagnosis	Bathing/Hygiene Self-Care Deficit related to musculoskeletal impairment as manifested by the inability to use hands effectively for performing hygiene independently.
Plan	**Goal** The patient will report feeling clean and refreshed after assistance with daily bathing and mouth care.

(continued)

NURSING CARE PLAN:
Bathing/Hygiene Self-Care Deficit *(Continued)*

Orders: 6/2

1. Bathe in bed after breakfast and before 1000.
2. Use patient's own castile soap.
3. Place small towel in rt. hand for assisting with drying face and chest.
4. Provide a gown with sleeves that fastens with snaps.
5. Apply deodorant and powder to underarms daily.
6. Turn toward the arm in traction for washing back and buttocks.
7. Provide mouth care after each meal as follows:
   - Wrap and tape washcloth around handle of toothbrush so patient can grasp it with fingers and thumb of right hand.
   - Apply toothpaste to toothbrush.
   - Set emesis basin and glass of water with straw on overbed table.

   _____ V. MILLER, RN

Implementation   6/3   0845   Brushed own teeth after breakfast. _____ L. COOK, LPN
(Documentation)   0900   Complete bed bath administered using castile soap. Able to assist with drying upper body. Hair under arms shaved. Deodorant and powder applied in axillae. Skin is pink, warm, and intact. No redness around edges of cast. Able to turn without difficulty to left side for back care. _____ L. COOK, LPN

Evaluation   0930   States, "I feel so much better about seeing my doctor and visitors after I've
(Documentation)   gotten cleaned up in the morning." _____ L. COOK, LPN

 FOCUS ON OLDER ADULTS

- Consider that older adults who neglect their hygiene and grooming may be manifesting a sign of depression.
- Older adults do not need to bathe as frequently as younger adults because they do not perspire as much and because they have a decrease in sebum production.
- Older adults may require assistance with hygiene due to joint changes. Long-handled bath sponges or hand-held shower attachments may help older adults remain independent.
- Older adults are much more receptive to hygiene measures if they are not rushed, chilled, or exposed while naked.
- Nonskid strips on the floor of bath tubs and showers along with strategically placed handles and grab rails help reduce the risk of falls for older adults when bathing.

- Soap is extremely drying to the skin; baby oil or mineral oil can be added to the water when administering a bed bath to an older adult.
- Lotions that contain alcohol are avoided because they tend to aggravate dry skin conditions that are prevalent among older adults.
- If older adults experience pruritus, or itching, their nails are kept short to avoid skin trauma from scratching.
- The skin of older adults is gently patted dry rather than rubbed vigorously with a towel.
- Older adults may have a diminished sense of temperature. They may draw bath water that is so hot it causes superficial burns. Therefore, it is best to check the temperature of the water with the wrist first before letting older adults step into the water.

(continued)

FOCUS ON OLDER ADULTS *(Continued)*

- Increasing oral fluid intake or adding humidity to the air may reduce the manifestations of dry skin.
- Clothing may need to be modified with Velcro closures, front zippers, or oversized buttons and button holes to facilitate an older adult's ability to dress and undress independently.
- Skin and nail problems on the lower extremities may be prevented by encouraging older adults to purchase sturdy shoes and replace or repair them as they become worn.
- It is best to thoroughly inspect the feet of older adult patients because they may have ulcerations of which they are unaware.
- Older adults have common benign skin lesions like *seborrheic keratoses* that appear as tan to black raised areas, commonly about the trunk,

and *senile lentigines*, brown, flat patches on the back of the hands, forearms, and face. However, some skin lesions may be precancerous or cancerous and their etiology should always be identified by a physician.
- Most older adults lose teeth because of periodontal disease.
- Impacted cerumen is often a cause of hearing loss among older adults. This condition may be treated by instilling commercial substances that moisten the cerumen like Debrox (Marion Laboratories, Kansas City, MO), instillations of 0.5 mL of mineral oil twice a day for 2 to 5 days, and irrigations of 3 ounces of 3% hydrogen peroxide mixed with a quart of warm water (Webber-Jones, 1992).

KEY CONCEPTS

- Hygiene refers to practices that promote health through personal cleanliness.
- Hygiene practices that most people perform regularly include bathing, shaving, oral hygiene, hair care, and nail care.
- It may be more appropriate for older adults to take a partial bath rather than a daily tub bath or shower because they do not perspire as much as young adults and soap tends further to dry their skin.
- Some advantages of towel and bag baths are that they: (1) add lubrication to the skin; (2) avoid friction, which preserves the integrity of the skin; (3) reduce the transmission of microorganisms from one part of the body to another; (4) save time; (5) provide more opportunity for self-care; and (6) tend to promote comfort because of the warmth of the liquid.
- Although shaving is a common hygiene practice, the use of a safety razor is contraindicated for patients who have clotting disorders, those receiving anticoagulants and thrombolytics, and those who may be depressed and suicidal.
- For oral hygiene, most dentists recommend using a soft-bristled toothbrush, tartar control toothpaste with fluoride, and waxed or unwaxed dental floss.
- The chief hazard in providing oral hygiene for unconscious patients is that they may aspirate liquid into their lungs. To prevent aspiration, unconscious patients are positioned on their side with their head lower than their body. Oral suction equipment is used to remove liquid from the mouth.

- To prevent damage, dentures are held over a plastic or towel-lined container and cold or tepid water is used.
- Hair tangles can be eliminated by applying hair conditioner, using a wide-toothed comb, and combing from the end of the hair toward the scalp.
- The physician is consulted on the possibility of referring nail care for patients with diabetes or those with poor circulation to a podiatrist.
- During daily hygiene it may be necessary to clean and care for visual or hearing devices such as eyeglasses, contact lenses, an artificial eye, or hearing aid.
- Patients who are unable to insert and care for contact lenses may wish to consider wearing eyeglasses, using a magnifying lens, or doing without.
- People who wear hearing aids may experience sound alterations due to dead or weak batteries, batteries that are not making full contact, corroded batteries, malposition within the ear, excessive volume, impacted cerumen, and dirty or damaged components.
- Infrared listening devices are an alternative to hearing aids. IRLDs convert sound into infrared light and then reconvert the light to sound through a receiver worn within a headset with earphones.

CRITICAL THINKING EXERCISES

- You have been assigned to two patients. One is a 75-year-old woman who is unconscious after a stroke; the other is a 38-year-old male mechanic who is being treated for an ulcer. How will their hygiene differ?

- How would you plan to provide a discussion on oral hygiene to a group of third-graders? What teaching methods might you use?

SUGGESTED READINGS

Brinkmann K. Why can't your patient hear you? RN January 1991;54:46–48.

Eliopoulos C. Gerontological Nursing. 3rd ed. Philadelphia: JB Lippincott, 1993.

Holder L. Hearing aids, handle with care. Nursing April 1982;12:64–67.

King PA, Longman AJ, Pergrin JV. Educating nursing home staff in lower extremity assessment and care. Geriatric Nursing November–December 1991;12:297–299.

Mahoney DF. Cerumen impaction: prevalence and detection in nursing homes. Journal of Gerontological Nursing April 1993;19:23–30.

McGovern M, Kuhn JK. Skin assessment of the elderly client. Journal of Gerontological Nursing April 1992;18:39–43.

NANDA nursing Diagnoses: Definitions and Classification 1994–1995. Philadelphia: North American Nursing Diagnosis Association, 1994.

Ruscin C, Cunningham G, Blaylock A. Foot care protocols for the older client. Geriatric Nursing July–August 1993;14:210–212.

Skewes S. No more bed baths! RN January 1994;57:34–35.

Walczak M, Bernstein AL, Senzer CL, Mohn N. Infrared listening device in a geriatric day center. Journal of Gerontological Nursing August 1993;19:5–9.

Webber-Jones J. Doomed to deafness? American Journal of Nursing November 1992;92:37–39.

Winkley GP, Brown JO, Stone TL. Interventions to improve oral care: the nursing assistant's role. Journal of Gerontological Nursing November 1993;19:47–48.

CHAPTER 17

Sleep and Rest

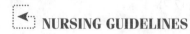

NURSING GUIDELINES

Facilitating Progressive Relaxation

SKILL

Giving a Back Massage

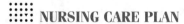

NURSING CARE PLAN

Sleep Pattern Disturbance

Key Terms

Bruxism
Circadian Rhythms
Diurnal
Drug Tolerance
Hypersomnolence
Hypnic Jerks
Hypnotics

Phototherapy
Polysomnography
Progressive Relaxation
Rapid Eye Movement
   Sleep
Rest
Sedatives

Insomnia
Jet Lag
Massage
Melatonin
Narcolepsy
Nocturnal Enuresis
Nocturnal Myoclonus
Nonrapid Eye Movement
   Sleep
Parasomnias
Paradoxical Sleep
Photoperiod

Sleep
Sleep Apnea/Hypopnea
   Syndrome
Sleep Diary
Sleep Latency
Sleep Rituals
Slow-wave Sleep
Somnambulism
Stimulants
Sundown Syndrome
Sunrise Syndrome
Tranquilizers

Learning Objectives

An understanding of the content within this chapter will be evidenced by the student's ability to:

- Differentiate between sleep and rest
- List at least five functions of sleep
- Name the two phases of sleep and describe their differences
- Describe the general trend in sleep requirements as people age
- Name 10 factors that affect sleep
- List four categories of drugs that affect sleep
- Name three tools that are used to assess sleep patterns
- Identify and describe four types of sleep disorders
- Discuss at least five techniques for promoting sleep
- Name two nursing measures that may be implemented to promote relaxation
- Discuss three unique characteristics of sleep among older adults

Sleep is a basic human need characterized as a state of arousable unconsciousness. **Rest** is a waking state during which there is a conscious effort to reduce activity and mental stimulation. Rest usually precedes sleep.

Although sleep requirements vary, alterations in sleep patterns can have serious physical and emotional consequences. This chapter describes the characteristics of sleep, factors that disturb it, and nursing measures for promoting sleep and rest.

FUNCTIONS OF SLEEP

Besides promoting emotional well-being, there is a belief that sleep enhances various physiologic processes. Although the exact mechanisms are not totally understood, the restorative functions of sleep may be inferred from the observable effects of sleep deprivation (Display 17-1).

Sleep, therefore, is thought to play a role in:

- Reducing fatigue
- Stabilizing moods
- Improving blood flow to the brain
- Increasing protein synthesis
- Maintaining disease-fighting mechanisms of the immune system
- Promoting cellular growth and repair
- Improving the capacity for learning and memory storage

SLEEP PHASES

Sleeping is divided into two phases: **nonrapid eye movement** (NREM) **sleep** and **rapid eye movement** (REM) **sleep**. These two phases were named after ob-

serving that there are periods during sleep when eye movements are either subdued or quite energetic.

Nonrapid eye movement sleep is also called **slow-wave sleep**, because during this phase electroencephalographic (EEG) waves appear as progressively slower oscillations. The REM phase of sleep is also referred to as **paradoxical sleep** because the EEG waves appear similar to those that are produced during periods of wakefulness (Fig. 17-1). Thus, NREM sleep has been characterized as quiet sleep and REM sleep as active sleep (Porth, 1994).

Sleep Cycles

During sleep, people pass back and forth through four distinct stages of NREM sleep and the REM phase of sleep. The characteristics and lengths of each phase are identified in Table 17-1.

Based on current research, NREM sleep always precedes REM sleep, the phase during which most dreaming occurs. Although the length of time spent in any one phase or stage varies according to age (Fig. 17-2) and other variables, most people cycle back and forth from stages 2, 3, and 4 of NREM to REM phases from four to six times during the night (Bullock & Rosendahl, 1992).

SLEEP REQUIREMENTS

Sleep requirements vary among different age groups. Despite individual differences, the need for sleep decreases with age (Table 17-2).

FACTORS AFFECTING SLEEP

The amount and quality of sleep can be affected by changes in the amount and intensity of light, activity, the environment, motivation, emotions and moods, food and beverages, illness, and drugs (Table 17-3).

Light

The sleep–wake cycle is influenced, among other things, by daylight and darkness, which occur once in every 24-hour period. Phenomena that cycle on a daily, or **diurnal**, basis are referred to as **circadian rhythms**, a term coined from combining two Latin words: *circa*, which means "about" and *dies* which means "day." Thus, drowsiness and sleeping correlate with the circadian rhythm of the setting sun and night. Wakefulness corresponds with sunrise and daylight.

Researchers (Rosenthal et al., 1984) suggest that the cycles of wakefulness followed by sleeping are linked to a photosensitive (light-sensitive) system involving

---

DISPLAY 17-1. *Effects of Chronic Sleep Deprivation*

- Reduced physical stamina
- Altered comfort such as headache and nausea
- Impaired coordination, especially of fine motor skills
- Loss of muscle mass and weight
- Increased susceptibility to infection
- Slower wound healing
- Decreased pain tolerance
- Poor concentration
- Impaired judgment
- Unstable moods
- Suspiciousness

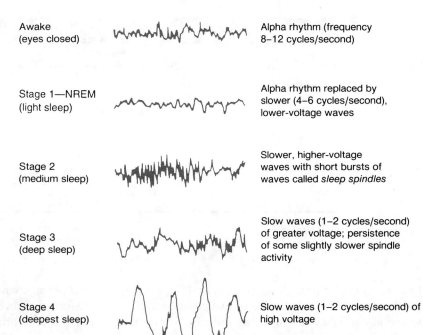

Awake (eyes closed) — Alpha rhythm (frequency 8–12 cycles/second)

Stage 1—NREM (light sleep) — Alpha rhythm replaced by slower (4–6 cycles/second), lower-voltage waves

Stage 2 (medium sleep) — Slower, higher-voltage waves with short bursts of waves called *sleep spindles*

Stage 3 (deep sleep) — Slow waves (1–2 cycles/second) of greater voltage; persistence of some slightly slower spindle activity

Stage 4 (deepest sleep) — Slow waves (1–2 cycles/second) of high voltage

Stage 1—REM ("dreaming sleep") — EEG similar to stage 1, but accompanied by episodic rapid eye movements, decreased muscle tone, and other physiological differences

FIGURE 17-1
Characteristic changes in electroencephalographic recordings during various stages of sleep. (Fuller J, Schaller-Ayers J: Health Assessment: A Nursing Approach, 2nd ed, p 39. Philadelphia, JB Lippincott, 1994)

TABLE 17-1. *Characteristics of Sleep Phases*

Sleep Phase	Length	Features
NREM	50–90 minutes	Deep, restful, dreamless sleep
Stage 1	A few minutes	Light sleep, easily aroused
		Gradual reduction in vital signs
Stage 2	10–20 minutes	Deeper relaxation
		Can be awakened with effort
Stage 3	15–30 minutes	Early phase of deep sleep
		Snoring
		Relaxed muscle tone
		Little or no physical movement
		Difficult to arouse
Stage 4	15–30 minutes; shortens toward morning	Deep sleep
		Sleepwalking, sleeptalking, and bedwetting may occur
REM	20-minute average; lengthens toward morning	Darting eye movements
		Very difficult to awaken
		Vivid, colorful, emotional dreams
		Loss of muscle tone; jaw relaxes; tongue may fall to the back of the throat
		Vital signs fluctuate
		Irregular respirations
		Pauses in breathing for 15–20 seconds
		Absence of snoring
		Muscle twitching
		Gastric secretions increase
		Men may have erections

NREM, nonrapid eye movement; REM, rapid eye movement.

TABLE 17-2. *Sleep Requirements*

Age	Total Sleep Time	Percentage in REM
Newborn	16–20 hours/day	50%
3 months to 1 year	14–15 hours/day	35%
Toddler	12 hours/night plus 1 or 2 naps	No data
Preschool	9–12 hours/night	No data
5 to 6 years	11 hours/night	20%
11 years	9 hours/night	No data
Adolescent	7–9 hours/night	25%
Adult	7–9 hours/night	20%–25%
Elderly	7–9 hours/night	13%–15%

REM, rapid eye movement.
Sundberg MC. Fundamentals of Nursing with Clinical Procedures. Boston: Jones and Bartlett Publishers, Inc., 1989, p. 861.

the eyes and the pineal gland in the brain (Fig. 17-3). In the absence of bright light, the pineal gland secretes a hormone called **melatonin** that induces drowsiness and sleep. Light activates receptors in the retina and travels through the brain to the pineal gland where it suppresses hormonal secretion.

Altering the amount and intensity of light tends to desynchronize the sleep–wake cycle. In support of this hypothesis, sleep disturbances have been noted to occur among shift workers, jet travelers, and those diagnosed with *seasonal affective disorder* (SAD), a type of cyclical mood disorder scientists believe is linked to a need for more exposure to sunlight.

SHIFT WORK

Shift workers are those who work evenings or nights or who alternately switch from one shift to another.

One of the characteristics of shift workers is that they are forced to reverse their sleep–wake cycles. However, the indoor lighting under which most shift workers are exposed is not bright enough to suppress melatonin. Consequently, many shift workers fight to stay awake, and statistics show that they are more prone to making errors and having job-related accidents (DeHart, 1993). According to Czeisler and colleagues (1990), most people who work night shifts never completely adapt to the reversal of day and night activities no matter how long the pattern is established.

JET TRAVEL

Jet travel causes a sudden change in the currently established **photoperiod**, or number of daylight hours, to which a person is accustomed. Consequently, travelers often describe having **jet lag**, a lay term for the emo-

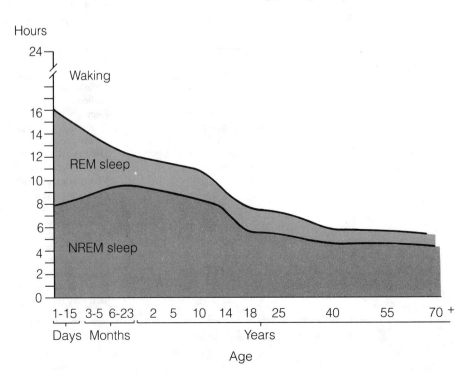

FIGURE 17-2
Sleep patterns according to age. (From Roftwang, Muzio, and Dement, 1966.) (Source: MR Rosenzweig and AL Leiman, Physiological Psychology (2nd ed.). New York: Random House, 1989.)

tional and physical changes experienced when arriving in a different time meridian.

Many jet travelers describe having difficulty falling or staying asleep. However, "jet lag" is more transient than shift work and, therefore, modifiable. Gillin and Byerley (1990) report that travelers may reestablish normal sleep–wake cycles, but that it takes a minimum of 1 day for each time zone that is crossed in an easterly direction and slightly less when traveling westerly.

SEASONAL AFFECTIVE DISORDER

Seasonal affective disorder is characterized by **hypersomnolence**, or increased sleep, lack of energy when awake, increased appetite accompanied by cravings for sweets, and weight gain. The symptoms have their onset during the darker winter months and spontaneously disappear as the number of daylight hours increase in the spring. In some ways the disorder resembles the hibernation patterns in bears and other animal species.

Some suggest that SAD may be due to an excess of melatonin. To counteract SAD symptoms, **phototherapy**, a technique for suppressing melatonin by stimulating light receptors in the eye, is prescribed.

To therapeutically manipulate the neurochemical changes in the brain, the artificial light used in phototherapy must be at least 2,000 to 2,500 *lux*, the equivalent of the bright light measured on a sunny, spring day (Varcarolis, 1990), and the daily light exposure must be between 2 to 6 hours to simulate the number of daylight hours during sunnier months (Display 17-2). Phototherapy usually relieves SAD symptoms within 3

to 5 days, but they may reoccur in the same amount of time if phototherapy is abruptly discontinued.

Activity

Activity, especially exercise, increases fatigue and the need for sleep. It appears that activity increases both REM and NREM sleep, especially the deep sleep of the fourth stage of NREM. However, if physical activity occurs just before bedtime, it may produce a stimulating rather than relaxing effect.

Environment

Most people sleep best in their usual environment. Because people tend to be creatures of habit, they develop a preference for a particular pillow, mattress, and blankets. There is also a tendency to adapt to the unique sounds within or near the place of residence, such as traffic, trains, and the hum of appliance motors or furnaces.

In addition, sleep may be induced by repeating certain habits, known as **sleep rituals**, before retiring. Sleep rituals may include eating a light snack, watching television, reading, and performing hygiene. Therefore, when the environment is altered or activities performed before bedtime are disturbed—as they may be while on vacation or in the hospital—the ability to fall asleep and remain asleep may be affected.

Motivation

When there is no particular reason to stay awake, sleep generally occurs easily. But if the desire to remain awake is strong, such as when a person wishes to participate in something interesting or important, the desire to sleep can be overcome.

TABLE 17-3. *Factors Affecting Sleep*	
Sleep-Promoting Factors	**Sleep-Suppressing Factors**
Darkness, dim light	Sunlight, bright light
Consistent sleep schedule	Inconsistent sleep schedule
Secretion of melatonin	Suppression of melatonin
Familiar sleep environment	Strange sleep environment
Optimum warmth and ventilation	Cold, hot, stuffy room
Perpetuation of sleep rituals	Disturbance of sleep rituals
Sedative, hypnotic drugs	Stimulant drugs
Depression	Depression, anxiety, worry
Relaxation	Activity
Satiation	Hunger, thirst
Proteins containing L-tryptophan	Protein-deficient diets
Excessive alcohol consumption	Metabolism of alcohol
Comfort	Pain, nausea, full bladder
Quiet	Noise
Effortless breathing	Difficulty breathing

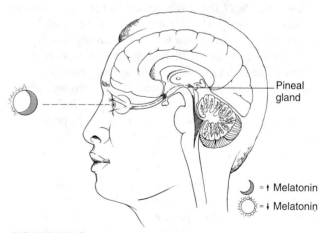

FIGURE 17-3
The sleep-wake cycle is influenced by a photosensitive light system.

DISPLAY 17-2. *Components of Phototherapy*

To relieve the symptoms of seasonal affective disorder, the patient:

- Initiates a schedule of full-spectrum* light exposure beginning in October–November
- Removes eyeglasses or contact lenses that have ultraviolet filters
- Sits within 3 feet of the artificial light for approximately 2 hours soon after awakening from sleep
- Glances at the light periodically but may engage in other activities such as reading or handiwork
- Repeats the exposure to light after sundown (to simulate extending the day-light hours) up to a cumulative time of 3 to 6 hours a day
- Continues the pattern of light exposure until spring

* Full-spectrum light simulates the energy of bright natural sunlight.

Emotions and Moods

Depressive disorders are classically associated with an inability to sleep or the tendency to sleep more than usual. Also, emotions such as anger, fear, anxiety, and dread may interfere with sleep. All are more than likely the result of changes in the types and amounts of neurotransmitters that affect the sleep–wake centers in the brain.

Sometimes sleeplessness can be conditioned. That is, anticipating sleeplessness, a characteristic pattern of some chronic insomniacs, may actually reinforce its occurrence—somewhat like a self-fulfilling prophecy. The expectation that the onset of sleep will be difficult increases the person's anxiety. The anxiety then floods the brain with stimulating chemicals that interfere with relaxation, an essential precursor to natural sleep.

Food and Beverages

Hunger or thirst often interferes with sleep. However, in the absence of these two, other factors, such as the consumption of particular foods and beverages, have been found to promote or inhibit the ability to sleep.

Sleep seems to be facilitated by a chemical, known as *L-tryptophan*. L-tryptophan is found in protein foods such as milk and dairy products. The recommendation to drink warm milk to induce sleep may have originally been an anecdotal observation of its hypnotic, or sleep-producing effect. Besides milk, L-tryptophan is also present in poultry, fish, eggs, and to some extent in plant sources of protein like legumes.

Alcohol is a depressive drug that promotes sleep, but it tends to reduce normal REM and deep sleep stages of NREM sleep. Furthermore, as alcohol is metabolized, stimulating chemicals that were blocked by the sedative effects of the alcohol tend to surge forth from neurons and may actually cause early awakening from sleep.

Beverages containing caffeine, a central nervous system stimulant, also tend to cause wakefulness. Caffeine is present in coffee, tea, chocolate, and most cola drinks.

Illness

Almost any illness is accompanied by stress, anxiety, and discomfort—any one of which can alter normal sleep patterns. Furthermore, if the ill person is in the hospital, other factors can contribute to sleep loss or fragmentation of sleep. These include being aroused by the noise from equipment, especially if it is continuous and monotonous; being awakened by nursing activities; and being disturbed by unfamiliar sounds such as loud talking, elevators, dietary carts, and housekeeping equipment.

In addition, there are several medical disorders whose symptoms may be aggravated at night or include a sleep disturbing component. For example, ulcers tend to be more painful during the night because hydrochloric acid is increased during REM sleep. In fact, pain of any kind is apt to be more distressing whenever there are few distractions. Also, conditions that are worsened by lying flat in bed, like some cardiac or respiratory diseases, may produce sleeplessness.

Drugs

Caffeine and alcohol, which have already been discussed, are nonprescription drugs that affect sleep. In addition, there are prescribed drugs that may promote or interfere with sleep. **Sedatives** and **tranquilizers** are drugs that produce a relaxing and calming effect. **Hypnotics** are those that induce sleep. **Stimulants** are those that excite structures in the brain, causing wakefulness (Table 17-4).

TABLE 17-4. *Drugs That Affect Sleep*

Drug Category	Drug Family	Example	Adverse Reactions
Sedatives	Barbiturates	Phenobarbital (Luminal*)	Sleepiness, lethargy, slowed respiratory rate, agitation, confusion
	Antihistamines	Diphenhydramine (Benadryl[†])	Sleepiness, dizziness, slowed reaction time, impaired coordination
	Antipsychotics	Haloperidol (Haldol[‡])	Sleepiness, postural hypotension, abnormal facial and mouth movements, stiff gait, dry mouth
Tranquilizers	Benzodiazepines	Alprazolam (Xanax[§])	Sleepiness, dry mouth, constipation, slowed heart rate, hypotension, liver damage
Hypnotics	Barbiturates	Pentobarbital (Nembutal[‖])	Same as phenobarbital, daytime drowsiness
	Nonbarbiturates	Temazepam (Restoril[¶])	Dizziness, lethargy during the day
Stimulants	Amphetamines	Dextroamphetamine (Dexedrine[#])	Insomnia, restlessness, anorexia, rapid heart rate
	Amphetamine-like	Methylphenidate (Ritalin**)	Nervousness, insomnia, rash, anorexia, nausea

* Winthrop Pharmaceuticals, New York, NY.
[†] Parke Davis, Morris Plains, NJ.
[‡] McNeil Pharmaceutical, Spring House, PA.
[§] Upjohn, Kalamazoo, MI.
[‖] Abbott Laboratories, North Chicago, IL.
[¶] Sandoz Pharmaceuticals, East Hanover, NJ.
[#] SmithKline Beecham, Philadelphia, PA.
** Ciba Pharmaceutical Co., Summit, NJ.

Unfortunately, sedative and hypnotics may have a paradoxical effect when administered to older adults—that is, they may tend to keep older adults awake rather than facilitate sleep. Also, people who take sedative and hypnotic drugs for a period of time tend to experience **drug tolerance**, or a diminished effect from the drug. Without realizing the danger, drug-tolerant people may increase the dose of the drug or the frequency of its administration to achieve the same effect first experienced at a lower dose. Increasing the dose or frequency may have life-threatening consequences. When sedatives, tranquilizers, and hypnotics are abruptly discontinued they may cause a period of intense stimulation that may interfere with sleep.

Some drugs, like diuretics, which increase the formation of urine, may awaken patients with a need to empty their bladder. For this reason, they are usually administered early in the morning so that the peak effect has diminished by bedtime.

SLEEP ASSESSMENT

Many people blame inadequate sleep for daytime fatigue, or they underestimate the actual amount of time they sleep. Therefore, a more accurate sleep pattern assessment may be obtained through sleep questionnaires, sleep diaries, and polysomnographic evaluation.

Questionnaires

Several questionnaires have been developed to help identify sleep patterns. Questionnaires are queries that are designed to obtain specific information, or they can be unstructured to allow people more freedom to respond. Sometimes the data are gathered during interviews, or the questions may be answered independently in the form of a self-report.

The following are examples of unstructured questions:

- When you think about your sleep, what kinds of impressions come to mind?
- Is there anything about your sleep that bothers you?
- What do you do to help yourself sleep well? (Floyd, 1993, p. 73)

Sleep Diary

A **sleep diary** is an account of sleeping and waking activities. Records may be compiled entirely by patients or by personnel in a sleep disorder clinic. The diary usually includes shaded blocks indicating sleep time, a description of daily activities during each 15-minute waking period, a 24-hour log of food and beverages that are consumed, and a list and time that medications are self-administered. Self-kept diaries usually cover a 2-week period of time.

Although sleep diaries are inexpensive and simple to compile, Rogers and colleagues (1993) found that self-maintained records varied in their accuracy and reliability. Therefore, sleep assessments ought to include other techniques for gathering data to ensure that sleep disorders and their etiologies are accurately identified.

Polysomnographic Evaluation

Polysomnography refers to the collective techniques used to obtain physiologic data during sleep. A polysomnographic evaluation involves analyzing electrical recordings of brain waves, muscle tone, and eye movements (Fig. 17-4). The diagnostic data are then compared to the patterns and characteristics of normal sleep cycles to help diagnose sleep disorders.

SLEEP DISORDERS

About 20% to 40% of adults report having sleeping problems (Dement & Mitler 1993). Most of the problems seem to be short-lived, but for some the sleep disorders are both chronic and serious. Some examples of sleep disorders from which millions of Americans suffer, but do not always seek treatment, include insom-

nia, narcolepsy, sleep apnea/hypopnea syndrome, and conditions referred to as parasomnias.

Insomnia

Insomnia is a condition characterized by difficulty falling asleep or staying asleep, or awakening early. Almost everyone has had insomnia. Most cases of insomnia resolve themselves in less than 3 weeks.

Chronic insomnia implies that sleep has been impaired for 3 weeks or longer (Gillin & Byerley, 1990). Although chronic insomnia may be treated with hypnotic drugs, it may be helpful to implement nonpharmacologic interventions initially.

Narcolepsy

Narcolepsy is a condition characterized by excessive sleepiness regardless of the amount of sleep that is obtained. This condition is not to be confused with hypersomnolence, which is excessive sleeping.

Although the diagnosis of narcolepsy usually requires polysomnographic evaluation, there are additional symptoms that help to distinguish it from other conditions that cause sleepiness. For example, the sleepiness of narcolepsy is usually accompanied by

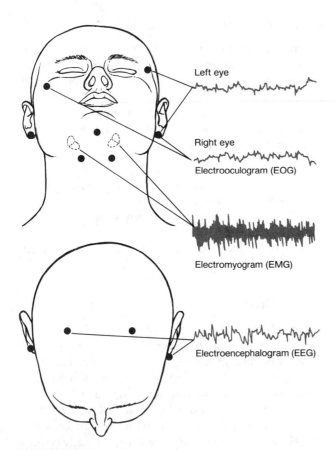

FIGURE 17-4
Normal sleep patterns and sleep disorders are evaluated by collecting physiologic data from electrical activity produced by the brain (EEG), muscles (EMG), and eyes (EOG). (Fuller J, Schaller-Ayers J: Health Assessment: A Nursing Approach, 2nd ed, p 392. Philadelphia, JB Lippincott, 1994)

◆ **PATIENT TEACHING FOR PROMOTING SLEEP**

Teach the patient or the family to do the following:
- Take diuretic drugs, if they are prescribed, early in the morning.
- Exercise regularly during the day, but not late in the evening.
- Resist napping during the day.
- Avoid alcohol, nicotine, and caffeine.
- Eat dairy products and other proteins daily.
- Modify the temperature and ventilation in the bedroom according to personal preferences.
- Use the bed and bedroom just for sleeping.
- Repeat your personal pattern of sleep rituals.
- Use earplugs or eyeshades to reduce environmental noise or light.
- Maintain a consistent sleep routine by always going to bed and arising at approximately the same time—even on weekends or days off.
- If the onset of sleep is delayed more than 20 to 30 minutes, get out of bed and do something else, like reading.
- Avoid using nonprescription or prescription sleeping pills unless they have been recommended by a physician.
- Follow labeled directions on any medications.

muscular weakness and brief periods of muscle paralysis just before sleep or when awakening. These two accompanying symptoms may result because people with narcolepsy experience REM sleep immediately or within 10 minutes after falling asleep. Because the REM phase includes loss of muscle tone, this may explain the abnormal muscular phenomena.

Narcoleptic symptoms tend to diminish with age in about a third of those affected. However, if the condition is untreated, there is a potential for endangering lives as a consequence of motor vehicle or occupational accidents. Prescribed stimulant drugs, such as methylphenidate (Ritalin; Ciba Pharmaceutical Co., Summit, NJ) or dextroamphetamine (Dexedrine; Smith Kline Beecham, Philadelphia, PA), often help to control the symptoms.

Sleep Apnea/Hypopnea Syndrome

Apnea is a cessation of breathing, whereas *hypopnea* is hypoventilation. **Sleep apnea/hypopnea syndrome** is a sleep disorder in which affected people stop breathing or their breathing slows for 10 seconds or longer, five or more times per hour (Dantzker & Steinberg, 1994; Prinz et al., 1990). During periods when ventilation is reduced, there is a drop in blood oxygenation. The accumulation of carbon dioxide and drop in oxygen causes those affected to awaken briefly throughout the night. Consequently, people with sleep apnea/hypopnea syndrome feel tired after having slept, or worse, their symptoms may cause a heart attack, stroke, or sudden death.

Sleep apnea is most prevalent among older adults, especially obese men who snore. The incidence of apneic episodes may be reduced by sleeping in other than the supine position, losing weight, and avoiding substances that depress respirations such as alcohol or sleeping medications. In severe cases, people with sleep apnea may wear a special breathing mask that keeps the alveoli within the lungs inflated at all times, or surgery may be performed on their airway.

Parasomnias

Parasomnias are activities that occur during sleep. In and of themselves, parasomnias are not life threatening. Some examples of parasomnias include **somnambulism**, or sleepwalking; **nocturnal enuresis**, or bedwetting; sleeptalking; **bruxism**, grinding of the teeth; and lower extremity muscular contractions called restless leg syndrome.

Restless leg syndrome, also known as **nocturnal myoclonus**, is characterized by periodic contractions of the ankles, knees, or hips that may awaken the person. A milder form, referred to as **hypnic jerks**, may occur just before the onset of true sleep while the person is extremely drowsy.

APPLICABLE NURSING DIAGNOSES

- Fatigue
- Sleep Pattern Disturbance
- Risk for Injury
- Impaired Gas Exchange
- Anxiety

NURSING IMPLICATIONS

After assessing evidence of altered sleep patterns, nurses may identify one or more of the nursing diagnoses listed under Applicable Nursing Diagnoses.

The accompanying Nursing Care Plan is an example of how the nursing process has been used in developing a plan of care for a patient with Sleep Pattern Disturbance. Sleep Pattern Disturbance is defined in the NANDA Taxonomy (1994) as a "disruption of sleeptime that causes discomfort or interferes with one's desired life-style."

Several sleep-promoting nursing measures, such as maintaining sleep rituals, reducing the intake of stimulating chemicals, promoting daytime exercising, and adhering to a regular schedule for retiring and awakening, have already been discussed. Two additional methods that may prove beneficial are assisting the patient with progressive relaxation exercises and providing a back massage.

Progressive Relaxation

Progressive relaxation is a therapeutic use of exercise in which a person actively contracts and then relaxes muscle groups. The technique is used to break the worry–tension cycle that interferes with relaxation.

Patients may eventually learn to perform progressive relaxation exercises independently using self-suggestion. Ultimately, some patients may even be able to omit the muscle contraction phase and go directly to progressively relaxing muscle groups.

NURSING GUIDELINES FOR FACILITATING PROGRESSIVE RELAXATION

- Select a room that is quiet, dimly lit, and provides privacy.
  Rationale: Reduces stimulation of the arousal center in the brain, which responds to noise, bright lights, and activity
- Encourage the patient to assume a comfortable position, which, more often than not, involves lying down or sitting.

Rationale: Provides external support for the body, which facilitates muscle relaxation
- Advise the patient to avoid talking and instead listen to the suggestions that will follow.
Rationale: Reduces performance anxiety, the anticipation of appearing incompetent or foolish, by encouraging a passive role
- Instruct the patient to close his or her eyes and consciously focus on breathing.
Rationale: Blocks visual stimuli and substitutes an alternative activity to help focus the patient's attention away from distracting thoughts and feelings
- Tell the patient to inhale deeply through the nose and exhale slowly from the mouth, and repeat the activity several times.

Rationale: Oxygenates the blood and brain, and reduces the heart rate
- Coach the patient to tighten the muscles in an area of the body, like the foot, and hold the position for at least 5 seconds.
Rationale: Depletes the level of stimulating neurotransmitters
- Direct the patient to relax the tensed muscles and focus on the pleasurable feeling.
Rationale: Directs the cortex's attention on the desired outcome and raises the person's sense of awareness
- Proceed with sequence after sequence of muscle contraction followed by relaxation until all muscle groups in the body have been exercised.

NURSING CARE PLAN:
Sleep Pattern Disturbance

Assessment

Subjective Data
States, "I feel so tired. It seems that it takes forever to fall asleep. It's been 2 weeks since I've gotten more than 4 hours of sleep. I'm so worried I'll never go home again."

Objective Data
63-year-old woman admitted to nursing home for intermediate care after repair of a fractured hip. Yawns frequently, naps rather than participating in activities. Asks for and receives barbiturate hypnotic each night, which is often repeated several hours later.

Diagnosis

Sleep Pattern Disturbance related to excessive stimulating neurochemicals secondary to anxiety over rehabilitation.

Plan

Goal
The patient will begin sleeping within 30 minutes of going to bed and remain asleep for a minimum of 6 hours within 10 days (by 3/15).

Orders: 3/5
1. Awaken patient at 0730, which is her usual time for rising.
2. Substitute decaffeinated coffee or tea at meals and offer an alternative for food items containing chocolate.
3. Discourage daytime napping for the next 5 days.
4. Supervise ambulation with a walker for at least 20 minutes three times a day, the last being no later than 1930.
5. Provide yogurt, vanilla pudding, custard, or some other diary product at approximately 2200.
6. Let patient stay up until 2330, which is her usual bedtime.
7. Hold sleeping medication and give a back massage instead. _____ J. HALEY, RN

Implementation
(Documentation)   3/5   1800–2300   Served decaffeinated coffee with supper. Peanut butter cookies substituted for chocolate brownie. At 1900, walked the length of the hall three times, which took 25 minutes. Ate a dish of vanilla ice cream at 2200. Assisted with hygiene and changing into gown and bathrobe. Watching television in room. _____ P. ROGERS, LPN

Evaluation
(Documentation)   3/5   2330   Assisted to bed._____ C. VARGAS, LPN
3/6   0000   Observed to be sleeping._____ C. VARGAS, LPN

TABLE 17-5. *Massage Techniques*

Technique	Description	Method
Effleurage	To skim the surface	The hands are used to make a circular pattern using long strokes over the massaged area.
Pétrissage	To knead	The skin is lifted and compressed or pulled in opposing directions.
Frôlement	To brush	The skin is lightly touched with the fingertips.
Tapotement	To tap	The skin is lightly struck with the sides of the hands.
Vibration	To set in motion	The skin is moved rhythmically with open or cupped palms, causing the tissue to quiver.
Friction	To rub	The skin is pulled from opposite directions using the thumbs and fingers.

Rationale: Leads to higher planes of relaxation
* Continue suggesting throughout the drill that the patient focus on "how relaxed" he or she feels, or to "note the feeling of weightlessness."
Rationale: Reinforces a relaxed physical response by suggesting verbal images
* Explain that as a numerical countdown commences, the patient can begin to move.
Rationale: Provides gradual termination of the relaxation period

Another technique that may promote sufficient relaxation to overcome muscular tension due to anxiety is to administer a back massage.

Back Massage

Massage involves stroking the skin, using a variety of techniques (Table 17-5), for the purposes of relaxing tense muscles and improving circulation (Skill 17-1). Massage may be performed using a variety of strok-

(text continues on page 346)

SKILL 17-1.
Giving A Back Massage

Suggested Action	Reason for Action
Assessment	
Observe if the patient is still awake 30 minutes after retiring for sleep.	Indicates a delay in the usual onset of sleep
Determine if the patient is experiencing pain, has a need for bladder or bowel elimination, is hungry, too warm or cold, or any other physical or environmental problem that may be easily overcome.	Eliminates all but psychophysiologic etiologies as the cause for sleeplessness
Check the patient's medical record to determine if there are any conditions for which a backrub would be contraindicated, like fractured ribs or back injury.	Demonstrates concern for the safety and comfort of the patient
Ask the patient if he or she would like a back massage.	Allows the patient an opportunity to participate in decision-making
Planning	
Obtain the following supplies: lotion or alternative substances like alcohol or powder if the patient's skin is oily.	Demonstrates organization and efficient time management
Use gloves if there are any open, draining lesions on the skin.	Provides a barrier against blood-borne microorganisms

(continued)

SKILL 17-1.
Giving A Back Massage (Continued)

Suggested Action	Reason for Action
Reduce environmental stimuli like bright lights and loud noise.	Decreases stimulation of the wake center in the brain
Implementation Pull the privacy curtain around the patient's bed.	Demonstrates respect for modesty
Raise the bed to an appropriate height to avoid bending at the waist.	Reduces back strain
Wash your hands; don gloves if appropriate.	Reduces the spread of microorganisms
Help the patient lie on his or her abdomen or side and untie the hospital gown or remove it completely.	Provides access to the back
Instruct the patient to breathe slowly and deeply in and out through an open mouth.Squirt a generous amount of lotion into your hands and rub them together.	Promotes ventilation and relaxationWarms the lotion
Place the entire surface of the hands on either side of the lower spine and move them upward over the shoulders and back again, using long, continuous strokes. Repeat the stroke pattern several times.	Uses *effleurage* to promote relaxation

Effleurage.

Apply firmer pressure with the upstroke and lighter pressure during the downstroke.	Enhances relaxation by alternating pressure and rhythm

(continued)

SKILL 17-1.
Giving A Back Massage *(Continued)*

Suggested Action	Reason for Action
Make smaller circular strokes up and down the length of the back with the thumbs.	Uses *friction* to improve blood flow and remove chemicals that accumulate in contracted muscles

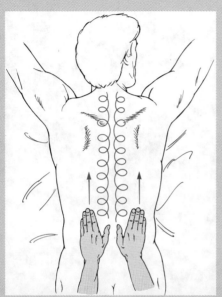

Friction.

Suggested Action	Reason for Action
Lift and gently compress tissue with the fingers starting at the base of the spine and ending at the neck and shoulder areas.	Uses *pétrissage* to increase the circulation of blood

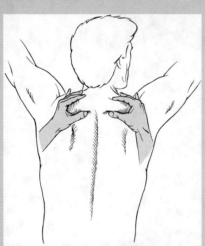

Pétrissage.

(continued)

SKILL 17-1.
Giving A Back Massage (Continued)

Suggested Action	Reason for Action
Pull the skin in opposite directions in a kneading fashion to lift and stretch the skin from the base of the spine to the shoulder areas.	Uses another pétrissage technique for reducing the tension in muscles and improving circulation

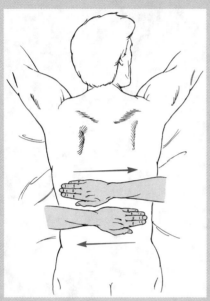

Kneading.

Suggested Action	Reason for Action
End the backrub by lightly stroking the length of the back, gradually lightening the pressure as the fingers are moved downward.	Uses *frôlement* to prolong the sensation of relaxation

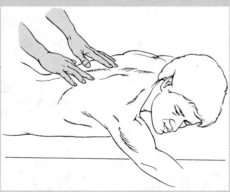

Frôlement

Suggested Action	Reason for Action
Lightly cover the patient and restore the bed to a lower position.	Extends the period of relaxation by reducing activity and may induce NREM sleep

(continued)

Suggested Action	Reason for Action

Evaluation
- Patient feels relaxed
- Sleep is promoted

Document
- Date and time of back massage
- Response of the patient

Sample Documentation

Date and Time   Unable to sleep. Assisted to bathroom to void. Light snack of graham crackers and milk provided. Back massaged for 10 minutes. Observed to be sleeping 20 minutes later. _____ **Signature, Title**

 FOCUS ON OLDER ADULTS

- Insomnia or hypersomnolence are often physical symptoms of underlying depression, which is quite common in older adults.
- Older adults tend to have more difficulty falling asleep, a problem called **sleep latency**. They also have fewer episodes of stage 3 and 4 NREM and their REM phases may be shorter. This may explain why some older adults feel tired even though they have slept an appropriate length of time (Hogstel, 1990).
- Use night lights rather than bright room lights if an older adult arises at night. Bright lights stimulate the brain and block efforts to resume sleeping.
- The National Institute of Aging recommends that sleep disorders experienced by older adults be managed without the use of hypnotic medications (Miller, 1993).
- Some older patients become confused at night, a condition referred to as **sundown syndrome** (Display 17-3). Others demonstrate **sunrise syndrome**, or early morning confusion, which may be caused by inadequate sleep or the effects of sedative and hypnotic drugs.
- Family members, especially spouses, may experience sleep disturbances if an older adult tends to wander at night, snores, or has restless leg syndrome.
- Hypnotic agents, when they are used, tend to have paradoxical effects when administered to older adults.

- Because REM sleep is reduced with the administration of hypnotic drugs, older adults are likely to experience nightmares if they are abruptly discontinued.
- Sleep cycles may remain disturbed for approximately 2 to 8 weeks after long-term use of hypnotic drugs has been stopped (Hogstel, 1990).
- Hypnotic drugs with a long *half-life*, the amount of time it takes to metabolize half of the drug dosage, may cause older adults to experience drug-induced lethargy, called a "hangover," the next day. Drugs such as triazolam (Halcion; Upjohn, Kalamazoo, MI), alprazolam (Xanax; Upjohn), oxazepam (Serax, Wyeth Laboratories, Philadelphia, PA), and zolpidem (Ambien) are hypnotics with short half-lives that may be tolerated better by older adults (Miller, 1993).
- Older adults, who have impaired physical mobility, may be helped to exercise by rocking in a rocking chair. Exercising in water, such as swimming pools, also is less taxing to painful joints for those with restricted range of motion.
- A foot massage may help some older adults relax before bedtime.
- Resting quietly for an hour or two in mid-morning and afternoon can restore energy among older adults without contributing to insomnia (Hogstel, 1990).

DISPLAY 17-3. *Characteristics of Sundown Syndrome*

- Alert and oriented during the day
- Onset of disorientation as the sun sets
- Disorganized thinking
- Restlessness
- Agitation
- Perseveration (ruminating over the same repetitive thought)
- Wandering about

ing techniques. Stimulating strokes such as tapotement and vibration are omitted if the purpose of the massage is to relax the patient.

KEY CONCEPTS

- Sleep is a basic human need characterized as a state of arousable unconsciousness. Rest is a waking state during which there is a conscious effort to reduce activity and mental stimulation.
- Among other things, sleep reduces fatigue, stabilizes moods, increases protein synthesis, promotes cellular growth and repair, and improves the capacity for learning and memory storage.
- There are two phases of sleep: nonrapid and rapid eye movement sleep. Nonrapid eye movement (NREM) sleep and its four subdivisions are characterized as a time when the body is active, but the brain is not. During rapid eye movement (REM) sleep, the body is physically inactive, but the brain is highly active.
- As humans age, they sleep fewer hours and spend less time in REM sleep. Newborns spend between 16 to 20 hours of each day sleeping, with approximately half of that in the REM phase. Older adults require 7 to 9 hours of sleep and spend only 13% to 15% of their sleep in the REM phase.
- The amount and quality of sleep can be affected by changes in circadian rhythms, activity, the environment, motivation, emotions and moods, food and beverages, illness, and drugs.
- There are four major categories of drugs that either promote or interfere with sleep. Sedatives and tranquilizers produce a relaxing and calming effect; hypnotics induce sleep; and stimulants excite structures in the brain, causing wakefulness.
- Sleep questionnaires, sleep diaries, and polysomnographic evaluations are techniques that are used to assess sleep patterns.

- Sleep may be promoted by (1) exercising regularly during the day, (2) avoiding alcohol, nicotine, and caffeine, (3) repeating one's personal pattern of sleep rituals, (4) going to bed and arising at approximately the same time every day, and (5) getting out of bed if sleep does not come easily and returning after some nonstimulating activity.
- To promote relaxation, which may facilitate the onset of sleep, nurses may assist patients with progressive relaxation exercises or provide a back massage.
- Older adults tend to have more difficulty falling asleep. They also have fewer episodes of stage 3 and 4 NREM and their REM phases may be shorter. This may explain why some older adults feel tired even though they have slept an appropriate length of time.

CRITICAL THINKING EXERCISES

- While working the night shift in a nursing home, you find an older adult patient wandering the halls. Discuss three reasons why the patient may be wandering and a nursing intervention for each.
- You have accepted responsibility for developing a sleep assessment tool. Identify what information would be important to include.

SUGGESTED READINGS

Bullock BL, Rosendahl PP. Pathophysiology, Adaptations and Alterations in Function. 3rd ed. Philadelphia: JB Lippincott, 1992.

Czeisler CA, Johnson MP, Duffy JF, Brown EN, Ronda JM, Kronauer RE. Exposure to bright light and darkness to treat physiologic maladaptation to night work. New England Journal of Medicine May 3, 1990;322:1253–1307.

Dantzker DR, Steinberg H. Pulmonary and critical care medicine. Journal of the American Medical Association June 1, 1994;271: 1709–1710.

DeHart RL. Limits and fatigue. Journal of the American Medical Association November 10, 1993;270:2230.

Dement WC, Mitler MM. It's time to wake up to the importance of sleep disorders. Journal of the American Medical Association March 24–31, 1993;269:1548–1549.

Floyd JA. The use of across-method triangulation in the study of sleep concerns in healthy older adults. Advances in Nursing Science December 1993; :70–80.

Fuller J, Schaller-Ayers J. Health Assessment: A Nursing Approach. 2nd ed. Philadelphia: JB Lippincott, 1994.

Gillin JC, Byerley WF. The diagnosis and management of insomnia. New England Journal of Medicine January 25, 1990;322:239–247.

Hensley M, Rodgers S. Shedding light on "SAD"ness. Archives of Psychiatric Nursing August 1987;1:230–235.

Hogstel MO. Geropsychiatric Nursing. St. Louis: CV Mosby, 1990.

Miller CA. Interventions for sleep pattern disturbances. Geriatric Nursing September–October 1993;14:235–236.

Morin GD. Seasonal affective disorder, the depression of winter: a literature review and description from a nursing perspective. Archives of Psychiatric Nursing 1990;4:182–187.

NANDA Nursing Diagnoses: Definitions and Classification 1994–1995. Philadelphia: North American Nursing Diagnosis Association, 1994.

Porth CM. Pathophysiology, Concepts of Altered Health States. 4th ed. Philadelphia: JB Lippincott, 1994.

Prinz PN, Vitiello MV, Raskind MA, Thorpy MJ. Geriatrics: sleep disorders and aging. New England Journal of Medicine August 23, 1990;323:520–525.

Rogers A, Caruso C, Aldrich M. Reliability of sleep diaries for assessment of sleep/wake patterns. Nursing Research 1993;42:368–371.

Rosenthal NE, Sack DA, Gillin C, et al. Seasonal affective disorder. Archives of General Psychiatry January 1984;41:72–80.

Scherer JC. Introductory Clinical Pharmacology. 4th ed. Philadelphia: JB Lippincott, 1992.

Stewart A. The sleep apnea/hypopnea syndrome. Canadian Nurse November 1991;87:25–27.

Varcarolis EM. Foundations of Psychiatric Mental Health Nursing. Philadelphia: WB Saunders, 1990.

CHAPTER 18

Comfort

NURSING GUIDELINES

Managing Pain

SKILLS

Making an Unoccupied Bed
Making an Occupied Bed
Preparing a Patient-Controlled Analgesia (PCA) Infuser
Operating a Transcutaneous Electrical Nerve Stimulation (TENS) Unit

NURSING CARE PLAN

Pain

Key Terms

Acupressure	Occupied Bed
Acupuncture	Pain
Acute Pain	Pain Management
Addiction	Pain Perception
Analgesic	Pain Threshold

Biofeedback
Chronic Pain
Comfort
Cutaneous Pain
Environmental Psychologist
Equianalgesic Dose
Hypnosis
Mattress Overlays
Neuropathic Pain
Nociceptors
Pain Tolerance
Patient-controlled Analgesia
Referred Pain
Somatic Pain
Suffering
Transcutaneous Nerve Stimulation
Unoccupied Bed
Visceral Pain

Learning Objectives

An understanding of the content within this chapter will be evidenced by the student's ability to:

- Name two factors that promote patient comfort
- Describe four ways that the patient environment is modified to promote comfort
- List four furnishings that are standard in each patient's room
- Give a general definition of pain
- Explain the difference between pain threshold and pain tolerance
- Describe the gate control theory of pain transmission
- Discuss how endogenous opioids reduce pain transmission
- Name at least five types of pain
- List five components of a comprehensive pain assessment
- Identify at least three occasions when a pain assessment ought to be performed and documented
- Name five techniques for managing pain

Timby BK: *Fundamental Skills and Concepts in Patient Care, Sixth Edition* © 1996 Lippincott-Raven Publishers

- Discuss the most common reason why patients request frequent administrations of pain-relieving drugs
- Explain what is meant by the term "placebo" and the basis for their positive effect
- Discuss at least two ways of modifying the care of older adults to ensure their comfort

Comfort refers to a state in which a person is relieved of distress. One of the factors that contributes to comfort is a safe, clean, and attractive environment. Therefore, this chapter addresses measures for ensuring that the setting for patient care is one that promotes a sense of well-being. And, because pain is probably the chief element that causes distress among patients, this chapter also provides information about pain and techniques for its relief.

THE PATIENT ENVIRONMENT

The term *environment*, as it is used here, refers to the room where the patient receives care, and the furnishings within it. Although most patients are unaware of the thought and consideration that now goes into designing their physical surroundings, it is an essential component of any new construction or remodeling project.

Patient Rooms

Patient rooms, which most resemble a bedroom, no longer appear as the bare, white, sterile environments of a few decades ago. Thanks to **environmental psychologists**, specialists who study how the environment affects behavior, patient rooms are now brighter, more colorful, and tastefully decorated. The wall and floor treatments, lighting, and mechanisms for maintaining climate control are not only conducive to comfort, but practical as well.

WALLS

Research indicates that various colors like blue and colors with blue tints, such as mauve and light green, promote feelings of relaxation (Bieren, 1961; Plack & Schick, 1974; Sharpe, 1975). Consequently, these color schemes are the preferred decor within health care settings and patient rooms. If they are not used exclusively, they are integrated into wallpaper trim and wall accent pieces such as framed pictures. Also, the prints that are selected as wall hangings often depict pastoral, country scenes primarily because they suggest peaceful imagery.

FLOORS

Because noise interferes with comfort, carpeting is now being used in the hallways and work stations of most health agencies. For functional purposes, most floors in patient rooms continue to have tile or linoleum surfaces to facilitate cleaning spills of blood and other body fluids.

LIGHTING

Adequate lighting, both natural and artificial, is important to the comfort of patients and nursing personnel. Newer buildings are being constructed with large window areas, atriums, skylights, and enclosed courtyards to facilitate exposure to sunlight as a technique for reducing stress.

Although bright artificial light may be best for health care workers, it may not be appreciated by patients. Therefore, most patient rooms are designed with multiple room lights in various locations with options for adjusting their intensity. Because sleep is promoted in dim light and darkness, yet injuries are more likely to occur in a dark and unfamiliar environment, many patient rooms have adjustable window shades and night lights near the floor.

CLIMATE CONTROL

Climate control refers to mechanisms for maintaining optimum temperature, humidity, and ventilation within a room.

Temperature and Humidity

Most patients are comfortable when the room temperature is between 68°F to 74°F (20°C–23°C). Newer buildings provide individual thermostats in each room for adjusting the temperature in the immediate environment according to the comfort level of the patient.

Humidity is the amount of moisture in the air; **relative humidity** is the ratio between the amount of moisture in the air and the greatest amount of water vapor the air can hold at a given temperature. At a relative humidity of 60%, the air contains 60% of its potential water capacity. A relative humidity of 30% to 60% ensures comfort for most patients.

If the environmental temperature becomes greater than the skin temperature, evaporation is the only mechanism for regulating body temperature; evaporation is reduced, however, when humidity levels rise because air that is almost or fully saturated with water cannot adequately absorb additional moisture. Therefore, instead of evaporating, sweat accumulates and drips from the skin.

To ensure patient comfort, many health care agencies are air conditioned. Electric fans and dehumidifiers, which are not always adequate substitutes, may be used where air conditioners are not available. In buildings where the air is dry, moisture can be added to the environment with a humidifier or by using a cool mist machine. However, some patients who have ineffective **thermoregulation**, an inability to maintain stable body temperature, may feel excessively warm or uncomfortably cool even when the temperature and humidity are within optimum ranges.

Ventilation

Ventilation refers to the movement of air. Opening windows or using ceiling fans are common techniques for circulating and replacing air in the home environment. However, open windows present a fire and safety hazard in hospitals and nursing homes, and ceiling fans blow dust and debris that may transport infectious microorganisms to other patients and staff. Consequently, ventilation is usually accomplished through a system of air ducts that circulate air in and out of each patient room.

Poorly ventilated rooms and buildings tend to harbor unpleasant odors. Removing soiled articles, emptying bedpans and urinals, and opening privacy curtains and room doors may help reduce odors in the patient's immediate environment. Another alternative is to use an air freshener or deodorant. In general, though, scented sprays tend to substitute one odor for another, and ill patients may find any strong smell disagreeable. It is also well to keep in mind that many patients find it offensive to receive care from nurses who are neglectful of oral and body hygiene, whose perfume is overpowering, or who smell of cigarette smoke.

Room Furnishings

Manufacturers of hospital furnishings attempt to design equipment that is both attractive yet serves a utilitarian purpose (Fig. 18-1). The bed and its components such as the mattress and pillow, chairs, the overbed table, and bedside stand must be safe, durable, and comfortable.

THE BED

Hospital beds are adjustable; that is, the height and position of the head and knees can be changed either electrically or manually. Adjusting the bed may promote comfort, enable self-care, or facilitate a therapeutic position (see Chap. 23). In most situations, hospital beds are kept in their lowest position except when patients are receiving nursing care.

Full or half side rails are usually attached to the bed frame. Currently there is controversy as to whether raised side rails are a risk or benefit because some patients try to climb over them. Side rails are now con-

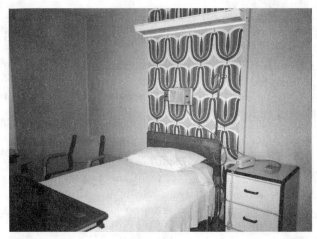

FIGURE 18-1
Hospital room. (Courtesy of Ken Timby.)

sidered a form of physical restraint in long-term care facilities, and their use must be justified (see Chap. 19).

Mattress

Many people equate comfort with the quality of their mattress. A good mattress adjusts to the shape of the body, yet supports it. A mattress that is too soft alters the alignment of the spine, causing some to awaken feeling sore from muscle and joint strain.

Hospital mattresses are usually made of tough materials that will withstand long-term use. Because mattresses are not sterilized between uses, they are usually covered with a waterproof coating that withstands cleansing with strong antimicrobial solutions.

Occasionally **mattress overlays**, layers of foam (Fig. 18-2) or other devices placed on top of the hospital mattress, are used to promote comfort or to keep the skin

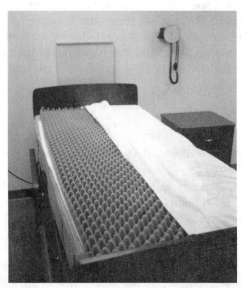

FIGURE 18-2
Egg crate mattress. (Courtesy of Ken Timby.)

intact when bedfast patients are relatively inactive (see Chap. 23).

Pillows

Pillows are primarily used for comfort, but they may also be used to elevate a part of the body, to relieve swelling, to promote breathing, or to help maintain a therapeutic position (see Chap. 23). Pillows may be stuffed with foam, kapok (a mass of silky fibers), or feathers.

Bed Linen

The linen that is used for most hospital beds includes a mattress pad, a bottom sheet, which is sometimes fitted, an optional drawsheet, which is placed beneath the patient's hips, a top sheet, spread, and pillow case. Some hospitals are using printed sheets to simulate a more home-like atmosphere.

To control expenses, bed linen may not be changed every day, but any linen that is wet or soiled is changed as frequently as necessary. Sometimes folded sheets or disposable, absorbent pads are used to avoid having to change the entire bed when it becomes soiled.

Skill 18-1 describes how to make an **unoccupied bed**, one that is empty. Skill 18-2 explains how to make an **occupied bed**, one in which the linen is changed while the patient remains in bed.

Privacy Curtain

A privacy curtain is a long fabric partition, mounted from the ceiling, that may be drawn completely around each patient's bed. The privacy curtain is used out of respect for patient dignity and modesty whenever it is necessary to examine or expose them for care. It may also be used to shield them from being observed while using a urinal or bedpan.

THE OVERBED TABLE

An overbed table is a portable, flat platform that can be positioned over the lap of a patient. The height of the table can be adjusted so that it may be used when the bed is in either a high or low position. The overbed table makes it convenient for the patient to eat while in bed and to perform personal hygiene or other activities requiring a flat surface. Nurses may also use the overbed table for holding equipment when providing patient care.

There is often a concealed compartment within the overbed table that may contain a mounted mirror and a place for personal items like a hair brush, comb, cosmetic bag, razor, or book.

THE BEDSIDE STAND

A bedside stand is actually a small cupboard. Most contain a drawer and two shelved compartments. The patient is free to place personal items in the drawer. The upper shelf is used to store the patient's bath basin, soap dish, soap, and a kidney-shaped basin called an *emesis basin*. The lower shelf is used to store a bedpan, urinal, and toilet paper. It is important to keep the elim-

(text continues on page 364)

SKILL 18-1
Making an Unoccupied Bed

Suggested Action	Reason for Action
Assessment	
Check the Kardex or nursing care plan to determine the patient's activity level.	Determines if the patient can be out of bed during bedmaking
Inspect the linen for moisture or evidence of soiling.	Indicates what and how much of the linen must be changed
Planning	
Plan to change the linen after the patient's hygiene needs have been met.	Reduces the potential for getting the clean linen wet or soiled
Wash your hands; use gloves if there is a potential for direct contact with blood, stool, or other body fluids.	Reduces the transmission of microorganisms
Bring necessary bed linen to the room.	Demonstrates organization and efficient time management

(continued)

SKILL 18-1
Making an Unoccupied Bed (Continued)

Suggested Action	Reason for Action
Place the clean linen on a clean, dry surface such as the back of a chair.	Reduces transmission of microorganisms to clean supplies

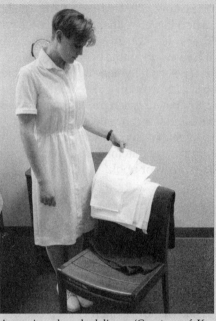

Arranging clean bed linen. (Courtesy of Ken Timby.)

Suggested Action	Reason for Action
Assist the patient from the bed.	Facilitates bedmaking
Implementation	
Raise the bed to a high position and lower all side rails.	Prevents back strain
Remove equipment attached to the bed linens such as the signal cord and drainage tubes, and check for personal items.	Avoids breakage, accidental spills, or loss of personal items
Loosen the bed linen from where it has been tucked under the mattress.	Facilitates removal or retightening
Fold any linen that may be reused and place it on a clean surface.	Promotes efficiency and orderliness

(continued)

SKILL 18-1
Making an Unoccupied Bed (Continued)

Suggested Action	Reason for Action
Roll linen that will be replaced so that the soiled surface is enclosed.	Reduces contact with sources of microorganisms

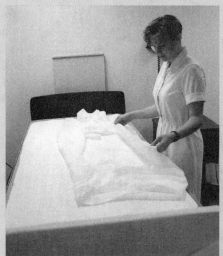

Enclosing soiled side of linen. (Courtesy of Ken Timby.)

Suggested Action	Reason for Action
Remove the soiled linen while holding it away from your uniform.	Prevents transferring microorganisms to your uniform and then to other patients

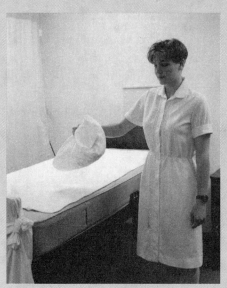

Avoiding contact with uniform. (Courtesy of Ken Timby.)

(continued)

SKILL 18-1
Making an Unoccupied Bed (Continued)

Suggested Action	Reason for Action
Place the soiled linen directly into a pillow case, laundry hamper, or self-made pouch from one of the removed sheets. *Do not place the soiled linen on the floor.*	Keeps the soiled linen from being further contaminated

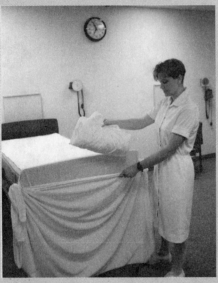

Placing soiled linen in temporary hamper. (Courtesy of Ken Timby.)

Suggested Action	Reason for Action
Remove gloves and wash your hands once the potential for contact with body secretions is no longer likely.	Facilitates use of the hands
Reposition the mattress so it is flush with the headboard.	Provides maximum foot room
Tighten any linen that will be reused.	Removes wrinkles, which promotes patient comfort

(continued)

SKILL 18-1
Making an Unoccupied Bed (Continued)

Suggested Action	Reason for Action
If the bottom sheet is in need of changing, center the longitudinal fold and open the layers of folded linen to one side of the bed.	Reduces back strain

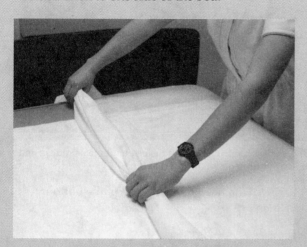

Centering the linen. (Courtesy of Ken Timby.)

If using a flat sheet, make sure that the flat edge of the hem is flush with the edge of the mattress at the foot end.	Prevents skin pressure and irritation

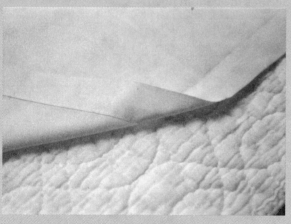

Positioning the hem. (Courtesy of Ken Timby.)

Tuck the upper portion of the sheet under the mattress, or if a fitted sheet is used, position the upper and lower corners of the mattress within the contoured corners of the sheet.	Anchors the bottom sheet

(continued)

Suggested Action	Reason for Action
Make a mitered or square corner at the top of the bed if a flat sheet is used.	Secures the bottom sheet

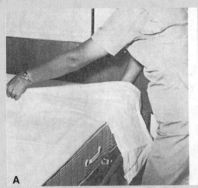
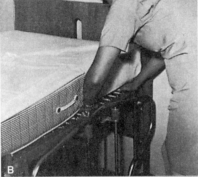
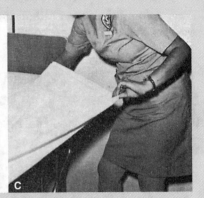

(*A*) Fold the edge of the sheet back on itself, forming a triangle; (*B*) tuck the edge hanging from the bed under the mattress; and (*C*) follow by tucking the remaining sheet under the mattress, preserving the mitered triangle at the corner.

If the patient is apt to soil the linen with urine or stool, fold a flat sheet horizontally, and tuck it in place approximately where the buttocks will be located. Do the same if a draw sheet is available.	Reduces the need to change all of the bottom linen
Position the top linen on one half of the bed at this time or wait until all of the bottom linen has been secured.	Saves time by reducing the number of moves about the bed
Move to the other side of the bed, pull the linen taut, and tuck the free edges beneath the mattress.	Secures the bottom linen

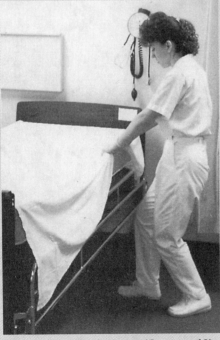

Pulling the bottom sheet taut. (Courtesy of Ken Timby.)

(continued)

SKILL 18-1
Making an Unoccupied Bed *(Continued)*

Suggested Action	Reason for Action
Center the top sheet and unfold it to one side, leaving sufficient length at the top for making a fold over the spread.	Provides a smooth edge next to the patient's neck
Add blankets if the patient wishes.	Demonstrates concern for the patient's comfort
Make a toe pleat by folding a small vertical or horizontal envelope of sheet near the bottom of the mattress.	Keeps pressure off the toes

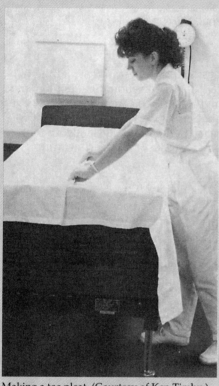

Making a toe pleat. (Courtesy of Ken Timby.)

Suggested Action	Reason for Action
Cover the top sheet with the spread, tuck the excess linen under the bottom of the mattress, and finish with a mitered or square corner.	Secures the top linen

(continued)

SKILL 18-1
Making an Unoccupied Bed (Continued)

Suggested Action	Reason for Action
Gather the pillow case as you would hosiery, and slip the case over the pillow.	Prevents contact between the pillow and your uniform

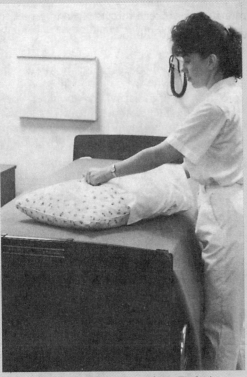

Covering the pillow. (Courtesy of Ken Timby.)

Suggested Action	Reason for Action
Place the pillow at the head of the bed with the open end away from the door and the seam of the pillowcase toward the headboard.	Presents a tidy view of the room from the hallway; prevents pressure on the skin around the head and neck

(continued)

SKILL 18-1
Making an Unoccupied Bed *(Continued)*

Suggested Action	Reason for Action
Fanfold or piefold the top linen toward the foot of the bed.	Facilitates returning to bed

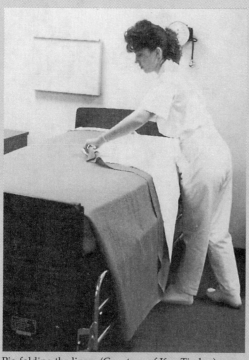

Pie-folding the linen. (Courtesy of Ken Timby.)

SKILL 18-1
Making an Unoccupied Bed *(Continued)*

Suggested Action	Reason for Action
Secure the signal device on or to the bed.	Ensures that the patient can request nursing assistance

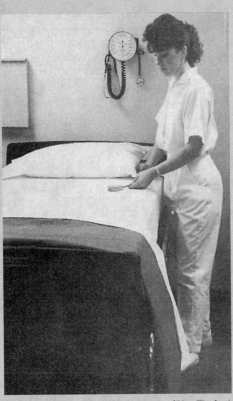

Attaching the signal cord. (Courtesy of Ken Timby.)

Suggested Action	Reason for Action
Adjust the bed to a low position.	Enables the patient to return to bed
Wash your hands.	Reduces the transmission of microorganisms

Evaluation
- The bed is clean and dry
- The linen is free of wrinkles
- The environment is orderly
- The patient feels comfortable

Document
- Date and time
- Characteristics of drainage if present
- Any unique measures taken to ensure patient comfort

Sample Documentation

Date and Time   Menses established. Bed linen changed while shower taken. Given a supply of sanitary napkins. Absorbent pad placed over bottom sheet. _____ **Signature, Title**

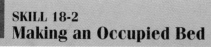

SKILL 18-2
Making an Occupied Bed

Suggested Action	Reason for Action
Assessment	
Check the Kardex or nursing care plan to confirm that the patient must remain in bed.	Demonstrates compliance with the plan for care
Assess the patient's level of consciousness, physical strength, breathing pattern, heart rate, and blood pressure.	Indicates a need for bed rest if abnormal findings are noted, regardless of whether it has been prescribed
Inspect the linen for moisture or evidence of soiling.	Indicates what and how much of the linen must be changed
Determine who might be available to assist if the patient is too weak or unable to cooperate.	Avoids injury and ensures the comfort and safety of the patient
Planning	
Plan to change the linen after the patient's hygiene needs have been met.	Reduces the potential for getting the clean linen wet or soiled
Wash your hands; use gloves if there is a potential for direct contact with blood, stool, or other body fluids	Reduces the transmission of microorganisms
Bring necessary bed linen to the room.	Demonstrates organization and efficient time management
Place the clean linen on a clean, dry surface such as the back of a chair.	Reduces transmission of microorganisms to clean supplies
Implementation	
Explain what you plan to do.	Informs the patient and promotes cooperation
Raise the bed to a high position.	Prevents back strain
Cover the patient with a bath blanket or leave the top sheet loosened, but in place.	Maintains warmth and demonstrates respect for modesty
Fold the top sheet or spread if it will be reused and place it on a clean surface.	Promotes efficiency and orderliness
Unfasten equipment attached to the bottom linen and check for personal items.	Avoids breakage, accidental spills, or loss of personal items
Loosen the bed linen from where it has been tucked under the mattress.	Facilitates removal or retightening
Lower the side rail on the side of the bed where you are standing and roll the patient toward the side rail on the far side of the bed.	Provides room for making the bed while ensuring the safety of the patient

(continued)

SKILL 18-2
Making an Occupied Bed (Continued)

Suggested Action	Reason for Action
Roll the soiled bottom sheets as close to the patient as possible.	Facilitates removal

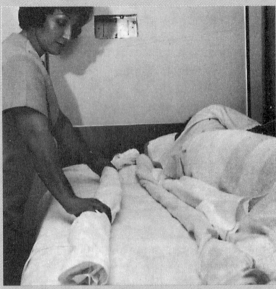

Changing linen on half of the bed.

Suggested Action	Reason for Action
Proceed to unfold and tuck the bottom sheet and drawsheet on the vacant side of the bed, as described in Skill 18-1.	Remakes half of the bed with clean linen
Fold the free edges of the sheet under the folded portion of the soiled sheets.	Keeps the clean sheet from becoming soiled; facilitates pulling the sheets from under the patient
Raise the side rail and move to the opposite side of the bed.	Prevents back strain
Lower the side rail in your new position and help the patient roll over the mound of sheets.	Helps reposition the patient on the clean side of the bed
Pull the soiled laundry close to the edge of the bed and the clean linen close beside it.	Reduces the mound of linen in the center of the bed
Remove the soiled linen and place it into a pillow case or pouch that is off the floor.	Keeps the soiled linen from becoming further contaminated

(continued)

SKILL 18-2
Making an Occupied Bed *(Continued)*

Suggested Action	Reason for Action
Pull the clean bottom sheet until it is unfolded from beneath the patient.	Promotes patient comfort

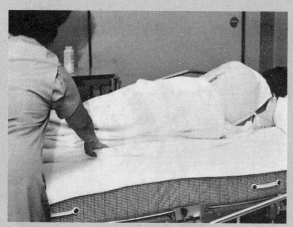

Pulling clean linen through.

Suggested Action	Reason for Action
Miter or square the upper corner of the sheet; pull and tuck the free edges under the mattress.	Secures the clean sheets
Assist the patient to the middle of the bed.	Ensures comfort and safety
Straighten or replace the top sheet, blankets, and spread; remove and replace the pillowcase if necessary.	Restores comfort and orderliness to the environment
Reposition the patient according to the therapeutic regimen or comfort.	Demonstrates compliance with the plan for care; shows concern for the patient's comfort
Lower the height of the bed and raise the remaining side rail if that is appropriate.	Reduces the potential for injury
Dispose of the soiled linen in a laundry hamper outside the room.	Restores order to the room and ensures that the linen is deposited where it will be collected for laundering
Wash your hands.	Reduces the transmission of microorganisms

Evaluation
- The bed is clean and dry
- The linen is free of wrinkles
- The environment is orderly
- The patient feels comfortable

Document
- Date and time
- Characteristics of drainage if present
- Measures taken to ensure patient comfort

Sample Documentation

Date and Time   Unresponsive even to painful stimuli. Complete bed bath given followed by linen change. Repositioned on L side with head at a 45° elevation. Full side rails raised. Bed in low position._____ **Signature, Title**

ination utensils separate from hygiene supplies to reduce the transmission of microorganisms. A carafe of water and drinking glass are often placed on top of the bedside stand.

CHAIRS

There is usually at least one chair per patient in each room. Hospital chairs usually are straight-backed to facilitate good postural support. The best sitting position is when the hips, knees, and ankles are all at 90° angles.

There may be one upholstered chair in each patient room. Although upholstered chairs are more comfortable, some patients find that rising from them is quite difficult.

However, no matter how comfortable the physical environment or how attractive and home-like the furnishings, recuperation may be sabotaged or prolonged by failing to relieve patients' pain adequately.

PAIN

Pain is an unpleasant sensation usually associated with disease or injury, but it also has an emotional component referred to as **suffering**. Because there is no effective method for validating or invalidating pain, Margo McCaffery (McCaffery & Beebe, 1989), a nursing expert on pain, probably defined pain best as being "whatever the person says it is, and existing whenever the person says it does."

Understanding how pain is produced and perceived, however, is essential to finding mechanisms for its relief.

Pain Transmission

The transmission of pain begins with some type of injury that stimulates nerve receptors called **nociceptors**. Nociceptors transmit the pain impulse using various neurochemicals over spinal pathways to the brain (Fig. 18-3).

Pain Perception

Pain perception, the conscious experience of discomfort, occurs when the pain threshold is reached. The **pain threshold** is the point at which the pain transmitting neurochemicals reach the brain, causing conscious awareness. Pain thresholds tend to be the same among healthy people. But for whatever reasons, people tolerate or bear the sensation of pain differently. **Pain tolerance** is the amount of pain a person endures once the threshold has been reached. Pain tolerance is often influenced by learned behaviors that are gender, age, and culture specific (see Chap. 6).

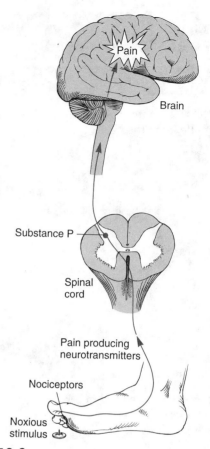

FIGURE 18-3
Pain transmission pathway.

Pain Theories

There are several theories that attempt to explain how pain is transmitted and the bases for pain-relieving mechanisms; no one theory seems to be all-encompassing. One that seems to have attracted a great deal of interest, however, is the gate control theory (Melzack & Wall, 1965).

GATE CONTROL THEORY

The **gate control theory** proposes that spinal pathways conduct several types of cutaneous (skin) sensations to the brain, but they can conduct only one at a time. When they are occupied in transmitting one sensation, the "gates" are closed to others (Fig. 18-4). The brain, therefore, does not perceive pain while it is preoccupied with other sensory input. This helps to explain how massage, vibration, pressure, heat, cold, and other nondrug mechanisms reduce pain perception.

Another mechanism for diminishing the perception of pain is endogenous opioids.

ENDOGENOUS OPIOIDS

Endogenous opioids are naturally produced, morphine-like chemicals called *endorphins, dynorphins,* and *enkephalins* that reduce pain. When released, they are

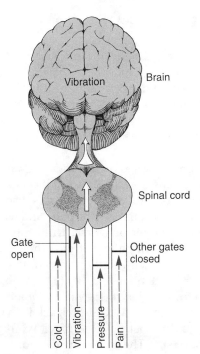

FIGURE 18-4
Gate-control theory.

thought to bind with sites on the nerve cell's membrane that block the transmission of pain-producing neurotransmitters (Fig. 18-5). They may also interfere with the nociceptive transmitter known as *substance P*, which is essential for continuing the transmission of the pain sensation from the spinal cord to the brain (Bullock & Rosendahl, 1992; Copstead, 1995).

Despite the accumulating knowledge about the physiology of pain, one of the unexplained phenomena is why there are different types of pain.

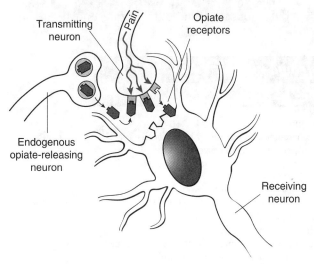

FIGURE 18-5
Mechanism of pain transmission and interference.

TYPES OF PAIN

Several types of pain have been described according to their source and duration. Sources of pain are differentiated as being either cutaneous, visceral, or neuropathic, whereas pain may be subdivided into acute and chronic depending on its duration.

Cutaneous Pain

Cutaneous pain originates at the skin level, and the depth of the trauma determines the type of sensation that is experienced. According to Bullock and Rosendahl (1992), damage confined to the epidermis produces sensations of itching and burning. At the dermis level, the pain is localized and superficial. Subcutaneous tissue injuries produce an aching, throbbing type of pain. **Somatic pain** is generated from deeper connective tissue structures such as muscles, tendons, and joints.

Visceral Pain

Visceral pain arises from internal organs that are diseased or injured. It tends, in some cases, to be referred or poorly localized. **Referred pain** is a term used to describe the discomfort that is perceived in a general area of the body, but not in the exact site where an organ is anatomically located (Fig. 18-6). Visceral pain also may be accompanied by other autonomic nervous system symptoms such as nausea, vomiting, pallor, hypotension, and sweating.

Neuropathic Pain

Neuropathic pain, also called functional or psychogenic, is pain with atypical characteristics. This type of pain is often experienced days, weeks, or even months after the source of the pain has been treated and resolved (Copstead, 1995). This leads some to speculate that there is a dysfunctional chemical message that is being transmitted to the brain.

One example of neuropathic pain is *phantom limb pain* and *phantom limb sensation*, in which people with amputated limbs perceive that the limb still exists and that disturbing sensations such as burning, itching, and deep pain are located in tissues that have been surgically removed.

Acute Versus Chronic Pain

Regardless of its source, pain may vary according to its duration. **Acute pain** has a short duration, whereas **chronic pain** lasts longer than 6 months. Either type may be intermittent, meaning there are periods of relief. However, duration is not the only characteristic that differentiates acute from chronic pain (Table 18-1).

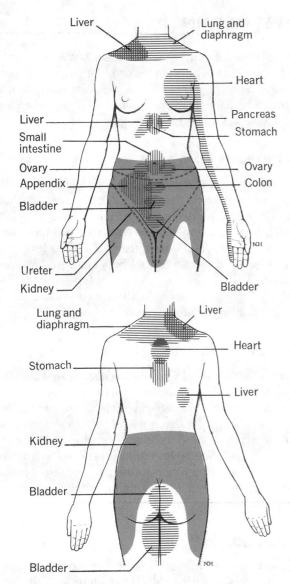

FIGURE 18-6
Areas of referred pain. (*Top*) Anterior view. (*Bottom*) Posterior view. (Chaffee, EE, & Lytle, IM: Basic Physiology and Anatomy, 4th ed., p. 266. Philadelphia: JB Lippincott, 1980)

PAIN ASSESSMENT

According to the American Pain Society (1992), "the most common reason for unrelieved pain in U.S. hospitals is the failure of staff to routinely assess pain and pain relief." Because there are no machines or laboratory tests that can measure pain, nurses are limited to the subjective information only patients can supply.

A full pain assessment includes the patient's description of its *onset*, *quality*, *intensity*, *location*, and *duration* (Table 18-2). In addition, nurses also ask what other symptoms accompany the pain, and what, if anything, makes it better or worse. Unfortunately, there are several groups of patients from whom assessment data cannot always be validly obtained (Display 18-1).

Pain disorder clinics ask patients to complete a self-assessment to help identify the unique qualities of their pain (Fig. 18-7). In the McGill-Melzack Pain Questionnaire, patients are instructed to check words that best describe their pain. The words are categorized according to the qualities of the pain, and are assigned a numeric value as well. The total score quantifies the severity of the patient's pain. By comparing changes in the number and types of word choices, therapists can evaluate whether patients are improving.

Assessment Techniques

The following are four techniques that may be used for quantifying a patient's pain intensity:

1. Using a *numeric scale*, patients are asked to select a number between 0 to 10 that best correlates with their pain, with 0 being the equivalent of no pain and 10 being the worst pain.
2. With a *word scale*, patients select from categories like none, little, mild, moderate, and severe.

TABLE 18-1. *Characteristics of Acute and Chronic Pain*	
Acute Pain	**Chronic Pain**
Recent onset	Remote onset
Symptomatic of primary injury or disease	Uncharacteristic of primary injury or disease
Specific and localized	Nonspecific and generalized
Severity is associated with the acuity of the injury or disease process	Severity is out of proportion to the stage of the injury or disease
Favorable response to drug therapy	Poor response to drug therapy
Requires less and less drug therapy	Requires more and more drug therapy
Diminishes with healing	Persists beyond healing stage
Suffering is decreased	Suffering is intensified
Associated with sympathetic nervous system responses like hypertension, tachycardia, restlessness, anxiety	Absence of autonomic nervous system responses; manifests depression and irritability

TABLE 18-2. *Components of Pain Assessment*

Characteristic	Description	Examples
Onset	The time or circumstances under which the pain became apparent	After eating, while shoveling snow, during the night
Quality	The sensory experiences and degree of suffering	Throbbing, crushing, agonizing, annoying
Intensity	The magnitude of the pain	None, slight, mild, moderate, severe; or numeric scale from 0 to 10
Location	The anatomic site	Chest, abdomen, jaw
Duration	Time span of pain	Continuous, intermittent, hours, weeks, months

3. A *linear scale* uses a line or continuum with one end labeled "no pain" and the other labeled "worst pain." Patients are asked to indicate where their pain fits on the line.
4. A *picture scale*, showing a series of faces from smiling to crying, may be used for children younger than 7 years of age.

Nurses also observe for pain behaviors, especially in patients who do not verbalize much about their pain. Clues that pain is being experienced include grimacing, lying still, and reluctance to breathe deeply, turn, or cough. In addition, autonomic nervous system responses may be apparent, such as tachycardia, hypertension, dilated pupils, perspiration, pallor, rapid and shallow breathing, urinary retention, reduced bowel motility, and elevated blood glucose levels. Patients with chronic pain, however, are not apt to manifest autonomic nervous system responses.

Assessment Standards

To ensure quality of care, Donovan and Miaskowski (1992) recommend that pain assessments be routinely performed, but not limited to:

DISPLAY 18-1. *Underassessed and Undertreated Pain Populations*

- Infants
- Children younger than 7 years of age
- Culturally diverse patients
- Mentally challenged (retarded) patients
- Patients with dementia (diminished brain function)
- Hearing- or speech-impaired patients
- Psychologically disturbed patients

- When patients are admitted
- After each potentially painful procedure or treatment
- At least once per shift when pain is an actual or potential problem
- When patients are at rest, as well as when involved in a nursing activity
- Before implementing a pain management intervention, like administering an **analgesic** (pain-relieving) drug, and 30 minutes after its implementation

All pain assessment findings are documented in the medical record.

PAIN MANAGEMENT

Pain management refers to the techniques used to prevent, reduce, or relieve pain. To demonstrate the importance of managing pain, the Joint Commission on Accreditation of Health Organizations (JCAHO) now requires evidence that the pain of terminally ill patients is being adequately treated (Donovan & Miaskowski, 1992). Also, as of 1992, the American Pain Society, working actively with the Agency for Health Care Policy and Research (AHCPR), a division of the United States Department of Health and Human Services, developed *Standards for the Relief of Acute Pain and Cancer Pain* (Display 18-2). The objective of this collaborative effort has been to improve the manner in which pain is assessed and controlled.

Approaches to Pain Management

There are four general approaches to pain management, any one or combination of which may be used in patient care (Table 18-3).

DRUG THERAPY

Nonopioid (non-narcotic), opioid (narcotic) drugs, and combinations of drug categories are a cornerstone

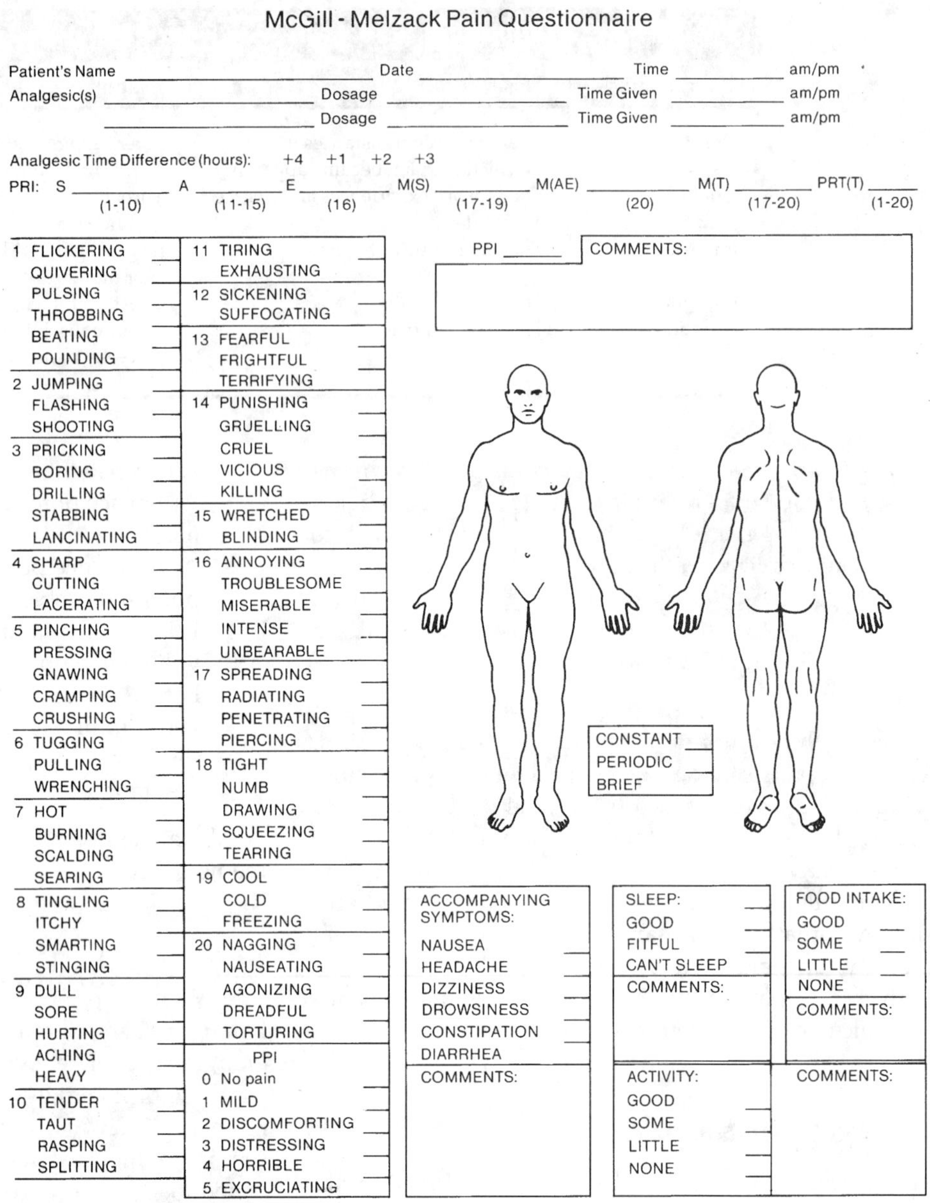

McGill - Melzack Pain Questionnaire

Patient's Name _____ Date _____ Time _____ am/pm
Analgesic(s) _____ Dosage _____ Time Given _____ am/pm
              _____ Dosage _____ Time Given _____ am/pm

Analgesic Time Difference (hours):   +4   +1   +2   +3

PRI: S _____ A _____ E _____ M(S) _____ M(AE) _____ M(T) _____ PRT(T) _____
         (1-10)   (11-15)   (16)   (17-19)   (20)   (17-20)   (1-20)

1 FLICKERING	11 TIRING
QUIVERING	EXHAUSTING
PULSING	12 SICKENING
THROBBING	SUFFOCATING
BEATING	13 FEARFUL
POUNDING	FRIGHTFUL
2 JUMPING	TERRIFYING
FLASHING	14 PUNISHING
SHOOTING	GRUELLING
3 PRICKING	CRUEL
BORING	VICIOUS
DRILLING	KILLING
STABBING	15 WRETCHED
LANCINATING	BLINDING
4 SHARP	16 ANNOYING
CUTTING	TROUBLESOME
LACERATING	MISERABLE
5 PINCHING	INTENSE
PRESSING	UNBEARABLE
GNAWING	17 SPREADING
CRAMPING	RADIATING
CRUSHING	PENETRATING
6 TUGGING	PIERCING
PULLING	18 TIGHT
WRENCHING	NUMB
7 HOT	DRAWING
BURNING	SQUEEZING
SCALDING	TEARING
SEARING	19 COOL
8 TINGLING	COLD
ITCHY	FREEZING
SMARTING	20 NAGGING
STINGING	NAUSEATING
9 DULL	AGONIZING
SORE	DREADFUL
HURTING	TORTURING
ACHING	PPI
HEAVY	0 No pain
10 TENDER	1 MILD
TAUT	2 DISCOMFORTING
RASPING	3 DISTRESSING
SPLITTING	4 HORRIBLE
	5 EXCRUCIATING

PPI _____   COMMENTS:

CONSTANT
PERIODIC
BRIEF

ACCOMPANYING SYMPTOMS:	SLEEP:	FOOD INTAKE:
NAUSEA	GOOD	GOOD
HEADACHE	FITFUL	SOME
DIZZINESS	CAN'T SLEEP	LITTLE
DROWSINESS	COMMENTS:	NONE
CONSTIPATION		COMMENTS:
DIARRHEA		
COMMENTS:	ACTIVITY:	COMMENTS:
	GOOD	
	SOME	
	LITTLE	
	NONE	

FIGURE 18-7
People with chronic pain may use this questionnaire or one like it to evaluate their pain.

of the treatment plan for managing pain, and nurses must be familiar with the indications for their use. The World Health Organization (1990) recommends following a three-tiered approach according to the patient's pain intensity and response to selected drug therapy (Fig. 18-8).

NURSING GUIDELINES FOR MANAGING PAIN

- Never doubt the patient's description of pain or need for relief.
  Rationale: Eliminates the possibility of bias, which may lead to withholding prescribed medication or undertreating the patient's symptoms
- Follow the written medical orders for administering pain medications.
  Rationale: Demonstrates compliance with nurse practice acts
- Administer pain-relieving drugs as soon as the need becomes evident.
  Rationale: Reduces needless suffering
- Consult the physician if the current drug therapy is not adequately controlling the patient's pain.
  Rationale: Demonstrates patient advocacy
- Collaborate with the physician on developing several pain management options based on combinations of drugs, alternative routes of drug administration, and dosing schedules.

DISPLAY 18-2. *Standards for the Relief of Acute Pain and Cancer Pain*

Standard I
Acute pain and cancer pain are recognized and effectively treated.

Standard II
Information about analgesics is readily available.

Standard III
Patients are informed on admission, both orally and in writing, that effective pain relief is an important part of their treatment, that their communication of unrelieved pain is essential, and that health professionals will respond quickly to their reports of pain.

Standard IV
Explicit policies for use of advanced analgesic technologies are defined.

Standard V
Adherence to standards is monitored by an interdisciplinary committee.

Reprinted with permission from American Pain Society, Principles of Analgesic Use in the Treatment of Acute Pain and Chronic Cancer Pain. Skokie, Illinois, 1992.

Rationale: Facilitates individualizing pain management

- Support the formation of an interdisciplinary pain management committee consisting of physicians, surgeons, nurses, pharmacists, anesthesiologists, and social workers who may be consulted on hard-to-manage pain problems.
  Rationale: Provides expertise from a variety of practitioners
- Administer pain medication before an activity that produces or intensifies pain.
  Rationale: Prevents pain, which is much easier than treating it
- Administer analgesic drugs on a scheduled basis rather than irregularly when the patient's pain is continuous.
  Rationale: Controls pain at lower levels of intensity
- Monitor for drug side effects such as respiratory depression, decreased levels of consciousness, nausea, vomiting, and constipation.
  Rationale: Demonstrates concern for the patient's safety and comfort
- Consult the professional literature or experts on the equianalgesic dose of a drug when changing from a parenteral (injectable) to an oral route. An **equianalgesic dose** is the adjusted oral dose that provides the same level of pain management as that provided when given by a parenteral route (Table 18-4).
  Rationale: Prevents undertreatment of pain as a result of changes in drug absorption or drug metabolism
- Change the patient's position, elevate a swollen limb to reduce swelling, loosen a tight dressing, and assist the patient with bowel or bladder elimination.
  Rationale: Reduces factors that intensify the pain experience
- Use nondrug interventions such as patient teaching, relaxation, music, biofeedback, imagery, and transcutaneous electrical nerve stimulation (TENS; discussed later) as additional techniques for pain management.
  Rationale: Reduces mild to moderate pain when used alone, or potentiates pain management outcomes when combined with drug therapy
- Space periods of rest between activities.
  Rationale: Prevents exhaustion, which reduces the patient's ability to cope with pain

In some cases, patients themselves are being given an opportunity to manage their own pain using intravenous infusion technology.

TABLE 18-3. *Approaches to Pain Management*

Approach	Intervention	Example(s)
Interrupting pain-transmitting chemicals at the site of injury	Local anesthetics, anti-inflammatory drugs	Procaine, lidocaine, aspirin, ibuprofen, acetaminophen, naproxen, indomethacin
Altering transmissions at the spinal cord	Intraspinal anesthesia and analgesia, neurosurgery	Epidural, caudal, rhizotomy, cordotomy, sympathectomy
Using gate-closing mechanisms	Cutaneous stimuli	Massage, acupuncture, acupressure, heat, cold, therapeutic touch, electrical stimulation
Blocking brain perception	Narcotics, nondrug techniques	Morphine, codeine, hypnosis, imagery, distraction

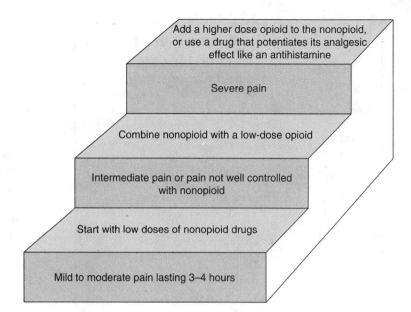

FIGURE 18-8
World Health Organization (WHO) analgesic ladder. (World Health Organization Expert Committee. Cancer pain relief and palliative care. WHO, Geneva, Switzerland, 1990)

Patient-Controlled Analgesia

Patient-controlled analgesia (PCA) is an intervention that allows patients to self-administer pain medication intravenously by using an infusion device. The infusion device is programed by the nurse so that the patient can receive a low drug dose at frequent intervals according to his or her level of discomfort (Skill 18-3). Once a dose is delivered, patients cannot readminister another dose for a safe period of time, which prevents overdoses.

The use of a PCA infuser has several advantages for both patients and nurses:

- Pain relief is rapidly experienced because the drug is delivered intravenously.
- Pain is controlled within a constant tolerable level (Fig. 18-9).

- Less narcotic is actually used because the patient's discomfort is continuously controlled with small doses.
- Patients are spared the discomfort of repeated injections.
- Anxiety is reduced because pain relief is not dependent on waiting while a nurse prepares and administers an injection.
- Drug side effects are reduced with smaller individual dosages and lower total dosages.
- Patients tend to ambulate and move about more, which reduces their potential for complications associated with immobility.
- Patients are able to take an active role in their pain management.
- PCA frees the nurse to carry out other nursing responsibilities.

Patient-controlled analgesia infusers are used primarily to relieve acute pain after surgery. However, this technology is finding its way into the home health arena, where it is being used by patients who have cancer.

NONDRUG INTERVENTIONS

There are several additional interventions that may assist with managing pain. Some, like education and TENS, can be easily implemented by nurses. Others, like acupuncture and acupressure, biofeedback, and hypnosis require consultation with people who have specialized training and expertise. These latter interventions are more likely to be used for patients with chronic pain or those for whom acute pain management techniques are unsuccessful or contraindicated.

TABLE 18-4. *Adult Equianalgesic Doses*		
Drug	Parenteral Dose	Oral Dose
Morphine sulfate	10 mg q 3–4 hr	30 mg q 3–4 hr
Meperidine (Demerol*)	100 mg q 3 hr	300 mg q 2–3 hr
Hydromorphone (Dilaudid†)	1.5 mg q 3–4 hr	7.5 mg q 3–4 hr
Pentazocine (Talwin*)	60 mg q 3–4 hr	150 mg q 3–4 hr

* Winthrop Pharmaceuticals, New York, NY.
† Knoll Pharmaceutical Co., Whippany, NJ.
Adapted from HHS/AHCPR Clinical Practice Guideline for Acute Pain Management: Operative or Medical Procedures and Trauma, Rockville, MD: Public Health Service, 1991.

SKILL 18-3
Preparing a Patient-Controlled Analgesia (PCA) Infuser

Suggested Action	Reason for Action
Assessment	
Check the written medical order for the use of a PCA infusion device, the prescribed drug, initial loading dose, the dose per self-administration, and the lockout interval.	Provides data for programming the infusion device
Check the patient's wristband.	Prevents medication errors
Assess what the patient understands about PCA.	Indicates the type and amount of teaching that must be provided
Check that the currently infusing intravenous (IV) solution is compatible with the prescribed analgesic.	Avoids incompatibility reactions
Planning	
Obtain the following equipment: infuser, PCA tubing, prefilled medication container.	Promotes organization and efficient time management
Plug the power cord into the electrical wall outlet.	Prolongs the life of the battery
Explain the equipment and how it functions.	Reduces anxiety and promotes independence
Implementation	
Wash your hands.	Reduces the transmission of microorganisms
Attach the PCA tubing to the assembled syringe.	Provides a pathway for delivering the medication

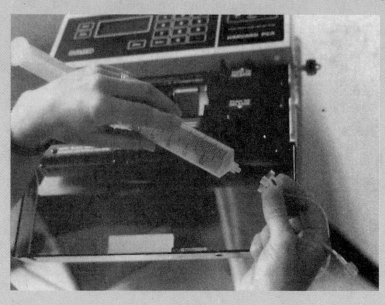

Connecting tubing. (Courtesy of Ken Timby.)

(continued)

SKILL 18-3
Preparing a Patient-Controlled Analgesia (PCA) Infuser (Continued)

Suggested Action	Reason for Action
Open the cover or door of the infuser and load the syringe into its cradle.	Stabilizes the syringe within the infuser

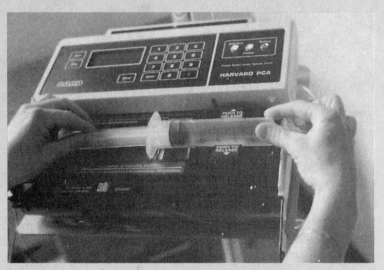

Loading the syringe. (Courtesy of Ken Timby.)

| Fill the PCA tubing with fluid. | Displaces air from the tubing |

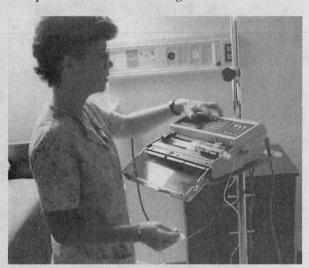

Purging air from tubing. (Courtesy of Ken Timby.)

(continued)

SKILL 18-3
Preparing a Patient-Controlled Analgesia (PCA) Infuser *(Continued)*

Suggested Action	Reason for Action
Connect the PCA tubing to the IV tubing.	Facilitates intermittent administration of medication
Assess the patient's pain.	Provides data from which to evaluate the drug's effectiveness
Set the volume for the prescribed loading dose and administer it to the patient.	Administers a slightly larger dose of the drug to establish a reduced level of pain rather quickly
Program the infuser according to the individual dose and lockout period.	Prevents overdosing
Close the security door and lock it with a key.	Prevents tampering

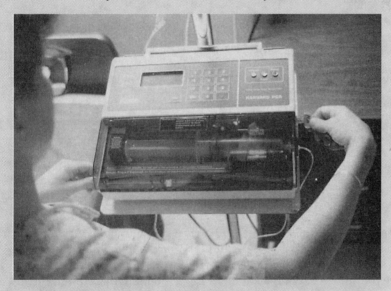

Locking the infuser. (Courtesy of Ken Timby.)

Instruct the patient to press and release the control button each time pain relief is needed.	Educates the patient on how to operate the equipment

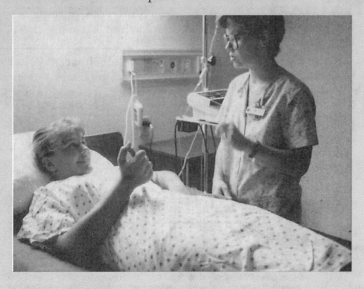

Explaining use. (Courtesy of Ken Timby.)

(continued)

SKILL 18-3
Preparing a Patient-Controlled Analgesia (PCA) Infuser (Continued)

Suggested Action	Reason for Action
Explain that a bell will sound when the infuser delivers medication.	Provides sensory reinforcement that the machine is working
Assess the patient's pain at least every 2 hours.	Complies with standards of care
Replace the medication syringe when it becomes empty.	Maintains continuous pain management
Change the primary IV solution container every 24 hours.	Complies with infection control policies

Evaluation
* The patient self-administers pain medication
* The patient's pain is controlled

Document
* Date and time
* Volume and type of analgesic solution
* Name of analgesic drug
* Initial pain assessment
* Loading dose
* Individual dose and time schedule
* Reassessments of pain
* Total volume self-administered per shift

Sample Documentation

Date and Time   30 mL syringe of saline c̄ 30 mg of morphine sulfate inserted within PCA pump. Describes pain around abdominal incision as continuous and stabbing. Rates the pain at a level of 7 on a scale of 0 to 10. Loading dose of 2 mg administered. Infuser programmed to deliver 0.1 mL—the equivalent of 0.1 mg at no more than 10-minute intervals. Rates pain at a level of 5 within 10 minutes after loading dose. Instructed and observed to self-administer a subsequent dose. _____ **Signature, Title**

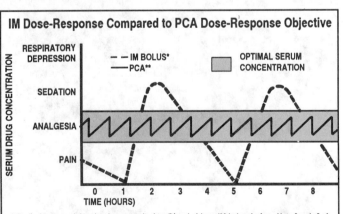

FIGURE 18-9

Pain is managed more effectively with patient-controlled analgesia (PCA) than with intramuscular (IM) analgesic administrations. (Adapted from White PF: Use of patient controlled analgesia infuser for the management of post-operative pain. In: Hormer M, Rosen M, Vickers MD, Eds. Patient-Controlled Analgesia. St. Louis, CV Mosby [Blackwell Scientific], 1985)

PATIENT TEACHING REGARDING PAIN AND ITS MANAGEMENT

Teach the patient or the family to do the following:
- Ask your doctor what to expect from the disorder or its treatment.
- Discuss pain control methods that have worked well or not so well before.
- Talk with your doctor and nurses about any concerns you may have about pain medicine.
- Identify any drug allergies you may have.
- Inform your doctor and nurses about other medicines you take in case they may interact with pain medications.
- Help your doctor and nurses "measure" your pain by reporting a number or word that best describes the pain.
- Ask for or take pain-relieving drugs when pain first begins or before an activity that causes pain.
- Set a pain control goal, such as having no pain worse than 4 on a scale of 0 to 10.
- Inform your doctor and nurses if the pain medication is not working.
- Perform simple techniques like abdominal breathing and jaw relaxation to increase your comfort.
- Consult with your doctor or nurses about the possibility of using cold or hot packs or other nondrug techniques that may enhance pain control.

Education

Educating patients about pain and methods for pain management supports the principle that patients who assume an active role in their treatment achieve positive patient outcomes sooner than others. Therefore, it is essential to include pain education whenever there is a realistic need for it.

Another point to stress during teaching is that patients should not expect to be totally pain free, but they should not have to endure severe pain either.

Transcutaneous Electrical Nerve Stimulation

Transcutaneous electrical nerve stimulation is a pain management technique that delivers bursts of electricity to the skin and underlying nerves (Skill 18-4). The electrical stimulus is perceived by the patient as being a pleasant tapping, tingling, vibrating, or buzzing sensation generated by a battery-powered stimulator.

Transcutaneous electrical nerve stimulation may be used intermittently for 15 to 30 minutes or longer

SKILL 18-4
Operating A Transcutaneous Electrical Nerve Stimulation (TENS) Unit

Suggested Action	Reason for Action
Assessment	
Check the written medical order for providing the patient with a TENS unit.	Demonstrates collaboration with the medical management of patient care
Ask the physician or physical therapist about the best location for electrode placement. Some possible variations include:	Optimizes pain management by individualizing electrode placement
• On or near the painful site	
• On either side of an incision	
• Over cutaneous nerves	
• Over a joint	
Read the patient's history to determine if there are any conditions for which the use of a TENS unit is contraindicated.	Demonstrates concern for the patient's safety
Check the patient's wristband.	Prevents errors
Assess what the patient understands about TENS.	Indicates the type and amount of teaching that must be provided

(continued)

SKILL 18-4
Operating A Transcutaneous Electrical Nerve Stimulation (TENS) Unit (Continued)

Suggested Action	Reason for Action
Planning	
Obtain the following equipment: TENS unit and two to four self-adhesive electrodes.	Promotes organization and efficient time management
Explain the equipment and how it functions.	Reduces anxiety and promotes independence
Establish a goal with the patient for the level of pain management desired.	Aids in evaluating the effectiveness of the intervention
Implementation	
Wash your hands.	Reduces the transmission of microorganisms
Peel the backing from the adhesive side of the electrodes.	Facilitates skin contact
Position each electrode flat against the skin.	Enhances contact with the skin for maximum effectiveness

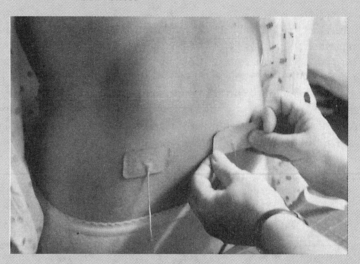

Attaching electrodes. (Courtesy of Ken Timby.)

Suggested Action	Reason for Action
Space the electrodes at least the width of one from the other.	Prevents the potential for burning caused by close proximity of the electrodes
Make sure the settings on the TENS unit are off.	Prevents premature stimulation to the skin
Attach the cord(s) from the electrodes to the outlet jack(s) on the TENS unit, much like a headset connects with a radio.	Completes the circuitry from the electrodes to the battery-operated power unit
Turn the amplitude (intensity) knob on to the lowest setting and assess if the patient can feel a tingling, buzzing, or vibrating sensation.	Helps acquaint the patient with the sensation produced by the TENS unit
Gradually increase the intensity to the point at which the patient experiences a mild or moderately pleasant sensation.	Adjusts intensity according to the patient's response—a high intensity does not always provide the most pain relief; in fact, it may cause discomfort, muscle contractions, or itching

(continued)

SKILL 18-4
Operating A Transcutaneous Electrical Nerve Stimulation (TENS) Unit (Continued)

Suggested Action	Reason for Action

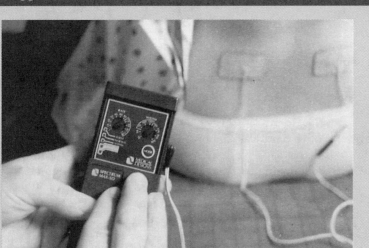

Adjusting the TENS settings. (Courtesy of Ken Timby.)

Suggested Action	Reason for Action
Set the rate (pulses per second) at a low rate and increase upward; a rate of 80 to 125 pulses per second is a conventional setting.	Adjusts the frequency of stimuli according to the patient's comfort and tolerance
Set the pulse width (the duration of each pulsation); a pulse width of 60 to 100 microseconds is usually used for acute pain; but 220 to 250 microseconds at higher amplitudes may be necessary for chronic or intense pain.	Provides wider and deeper stimulation as the pulse width increases
Turn the unit off when a sufficient level of pain relief occurs and turn it back on when pain reappears.	Tests whether the TENS unit may be sufficient for intermittent rather than continuous use
Turn off the unit and remove the cord from the outlet jacks before bathing the patient.	Reduces hazards from potential contact of electrical equipment with water
Remove the electrode patches periodically to inspect the skin; reapply electrodes if they become loose.	Aids in skin assessment
Slightly change the position of the electrodes if skin irritation develops.	Promotes the integrity of the skin
Replace or recharge the batteries as needed.	Maintains function of the unit

Evaluation
- Pain is managed at the goal set by the patient
- Activity is increased
- Less pain medication is required
- Emotional outlook is improved

Document
- Date and time
- Initial pain assessments
- Location of electrodes

(continued)

SKILL 18-4
Operating A Transcutaneous Electrical Nerve Stimulation (TENS) Unit *(Continued)*

Suggested Action	Reason for Action

- Power settings
- Length of time TENS unit is in use
- Reassessments of pain 30 minutes after application of unit and at least once per shift
- Time when TENS is stopped or discontinued

Sample Documentation

Date and Time   Selects the word "severe" from a pain scale of none to severe. Pain is described as "piercing" and continuous. Points to lower spine when asked to identify location of pain. Electrodes placed to the immediate R. and L. of the lumbosacral vertebrae. TENS unit initially set at a rate of 80 pulses per second and a pulse width of 60 microseconds. Used for 30 minutes, at which time rated pain at "moderate." Rate increased to 100 pulses per second with a pulse width of 150. _____ **Signature, Title**

whenever the patient feels a need for it, or on a continuous basis. TENS has been used for patients with chronic pain for some time. More recently, surgical patients are using it. Reports of its effectiveness range from useless to fantastic.

No one is sure how TENS works. Some think the gate control theory explains its effectiveness. Supposedly, the transmission of electrical stimuli over larger myelinated nerves takes precedence over the transmission of pain-producing stimuli to the brain. Others think TENS stimulates the body to release endogenous opioids, whereas others suggest that its success is based on the power of suggestion.

There are several advantages to TENS. It is a nonnarcotic, noninvasive agent without toxic effects. However, it is contraindicated for pregnant women because its effect on the unborn fetus has not been determined. Also, people using cardiac pacemakers (especially the demand type of pacemaker), patients prone to irregular heartbeats, and those having had previous heart attacks are not candidates for TENS.

Acupuncture and Acupressure

Acupuncture is a pain management technique in which long, thin needles are inserted into the skin. **Acupressure** uses tissue compression, rather than needles, to reduce pain. The location for pressure and needle placement is based on 2,000-year-old traditions practiced in Chinese medicine.

Both techniques have been demonstrated to prevent or relieve pain, but their exact analgesic mechanisms are not completely understood. Some speculate that these techniques stimulate the body's production of endogenous opioids. Another theory is that the twisting, vibration, or pressure are forms of cutaneous stimuli

that close the gates to pain-transmitting neurochemicals. Although acupuncture and acupressure are primarily practiced in Asiatic countries, they are becoming more accepted as legitimate forms of pain therapy in the United States.

Biofeedback

Biofeedback is an adjunct to traditional pain-relieving techniques in which a person learns to control or alter some physiologic phenomenon like pain, hypertension, headache, a racing heart, or seizures. Many of the bothersome symptoms that patients wish to alleviate are associated with or aggravated by sympathetic nervous system stimulation.

Initially, the patient is attached to a physiologic sensing instrument like a pulse oximeter or electromyography machine. The instrument produces a visual or audible signal that correlates with the person's heart rate, skin temperature, tension in muscles, and so on. The patient is encouraged to reduce the signal using whatever mechanism he or she can. Usually this is accomplished by physically relaxing the body.

Patients receive "feedback" from the machine, indicating how well they are accomplishing the goal. Eventually, patients may learn to control their symptoms without the assistance of the biofeedback equipment, using self-suggestion alone.

Hypnosis

Hypnosis is a technique in which a person assumes a trance-like state during which perception and memory are altered. During hypnosis, a suggestion may be made that a person's pain will be eliminated or the sensation will be experienced in a more pleasant way.

Although self-hypnosis is possible, more often it is facilitated with the help of a hypnotherapist, some of whom are physicians, dentists, and psychologists. Clinical hypnotherapists receive special clinical training and are certified members of organizations such as the American Society of Clinical Hypnosis or the International Society for Medical and Psychological Hypnosis.

NURSING IMPLICATIONS

Patients who experience discomfort are likely to have one or more of the nursing diagnoses listed in the accompanying Applicable Nursing Diagnoses.

The Nursing Care Plan in this chapter is an example of how the steps in the nursing process have been fol-

APPLICABLE NURSING DIAGNOSES

- Pain
- Chronic Pain
- Anxiety
- Fear
- Ineffective Individual Coping
- Knowledge Deficit: Pain Management

NURSING CARE PLAN:
Pain

Assessment

Subjective Data
States, "It feels like a semi-truck is parked on my chest. I know I must be having a heart attack." Indicates that pain measures 10 on a scale of 1 to 10.

Objective Data
55-year-old man brought to Emergency Department from work. Holds hands over L. precordial area. Rubs L. arm. Perspires profusely. Startles when staff enter room. Pulse is 108 beats/min and irregular. Blood pressure is 148/92. Respirations are 30/min. Elevated ST segment on cardiac rhythm strip.

Diagnosis
Pain related to possible reduction in oxygen to myocardium.

Plan

Goal
That patient will report that his pain is reduced to ≤7 using a 0–10 scale by 9/20.

Orders: 9/19
1. Maintain bed rest.
2. Administer 50% oxygen continuously by mask.
3. Explain all procedures and routines before being performed.
4. Allow wife to remain at bedside as desired.
5. Administer prescribed analgesic as needed. _____ R. VERCLER, RN

Implementation
(Documentation)   9/19
1400   Face mask applied and oxygen administered at 6 liters per minute. Respirations 28 and labored. Placed in high Fowler's position. _____ N. DUNN, RN
1415   States, "I feel tightness and aching from my chest into my neck and L. arm. It's still a 10; please do something." _____ N. DUNN, RN
1420   Nitroglycerin tab given sublingually. Instructed to let tablet remain under tongue for absorption. Explained there may be tingling in the area of the tablet, a headache, and a warm, flushed feeling associated with absorption, but the medication will help more blood get to the heart muscle. Advised to remain in bed for the time being. Wife at bedside holding hands. _____ N. DUNN, RN
1435   1000 mL D5W started IV in L. hand with a #18 angiocath. Running at a keep open rate. No pain relief from nitroglycerin. _____ N. DUNN, RN
1445   Morphine sulfate 4 mg given IV push for chest pain. _____ N. DUNN, RN

Evaluation
(Documentation)
1500   States, "My pain is starting to ease up. It's about an 8½ right now." _____ N. DUNN, RN

lowed when planning the care of a patient with a nursing diagnosis of Pain. Pain is defined in the NANDA taxonomy (1994) as "A state in which an individual experiences and reports the presence of severe discomfort or an uncomfortable sensation."

Despite all the knowledge nurses acquire about pain and its management, one of the leading factors that interferes with adequate pain management is the fear of contributing to patient addiction.

Addiction

Addiction, or psychological dependence, according to the American Pain Society (1992), is "a pattern of compulsive drug use characterized by a continued craving for an opioid and the need to use the opioid for effects other than pain relief." Research conducted by Porter and Jick (1980) found only four cases of addiction among over 12,000 pain patients they studied. These statistics indicate that the fear of addiction is greater than the actual reality.

Unfortunately, nurses often infer that requests for frequent administrations of narcotics are motivated by a patient's desire to experience the drug's pleasant effects. In fact, the patient's currently prescribed dose or frequency of medication administration is probably not sufficient to control the pain. Consequently, nurses may undertreat the patient's pain, or they may convince physicians to prescribe placebos.

Placebos

A **placebo** is an inactive substance given as a substitute for drug therapy. Studies have shown that placebos can relieve pain, especially when patients have confidence in their health care providers. The patient–nurse or patient–physician trust relationship has probably more to do with the efficacy of placebos than any other factor.

 FOCUS ON OLDER ADULTS

- Older adults who must move to a nursing or retirement home may feel more comfortable with their own bed, furnishings, and personal mementos.
- Older adults often feel more comfortable when the environment is kept warmer than usual.
- Complaints of pain among older adults may be a camouflage for feelings of depression.
- Pain is often underreported among older adults because they believe that pain is a normal part of aging.
- Because older adults experience physical degeneration and more chronic diseases, they are at higher risk for experiencing pain.
- Older adults tend to respond atypically to acute pain because cutaneous age-related changes reduce the transmission of pain stimuli to the brain.
- Besides the standard questions asked during pain assessment, older adults are encouraged to identify how the pain interferes with their daily functions.
- The pain tolerance of older adults is usually decreased because they have less energy to cope with pain and because their pain tends to be chronic.
- Pain may be unnecessarily endured by older adults because they do not want to be perceived as a nuisance or bother.

- The oral route is the preferred route for analgesic drug administration.
- Older adults are more sensitive than others to narcotics. They are more likely to experience both higher peak and longer durations of pain relief (Jacox et al., 1992).
- Meperidine (Demerol) and pentazocine (Talwin) tend to cause mental disturbances even at relatively low doses when administered to older adults (Eliopoulos, 1993).
- The manifestation of analgesic drug side effects is often more dramatic in older adults. Common adverse effects include confusion and disorientation, gastritis, constipation, urinary retention, and blurred vision.
- Pain management may be enhanced among older adults by the administration of antidepressants, anticonvulsants, alcohol, or stimulants such as caffeine and methylphenidate (Ritalin; Ciba Pharmaceutical Co., Summit, NJ) (Carnevali & Patrick, 1993).
- Unrelenting pain, like that associated with cancer, can lead to sleep deprivation, poor nutrition, decreased social interactions, feelings of helplessness, and consideration of suicide.
- Vascular pain, a problem experienced by many older diabetics, is often described as "burning."

Consequently, it is a fallacy to assume that patients who respond to placebos are addicted, malingerers, or imagining their pain. Furthermore, using deception is considered an unethical practice (American Pain Society, 1992).

KEY CONCEPTS

- Two factors that contribute to comfort are a safe, clean, and attractive environment and relief from pain.
- To promote patient comfort in modern hospitals, (1) the walls and room decor are more colorful, (2) carpeting is used to reduce noise, (3) there is more attention to increasing the amount of natural sunlight, and (4) the climate within the environment is more adequately controlled.
- The furnishings that are standard in all patient rooms include the bed, the overbed table, the bedside stand, and at least one chair.
- Pain is an unpleasant sensation usually associated with disease or injury.
- Pain threshold is the point at which pain-transmitting neurochemicals reach the brain and cause conscious awareness. Pain tolerance, on the other hand, is the amount of pain a person endures once the threshold has been reached.
- The gate control theory proposes that although there are several pathways for transmitting cutaneous information to the brain, the gates to all but one pathway close, permitting only a single stimulus to be transmitted at a time.
- Endogenous opioids are naturally produced chemicals with morphine-like properties. It is believed that these chemicals bind at nerve receptor sites and block the transmission of pain producing neurotransmitters.
- There are many types of pain, some of which include cutaneous pain, somatic pain, visceral pain, referred pain, neuropathic pain, acute pain, and chronic pain.
- When assessing pain, it is essential to ask the patient for a description of its onset, quality, intensity, location, and duration.
- A pain assessment is performed at least on admission, once per shift when pain is an actual or potential problem, and before and after implementing a pain management intervention.
- Techniques for managing pain include administering analgesic drugs, assisting with PCA, educating patients about pain and its control, and using nondrug interventions like TENS, acupuncture and acupressure, biofeedback, and hypnosis.
- Patients often request frequent administrations of pain-relieving medications because their currently prescribed dose or the schedule for its administration is probably not sufficient to control the pain.
- A placebo is an inactive substance given as a substitute for an actual drug. The positive effect some patients experience from placebos is probably the result of the trust they feel in the physician or nurse.
- To ensure the environmental comfort of older adults, nurses may advocate that they be allowed to bring their own bed, furnishings, and personal mementos when admitted to a nursing home. To promote physical comfort, nurses assess for pain more actively because older adults may not verbalize about their pain or ask for treatment.

CRITICAL THINKING EXERCISES

- Discuss factors in the health care environment that are likely to contribute to distress and measures that can prevent or relieve them.
- Assume you are a member of a committee involved in the plans for remodeling a patient care unit. Discuss recommendations that you would make.
- Recall a personal experience involving pain. Describe factors that intensified the pain and measures, other than using medications, that relieved it. Discuss how this information can be applied to restoring comfort among patients who are experiencing pain.

SUGGESTED READINGS

Agency for Health Care Policy and Research. Pain Control After Surgery, a Patient's Guide. Publication No.92-0021. Silver Spring, MD: Publications Clearinghouse, 1992.

American Pain Society. Principles of Analgesic Use in the Treatment of Acute Pain and Cancer Pain. 3rd ed. Skokie, IL: 1992.

Bieren F. Color Psychology and Therapy. Secaucus, NJ: University Books, 1961.

Bullock BL, Rosendahl PP. Pathophysiology: Adaptations and Alterations in Function. 3rd ed. Philadelphia: JB Lippincott, 1992.

Carnevali DL, Patrick M. Nursing Management for the Elderly. 3rd ed. Philadelphia: JB Lippincott, 1993.

Copstead LC. Perspectives on Pathophysiology. Philadelphia: WB Saunders, 1995.

Cushing M. Pain management on trial. American Journal of Nursing February 1992;92:21, 23.

Donovan MI, Miaskowski C. Striving for a standard of pain relief. American Journal of Nursing March 1992;92:106–107.

Eliopoulos C. Gerontological Nursing. 3rd ed. Philadelphia: JB Lippincott, 1993.

McCaffery M, Beebe A. Pain: Clinical Manual for Nursing Practice. St. Louis: CV Mosby, 1989.

Melzack R, Wall PD. Pain mechanisms: a new theory. Science 1965;150:971–974.

Plack JJ, Schick J. The effects of color on human behavior. Journal of the Association for Study in Perception 1974;9:4–16.

Porter J and Jick H. Addiction rare in patients treated with narcotics. New England Journal of Medicine January 10, 1980;302:123.

Sharpe DT. The Psychology of Color and Design. Lanham MD: Littlefield Adams, Division of Rowman and Littlefield Publishers, Inc. 1975.

World Health Organization Expert Committee. Cancer pain relief and palliative care. Geneva, Switzerland: World Health Organization, 1990.

CHAPTER 19
Safety

Learning Objectives

An understanding of the content within this chapter will be evidenced by the student's ability to:

- Give an example of one common injury that predominates at each stage of development from infancy through older adulthood
- Name five injuries that are caused by environmental hazards
- List four broad responsibilities that are incorporated into most fire plans
- Name four types of fire extinguishers and the type of fires for which each is best used
- Discuss three methods for preventing burns
- Name three common causes of asphyxiation
- Discuss three methods for preventing drowning
- Explain why humans are susceptible to electrical shock
- Discuss three methods for preventing electrical shock
- Name at least six substances that commonly are associated with poisonings
- Discuss three methods for preventing poisonings
- Explain why older adults are prone to falling
- Discuss the benefits and risks of using physical restraints
- Explain the basis for enacting restraint legislation
- Differentiate between a restraint and restraint alternative
- Give at least four criteria for applying a physical restraint
- Describe two areas of concern if an accident happens

Safety refers to measures that prevent accidents, or unintentional injuries. This chapter deals with environmental hazard factors that place patients at risk for injury, and the nursing measures that may be used to keep them safe.

AGE-RELATED SAFETY FACTORS

No age group is immune to accidental injury. However, there are distinctive differences among various age groups that contribute to their risks for injury.

Infants must rely on the safety consciousness of their adult caretakers. Therefore, they are vulnerable to falls from changing tables or to injury when unrestrained in automobiles. Toddlers are naturally curious, more mobile than infants, and fail to understand the danger of climbing. Consequently, they are often the victims of accidental poisoning, falling from high chairs or down stairs, and drowning in unbarricaded swimming pools. School-aged children are physically active, which makes them prone to play-related injuries. Many adolescents experience sports-related injuries because they participate in physically challenging activities—sometimes without adequate protective equipment—before their musculoskeletal systems can withstand the stress. Adolescents also tend to be impulsive and take risks as a result of peer pressure. The types of injuries to which adults are prone are also unique to their social and developmental characteristics (Table 19-1).

ENVIRONMENTAL HAZARDS

Environmental hazards are potentially dangerous conditions in the physical surroundings that may alter the health and well-being of people if they are not safely managed. Some examples of injuries that are caused by environmental hazards include thermal burns, asphyxiation, electrical shock, poisoning, and falls.

Burns

A **thermal burn** is a type of skin injury caused by flames, hot liquids, or steam. Burns may also result from contact with caustic chemicals (eg, lye), electric wires, or lightning.

Despite the ban on tobacco smoking in health care facilities, it still accounts for a major share of fires (Fig. 19-1). Some attribute this to the fact that secretive smokers tend quickly to discard smoldering cigarette butts rather than risk being discovered. Home fires, on the other hand, often occur when smokers fall asleep with a burning cigarette or when children play with matches or lighters.

TABLE 19-1. Age-Related Factors Affecting Adult Safety

Adult Group	Contributing Factors	Common Types of Injuries
Young adults	Alcohol and drug abuse Emancipation from parental supervision Naïveté about workplace hazards	Motor vehicle accidents Boating accidents Head and spinal cord injury Eye injuries, chemical burns, traumatic amputations, soft tissue and back injuries
Middle-aged adults	Failure to use safety devices Overexertion and fatigue Disregard for use of seat belts and car safety harnesses Lack of expertise in performing home maintenance or repairs	Physical trauma (see above) Burns and asphyxiation related to nonfunctioning smoke, heat, and carbon monoxide detectors
Older adults	Visual impairment Urinary urgency Postural hypotension Reduced coordination Impaired mobility Inadequate home maintenance Mental confusion Impaired temperature regulation	Falls Poisoning/medication errors Hypothermia and hyperthermia Scalds and burns

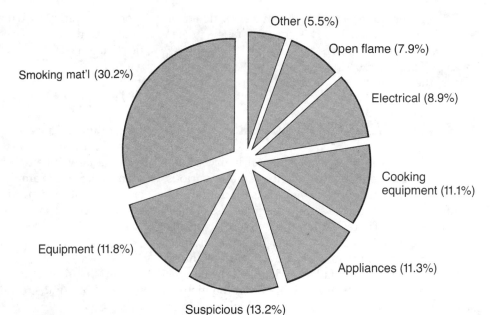

FIGURE 19-1
Smoking statistics as collected by the National Fire Protection Association.

BURN PREVENTION

Because many adults become complacent about safety hazards, it may be appropriate to review burn prevention measures with patients who are treated for thermal-related accidents.

Most fire codes require that public buildings, which include hospitals and nursing homes, have a functioning sprinkling system. Sprinkling systems help to control the fire and limit structural damage. The prevention or limitation of burn injuries in a health care

---

 PATIENT TEACHING REGARDING BURN PREVENTION

Teach the patient or the family to do the following:
- Change the batteries in smoke, heat, and carbon monoxide detectors at least every year.
- Equip the home with at least one fire extinguisher.
- Develop an evacuation plan (and an alternate escape route) and a place for family members to meet after exiting a burning home or apartment.
- Practice the evacuation plan periodically.
- Keep all windows and doors barrier free.
- Identify the location of exits when staying in a hotel.
- Use stairs rather than an elevator if a building is on fire.
- Close doors behind you when exiting.
- Never run if clothing is on fire; instead, stop, drop, and roll.
- Never return to a burning building, regardless of whom or what has been left inside.
- Go to a neighbor's home to call the fire department or 911 operator.
- Never smoke when sleepy.
- Use safety matches, rather than a lighter, which children are less likely to ignite.

- Purchase clothing, especially sleepwear, that is made from flame-resistant fabrics.
- Feel if the surface of a door is hot before opening it.
- Crawl on the floor if the environment is smoke filled.
- Dispose of rags that have been saturated with chemical solvents.
- Keep items away from the pilot lights on the furnace, water heater, or clothes dryer.
- Avoid storing gasoline, kerosene, turpentine, or other flammable substances.
- Go to public fireworks displays rather than let children light their own.
- Do not overload electrical outlets or circuits.
- Set thermostats on hot water heaters for less than 120°F (48.8°C).
- Keep cords to coffee pots, electric frying pans, or other small cooking appliances higher than can be reached by a young child.
- Flush the skin with copious amounts of water if there is contact with caustic chemicals.
- Take cover indoors when the weather is threatening or lightning is observed.

institution depends on all employees knowing and following the agency's fire plan.

FIRE PLANS

A **fire plan** is a procedure that is followed in the event that a fire occurs. Personnel in hospitals and other agencies where patients are housed practice periodic fire drills to prepare for an actual evacuation, should it become necessary.

The National Fire Protection Association recommends using the acronym RACE, which stands for **R**escue, **A**larm, **C**onfine (the fire), and **E**xtinguish, to identify the essential steps in fire rescue proceedings. Most fire plans include the following:

- Keep fire doors closed at all times.
- Identify the location of the fire.
- Evacuate patients from the room where the fire is located.
- Inform the switchboard operator, who will then alert personnel using a designated code over the public address system and notify the fire department.
- Return to the nursing unit when an alarm sounds.
- Clear the halls of visitors and equipment.
- Close all the doors to patient rooms and wait for further directions.
- Place moist towels or bath blankets at the threshold of doors where smoke is escaping.
- Use an appropriate fire extinguisher, if necessary (Table 19-2).

NURSING GUIDELINES FOR USING A FIRE EXTINGUISHER

- Know the location of each type of fire extinguisher.
  Rationale: Minimizes response time
- Free the extinguisher from its enclosure.
  Rationale: Ensures portable use of the extinguisher
- Remove the pin that locks the handle.
  Rationale: Prepares the extinguisher for use
- Aim the nozzle near the edge, not the center, of the fire.
  Rationale: Contains the fire
- Move the nozzle from side to side.
  Rationale: Increases the effectiveness of fire control
- Avoid skin contact with the contents of the fire extinguisher.
  Rationale: Reduces potential for injury
- Return the extinguisher to the maintenance department for replacement or refilling.
  Rationale: Ensures preparation for future use

If an evacuation is necessary, it is helpful to lead ambulatory patients, hand in hand, down a stairwell to a safe location. Nonambulatory patients may be pulled on mattresses or sheets. Infants and small children may be carried.

Asphyxiation

Asphyxiation refers to an inability to breathe. Asphyxiation may be caused by any number of reasons, such as airway obstructions (see Chap. 37), inhaling noxious gases like smoke or carbon monoxide, or drowning.

SMOKE INHALATION

Smoke is sometimes more deadly than the fire with which it is associated. To avoid death and serious injury, many single- and multiple-family residential buildings are equipped with smoke detectors. However, people sometimes dismantle their smoke detector when it begins to emit an audible alarm signaling low battery power, and then fail to replace the batteries.

CARBON MONOXIDE

Carbon monoxide (CO) is an odorless gas released during the incomplete combustion of carbon products such as fossil fuels—kerosene, natural gas, wood, and coal—the common substances used to heat homes. When carbon monoxide is inhaled, it binds with hemoglobin and interferes with the oxygenation of cells. Without adequate ventilation, the consequences can be lethal.

Because carbon monoxide can be present in the absence of smoke, it is advisable that everyone install detectors that sense and alert home dwellers to its presence. All alarms should be investigated by fire department personnel.

Without detectors, victims are often unaware of carbon monoxide's presence and mistake its effects as flu-like symptoms. As their condition deteriorates, mental confusion ensues, and they lapse into coma, followed by death.

DROWNING

Drowning refers to a condition in which fluid occupies the airway and interferes with ventilation. Accidental drownings tend to occur during water activities such as fishing, boating, swimming, and water-skiing. Some incidences are linked with alcohol abuse, which often interferes with good judgment and promotes risk taking. Other drowning victims may be nonswimmers or those who overestimate their stamina. However, drownings may also occur within the home or health care environment.

TABLE 19-2. *Types of Fire Extinguishers*

Type	Contents	Use
Class A	Water under pressure	Burning paper, wood, cloth
Class B	Carbon dioxide	Fires caused by gasoline, oil, paint, grease, and other flammable liquids
Class C	Dry chemicals	Electrical fires
Class ABC (combination extinguisher)	Graphite	Fires of any kind

Young children are often the victims of home drownings when they are left momentarily in a bathtub or with access to a swimming pool. Although the potential for drowning in a health care institution is statistically remote, it is not impossible. Consequently, any helpless or cognitively impaired patient—young or old—is never left alone in a tub of water, regardless of its depth.

Victims of cold water drownings are more apt to be resuscitated. Their lowered metabolism conserves oxygen, which is an advantage over those who succumb in warm water (see Chap. 11). Prevention, however, is far better than having to treat drowning victims.

Drowning Prevention

Everyone should learn to swim but never swim alone, wear approved flotation devices, and avoid drinking alcohol when participating in water-related activities. Waterways are often patrolled, but if not, a designated law enforcement officer should be notified if boaters appear unsafe. In the case of bathing, children should be removed from the water rather than left unattended; swimming pools should be fenced and locked when adults are not available for supervision.

RESUSCITATION

In the event that someone is pulled unconscious from the water or is asphyxiated from some other cause, cardiopulmonary resuscitation (CPR), if begun immediately, may be lifesaving (see Chap. 37). Current CPR certification is often an employment requirement for nursing personnel. It also is becoming a common hospital practice to teach one or both new parents how to administer infant CPR (Fig. 19-2).

Electrical Shock

Electrical shock is the discharge of electricity through the body. The body is quite susceptible to electrical shock because it is composed of water and electrolytes, both of which are good conductors of electricity. A *conductor* is a substance that facilitates the flow of electrical current, whereas an *insulator* is a substance that contains electrical currents so they do not scatter. Electrical cords are covered with rubber or some other insulating substance.

Macroshock, if it occurs, is the harmless distribution of low-amperage electricity over a large area of the body. Macroshock is experienced as a slight tingling. **Microshock** can result from low-voltage but high-amperage electricity. Microshock is not usually felt by people with intact skin. Intact skin helps to prevent shock and injury because it offers resistance or acts as a barrier between the electrical current and the water and electrolytes within. But, if the skin is wet or its integrity has been impaired, the electrical current may be fatal, especially if delivered directly to the heart.

SHOCK PREVENTION

The potential for electrical shock can be reduced by using grounded equipment. A *ground* diverts leaking electrical energy to the earth. Grounded equipment contains a three-pronged electrical plug.

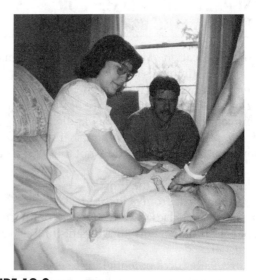

FIGURE 19-2
Parents being taught cardiopulmonary resuscitation as part of discharge planning. (Courtesy of Ken Timby.)

In addition to using grounded equipment, there are other safety measures that are employed for preventing electrical shock:

- Never use an adaptor to bypass a grounded outlet.
- Make sure all outlets and switches have cover plates.
- Plug all electrical machines used for patient care into outlets within a range of 12 feet of one another or within the same cluster of wall outlets (Berger & Williams, 1992; Sundberg, 1989).
- Discontinue and disconnect all electrical machines once they are no longer necessary.
- Discourage patients from resting electric hair dryers, curling irons, or razors on or near a sink that contains water.
- Replace and avoid using any electrical machine with a frayed or cracked cord, or if the plug has exposed wires.
- Grasp the plug, not the cord, to remove it from its outlet.
- Avoid extension cords.
- Report macroshocks to the engineering department.
- Clean liquid spills as soon as possible.
- Stand clear of the patient and bed when cardiac defibrillation is being performed.

Poisoning

Poisoning is an injury caused by the ingestion, inhalation, or absorption of a toxic substance. Poisonings are more prevalent in homes than health care institutions. More often than not, accidental poisonings occur among toddlers, and usually involve the ingestion of substances that are located in the bathroom or kitchen (Display 19-1). Unfortunately, of those children treated for accidental poisoning, about half have a repeat episode within 1 year (Smith et al., 1982).

There are fewer poisonings in hospitals and other places where patients are cared for because medications are kept locked. Furthermore, law requires that chemicals like liquid antiseptics intended for external use be kept separate from other drugs. This is not to imply that poisonings never occur in health care institutions! One could consider medication errors (see Chap. 32) in which the wrong medication or dose is administered to the wrong patient as a form of poisoning.

POISON PREVENTION

Educating curious children is not the only way to prevent childhood poisoning, although it certainly is one component. Because toddlers cannot read, poison control centers offer stickers (Fig. 19-3) for educational and

DISPLAY 19-1. *Common Substances Associated With Childhood Poisonings*

Drugs: aspirin, acetaminophen, vitamins with iron, antidepressants, sedatives, tranquilizers, antacid tablets, diet pills, laxatives

Cleaning Agents: bleach, toilet bowl or tank disks, detergents, drain cleaners

Paint Solvents: turpentine, kerosene, gasoline

Heavy Metals: lead paint chips

Chemical Products: glue, shoe polish, antifreeze, insecticides

Cosmetics: hair dye, shampoo, nail polish remover

Plants: mistletoe berries, rhubarb leaves, foxglove, castor beans

prevention purposes. Parents are encouraged to place these stickers on toxic substances and explain to their children that any container displaying a sticker is to be left untouched. Often, however, the more effective approach is to educate parents on how to reduce or eliminate the availability of potentially dangerous substances.

In the event that an adult may not be able to self-administer medications as they have been prescribed, there are containers that may be prefilled by a responsible person (Fig. 19-4).

TREATMENT FOR POISONINGS

Whenever a poisoning is suspected, initial treatment involves maintaining breathing and cardiac function. After this is ensured, there is an attempt to identify

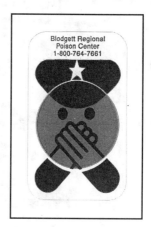

FIGURE 19-3
This sticker provided by poison control centers may prevent young children from being poisoned.

PATIENT TEACHING FOR PREVENTING CHILDHOOD POISONING

Teach parents or caretakers to do the following:
- Install latches on cupboard doors that cannot be opened easily by a child.
- Request childproof caps on all prescription medications; purchase chemicals and nonprescription drugs that have tamperproof lids.
- Flush old medications down the toilet.
- Never transfer a toxic substance to a container usually used for food.
- Avoid implying that medications are "candy" or that they taste "yummy."

- Forgo keeping drugs in a purse.
- Remind grandparents or babysitters to "child-proof" toxic substances within their homes.
- Check with a pediatric nurse about house-plants that are nontoxic.
- Keep the home well ventilated when using an aerosol or substance that leaves lingering fumes in the air.

what has been ingested, how much was taken, and approximately how long ago the incident occurred.

Definitive treatment depends on the specific substance, the condition of the patient, and if the substance is still in the stomach or is at the point of being absorbed. In cases of commercial products that contain multiple ingredients, the poison control center may need to be consulted. Otherwise, treatment may follow the course of a simple decision tree (Fig. 19-5).

Falls

Falls, more than any other injury discussed thus far, are the most prevalent accident experienced by older adults, and they have the most serious consequences

for this age group as well. Approximately 172,000 older adults sustain fractured hips each year, and 9,500 adults older than 65 years of age die from complications associated with a fall (Jech, 1992). Many who live face years of disability, impaired mobility, and pain.

CONTRIBUTING FACTORS

Older adults are more prone to falling for several reasons. Many have age-related changes such as visual impairments and disorders that affect gait, balance, and coordination. Some take medications that lower blood pressure, causing them to feel dizzy on rising. Others experience urinary urgency and rush to reach the toilet.

Besides chronic health problems, there are other social and environmental factors that influence the high

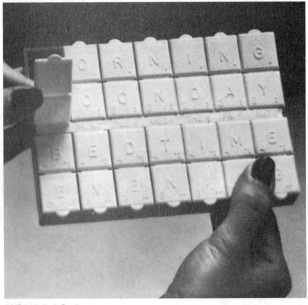

FIGURE 19-4
A pill organizer may help reduce the incidence of medication overdoses. (Courtesy of Apex Medical Corp, Bloomington, MN.)

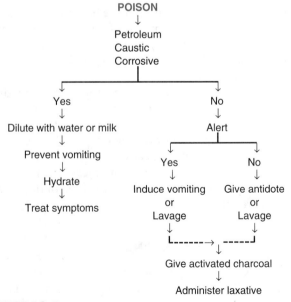

FIGURE 19-5
Decision tree for treating ingested poisons.

incidence of falls in older adults. For example, their choice in footwear sometimes places them at risk. Older adults often wear slippers to accommodate the fact that their feet tend to swell. Although slippers provide more comfort, are less expensive, and are less tiring to put on than shoes, they do not offer much support or traction with the floor. In addition, clutter may accumulate because some older adults resist discarding items that they feel are still functional even though they are infrequently used.

When hospitalized, older adults face added risks such as being in an unfamiliar environment. They are also forced to rely on nursing assistance for mobility—assistance that sometimes is not as expeditious as it could be. Changed health status and the administration of different drugs also may result in temporary confusion and poor judgment in the hospitalized older adult.

FALL ASSESSMENT

Because falls occur so frequently among the elderly, it is reasonable to believe that some falls could be prevented by determining which patients are at greater risk. Many long-term agencies have developed or adopted assessment tools for this purpose (Fig. 19-6). Most tools score risk factors to predict which patients require fall prevention protocols.

FALL PREVENTION

Fall prevention approaches may differ depending on whether older adults are living at home or are residents in a health care facility. Therefore, selected measures for preventing falls are modified according to the individual patient's circumstances.

Older adults may be advised to have a list of emergency numbers posted by the phone. Another suggestion for those who live alone is to become part of a daily phone tree. Then, if a call goes unanswered, it alerts someone to investigate if help is needed.

Unfortunately, when older adults are admitted to health care agencies, the interventions used for preventing falls are not always as dignified as those available at home, because too often they include the use of physical, and in some cases chemical, restraints.

RESTRAINTS

Physical restraints "are any manual method or physical or mechanical device, material or equipment attached or adjacent to the resident (patient's) body that the individual cannot remove easily, which restricts freedom of movement or normal access to one's body" (Federal Register, 1989). Examples of restraints include full bed rails that are raised; leg, arm, waist, and vest cloth restraints; wheelchair safety bars, chairs that prevent rising, and even tucking patients in so tightly with sheets that they cannot move.

Although the use of restraints is intended to prevent falls and other injuries, their risks, in many cases, may outweigh their benefits. Research indicates that patients who are restrained become increasingly confused, experience chronic constipation and incontinence, are prone to increased infections (eg, pneumonia) and pressure sores, and progressively decline in their ability to perform activities of daily living (Varone et al., 1992). Even more distressing is the finding that restrained patients are eight times more likely to die during hospitalization than patients who are unrestrained (Lofgren et al., 1989).

Restraint Legislation

After it was found that the use of physical restraints ranged from 25% to 84% among residents in surveyed health care institutions in the United States (Varone et al., 1992), it was obvious that there was a need to control their indiscriminate use. Consequently, federal legislation addressing the use of restraints was passed within the Omnibus Budget Reconciliation Act (OBRA) in 1987 (Display 19-2). Compliance with the law became effective in 1990, but it applies only to long-term facilities like nursing homes, not acute care institutions such as hospitals.

One result of the OBRA legislation has been the development of restraint alternatives to prevent falls and other injuries.

DISPLAY 19-2. *OBRA Legislation Addressing Restraints*

The Omnibus Reconciliation Act (OBRA) of 1987 specifies that:

The resident (patient) has the right to be free from any physical restraints imposed or psychoactive drug administered for purposes of discipline or convenience, and not required to treat the resident's (patient's) medical symptoms. . . . Restraints may only be imposed to ensure the physical safety of the resident or other residents and only upon the written order of a physician that specifies the duration and the circumstances under which the restraints are to be used (except in emergency situations which must be addressed in the facility's restraint policy).

Patient's Name:	Prepared By: *(Signature and Title)*	Date:

INSTRUCTIONS: This assessment is to be completed on all patients age 70 and older or if a fall occurs.

1. Check applicable items, indicate points at right. Refer to definitions on back of this sheet.

2. Add points and note total score below.

I.   AGE   ☐ (1 pt.) 80 or more years old   ☐ (2 pts.) 70-79 years old pts.   _____ pts.

II.   MENTAL STATUS   ☐ (0 pts.) Oriented at all times or comatose   ☐ (2 pts.) Confusion at all times   ☐ (4 pts.) Intermittent confusion   _____ pts.

III.   DAY NUMBER OF STAY   ☐ (0 pts.) Over 3 days   ☐ (2 pts.) Up to 3 days   _____ pts.

IV.   ELIMINATION   ☐ (0 pts.) Independent and continent   ☐ (1 pt.) Catheter and/or ostomy   ☐ (3 pts.) Elimination with assistance   ☐ (5 pts.) Independent and incontinent   _____ pts.

V.   HISTORY OF FALLING WITHIN THE PAST SIX MONTHS   ☐ (0 pts.) No history   ☐ (2 pts.) Has fallen 1 or 2 times before   ☐ (5 pts.) Multiple history of falling   _____ pts.

VI.   VISUAL IMPAIRMENT (1 pt.)   _____ pts.

VII.   CONFINED TO CHAIR (3 pts.)   _____ pts.

VIII.   DROP IN SYSTOLIC BLOOD PRESSURE of 20mm Hg or more between lying and standing   ☐ (2 pts.)   _____ pts.

IX.   GAIT AND BALANCE
Assess patient's gait while: 1) Standing in one spot with both feet on the ground for 30 seconds without holding onto something; 2) Walking straight forward; 3) Walking through a doorway; 4) Walking while making a turn. NOTE:Check for any yes answer.

☐ (1 pt.) Wide base of support   ☐ (1 pt.) Lurching, swaying or slapping gait
☐ (1 pt.) Loss of balance while standing   ☐ (1 pt.) Gait pattern changed when walking through doorway
☐ (1 pt.) Balance problems when walking   ☐ (1 pt.) Jerking or instability when making turns
☐ (1 pt.) Decrease in muscular coordination   ☐ (1 pt.) Use of assistive devices (cane, walker, furniture, etc)   _____ pts.

X.   MEDICATIONS

☐ Alcohol Anesthetic   ☐ Antihistamine   ☐ Antihypertensives   ☐ Antiseizure/Antiepileptic
☐ Benzodiazeplines   ☐ Cathartics   ☐ Diuretics   ☐ Hypoglycemic agents   ☐ Narcotics
☐ Psychotrophics   ☐ Sedatives/Hypnotics   ☐ Other (specify)

From the above medication groups, indicate how many the patient is currently taking, or took prior to admission.
☐ (0 pts.) No medications   ☐ (1 pt.) 1 medication   ☐ (2 pts.) 2 or more medications
☐ With a change of medication and/or dosage in the past five days, add 1 point to the medication score.   _____ pts.

A score of ten (10) or above indicates a risk of falling: USE STANDARDIZED CARE PLAN.   **TOTAL SCORE**   _____ pts.

© 1993 Posey Co. ● Posey and the familiar Posey flower logo are registered trademarks of the J.T. Posey Co.

FIGURE 19-6
Fall assessment tool.

Restraint Alternatives

A **restraint alternative** is a protective or adaptive device that promotes patient safety and postural support, but which the patient can release independently. Restraint alternatives are usually appropriate for patients who tend to need repositioning to maintain their body alignment or improve their independence and functional status. Some examples include seat inserts or gripping materials that prevent sliding, support pillows, seat belts or harnesses with front-releasing Velcro or buckle closures, and commercial or home-made tilt wedges (Fig. 19-7). However, if a patient does not know how or is unable to release the restraint alternative, it is then considered a restraint.

Other supplementary measures may also reduce the need for restraints. Personnel are encouraged to improve gait training, provide physical exercise, reorient patients, encourage assistive ambulatory devices such as walkers and hall rails, and use electronic seat and bed monitors that sound an alarm when patients get up without assistance. Before entertaining the use of physical restraints, the patient's response to other alternatives is observed and documented.

Teach the patient or the family to do the following:
- Keep the environment well lit.
- Install and use handrails on stairs inside and outside the home.
- Place a strip of light-colored adhesive tape on the edge of each stair, making them easy to see.
- Avoid scatter rugs.
- Keep extension cords next to the wall.
- Omit waxing the floor.
- If slippers are worn, make sure they have non-skid soles.
- Keep pathways clutter-free.
- Wear short robes without cloth belts that may loosen and tangle in your feet.
- Use a cane or walker if it has been prescribed.
- Replace the tip on a cane as it wears down.
- Postpone going outside when the weather is icy, wet, or snowy.
- Ask someone for their seat if none is available on public transportation.
- Add grab bars in the shower and near the toilet.
- Place a nonskid mat or decals on the floor of the tub or shower.
- Use soap on a rope or a suspended container of liquid soap when bathing to prevent slipping on a loose soap bar.
- Use a flashlight or nightlight when it is dark.
- Make sure that pets are not underfoot.
- Mop up all spills immediately.
- Use a long-handled tong to reach high objects rather than climbing on a chair.

Restraint Criteria

The spirit of the OBRA restraint law is to promote safety without restricting personal freedom unnecessarily. It is not intended to prohibit their use entirely. The law is very clear, however, that restraints may not be used for the convenience of nursing personnel or as a disciplinary measure.

When restraints are necessary, there must be documented evidence that their use is justified. In general, restraints may be validly used when a patient:

- Has a history of previous falls or may experience life-threatening consequences if a fall were to occur
- Has demonstrated risks to safety or a potential compromise in functional ability during previous trials with restraint alternatives
- Is physically or mentally impaired to such an extent that he or she could not maintain his or her own safety

- May need restriction of movement temporarily during a life-threatening event that requires treatment

The best decisions and outcomes regarding restraints usually occur when there is collaboration among staff, the patient, and the patient's family. The goal is to use the least restrictive type of device possible and to continue providing measures that may enable the patient to function restraint-free in the future.

Using Restraints

After an appropriate assessment and, in some cases, after discussing the assessment findings with the patient and family, the physician is ultimately responsible for writing a medical order prescribing the use of restraints. A new order is required for each restraining episode. In addition, hospitals are required by the Joint Commission on Accreditation of Healthcare Organizations (JCAHO) to have a written restraint policy or procedure and demonstrate evidence that the policy is followed. To ensure that restraints are applied and used appropriately, follow the suggested actions in Skill 19-1.

NURSING IMPLICATIONS

It is essential that nurses recognize safety hazards and identify those patients who are at greatest risk for accidents. Once the data have been gathered, several nursing diagnoses may be identified.

The accompanying Nursing Care Plan is an example of interventions that have been planned for a patient with a nursing diagnosis of Risk for Trauma. This diagnosis is defined in the NANDA taxonomy (1994) as "Accentuated risk of accidental tissue injury, e.g., wound, burn, fracture."

Despite appropriate assessments and plans for preventing unintentional injuries, accidents still occur. And, when they do, the nurse's first concern is for the safety and care of the patient, and second, for the potential for legal allegations of malpractice. Therefore, when

(text continues on page 399)

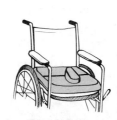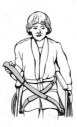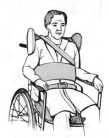

FIGURE 19-7
Restraint alternatives.

SKILL 19-1
Using Physical Restraints

Suggested Action	Reason for Action
Assessment	
Assess the patient's physical and mental status for signs suggesting dangerousness to self or others.	Provides data for determining the need for physical restraints
Consult with staff and family on options other than the use of restraints.	Supports the principle of using less restrictive approaches initially
Observe the patient's response to alternative measures.	Determines the need to revise the current plan for care
Check the chart for a physician's order for the use of restraints.	Complies with Joint Commission on Accreditation of Healthcare Organizations (JCAHO) requirements
Review the agency's restraint policy or procedure if there is no current medical order.	Follows standards for care
Assess the patient's skin and circulation.	Provides a baseline of information for future comparisons
Inspect the restraint that will be used and avoid any that are in poor condition.	Ensures safety
Planning	
Obtain a current order for the use of physical restraints if it appears they are necessary.	Complies with JCAHO guidelines
Choose a restraint that is compatible with the size of the patient.	Prevents injury
Approach the patient slowly and calmly. Speak in a soft but controlled voice.	Reduces agitation
Use the patient's name and make eye contact.	Helps to secure the patient's attention
Explain the reasons that restraint is necessary.	Promotes understanding and cooperation
Reassure the patient that the restraints will be discontinued when the possibility for harm no longer exists.	Indicates criteria for releasing restraints
Plan to remove or loosen the restraint(s) at time periods established by agency policy to assess circulation, provide joint mobility, give skin care, assist with elimination, offer food and fluids, and evaluate if circumstances continue to warrant use of the restraint(s).	Demonstrates attention to basic physiologic and safety needs; supports the principle that restraints are not applied longer than necessary
Implementation	
Place the patient in a position of comfort and in proper body alignment (see Table 19-3).	Maintains functional position and reduces discomfort
Protect any bony prominences or fragile skin that may be injured by a restraint.	Reduces or prevents unnecessary injury

(continued)

SKILL 19-1
Using Physical Restraints *(Continued)*

Suggested Action	Reason for Action

Upper Extremity Restraints

Apply mitts rather than wrist restraints, if possible.

Maintains freedom to move elbows and shoulders

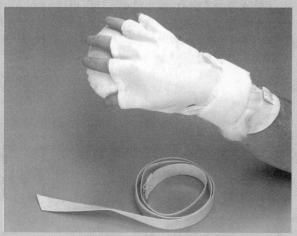

Hand mitts can be applied with or without ties. (Courtesy of the J. T. Posey Co., Arcadia, CA.)

Use soft cloth restraints instead of stiff leather.

Promotes skin integrity

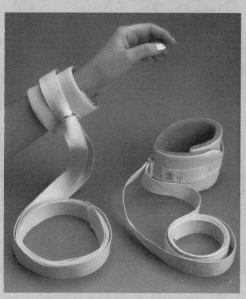

Soft wrist restraints. (Courtesy of the J. T. Posey Co., Arcadia, CA.)

Provide as much length as possible without allowing the potential for pulling at tubes or other treatment devices.

Facilitates movement

(continued)

SKILL 19-1
Using Physical Restraints (Continued)

Suggested Action	Reason for Action
Wheelchair Restraints Avoid back cushions if possible.	Creates the potential for slack if they become dislodged
Make sure the patient's hips are flush with the back of the chair.	Promotes good posture and skeletal alignment
Apply belts snugly over the thighs with at least a 45° angle between the belt and knees.	Minimizes sliding up toward the ribs and compromising breathing

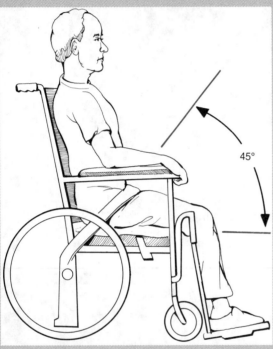

With the lap strap at a 45° angle to the knees, the hips are held toward the back of the chair.

Suggested Action	Reason for Action
Apply vests with Velcro or zipper closures at the back; use criss-crossing vests with front closures only on docile patients.	Keeps fasteners out of reach; prevents strangulation
Support the feet on footrests.	Reduces pressure behind the knees and promotes circulation of blood

(continued)

SKILL 19-1
Using Physical Restraints *(Continued)*

Suggested Action	Reason for Action
Tie restraints under the chair, not behind the back.	Prevents suffocation if the patient should slide downward

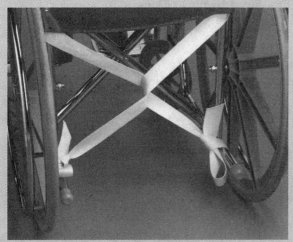

Restraint ties are secured beneath the chair. (Courtesy of the J. T. Posey Co., Arcadia, CA.)

Suggested Action	Reason for Action
Use a quick-release knot when tying any type of restraint.	Facilitates removal should the patient's safety become compromised

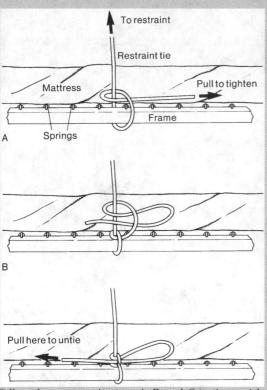

Follow the sequence in steps A, B, and C to tie a quick-release knot.

(continued)

SKILL 19-1
Using Physical Restraints (Continued)

Suggested Action	Reason for Action
Keep the patient in sight whenever restraints are used.	Aids in monitoring the patient's safety
Never restrain a patient to a toilet.	Prevents drowning or falls
Bed Restraints	
Position the patient in the center of the mattress.	Allows maximum movement and proper body alignment
Use full side rails and maintain them in an "up" position while the patient is restrained.	Prevents injury from slipping between or below half rails
Apply side rail covers or pad the rails with soft bath blankets if the patient is extremely restless.	Reduces the potential for becoming caught or injured within the open spaces of the rails
Apply belt restraints snugly at the waist but with enough room to slide an open hand between the device and the patient.	Ensures ventilation
Secure the straps to the moveable part of the bed frame, not the side rails or stationary frame.	Prevents sliding and chest compression

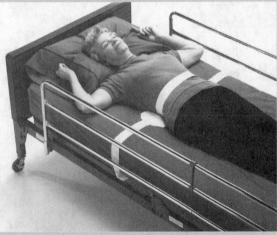

The restraint ties are secured to the moveable portion of the bed frame. (Courtesy of the J. T. Posey Co., Arcadia, CA.)

Monitor aggressive, agitated, or restless patients frequently.	Promotes patient safety

Evaluation
- Restraint(s) are applied correctly
- No injuries occur
- Restraints are released according to policy
- Basic needs are met
- Restraints are discontinued when no longer needed

Document
- Assessment findings that indicate a need for restraint
- Types of restraint alternatives and the patient's response

(continued)

Suggested Action	Reason for Action

- Condition of skin, circulation, sensation, and joint mobility before restraint application
- Type of restraint applied
- Communication with physician and responsible family member
- Frequency of release and assessment findings
- Nursing measures used to promote skin integrity and joint flexibility, and meet nutritional and elimination needs
- Assessments indicating an ongoing need for restraint(s)

Sample Documentation

Date and Time — Pulling on urinary catheter. Reminded to leave catheter alone. Placed close to nursing station so as to intervene quickly and given a skein of yarn to wrap as a ball to distract patient from catheter. Continues to tug at catheter. Catheter is patent, but urine now appears bloody. Order obtained for soft cloth wrist restraints. Skin over wrists is intact, no edema, full mobility, fingers are warm and pink, can differentiate sharp from dull sensation. Restraints secured to arms of wheelchair. Daughter notified of need to use restraints at this time and concurs with treatment plan.

_____ **Signature, Title**

 FOCUS ON OLDER ADULTS

- Older adults are at higher risk for accidents because of age-related changes such as those affecting mobility, balance, and sensory organs.
- The U.S. Consumer Product Safety Commission estimates that over 734,000 adults aged 65 years and older are treated per year for injuries with products they use everyday; 6,800 of those injuries are associated with rugs and runners that tend to slide.
- Osteoporosis, a softening of the bones, makes older adults, especially women, at higher risk for fractures should a fall occur.
- Some older adults develop an exaggerated fear of falling that may inhibit them from pursuing activities that enhance their quality of life.
- Murphy and Isaacs (1982) described a condition called "post-fall syndrome" that is characterized by a distinct gait attributed more to being overly cautious than from prior injury.
- Restraining older adults can be just as detrimental as the consequences of a fall.
- Hospitalizations are twice as lengthy for those who fall compared to those who do not, and 47% of those who are hospitalized for falling eventually become transferred to a nursing home (Miller, 1990).

- To prevent wandering out of doors, it may be helpful to disguise a door by covering it with a full-length curtain or with wallpaper that is the same as that on adjacent walls.
- Any older adult who is apt to wander away should wear an identification bracelet that includes a phone number.
- It may be helpful to photograph all residents in an extended care facility for the purposes of search and identification.
- During each day's assessment, it may be important to document a description of what a potential wanderer is wearing so that they may be identified more easily.
- Reflective tape placed on the floor may be helpful in identifying the path to the bathroom for older adults who get up at night.
- To distract patients from attempts to pull out tubes or interfere with other treatment measures, they may be kept busy with stringing large wooden beads or buttons or sorting items. Care must be taken that the objects will not be swallowed or inhaled.
- Responsible caretakers of older adults may benefit from being relieved for periods of times either by other family members or by community volunteers.

TABLE 19-3. *Basic Wheelchair Positioning Principles*

Structure	Front View	Side View
Head	Head/neck centered over trunk midline	Head/ear centered over hip
Shoulders	Level in horizontal line	Top of shoulder over hip
Trunk	Sternum is perpendicular to center of pelvis	Spine is perpendicular to hip
Pelvis	Tops of hips are level in horizontal line	Lumbar curve is preserved
Thighs	Knees are level in horizontal line	Hip and knee are level in horizontal line
Knees	Knees are not touching; legs are perpendicular to floor	Knees are bent 90°; edge of seat is 3 inches from knee crease
Feet	Great toes and fifth toes level in horizontal line	Heel and forefoot positioned on footplate; ankle in neutral position

Pang J. Proper patient positioning in wheelchairs. Nursing Update Winter 1994;5(1):2. With permission from J. T. Posey Co., Arcadia, CA.

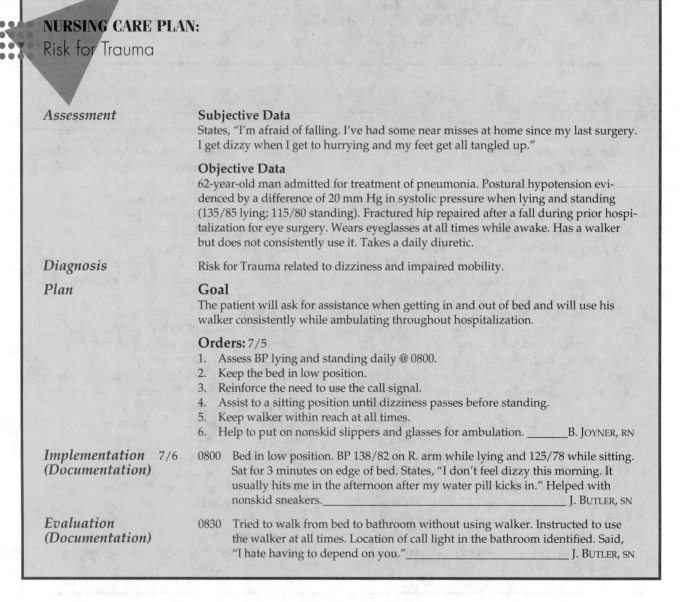

NURSING CARE PLAN:
Risk for Trauma

Assessment

Subjective Data
States, "I'm afraid of falling. I've had some near misses at home since my last surgery. I get dizzy when I get to hurrying and my feet get all tangled up."

Objective Data
62-year-old man admitted for treatment of pneumonia. Postural hypotension evidenced by a difference of 20 mm Hg in systolic pressure when lying and standing (135/85 lying; 115/80 standing). Fractured hip repaired after a fall during prior hospitalization for eye surgery. Wears eyeglasses at all times while awake. Has a walker but does not consistently use it. Takes a daily diuretic.

Diagnosis

Risk for Trauma related to dizziness and impaired mobility.

Plan

Goal
The patient will ask for assistance when getting in and out of bed and will use his walker consistently while ambulating throughout hospitalization.

Orders: 7/5
1. Assess BP lying and standing daily @ 0800.
2. Keep the bed in low position.
3. Reinforce the need to use the call signal.
4. Assist to a sitting position until dizziness passes before standing.
5. Keep walker within reach at all times.
6. Help to put on nonskid slippers and glasses for ambulation. _____B. JOYNER, RN

Implementation   7/6
(Documentation)

0800   Bed in low position. BP 138/82 on R. arm while lying and 125/78 while sitting. Sat for 3 minutes on edge of bed. States, "I don't feel dizzy this morning. It usually hits me in the afternoon after my water pill kicks in." Helped with nonskid sneakers._____ J. BUTLER, SN

Evaluation
(Documentation)

0830   Tried to walk from bed to bathroom without using walker. Instructed to use the walker at all times. Location of call light in the bathroom identified. Said, "I hate having to depend on you."_____ J. BUTLER, SN

APPLICABLE NURSING DIAGNOSES

- Risk for Injury
- Risk for Trauma
- Impaired Physical Mobility
- Sensory/Perceptual Alteration: Visual
- Altered Thought Processes
- Impaired Home Maintenance Management

responding to a situation involving an accident and potential injury, it is appropriate to do the following:

- Check the patient's condition immediately.
- Call for help if the patient is in danger.
- Comfort and reassure the patient.
- Avoid moving the patient until it is safe to do so.
- Report the accident and assessment findings to the physician.
- Complete an incident report as soon as the patient is stabilized (see Chap. 3).

KEY CONCEPTS

- Accidental injuries vary according to the stages of development. Because infants must rely on their caretakers, they are susceptible to falls. Poisonings are common among toddlers. School-aged children sustain play-related injuries, and adolescents are often the victims of sports-related injuries. Young adults are commonly involved in motor vehicle accidents. Middle-aged adults experience a variety of physical trauma, such as back injuries. Falls are quite common among older adults.
- Environmental hazards often contribute to injuries such as burns, asphyxiation, electrical shock, poisoning, and falls.
- Most fire plans incorporate the following four steps: (1) rescue those in danger; (2) sound an alarm; (3) confine the fire; and (4) extinguish the blaze.
- There are class A, B, C, and ABC fire extinguishers. Class A extinguishers are used for paper, wood, and cloth fires. Class B extinguishers are used on fuels and flammable liquids. Electrical fires are controlled with class C extinguishers. A class ABC extinguisher can be used on any type of fire.
- Some methods of preventing burns include installing and maintaining smoke detectors, developing and practicing a fire evacuation plan, and never returning to a burning building.
- Asphyxiation is commonly caused by smoke inhalation, carbon monoxide poisoning, and drowning.

- Drownings can be prevented by never swimming alone, wearing approved flotation devices, and avoiding alcohol consumption.
- People are susceptible to injury from electrical shock because the human body is predominantly composed of water and electrolytes, which are good conductors of electrical current.
- Electrical shock may be prevented by always using grounded equipment, making sure all cover plates are intact, and replacing equipment with frayed electrical cords.
- Some substances that are commonly implicated in poisonings include chemicals like drugs, cleaning agents, paint solvents, heavy metals, cosmetics, and those found in plants.
- Poisonings may be prevented by using childproof caps on medications, installing latches on storage cupboards, and never transferring a toxic substance to a container associated with food.
- Older adults are prone to falling because they often have gait and balance problems caused by age-related changes, visual impairment, postural hypotension, and urinary urgency.
- Although physical restraints prevent falls, they create concomitant risks for constipation, incontinence, increased infections like pneumonia, pressure sores, and a progressive decline in the ability to perform activities of daily living.
- The excessive and sometimes unnecessary use of physical restraints led to the passage of legislation concerning their use.
- Restraints are devices that restrict movement; restraint alternatives are protective and adaptive devices that can be independently removed by patients.
- Restraints may be justified when patients have a history of previous falls or may experience life-threatening consequences, when there has been a less-than-desired response with restraint alternatives, when patients are seriously impaired mentally or physically, or if their movement must be restricted during a life-threatening event.
- When an accident occurs, the nurse's first concern is for the safety and condition of the patient, and second, for the potential for legal allegations of malpractice.

CRITICAL THINKING EXERCISES

- When discharging an older adult to the care of a family member, what safety measures would be appropriate to include during discharge instructions?
- How might you prevent falls in a patient who demonstrates an unsteady gait without resorting to the use of restraints?

SUGGESTED READINGS

Berger KJ, Williams MB. Fundamentals of Nursing, Collaborating for Optimal Health. Norwalk, CT: Appleton & Lange, 1992.

Brady R, Chester FR, Pierce LL, Salter JP, Schreck S, Radziewicz R. Geriatric falls: prevention strategies for the staff. Journal of Gerontological Nursing September 1993;19:26–32.

Federal Register, February 2, 1989;54(21).

Ginter SF, Mion LC. Falls in the nursing home: preventable or inevitable? Journal of Gerontological Nursing November 1992;18: 43–47.

Jackson DB, Saunders RB. Child Health Nursing: A Comprehensive Approach to the Care of Children and Their Families. Philadelphia: JB Lippincott, 1993.

Jech AO. Preventing falls in the elderly. Geriatric Nursing January–February 1992;13:43–44.

Kallmann SL, Denine-Flynn M, Blackburn DM. Comfort, safety, and independence: restraint release and its challenges. Geriatric Nursing May–June 1992;13:143–148.

Krenzelok EP. The contemporary management of poisoning emergencies. Journal of Practical Nursing March 1992;42:24–31.

Lofgren RP, MacPherson DS, Granieri R, Myllenbeck S, Sprafka JM. Mechanical restraints on the medical wards: are protective devices safe? American Journal of Public Health June 1989;79:735–738.

Miller CA. Nursing Care of Older Adults: Theory and Practice. Glenview, IL: Scott, Foresman/Little, Brown Higher Education, 1990.

Murphy J, Isaacs B. The post-fall syndrome. Gerontology 1982;28: 265–270.

NANDA Nursing Diagnoses: Definitions and Classification 1994–1995. Philadelphia: North American Nursing Diagnosis Association, 1994.

Press MM. Restraints—protection or abuse? Canadian Nurse December 1991;87:29–30.

Smith MJ, Goodman JA, Ramsey NL, Pasternack SB. Child and Family: Concepts of Nursing Practice. New York: McGraw-Hill, 1982.

Sundberg MC. Fundamentals of Nursing With Clinical Procedures. 2nd ed. Boston: Jones and Bartlett, 1989.

United States Consumer Product Safety Commission. Safety for Older Adults. Washington, DC:

Varone L, Tappen R, Dixon-Antonio E, Gonzales I, Glussman B. To restrain or not to restrain? The decision-making dilemma for nursing staff. Geriatric Nursing September–October 1992;13:269–272.

CHAPTER 20

Oxygenation

NURSING GUIDELINES

The Safe Use of Oxygen

SKILLS

Using a Pulse Oximeter
Administering Oxygen
Maintaining a Water-Seal Drainage System

NURSING CARE PLAN

Ineffective Breathing Pattern

Key Terms

Learning Objectives

An understanding of the content within this chapter will be evidenced by the student's ability to:

- Differentiate between ventilation and respiration
- Name two methods for assessing the oxygenation status of patients at the bedside
- List at least five signs of inadequate oxygenation
- Name two nursing interventions that can be used to improve ventilation and oxygenation
- Identify four items that may be needed when providing oxygen therapy
- Name four sources for supplemental oxygen
- List five common oxygen delivery devices
- Discuss two hazards that accompany the administration of oxygen
- Describe two additional therapeutic techniques that relate to oxygenation
- Discuss at least two facts concerning oxygenation that affect the care of older adults

xygen is essential for almost every form of animal and plant life. It is used by each cell of the body to metabolize nutrients and produce energy. Without oxygen, cell death occurs rapidly.

This chapter describes the bedside procedures for monitoring oxygen content of the blood, types of equipment used in oxygen therapy, and the skills needed to maintain respiratory function.

OXYGENATION

Oxygenation depends on ventilation and respiration. **Ventilation** is the act of moving air in and out of the lungs. **Respiration** refers to the mechanisms by which oxygen is delivered to the cells. **External respiration** involves the exchange of oxygen from the alveoli to the blood. After being transferred to the blood, the major portion of oxygen becomes attached to the hemoglobin molecules and a smaller portion diffuses into the plasma. **Internal respiration** is the transfer of oxygen from hemoglobin across cellular membranes.

If anything interferes with the act of breathing or the diffusion of oxygen, the consequences may be life-threatening. Therefore, nurses must be able to assess each patient's oxygenation status.

ASSESSING OXYGENATION

The quality of oxygenation can be determined at the bedside by both physical assessment and pulse oximetry.

Physical Assessment

Oxygenation may be assessed by observing the patient's respiratory rate, breathing pattern, chest symmetry, and auscultating lung sounds (see Chap. 12). Other pertinent assessments include heart rate, level of consciousness, and the color of the skin, mucous membranes, and nailbeds.

Analyzing physical assessment data may help to identify signs of **hypoxemia**, insufficient oxygen within arterial blood, and **hypoxia**, inadequate oxygen at the cellular level (Display 20-1).

Pulse Oximetry

Pulse oximetry refers to the technique for measuring the oxygen saturation of blood (Skill 20-1). **Oxygen saturation**, or SaO_2, is the percentage of oxygen that is bound to hemoglobin. In normal, healthy adults, the normal oxygen saturation is 95% to 100%.

Oxygen saturation is monitored with a device called a pulse oximeter. A pulse oximeter is composed of a

---

DISPLAY 20-1. *Common Signs of Inadequate Oxygenation*

- Restlessness
- Rapid, shallow breathing
- Rapid heart rate
- Sitting up to breathe
- Nasal flaring
- Use of accessory muscles
- Hypertension
- Confusion, stupor, coma
- Cyanosis of the skin, lips, and nailbeds

---

sensor and a microprocessor. Red and infrared light is emitted from one side of the sensor, which is attached to a finger (Fig. 20-1), toe, earlobe, or bridge of the nose. The opposite side of the sensor detects the amount of light that is absorbed by hemoglobin. The microprocessor then computes the information and displays it on a machine at the bedside.

A sustained level of less than 90% is cause for concern. If the SaO_2 remains below 70%, oxygen therapy of one kind or another is needed. However, various factors may affect the accuracy of the displayed information (Table 20-1). After troubleshooting the equipment, concomitant physical assessments and laboratory arterial blood gas measurements may help to confirm the significance of the displayed findings.

PROMOTING OXYGENATION

Oxygenation can be promoted by using positioning and breathing techniques.

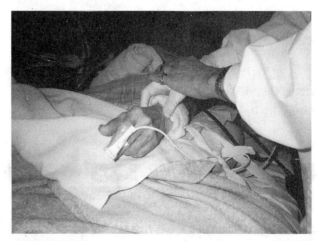

FIGURE 20-1

An adhesive oximeter sensor. (Courtesy of Ken Timby.)

SKILL 20-1
Using a Pulse Oximeter

Suggested Action	Reason for Action
Assessment	
Assess potential sensor sites for the quality of circulation, presence of edema, tremor, restlessness, nail polish, or artificial nails.	Determines where sensor is best applied
Review the medical history for data indicating vascular or other pathology like anemia or carbon monoxide inhalation.	Suggests that data from oximeter may be unreliable
Check prescribed medications for vasoconstrictive effects.	Suggests that data from oximeter may be unreliable
Determine how much the patient understands about pulse oximetry.	Indicates the need for and type of teaching
Planning	
Explain the procedure to the patient.	Reduces anxiety and promotes cooperation
Obtain equipment.	Promotes organization and efficient time management
Implementation	
Wash your hands.	Reduces the transmission of microorganisms
Position the sensor so that the light emission is directly opposite the detector.	Ensures accurate monitoring

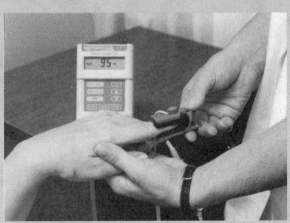

Spring-tension sensor and microprocessor. (Courtesy of Ken Timby.)

Suggested Action	Reason for Action
Attach the sensor cable to the machine.	Connects the sensor with the microprocessor
Observe the numeric display, audible sound, or waveform on the machine.	Indicates that the equipment is functioning
Set the high and low alarms according to the manufacturer's directions.	Alerts the nurse to check the patient
Move an adhesive finger sensor every 4 hours and a spring-tension sensor every 2 hours.	Prevents skin breakdown

(continued)

SKILL 20-1
Using a Pulse Oximeter (Continued)

Suggested Action	Reason for Action

Evaluation
- SaO_2 measurements remain within 95%–100%
- No evidence of hypoxemia or hypoxia

Document
- Normal SaO_2 measurements once a shift unless ordered otherwise
- Abnormal SaO_2 measurements when they are sustained
- Nursing measures to improve oxygenation if SaO_2 levels fall below 90% and are prolonged
- Person to whom abnormal measurements have been reported and outcome of communication
- Removal and relocation of the sensor
- Condition of the skin at the sensor site

Sample Documentation

Date and Time SaO_2 remains constant at 95%–98%. Respirations unlabored. Skin under sensor is intact. Spring-tension sensor changed from L. index finger to R. index finger.

_____ **Signature/Title**

Positioning

Unless contraindicated by their condition, hypoxic patients are placed in a high Fowler's position (see Chap. 23). This upright, seated position eases breathing by causing the abdominal organs to descend away from the diaphragm. As a result, the lungs potentially can fill with a greater volume of air.

As an alternative, patients who find breathing difficult may benefit from a variation of the Fowler's position called the **orthopneic position**. When the orthopneic position is used, the patient is seated and the arms are supported on pillows or the arm rests of a chair (Fig. 20-2). The orthopneic position also allows room for maximum chest expansion and provides comfort while resting or sleeping.

Breathing Techniques

Breathing techniques such as deep breathing, pursed-lip, and diaphragmatic breathing help patients to breathe more efficiently.

DEEP BREATHING

Deep breathing is a technique for maximizing ventilation. By taking in a large volume of air, a greater number of alveoli tend to fill, thus improving gas exchange.

Deep breathing is therapeutic for patients who breathe shallowly, like those who are inactive or in pain. To encourage deep breathing, the patient is instructed to take in as much air as possible, hold the breath briefly, and exhale slowly. In some cases it may be helpful to use an incentive spirometer.

Incentive Sprirometry

Incentive spirometry is a technique for measuring the volume of air that a patient inhales. Spirometers are useful for evaluating the effectiveness of the patient's efforts at deep breathing. They also provide a visual reinforcement, or incentive, to reach a specific volume-related goal.

Although spirometers are constructed in different ways, all are calibrated in at least 100 mL increments and provide some visual cue as to how much air has been inhaled. Some use a light to indicate the inspired volume (Fig. 20-3). Others operate in such a way as to raise lightweight balls within a calibrated column.

PURSED-LIP BREATHING

Pursed-lip breathing is a form of controlled ventilation in which the expiration phase is consciously pro-

TABLE 20-1. *Factors That Interfere With Accurate Pulse Oximetry*

Factor	Cause(s)	Remedy
Movement of the sensor	Tremor	Relocate sensor to another site
	Restlessness	
	Loss of adhesion	Replace sensor or tape in place
Poor circulation at the sensor site	Peripheral vascular disease	Change the sensor location or type of sensor
	Edema	
	Tourniquet effect from a taped sensor	Loosen or change sensor location
	Vasoconstrictive drug effects	Discontinue oximetry temporarily
Light barrier	Nail polish	Remove polish
	Thick toenails	Relocate sensor
	Acrylic nails	Remove nail
Extraneous light	Direct sunlight or bright room light	Cover the sensor with a towel
Hemoglobin saturation with other substances	Carbon monoxide poisoning	Discontinue oximetry temporarily

longed. If done correctly, it helps to eliminate carbon dioxide, thus freeing oxygen binding sites on the hemoglobin molecule. Pursed-lip breathing and diaphragmatic breathing are especially helpful for patients who have chronic lung diseases, like emphysema.

Pursed-lip breathing is performed by:

- Inhaling slowly through the nose while counting to three
- Pursing the lips as though to whistle
- Contracting the abdominal muscles
- Exhaling through pursed lips for a count of six or more

Expiration should last two to three times longer than inspiration. Not all patients can reach this goal initially, but with practice the length of expiration may increase.

DIAPHRAGMATIC BREATHING

Diaphragmatic breathing, also called *abdominal breathing*, promotes the use of the diaphragm, rather than upper chest muscles, to breathe. When diaphragmatic breathing is used, the respiratory rate decreases but the volume of air that is exchanged during inspiration and expiration increases.

When performing diaphragmatic breathing, the patient is taught to do the following:

- Place one hand on the abdomen and the other on the chest.
- Inhale slowly and deeply through the nose while letting the abdomen rise more so than the chest.
- Purse the lips.
- Contract the abdominal muscles.
- Press inward and upward with the hand on the abdomen.
- Repeat for a full minute; rest for at least 2 minutes.
- Practice the breathing exercises at least twice a day for a period of 5 to 10 minutes.
- Progress to doing diaphragmatic breathing while being active.

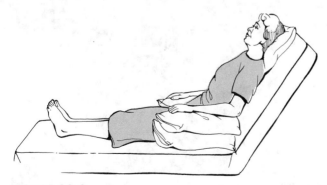

FIGURE 20-2
Orthopneic position.

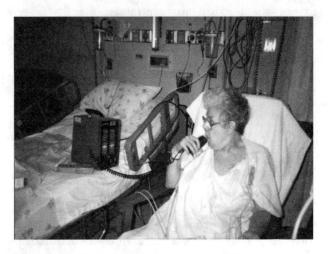

FIGURE 20-3
Using an incentive spirometer. (Courtesy of Ken Timby.)

PATIENT TEACHING FOR USING AN INCENTIVE SPIROMETER

Teach the patient to do the following:
- Sit upright unless contraindicated.
- Identify the mark indicating the goal for inhalation.
- Exhale normally.
- Insert the mouthpiece, sealing it between the lips.

- Inhale slowly until the predetermined volume has been reached.
- Hold the breath for 2 to 6 seconds.
- Exhale normally.
- Repeat the exercise 10 to 20 times per hour while awake, or as prescribed by the physician.

When positioning and breathing techniques are inadequate for keeping the blood adequately saturated with oxygen, oxygen therapy may be necessary.

OXYGEN THERAPY

Oxygen therapy is a therapeutic intervention for improving cellular oxygenation by administering more oxygen than the 21% that exists in the atmosphere. Oxygen therapy requires an oxygen source; a flowmeter; in some cases, humidification; and an oxygen delivery device.

Oxygen Sources

Oxygen can be supplied from any one of four sources. It may be dispensed from a wall outlet, portable tank, liquid oxygen unit, or oxygen concentrator.

WALL OUTLET

Most modern health care facilities have been constructed so as to supply oxygen through a wall outlet located in each patient's room. The outlet is connected to pipes that lead to a large central reservoir that is kept filled with oxygen.

However, when oxygen is not piped to individual rooms, or in cases where the patient needs to leave the room temporarily, oxygen may be provided in portable tanks.

PORTABLE TANKS

Oxygen may be stored in tanks resembling steel cylinders (Fig. 20-4) that hold various volumes under extreme pressure. A large tank of oxygen is pressurized at 2,000 pounds per square inch. Therefore, tanks are delivered with a protective cap to prevent accidental force against the tank outlet. Any accidental force applied to a partially opened outlet could cause the tank to take off like a rocket, with disastrous results. There-

fore, oxygen tanks are transported and stored while strapped to a wheeled carrier.

Before oxygen is administered from a portable tank, the tank must be *cracked* to clear the outlet of dust and debris. Cracking is done by turning the tank valve slightly to allow a brief release of pressurized oxygen. The force causes a loud hissing noise, which may be frightening. Therefore, it is best to crack the tank away from the patient's bedside.

LIQUID OXYGEN UNIT

Liquid oxygen units (Fig. 20-5), which are small, lightweight, and portable, convert cooled liquid oxygen to a gas by passing it through heated coils. These units are used primarily by ambulatory home patients because they allow greater mobility, both within and away from their residence. Each unit holds approximately 4 to 8 hours' worth of oxygen. However, liquid oxygen is comparatively more expensive, may leak during warm weather, and the outlet may become occluded by frozen moisture.

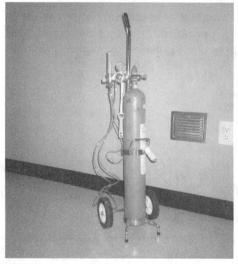

FIGURE 20-4
Portable oxygen tank. (Courtesy of Ken Timby.)

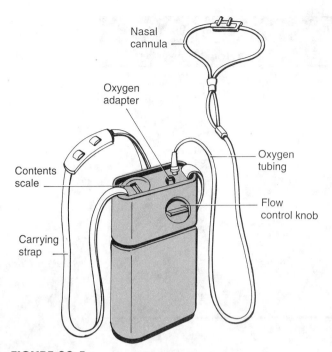

FIGURE 20-5
Liquid oxygen unit.

OXYGEN CONCENTRATOR

An **oxygen concentrator** (Fig. 20-6) is a machine that collects and concentrates oxygen from room air and stores it for patient use. An oxygen concentrator eliminates the need for a central reservoir of piped oxygen or the use of bulky tanks that must be constantly replaced. This type of oxygen source is being used more and more in home health care and long-term care facilities, primarily because of its convenience and economy.

Although it is more economical than other sources of oxygen in portable tanks, the device does increase

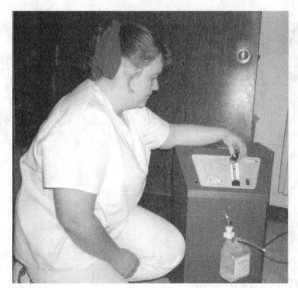

FIGURE 20-6
Oxygen concentrator. (Courtesy of Ken Timby.)

the patient's electric bill somewhat. Other disadvantages include that it generates heat from its motor and produces an unpleasant odor or taste if the filter is not cleaned regularly. Also, patients must have a secondary source of oxygen available in case of a power failure.

To determine how much oxygen is being administered, a flowmeter must be attached to the oxygen source.

Flowmeter

A **flowmeter** (Fig. 20-7) is a metered gauge that attaches to the oxygen source. It is used to regulate the number of liters of oxygen delivered to the patient. To adjust the rate of flow, the nurse turns the dial until the indicator is directly beside the prescribed amount.

The physician prescribes the amount of oxygen, sometimes referred to as the **fraction of inspired oxygen** or FiO_2, based on the condition of the patient. The Joint Committee for Accreditation of Healthcare Organizations (JCAHO) requires that oxygen be prescribed in percentage rather than liter flow. However, nurses may find that physicians continue to prescribe the amount in liters per minute (L/minute). Depending on the oxygen delivery device, the same liters per minute may provide different percentages (Table 20-2).

Humidification

Oxygen is drying to the mucous membranes. Therefore, oxygen is humidified, in most cases, when over 4 L/minute is administered for an extended period of

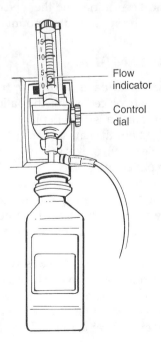

FIGURE 20-7
An oxygen flowmeter with humidification bottle attached.

TABLE 20-2. *Conversion Equivalents for Oxygen Therapy*

Delivery Method	L/min	Equivalent Percentage
Nasal cannula	2	28
	4	36
	6	44
Simple mask	5	40
	6–7	50
	7–8	60
Partial rebreather mask	6	35
	8	45–50
	10	60
Nonrebreather mask	6	55–60
	8	60–8
	10	80–90
Venturi mask		
Color code: Blue	4	24
Color code: Yellow	4	28
Color code: White	6	31
Color code: Green	8	40

time. To do this, a humidifier bottle is filled with distilled water and attached to the flowmeter (see Fig. 20-7). The water level is checked daily and refilled as needed by a respiratory therapist or nurse.

Common Delivery Devices

Oxygen can be administered in several ways. Common delivery devices include a nasal cannula, masks, face tent, tracheostomy collar, or T-piece. The device that is used usually depends on the patient's oxygenation status, physical condition, and the type of device that can best deliver the appropriate amount of oxygen.

NASAL CANNULA

A **nasal cannula** is a hollow tube with ½-inch prongs that are placed within the patient's nostrils (Fig. 20-8). The cannula is held in place by either wrapping the tubing about the ears and adjusting the fit beneath the chin (Fig. 20-9), or it is secured with an elastic band about the patient's head.

Because a nasal cannula provides a means of administering low percentages of oxygen, it is ideal for patients who are not extremely hypoxic or who have chronic lung diseases. High percentages of oxygen are contraindicated for patients with chronic lung disease because, having adapted to excessive levels of retained carbon dioxide, their drive to breathe is stimulated by low blood oxygen levels. Consequently, if patients with chronic lung disease receive more than 2 to 3 liters of oxygen over a sustained period of time, their respiratory rate may slow or even stop.

MASKS

Oxygen may be delivered with one of several different types of masks such as a simple, partial rebreather, nonrebreather, and Venturi mask (Fig. 20-10). When administering oxygen by mask, it is delivered at no less than 5 L/minute.

Simple Mask

A **simple mask** fits over the nose and mouth and is held in place by an elastic strap. The simple mask as well as other types of masks facilitates administering higher levels of oxygen than possible with a cannula. However, the efficiency of any mask is affected by how

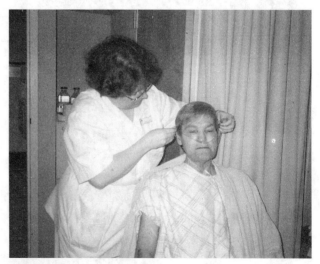

FIGURE 20-8
Applying a nasal cannula. (Courtesy of Ken Timby.)

into the atmosphere through small ports in the mask (Fig. 20-11). Because the initial portion of exhaled air comes directly from the upper airways, it contains oxygen but no carbon dioxide. Therefore, every breath provides a much larger concentration of oxygen than could be delivered with a simple mask.

Nonrebreather Mask

A **nonrebreather mask** is similar to a partial rebreather mask except that *all* the exhaled air leaves the mask rather than partially entering the reservoir bag. Consequently, it is possible to administer an FiO_2 of 90% to 100%. Obviously, patients who require such high concentrations of oxygen are usually critically ill and may eventually need mechanical ventilation.

Humidification is *not* used whenever a mask with a reservoir bag is used despite the high concentrations of oxygen. Also, patients with partial and nonrebreather masks must be monitored closely to ensure that the reservoir bag remains partially inflated at all times.

Venturi Mask

A **Venturi mask**, sometimes called a Venti mask, has a large ringed tube that extends from the mask. Adapters within the tube that may be color-coded or regulated by a dial system, permit only specific amounts of room air to mix with the oxygen. This feature makes the Venturi mask advantageous for administering precise amounts of oxygen.

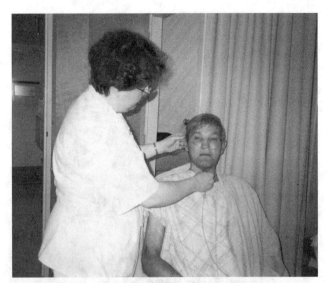

FIGURE 20-9
Adjusting the cannula. (Courtesy of Ken Timby.)

well it fits the face. Without a good seal, the oxygen may leak from the mask, thus diminishing its concentration.

There are other problems associated with masks as well. All oxygen masks interfere with eating and make communication difficult. Also, some patients become anxious when their nose and mouth are covered because it creates for them a feeling of suffocating. Skin care also becomes a priority because masks create pressure and trap moisture.

Partial Rebreather Mask

A **partial rebreather mask** is attached to a reservoir bag. During expiration, the first one third of exhaled air enters the reservoir bag, while the remainder is vented

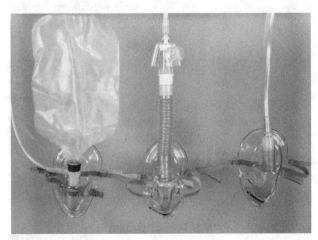

FIGURE 20-10
From left to right: Simple oxygen mask, Venturi mask, partial rebreather mask that can be converted to a nonrebreather mask. (Courtesy of Ken Timby.)

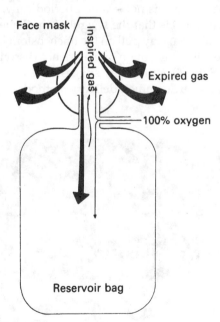

FIGURE 20-11
Patterns of air flow with a partial rebreather mask. (The Lippincott Manual of Nursing Practice, 5th ed, p 220. Philadelphia, JB Lippincott, 1991)

FACE TENT

A **face tent** (Fig. 20-12) delivers oxygen without the discomfort of a mask. Because the face tent is open and loose around the face, patients are less likely to feel claustrophobic. An added advantage is that a face tent can be used for patients with facial trauma or burns. Unfortunately, the amount of oxygen patients actually receive may be inconsistent with what is prescribed because of environmental losses.

TRACHEOSTOMY COLLAR

A **tracheostomy collar** (Fig. 20-13) is a device that is applied about a patient's neck to cover a tracheostomy, an opening into the trachea through which a patient breathes (see Chap. 36). Because the warming and moisturizing functions of the nose are bypassed, a tracheostomy collar provides a means for both oxygenation and humidification. The moisture that collects, however, tends to saturate the gauze dressing, making it necessary to change it frequently.

T-PIECE

A **T-piece** (Fig. 20-14) is similar to a tracheostomy collar except that the device fits securely onto a tracheostomy tube or endotracheal tube. Although the gauze around the tracheostomy usually remains dry, the moisture that collects within the tubing tends to condense and may enter the airway during position changes if it is not drained periodically. Another disadvantage is that the weight of the T-piece, or its manipulation, may pull on the tracheostomy tube, causing the patient to cough or experience discomfort.

Skill 20-2 provides suggestions for administering oxygen by common delivery methods.

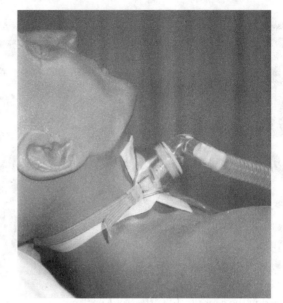

FIGURE 20-13
Tracheostomy collar. (Courtesy of Ken Timby.)

Additional Delivery Devices

There are other methods for delivering oxygen, but they are not as commonly used. Occasionally, oxygen may be delivered via a nasal catheter, oxygen tent, or transtracheal catheter.

NASAL CATHETER

A **nasal catheter** is a tube that is inserted through the nose into the posterior nasal pharynx (Fig. 20-15). However, because the catheter tends to be irritating and annoying to patients, it is not often used.

If a catheter is prescribed, the nurse secures it to the nose to avoid displacement and cleans the nostril with

(text continues on page 414)

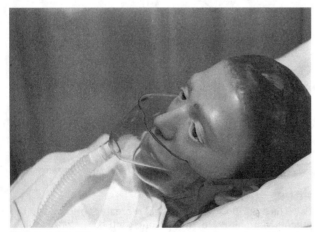

FIGURE 20-12
Face tent. (Courtesy of Ken Timby.)

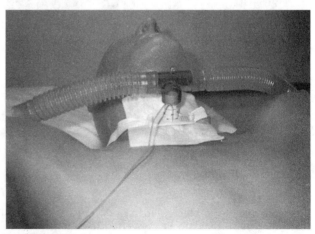

FIGURE 20-14
T-piece. (Courtesy of Ken Timby.)

SKILL 20-2
Administering Oxygen

Suggested Action	Reason for Action
Assessment	
Perform physical assessment techniques that focus on oxygenation.	Provides a baseline for future comparisons
Monitor the SaO₂ level with a pulse oximeter.	Provides a baseline for future comparisons
Check the medical order for the type of oxygen delivery device, liter flow or percentage prescribed, and whether the oxygen is to be administered continuously or only as needed.	Ensures compliance with the plan for medical treatment
Note if a wall outlet is available, or if another type of oxygen source must be obtained.	Promotes organization and efficient time management
Determine how much the patient understands about oxygen therapy.	Indicates the need for and type of teaching that must be done
Planning	
Obtain equipment, which usually includes a flowmeter, delivery device, and in some cases a humidification bottle.	Promotes organization and efficient time management
Contact the respiratory therapy department for equipment, if that is agency policy.	Follows interdepartmental guidelines
Crack the portable oxygen tank, if that is the type of oxygen source being used.	Prevents alarming the patient
Explain the procedure to the patient.	Decreases anxiety and promotes cooperation
Post a "No Smoking" sign on the patient's door.	Demonstrates concern for safety
Implementation	
Wash your hands.	Reduces the transmission of microorganisms
Assist the patient to a Fowler's or alternate position.	Promotes ventilation
Attach the flowmeter to the oxygen source.	Provides a means for regulating the prescribed amount of oxygen

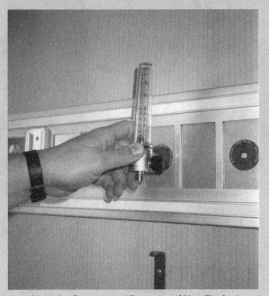

Attaching the flowmeter. (Courtesy of Ken Timby.)

(continued)

SKILL 20-2
Administering Oxygen (Continued)

Suggested Action	Reason for Action
Fill a humidifier bottle with distilled water to the appropriate level if administering 4 or more L/minute.	Moisturizes mucous membranes
Connect the humidification bottle to the flow-meter.	Provides a pathway through which the oxygen will be humidified

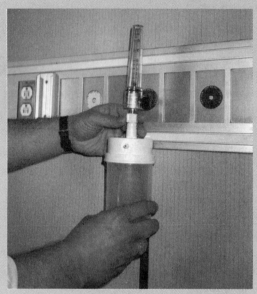

Connecting the humidification bottle. (Courtesy of Ken Timby.)

Suggested Action	Reason for Action
Insert the appropriate color-coded valve or dial the prescribed percentage if a Venturi mask is being used.	Regulates the FiO_2

(continued)

SKILL 20-2
Administering Oxygen (Continued)

Suggested Action	Reason for Action
Attach the distal end of the tubing from the oxygen delivery device to the flowmeter or humidification bottle.	Provides a pathway for oxygen from its source to the patient

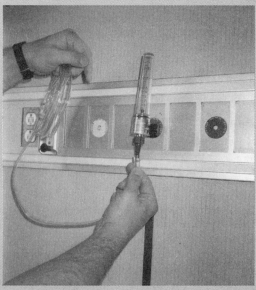

Attaching tubing from the delivery device. (Courtesy of Ken Timby.)

Turn on the oxygen by adjusting the flowmeter to the prescribed volume.	Fills the delivery device with oxygen-rich air
Verify that bubbles appear in the humidification bottle, if one is used, or that air is felt at the proximal end of the delivery device.	Indicates that oxygen is being released
Make sure that if a reservoir bag is used, it is partially filled and remains that way throughout oxygen therapy.	Prevents asphyxiation
Attach the delivery device to the patient.	Provides oxygen therapy
Drain any tubing that collects condensation.	Maintains a clear pathway for oxygen and prevents accidental aspiration when turning a patient
Remove the oxygen delivery device and provide skin, oral, and nasal hygiene at least every 4 to 8 hours.	Maintains intact skin and mucous membranes; reduces the growth of microorganisms
Reassess the patient's oxygenation status at least once per shift.	Indicates how well the patient is responding to oxygen therapy
Notify the physician if the patient manifests signs of hypoxemia or hypoxia despite oxygen therapy.	Demonstrates concern for patient safety

(continued)

SKILL 20-2
Administering Oxygen (Continued)

Suggested Action	Reason for Action

Evaluation

- Respiratory rate is within 12 to 24 breaths per minute at rest.
- Breathing is effortless
- Heart rate is <100 bpm
- Is alert and oriented
- Skin and mucous membranes are normal color
- SaO_2 is ≥90%
- FiO_2 and delivery device correspond to medical order

Document
- Assessment data
- Percentage of oxygen administration
- Type of delivery device
- Length of time in use
- Response of the patient to oxygen therapy

Sample Documentation

Date and Time   Restless, pulse rate 120, resp. rate 32 with nasal flaring. Placed in high Fowler's position. SaO_2 at 85%–88%. Simple mask applied with administration of oxygen at 5 L/min. After 15 min. of oxygen therapy is less agitated, pulse rate 100, respiratory rate 28, no nasal flaring noted. SaO_2 at 90%–92%. Oxygen continues to be administered. _____ **Signature, Title**

a cotton applicator on a regular basis to remove dried mucus.

OXYGEN TENT

An **oxygen tent** is a clear plastic enclosure that provides cooled, humidified oxygen. Oxygen tents, if used, are more likely employed in the care of active, toddler-aged children. Children this age are less likely to keep a mask or cannula in place, yet may require oxygenation and humidification for respiratory conditions such as croup or bronchitis. A face hood may be used for less active infants.

When caring for a child in an oxygen tent, it is essential to keep the edges of the tent tucked securely beneath the mattress and to limit opening the zippered access ports so that oxygen does not escape too freely.

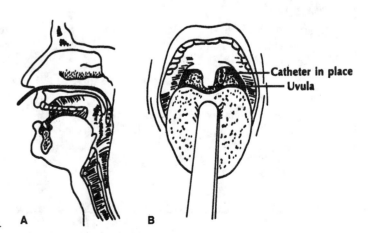

FIGURE 20-15
Nasal catheter placement.

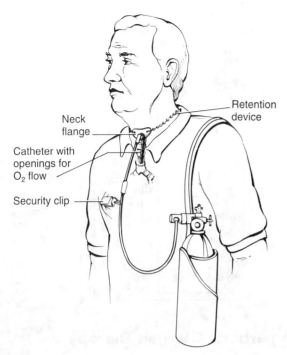

FIGURE 20-16
Transtracheal oxygen administration.

TRANSTRACHEAL OXYGEN

Some patients who require long-term oxygen therapy may prefer its administration through a transtracheal catheter (Fig. 20-16). This device is less noticeable than a nasal cannula, and because the patient may be adequately oxygenated with lower liter flows, the costs of replenishing the oxygen source may be decreased.

Before transtracheal oxygen can be used, a temporary tube or **stent** is inserted into a surgically created

---

◀ **NURSING GUIDELINES FOR THE SAFE USE OF OXYGEN**

- Post "No Smoking" signs wherever oxygen is stored or in use.
  Rationale: Warns others of potential fire hazard
- Prohibit the burning of candles during religious rites.
  Rationale: Eliminates a source of open flames
- Check that electrical devices have a three-pronged plug (see Chap. 19).
  Rationale: Provides a ground for leaking electricity
- Inspect electrical equipment for the presence of frayed wires or loose connections.
  Rationale: Avoids sparks or uncontrolled pathway for electricity
- Avoid petroleum products, aerosol products like hair spray, and products containing acetone such as nail polish remover, where oxygen is used.

Rationale: Prevents potential for igniting flammable substance
- Secure portable oxygen cylinders to rigid stands.
  Rationale: Prevents rupturing the tank
- Avoid synthetic fabrics.
  Rationale: Reduces potential for static electricity

---

opening and remains there until the wound heals. Thereafter, the stent is removed and the catheter is inserted and held in place by a necklace-type chain. Patients are taught how to clean the tracheal opening and catheter—a procedure that is done several times a day. During cleaning, patients can administer oxygen with a nasal cannula.

Regardless of what device is used to deliver oxygen, its administration involves potential hazards.

OXYGEN HAZARDS

There are two major hazards involved in administering oxygen. First, and foremost, is its capacity to support fires; second, it has the potential for causing oxygen toxicity.

Fire Potential

Oxygen itself does not burn, but it does support combustion. In other words, it contributes to the burning process. Therefore, it is necessary to control all possible sources of open flames or ungrounded electricity.

Oxygen Toxicity

Oxygen toxicity refers to lung damage that develops when oxygen concentrations of over 50% are administered longer than 24 to 48 hours. The exact mechanism by which hyperoxygenation damages the lungs is not definitely known. Once it develops, however, it is difficult to reverse. Unfortunately, the early symptoms are quite subtle (Display 20-2). The best prevention is to administer the lowest FiO_2 possible for the shortest amount of time.

RELATED OXYGENATION TECHNIQUES

There are two additional techniques that relate to oxygenation. One involves the use of a water-seal drainage system and the other involves using hyperbaric oxygen therapy.

Water-Seal Drainage

Water-seal drainage refers to a technique for evacuating air or blood from the pleural cavity, restoring neg-

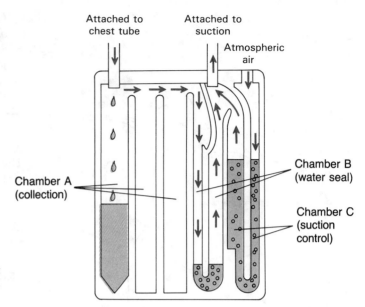

FIGURE 20-17
A three-chambered water-seal drainage system. (Earnest VV: Clinical Skills in Nursing Practice, 2nd ed, p 760. Philadelphia, JB Lippincott, 1992)

ative intrapleural pressure, and reinflating the lung. Patients who require water-seal drainage have one or two chest tubes that connect to the drainage system.

Several commercial companies provide equipment for water-seal drainage. All of them are similar in that they consist of a three-chambered system (Fig. 20-17). One chamber collects blood or acts as an exit route for pleural air. A second compartment holds water, which prevents atmospheric air from reentering the pleural space—hence the origin of the term "water seal." A third chamber, if used, facilitates adding suction, which may speed the evacuation of blood or air.

One of the most important principles when caring for patients with water-seal drainage is that the chest tube(s) must never be separated from the drainage system unless it is clamped. Even then, the tube may be clamped only for a brief amount of time. Additional nursing responsibilities are included in Skill 20-3.

Hyperbaric Oxygen Therapy

Hyperbaric oxygen therapy consists of delivering 100% oxygen at three times the normal atmospheric pressure within an airtight chamber (Fig. 20-18). Treatments, which last approximately 90 minutes, may be repeated over days, weeks, or months of therapy. Providing pressurized oxygen increases the oxygenation of blood plasma from a normal level of 80 to 100 mm Hg to more than 2,000 mm Hg (Collison, 1993). Oxygen toxicity is avoided by providing patients with brief periods during which they breathe room air.

Hyperbaric oxygen therapy helps regenerate new tissue at a faster rate, and thus its most popular use is for promoting wound healing. However, it is also used for treating carbon monoxide poisoning, gangrene associated with diabetes or other conditions of vascular insufficiency, decompression sickness experienced by deep sea divers, anaerobic infections (especially those

(text continues on page 422)

DISPLAY 20-2. _Signs and Symptoms of Oxygen Toxicity_

- Nonproductive cough
- Substernal chest pain
- Nasal stuffiness
- Nausea and vomiting
- Fatigue
- Headache
- Sore throat
- Hypoventilation

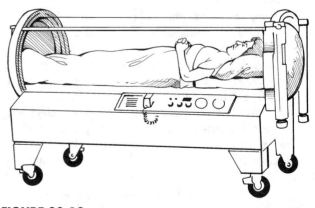

FIGURE 20-18
A one-person, or monoplace, hyperbaric oxygen chamber.

SKILL 20-3
Maintaining a Water-Seal Drainage System

Suggested Action	Reason for Action
Assessment	
Review the patient's medical record to determine the condition that necessitated inserting a chest tube.	Indicates whether to expect air, bloody drainage, or both
Determine if the physician has inserted one or two chest tubes.	Helps direct assessment
Note the date of chest tube(s) insertion.	Provides a point of reference for evaluating assessment data
Check the medical orders to determine if the drainage is being collected by gravity or with the addition of suction, and, if so, how much.	Provides guidelines for carrying out medical treatment
Planning	
Arrange to perform a physical assessment of the patient and equipment as soon as possible after receiving report.	Establishes a baseline and early opportunity for troubleshooting abnormal findings
Locate a roll of tape and container of distilled water.	Facilitates efficient time management for general maintenance of the drainage system
Implementation	
Introduce yourself to the patient and explain the purpose of the interaction.	Reduces anxiety and promotes cooperation
Wash your hands.	Reduces the transmission of microorganisms
Check to see that a pair of hemostats, instruments for clamping, are at the bedside.	Facilitates checking for air leaks in the tubing or clamping the chest tube in the event the drainage system must be replaced
Turn off the suction regulator, if one is used, before assessing the patient.	Eliminates noise that may interfere with chest auscultation
Assess the patient's lung sounds; expect that no lung sounds will be heard where the lung is deflated.	Provides a baseline for future comparisons
Inspect the dressing for signs that it has become loose or saturated with drainage.	Indicates a need for changing the dressing (see Chap. 28)
Palpate the skin around the chest tube insertion site to feel and listen for air crackling in the tissues.	Indicates subcutaneous air leak

(continued)

SKILL 20-3
Maintaining a Water-Seal Drainage System (Continued)

Suggested Action	Reason for Action
Inspect all connections to determine that they are taped and secure.	IIndicates appropriate care has been performed

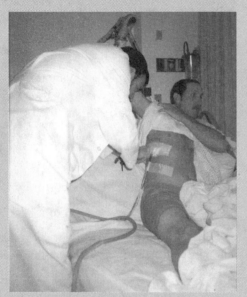

Palpating for air bubbles. (Courtesy of Ken Timby.)

Suggested Action	Reason for Action
Reinforce connections where the tape may be loose.	Prevents accidental separation
Check that all of the tubing is unkinked and hangs freely into the drainage system.	Ensures evacuation of air and bloody drainage
Observe the fluid level in the water-seal chamber to see if it is at the 2-cm level.	Maintains the water seal
Add distilled water to the appropriate mark indicated by the manufacturer if the fluid level is below standard.	Ensures water seal

(continued)

SKILL 20-3
Maintaining a Water-Seal Drainage System (Continued)

Suggested Action	Reason for Action
Note if the water is tidaling, that is, rising and falling with each respiration.	Indicates that the tubing is unobstructed and the lung has not completely inflated

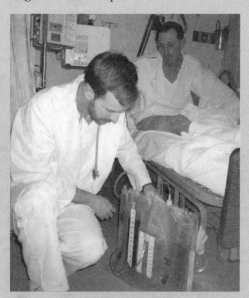

Watching for tidaling. (Courtesy of Ken Timby.)

Suggested Action	Reason for Action
Observe for the presence of continuous bubbling in the *water-seal chamber*.	Indicates an air leak in the tubing or at a connection; *constant bubbling is expected in the suction control chamber*
If constant bubbling is observed, clamp the hemostats at the chest and a few inches away and observe if the bubbling stops; continue releasing and reapplying the hemostats toward the drainage system until the bubbling stops.	Provides a means for determining the location of an air leak within the tubing
Apply tape around the tube above where the last clamp was applied when the bubbling stopped.	Seals the origin of the air leak

(continued)

SKILL 20-3
Maintaining a Water-Seal Drainage System (Continued)

Suggested Action	Reason for Action
Note if the water level in the suction chamber is at 20 cm.	Determines appropriate water level for suction

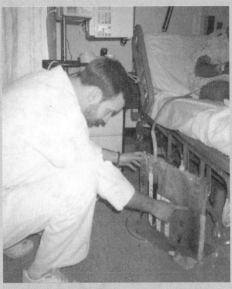

Noting water levels. (Courtesy of Ken Timby.)

Suggested Action	Reason for Action
Add distilled water to the appropriate mark in the suction control chamber if it has evaporated.	Maintains appropriate amount of suction

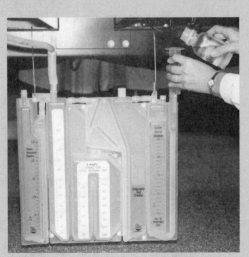

Adding water to the suction control chamber. (Courtesy of Ken Timby.)

Suggested Action	Reason for Action
Regulate the suction so that it produces *gentle* bubbling.	Prevents rapid evaporation and unnecessary noise
Observe the nature and amount of drainage in the collection chamber.	Provides comparative data; more than 100 mL/hour or bright red drainage is reported

(continued)

SKILL 20-3
Maintaining a Water-Seal Drainage System *(Continued)*

Suggested Action	Reason for Action
Keep the drainage system below the chest.	Maintains gravity flow of drainage
Position the patient so as to avoid compressing the tubing.	Facilitates drainage
Curl and secure excess length of tubing on the bed.	Avoids dependent loops
Milk the tubing, a process of compressing and stripping the tubing to move stationary clots, only if absolutely necessary.	Creates extremely high negative intrapleural pressure, and therefore is never done routinely
Encourage coughing and deep breathing at least every 2 hours while awake.	Promotes lung reexpansion
Instruct the patient to move about in bed, ambulate while carrying the drainage system, and exercise the shoulder on the side of the drainage tube.	Prevents hazards of immobility and maintains joint flexibility
Never clamp the chest tube for an extended period of time (it is safe to clamp it briefly, for example when changing the entire drainage system).	Predisposes to development of a **tension pneumothorax**, extreme air pressure within the lung when there is no avenue for escape
Insert a separated chest tube within water until it can be reattached and secured to the drainage system.	Provides a temporary water seal
Prevent air from entering the tube insertion site, if the tube should be accidentally pulled out.	Reduces the amount of lung collapse
Mark the drainage level on the collection chamber at the end of each shift. *Never empty the drainage container.*	Contributes to data concerning fluid loss without the risk of recollapsing the lung

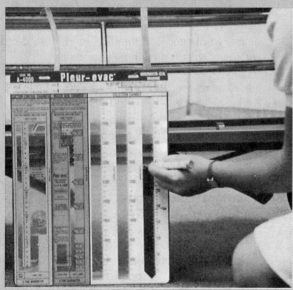

Marking drainage level. (Courtesy of Ken Timby.)

(continued)

SKILL 20-3
Maintaining a Water-Seal Drainage System (Continued)

Suggested Action	Reason for Action

Evaluation
- No evidence of respiratory distress
- Dressing is dry and intact
- Equipment is functioning appropriately
- Water is at recommended levels

Document
- Assessment findings
- Care provided
- Amount of drainage during period of care

Sample Documentation

Date and Time Upper and lower chest tubes connected to water-seal drainage system. Normal lung sounds heard throughout chest except in apex and base of left lung where chest tubes are inserted. Tidaling still observed in water-seal chamber. 20 cm of suction maintained. Dark red chest tube drainage measures a scant 50 mL. Ambulated in hall while disconnected from suction. Performed full range of motion with left shoulder. _____ **Signature, Title**

that occur among burn patients), and a host of other medical conditions.

NURSING IMPLICATIONS

Nurses assess the oxygenation status of patients on a day-by-day and shift-by-shift basis. Therefore, it is not unusual to identify any one or several of the nursing diagnoses listed in Applicable Nursing Diagnoses among patients who are experiencing hypoxemia or hypoxia.

Abnormal assessment findings often lead to collaboration with the physician and the prescription for oxygen therapy. The accompanying Nursing Care Plan has been developed to illustrate how the nursing process applies to a patient with the nursing diagnosis of Inef-

APPLICABLE NURSING DIAGNOSES

- Ineffective Breathing Pattern
- Ineffective Airway Clearance
- Impaired Gas Exchange
- Anxiety
- Risk for Injury

FOCUS ON OLDER ADULTS

- Older adults often manifest age-related changes that compromise ventilation and respiration, such as calcification of rib cartilage, skeletal changes in the spine and ribs, reduced numbers of alveoli, less elastic recoil of the lungs, weakened cough reflex, and more dead air space within the lungs (Eliopoulos, 1993).
- Inactive older adults are at higher risk for respiratory infections because they breathe shallowly.
- Older adults who have lost weight and the subcutaneous fat within their cheeks may not receive the prescribed amounts of oxygen by mask because of an inadequate facial seal.
- Older adults should have a liberal fluid intake, unless contraindicated, to keep their mucous membranes moist.
- Those who require home use of oxygen need to be encouraged to continue socializing with others outside their home to avoid becoming isolated and depressed.
- Older adults should receive influenza vaccine on a yearly basis; one dose of pneumococcal pneumonia vaccine is effective for a lifetime of protection.

NURSING CARE PLAN:
Ineffective Breathing Pattern

Assessment	**Subjective Data** States, "It seems so hard for me to get my breath. I can't work in my flower garden because I get winded when I try to do any gardening. I can't sleep lying down because I can't breathe except sleeping in a chair." **Objective Data** 55-year-old woman with a history of smoking 1–2 packs of cigarettes daily for 30 years. Respiratory rate is rapid and shallow at 40 breaths per minute. Using accessory muscles to breathe. Barrel chest noted with diminished lung sounds bilaterally.
Diagnosis	Ineffective Breathing Pattern related to retention of carbon dioxide secondary to chronic pulmonary damage from long-term cigarette smoking.
Plan	The patient will demonstrate an effective breathing pattern by 5/10 as evidenced by a respiratory rate no greater than 32 while performing mild activity such as bathing face, arms, and chest.

Orders: 4/28
1. Provide periods of rest between activities.
2. Elevate the head of the bed up to 90°
3. Teach how to perform diaphragmatic and pursed-lip breathing and practice same at least b.i.d.
4. Administer oxygen per nasal cannula at 2 L/minute as prescribed by the physician if SaO_2 falls below 90% and is sustained there.
5. Explore nicotine cessation therapy with transdermal skin patches
—————————————————————————————— R. ANTONIO, RN

Implementation (Documentation)   4/28   1000   Washed upper body and then provided 15 minutes of rest. Respiratory rate at 40 breaths per min. Placed in high Fowler's position. Pulse oximeter shows SaO_2 of 86%. 2 L of oxygen administered per nasal cannula. Discontinued after 30 min. when SaO_2 measured 90%. ———————————— S. LUNCEFORD, LPN

1030   Demonstrated diaphragmatic and pursed-lip breathing. Having difficulty performing breathing exercises while lying down. Head raised and technique practiced again. Tolerance and performance improves in seated position.
—————————————————————————————— S. LUNCEFORD, LPN

fective Breathing Pattern. This diagnostic category is defined in the NANDA taxonomy (1994) as "A state in which an individual's inhalation and/or exhalation pattern does not enable adequate pulmonary inflation or emptying."

KEY CONCEPTS

- Ventilation is the act of moving air in and out of the lungs. Respiration refers to the mechanisms by which oxygen is delivered to the cells.

- The oxygenation status of patients can be determined at the bedside by performing focused physical assessments and using pulse oximetry.
- Five signs of inadequate oxygenation include restlessness, rapid breathing, rapid heart rate, sitting up to breathe, and use of accessory muscles.
- Oxygenation can be improved by positioning patients so as to elevate the head and chest and teaching them to perform breathing exercises.
- When oxygen therapy is prescribed, nurses need to obtain a source for the oxygen, a flowmeter, an oxygen delivery device, and, in some cases, a humidification bottle.

- Oxygen may be supplied through a wall outlet, in portable tanks, within a liquid oxygen unit, or with an oxygen concentrator.
- Most patients receive oxygen therapy through a nasal cannula, any one of several types of masks, or a face tent. Those who have had an opening created in their trachea may receive oxygen through a tracheostomy collar or T-piece.
- Whenever oxygen is administered, nurses must be concerned about two hazards: the potential for fire and oxygen toxicity.
- Older adults have unique respiratory risk factors for several reasons. For example, they often have age-related physical changes that compromise ventilation and respiration, and approximately 80% of the elderly population has some degree of chronic lung disease.

CRITICAL THINKING EXERCISES

- Discuss the differences between oxygen therapy in a health care setting and that in a home environment.
- Of the four methods of supplying oxygen, list them in order from most advantageous to least. Explain the reasons for the order in which you have ranked them.

SUGGESTED READINGS

Collison L. Hyperbarics, when pressuring patients helps. RN March 1993;56:42–48.

Coull A. Making sense of pulse oximetry. Nursing Times August 1992;88:42–43.

Eliopoulos C. Gerontological Nursing. 3rd ed. Philadelphia: JB Lippincott, 1993.

Ellstrom J. What's causing your patient's respiratory distress? Nursing November 1990;20:57–61

Finesilver C. Perfecting the art of respiratory assessment. RN February 1992;55:22–29.

Gift AG, Pugh LC. Dyspnea and fatigue. Nursing Clinics of North America June 1993;28:373–384.

Jacobson A. Prone to oxygenate. American Journal of Nursing August 1993;93:20.

Kuhn JK, McGovern M. Respiratory assessment of the elderly. Journal of Gerontological Nursing May 1992;18:40–43.

McConnell EA. Performing pursed-lip breathing. Nursing December 1992;22:18.

McConnell EA. Teaching your patient to use an incentive spirometer. Nursing February 1993;23:18–20.

NANDA Nursing Diagnoses: Definitions and Classifications 1994–1995. Philadelphia: North American Nursing Diagnosis Association, 1994.

Sonnesso G. Are you ready to use pulse oximetry? Nursing August 1991;21:60–64.

Steismeyer JK. A four-step approach to pulmonary assessment. American Journal of Nursing August 1993;93:22–28, 31.

Witta K. When gauging respiratory status is critical. RN November 1993;56:40–45.

UNIT VI
Preventing Infection

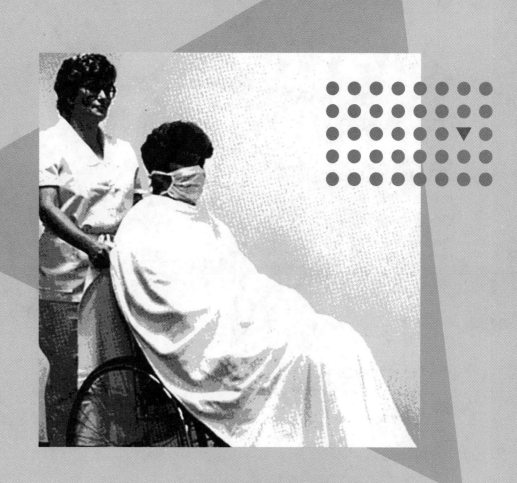

CHAPTER 21
Asepsis
CHAPTER 22
Infection Control

CHAPTER 21

Asepsis

Key Terms

Antibiotics	Nosocomial Infections
Antimicrobial Agents	Opportunistic Infections
Antiseptics	Pathogens
Asepsis	Port of Entry
Aseptic Techniques	Reservoir
Concurrent Disinfection	Resident Microorganisms
Disinfectants	Spore

Exit Route	Sterilization
Handwashing	Surgical Asepsis
Infectious Process Cycle	Susceptible Host
Medical Asepsis	Terminal Disinfection
Microorganisms	Transient Microorganisms
Nonpathogens	Transmission
Normal Flora	

Learning Objectives

An understanding of the content within this chapter will be evidenced by the student's ability to:

- Describe microorganisms
- Differentiate between nonpathogens and pathogens, resident, transient, aerobic, and anaerobic microorganisms
- Name six components of the infectious process cycle
- Discuss two mechanisms by which some microorganisms have adapted to ensure their survival
- Explain the meaning of the term "nosocomial infection"
- Discuss the concept of asepsis and differentiate between medical and surgical asepsis
- Identify at least three principles of medical asepsis
- List five examples of medically aseptic practices
- Name three techniques for sterilizing equipment
- Identify at least three principles of surgical asepsis
- List at least three nursing activities that require the application of principles of surgical asepsis

Microorganisms, or what most people call germs, are living animals or plants that are so small they cannot be seen except with a microscope. What they lack in size, they make up for in numbers. Microorgan-

are literally everywhere. They are in the air, soil, ater, as well as on and within virtually everything and everyone.

Nonpathogens are generally harmless microorganisms, whereas **pathogens** have a high potential for causing infections and contagious diseases. Because preventing disease is one of the priorities in nursing, this chapter addresses how microorganisms survive and the mechanisms, referred to as **aseptic techniques**, that are used to reduce or eliminate their presence.

MICROORGANISMS

Microorganisms like bacteria, viruses, fungi, yeasts, molds, rickettsiae, and protozoa share a common characteristic with other species that inhabit the earth: they all need a favorable environment in which to thrive.

Although each type of microorganism is unique, some conditions that promote the survival of most, but not all, include warmth, darkness, oxygen, water, and nourishment. One has only to look at the list to realize that humans are optimal hosts for supporting the growth and reproduction of microorganisms. However, by interfering with the conditions that facilitate their invasion, many humans can be spared from acquiring minor to life-threatening infections.

INFECTIOUS PROCESS CYCLE

The **infectious process cycle** (Fig. 21-1) is a sequence of circumstances—all of which must be present—for the development of an infection. To transmit an infection, the following are required: (1) an infectious agent, (2) a reservoir for growth and reproduction, (3) an exit route from the reservoir, (4) a method for transmission, (5) a port of entry, and (6) a susceptible host.

Infectious Agents

All microorganisms, whether classified as pathogens or nonpathogens, must be considered infectious agents. However, it is true that some are less dangerous than others. Just as other animal species coexist *symbiotically*, that is, for mutual benefit, there are some microorganisms, called **normal flora**, that reside in and on humans.

Unless and until the supporting host becomes weakened, normal flora remain in check. But, if the host's defenses are weakened, even benign microorganisms take advantage of the situation and produce what are termed **opportunistic infections**. More often than not,

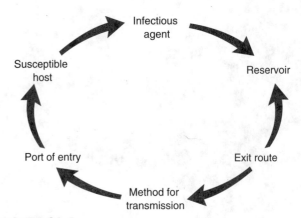

FIGURE 21-1
The infectious process cycle.

however, infections are caused by pathogenic microorganisms that by their very nature invade tissues and organs of the body, producing infections and contagious diseases (Display 21-1).

ADAPTATION

Unfortunately, many pathogens have developed the ability to adapt to hostile environments and unfavorable living conditions. Their adaptability has ensured their survival, and therefore, they continue to pose a threat to humankind.

One example of biologic adaptation is the capacity of some microorganisms to form spores. A **spore** is a microorganism that has temporarily altered its physical form so as to remain alive, but inactive, until conditions are favorable for resuming growth and reproduction. Consequently, spores are more difficult to destroy than their more biologically active counterparts. Another example of adaptation is the resistance many microorganisms are developing to antibiotics that once were quite effective (Shovein & Young, 1992).

DISPLAY 21-1. *Common Infectious Disorders*

Tuberculosis	Gonorrhea
Common cold	Tonsillitis
Hepatitis A and B	Herpes
AIDS	Influenza
Pneumonia	Wound infections
Meningitis	Boils
Measles	Diarrhea
Chickenpox	

Reservoir

A **reservoir** is the place on which, or in which, microbes grow and reproduce. Microorganisms survive in various reservoirs. Some prefer inhabiting living tissue, such as within the superficial crevices of the skin, on shafts of hair, in open wounds, in the bloodstream, inside the lower digestive tract, in nasal passages, and so on. Some grow abundantly in stagnant water or on uncooked and unrefrigerated food. They are present in intestinal excreta and the organic material in the earth. Although some, called *aerobic microorganisms*, depend on oxygen, there are others, called *anaerobic microorganisms*, that live in reservoirs without it.

Exit Route

The **exit route** is the manner in which microorganisms leave their original reservoir, thus enabling them to continue the cycle of infection. When present in or on humans, microorganisms are displaced when handling or touching objects or whenever blood, body fluids, secretions, and excretions are released. In the environment, weather-related factors may provide a mechanism for escape, such as through flooding and soil erosion.

Transmission

Transmission refers to the manner in which infectious microorganisms move from one source to another. Microorganisms are transferred to a secondary location by one of five routes: contact, droplet, airborne, vehicle, and vector-borne transmission (Table 21-1).

Port of Entry

The **port of entry** is the site at which the microorganisms find a way on or into the new host. One of the most common ports of entry is through openings in the skin or mucous membranes. However, microorganisms may also be inhaled, swallowed, introduced into the bloodstream, or transferred by contaminated instruments.

Susceptible Host

A **susceptible host** is one whose natural body defenses are weakened in some way (Display 21-2). Patients are prime candidates for infections because their health is already compromised in some way. Furthermore, health care institutions are teeming reservoirs of microorganisms because of the sheer numbers of sick people who are there. Add to this the numbers of caretakers, equipment, and treatment devices, all of which are in constant flux, and it is easy to understand why infection control is a major concern in patient care. Thus, it is important to understand and practice methods that will prevent hospital-acquired infections, known as **nosocomial infections**.

ASEPSIS

Asepsis is a term that refers to practices that decrease or eliminate infectious agents, their reservoirs, and vehicles for transmission. Two forms of asepsis, medical asepsis and surgical asepsis, are used to accomplish this goal.

TABLE 21-1. *Methods of Transmission*

Route	Description	Example
Contact transmission		
Direct contact	Actual physical transfer from one infected person to another	Sexual intercourse with an infected person
Indirect contact	Contact between a susceptible person and a contaminated object	Use of a contaminated needle for administering an injection
Droplet transmission	Transfer of moist particles from an infected person who is within a radius of 3 feet	Inhalation of droplets released during sneezing, coughing, or talking
Airborne transmission	Movement of microorganisms attached to evaporated water droplets or dust particles that have been suspended and carried over distances greater than 3 feet	Inhalation of spores
Vehicle transmission	Transfer of microorganisms present on or in contaminated items like food, water, medications, devices, and equipment	Consumption of water contaminated with microorganisms
Vector transmission	Transfer of microorganisms from an infected animal carrier	Diseases spread by mosquitoes, fleas, ticks, and so on

Medical Asepsis

Medical asepsis is also called *clean technique*. It involves those practices that confine or reduce the presence of microorganisms.

PRINCIPLES OF MEDICAL ASEPSIS

Being aware of the principles of medical asepsis can help interrupt the infectious process cycle and thus reduce the transmission of microorganisms. Some principles include the following:

- Microorganisms exist everywhere except on sterilized equipment.

- Frequent handwashing and maintaining intact skin are the best methods for reducing the transmission of microorganisms.
- Blood and body substances are considered major reservoirs of microorganisms.
- Barriers like gloves, gown, mask, goggles, and hair and shoe covers are garments that, when worn, interfere with the transmission of microorganisms.
- Keeping the environment clean reduces the number of microorganisms.
- Certain areas in the environment, like the floor, toilet, and the inside of sinks, are considered more contaminated than other areas.
- The transmission of microorganisms is reduced by flushing body substances, using antimicrobial cleaning agents, containing soiled items in covered containers, and controlling gusts of air currents.

MEDICAL ASEPTIC PRACTICES

Examples of medical aseptic practices include using antimicrobial agents, performing handwashing, wearing hospital garments, confining and containing soiled materials appropriately, and keeping the environment as clean as possible. Actual transmission control measures are discussed in more detail in Chapter 22.

Antimicrobial Agents

Antimicrobial agents are chemicals that limit the numbers of infectious microorganisms by destroying or suppressing their growth (Table 21-2). Some antimi-

TABLE 21-2. *Antimicrobial Agents*

Type	Mechanism	Example	Use
Soap	Lowers the surface tension of oil on the skin, which holds microorganisms; facilitates removal during rinsing	Dial, Safeguard	Hygiene
Detergent	Same as soap, except detergents do not form a precipitate when mixed with water	Dreft, Tide	Sanitizing eating utensils, laundry
Alcohol	A 70% concentration injures the protein and lipid structures in the inner cellular membrane of some microorganisms	Isopropanol, ethanol	Cleansing skin, instruments
Iodine	Damages the inner cell membrane of microorganisms and disrupts their enzyme functions; not effective against *Pseudomonas*, a common wound pathogen	Betadine	Cleansing skin
Chlorine	Interferes with microbial enzyme systems	Bleach, Clorox	Disinfecting water, utensils, blood spills
Chlorhexidine	Damages the inner cell membrane of microorganisms, but is ineffective against spores and most viruses	Hibiclens	Cleansing skin and equipment
Mercury	Alters microbial cellular proteins	Merthiolate, Mercurochrome	Disinfecting skin
Glutaraldehyde	Inactivates cellular proteins of bacteria, viruses, and microbes that form spores	Cidex	Sterilizing equipment

crobials are used to clean equipment, the surfaces of furnishings, and inanimate objects. Others are applied directly to the skin or administered internally. Examples of antimicrobial agents include antiseptics, disinfectants, and antibiotics.

Antiseptics. **Antiseptics**, also known as *bacteriostatic agents*, are chemicals like alcohol that inhibit, but do not completely kill, microorganisms. Antiseptics are usually applied to the skin or mucous membranes. They may also be used as cleansing agents.

Disinfectants. **Disinfectants**, also known as *germicides* and *bactericides*, actually destroy active microorganisms, but not spores. Phenol, household bleach, and formaldehyde are examples of disinfectants. However, because they are so strong chemically, they are rarely applied to the skin. Instead, they are used to kill and remove microorganisms from equipment, supplies, floors, walls, and so on.

Antibiotics. **Antibiotics** are drugs whose chemical components alter the metabolic processes of microorganisms, with the exception of viruses, in such a way as to damage or destroy them. Antibiotics may be applied to the skin in the form of ointments, or they may be administered internally.

Handwashing
Handwashing is an aseptic practice that removes transient and resident microorganisms from the hands by scrubbing the skin with soap, water, and friction (Skill 21-1).

Resident microorganisms are generally non-pathogens that are constantly present on the skin.

Transient microorganisms are generally pathogens that are picked up during brief contact with contaminated reservoirs. Transient microorganisms are more pathogenic, but they are more easily removed during handwashing. However, transients tend to cling to carved grooves in metal rings, around the facets in gems, at the margins of chipped fingernail polish, and under long fingernails. Therefore, these conditions are avoided when caring for patients. Furthermore, if handwashing is not conscientiously practiced, transient microorganisms can become residents, thereby increasing the potential for transmitting infection to oneself and others.

According to the Centers for Disease Control and Prevention, to be reasonably effective, lathered hands must be vigorously rubbed together for at least 10 seconds and rinsed under a stream of running water. More time is advised if the hands are visibly soiled, before assisting with a surgical procedure (Table 21-3), or before caring for a newborn or immunosuppressed patient.

Although handwashing never totally eliminates microorganisms from the skin, there are certain times when handwashing is more important than others (Display 21-3). And, considering how much the hands are used during the course of patient care, it should come as no surprise that *handwashing is the single most effective way to prevent infections.*

Hospital Garments
There are various garments that reduce the transfer of microorganisms between personnel and patients. They include uniforms, scrub suits or gowns, masks,

(text continues on page 435)

SKILL 21-1
Handwashing

Suggested Action	Reason for Action
Assessment	
Review the medical record, to determine if it is appropriate to perform handwashing for longer than 10 seconds.	Indicates if the procedure requires modification to protect immunosuppressed patients
Check that there is sufficient soap and paper towels near the sink and that a waste receptacle is nearby.	Promotes effective handwashing and disposal of paper towels
Planning	
Explain the purpose for handwashing to the patient.	Reinforces and demonstrates a concern for patient safety
Remove all jewelry except for a plain, smooth wedding band; roll up long sleeves.	Facilitates removing transient and resident microorganisms

(continued)

SKILL 21-1
Handwashing (Continued)

Suggested Action	Reason for Action
Implementation	
Turn on the flow of water using faucet handles, knee, elbow, or foot controls.	Serves as a wetting agent and facilitates lathering

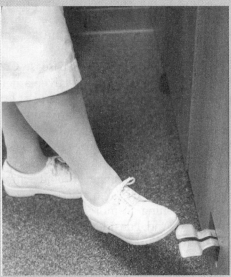

Using foot controls. (Courtesy of Ken Timby.)

Wet your hands with comfortably warm water from the wrists toward the fingers.	Allows water to flow from the least contaminated area to the most contaminated

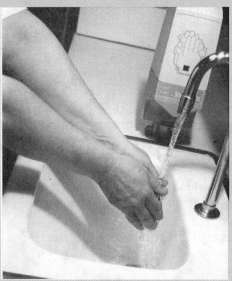

Wetting hands. (Courtesy of Ken Timby.)

Avoid splashing water from the sink onto your uniform.	Prevents transferring microorganisms to clothing

(continued)

SKILL 21-1
Handwashing (Continued)

Suggested Action	Reason for Action
Dispense about a teaspoon of liquid soap into your hands or wet a cake of bar soap.	Provides an agent for emulsifying body oils and releasing microorganisms
Work the soap into a lather.	Expands the volume and distribution of the soap; begins to soften the keratin layer of the skin

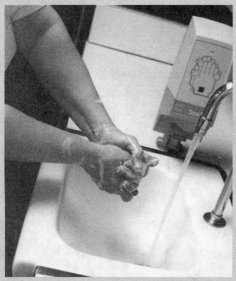

Working up a lather. (Courtesy of Ken Timby.)

Rinse the bar soap, if used, and replace it within the soap dish.	Flushes microorganisms from the surface of the soap
Rub the soap lather over all the surfaces of the hands, especially between fingers and over the knuckles as well as under the fingernails.	Frees microorganisms that are lodged in creases and crevices
Continue scrubbing from 10 seconds to as long as 2 minutes or longer, depending on the potential for contamination with microorganisms.	Ensures effectiveness

(continued)

SKILL 21-1
Handwashing *(Continued)*

Suggested Action	Reason for Action
Rinse the soap from your hands by letting the water run from the wrists toward the fingers.	Avoids transferring microorganisms to cleaner areas

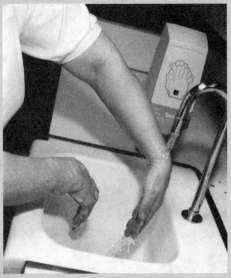

Rinsing hands. (Courtesy of Ken Timby.)

Suggested Action	Reason for Action
Stop the flow of water if it is controlled by a foot, knee, or elbow lever.	Terminates the flow of water without recontaminating the hands
Hold your hands lower than your wrists.	Promotes drainage by gravity flow toward the fingers
Dry your hands thoroughly with paper towels.	Prevents chapping
Turn the hand controls of the faucet off using a paper towel.	Prevents recontamination of clean hands

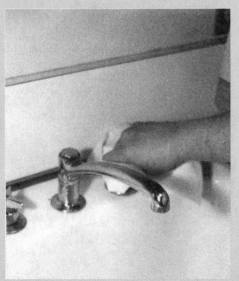

Turning off hand controls. (Courtesy of Ken Timby.)

Suggested Action	Reason for Action
Apply hand lotion from time to time.	Maintains the integrity of the skin

(continued)

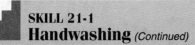

SKILL 21-1
Handwashing *(Continued)*

Suggested Action	Reason for Action
Evaluation	
• Handwashing has met time requirements	
• Hands are clean	
Document	
Because handwashing is performed so frequently, it usually is not documented, but it is expected as a standard for care among all health care personnel.	

gloves, hair and shoe covers, and, in some cases, protective eyewear. Some of these items are worn when caring for any patient regardless of his or her diagnosis or presumed infectious status (see section on Standard Precautions, Chap. 22).

Uniforms. Usually uniforms are worn only while working with patients. Some nurses wear a clean laboratory coat over their uniform to reduce the spread of microorganisms onto or from the surface of clothing worn from home. When caring for patients, a plastic apron or cover gown can be worn over the uniform if there is a potential for soiling with blood or body fluids from patients. If a cover is not worn, care is taken to avoid touching the uniform with any soiled items, like bed linen.

After working, the uniform is changed as soon as possible. This practice helps to avoid exposing others such as one's family or others in public places to microorganisms that may be present on work clothing.

Scrub Suits and Gowns. Scrub suits and gowns are hospital garments that are worn by personnel in lieu of a traditional uniform. They may be provided for employees who work in various departments like the nursery, operating room, and delivery room. Their use helps shield patients from the microorganisms that health care personnel bring with them on clothing worn from home.

Personnel change into this type of outerwear immediately after they arrive for work. Cover gowns are worn over the scrub attire when leaving the department for coffee or lunch breaks.

Masks. Masks are items that cover the nose and mouth (Fig. 21-2). They are worn by hospital personnel to protect patients from droplet transmission of microorganisms. Masks may also be used as a barrier against inhaling microorganisms spread by droplet and airborne transmission. To prevent the transmission of infectious agents that cause tuberculosis, the Centers for Disease Control and Prevention (1994) recommends wearing a high-efficiency mask called a *particulate air filter respirator* (Fig. 21-3).

To be effective, certain guidelines for wearing masks are followed.

TABLE 21-3. *Differences Between Handwashing and a Surgical Scrub*

Handwashing	Surgical Scrub
Plain wedding band may be worn	Rings and watch are removed
Faucets with hand controls may be used	Faucets are regulated with foot, knee, or elbow controls
Liquid or bar soap may be used	Liquid soap is used
Washing lasts 10 seconds to 2 minutes	Initial scrub is done for 10 minutes
Hands are held below the level of the elbows during washing, rinsing, and drying	Hands are held higher than the elbows during washing, rinsing, and drying
Areas beneath fingernails are washed	Areas beneath fingernails are cleaned with an orange stick
Friction is produced by rubbing the hands together	Friction is produced by scrubbing with a hand brush
Hands are dried with paper towels and the paper is used to turn off hand-regulated faucet controls	Hands are dried with sterile towels
Clean gloves may be donned if the nurse has open skin or if there is a potential for contact with blood or body fluids	Sterile gloves are donned immediately after the hands are dried

DISPLAY 21-3. *Handwashing Guidelines*

Handwashing should be performed:

- When arriving and leaving work
- Before and after contact with each patient
- Before and after equipment is handled
- Before and after gloving
- Before and after specimens are collected
- Before preparing medications
- Before serving trays or feeding patients
- Before eating
- After toileting, hair combing, or other hygiene
- After cleaning a work area

Gloves. Clean gloves, sometimes called examination gloves, are used in the following circumstances:

- As a barrier to prevent direct hand contact with blood, body fluids, secretions, excretions, mucous membranes, and nonintact skin
- As a barrier to protect patients from microorganisms that may be transmitted from nursing personnel when performing procedures or care involving contact with the patient's mucous membranes or nonintact skin
- When there may be a potential indirect transfer of microorganisms from one patient or object to another patient during subsequent nursing care

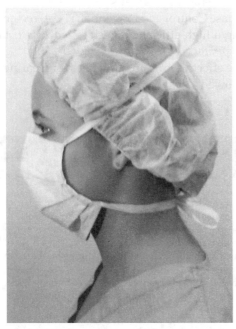

FIGURE 21-2
Face mask and hair cover. (Courtesy of Ken Timby.)

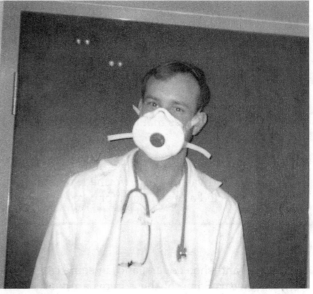

FIGURE 21-3
Particulate air filter respirator. (Courtesy of Ken Timby.)

NURSING GUIDELINES FOR USING A MASK OR FILTER RESPIRATOR

- Wear a mask if there is a risk for coughing or sneezing within a radius of 3 feet.
  Rationale: Blocks the route of exit
- Wear a mask or filter respirator if there is a potential for acquiring diseases through droplet or airborne transmission.
  Rationale: Blocks the port of entry
- Position the mask or respirator so it covers the nose and mouth.
  Rationale: Provides a barrier to nasal and oral ports of entry
- Tie the upper strings of a mask snugly at the back of the head and the lower strings at the back of the neck.
  Rationale: Reduces exit and entry routes for microorganisms
- Avoid touching the mask or respirator once it is in place.
  Rationale: Prevents transferring microorganisms to the hands
- Change the mask or respirator every 20 to 30 minutes or when it becomes noticeably damp.
  Rationale: Preserves effectiveness
- Touch only the strings of the mask or the respirator strap during its removal.
  Rationale: Avoids contact with areas that have major contamination
- Discard used masks or respirators into a lined or waterproof waste container.

Rationale: Reduces the transmission of micro-organisms to others
- Perform handwashing after removing a mask or respirator
Rationale: Removes microorganisms from the hands

Types of Gloves. Examination gloves are usually made of latex or vinyl, although there are other types of gloves under development. Both latex and vinyl gloves are equally protective with nonvigorous use, but latex gloves have some added advantages. They stretch and mold to fit the wearer almost like a second layer of skin, thus permitting greater flexibility with movement. And, perhaps most important, they have the capacity to reseal tiny punctures.

Unfortunately, some nurses and patients are allergic to latex. Reactions vary and may range from annoying symptoms like skin rash, flushing, itching, watery eyes, and nasal stuffiness, to others that are more life threatening, like swelling of the airway and low blood pressure. Those nurses who are particularly sensitive to latex may work with their nursing supervisors on purchasing a supply of gloves made from alternative synthetics, or they may wear a double pair of vinyl gloves when there is a high risk for contact with blood or body fluids.

Removing Gloves. Gloves, especially those made of vinyl, which is not as protective after 5 minutes of wear, are changed if they become perforated, after brief use, and between the care of patients. By following aseptic techniques, gloves are removed without directly touching their more contaminated outer surface.

NURSING GUIDELINES FOR REMOVING GLOVES

- Grasp one of the gloves at the upper, outer edge at the wrist (Fig. 21-4).
Rationale: Maintains a barrier between contaminated surfaces
- Stretch and pull the upper edge of the glove downward while inverting the glove as it is removed (Fig. 21-5).
Rationale: Encloses the soiled surface, thus interfering with a potential exit route
- Insert the fingers of the ungloved hand within the inside edge of the remaining glove (Fig. 21-6).
Rationale: Provides direct contact with the cleaner surface of the glove
- Pull the second glove inside out while enclosing the first glove within the palm.

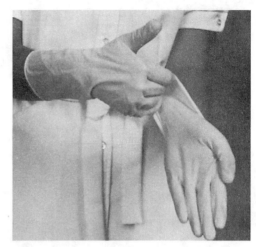
FIGURE 21-4
Pulling at cuff.

Rationale: Restricts the reservoir of microorganisms
- Place the gloves within a lined waste container.
Rationale: Confines the reservoir of microorganisms
- Perform handwashing immediately after gloves are removed.
Rationale: Removes transient and resident microorganisms that may have proliferated within the warm, dark, moist environment inside the gloves

Hair and Shoe Covers. Hair and shoe covers are items that reduce the transmission of pathogens that may be present on loose, falling hair or on shoes. These garments are usually worn during surgical procedures or when a baby is delivered.

When shoe covers are used, they are fastened so as to cover the open ends of pant legs. Hair covers, when

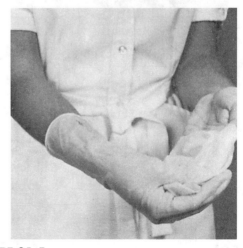
FIGURE 21-5
Inverting the glove.

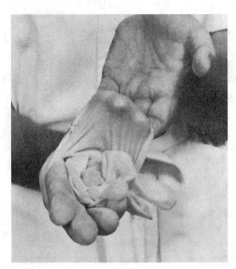

FIGURE 21-6
Enclosing contaminated surfaces.

worn properly, envelop the entire head. There are specially designed head covers that resemble a cloth or paper helmet for men who may have beards or long sideburns.

Even though hair covers are not required during the course of general nursing care, as a medically aseptic practice, health care workers keep their hair short or contained with a hair clip, rubber band, or by some other means.

Protective Eyewear. Protective eyewear such as goggles is worn when there is a possibility that body fluids will splash into the eyes. If only goggles are available,

they are used with a mask, or a multipurpose face shield may be used (Fig. 21-7).

Confining Soiled Articles

There are several medically aseptic practices used in hospitals that confine and contain reservoirs of microorganisms, especially those present on soiled equipment and supplies. They include using designated clean and dirty utility rooms and varieties of waste receptacles.

Utility Rooms. There are usually at least two utility rooms on each nursing unit. One is designated a clean room, whereas the other is considered dirty. It is essential that nursing personnel avoid placing soiled articles within the clean utility room.

The dirty or soiled utility room often contains covered waste receptacles, at least one large laundry hamper, and a flushable hopper. This room may also house equipment for testing stool or urine. A sink may be located within the soiled utility room to rinse grossly contaminated equipment as well as provide an opportunity for handwashing.

Waste Receptacles. One has only to look about to find a variety of measures used temporarily to contain soiled articles until they can be more permanently disposed. For example, most patients have a paper bag at their bedside for tissues or other small, burnable items. Waste baskets are usually plastic lined. Suction and drainage containers are kept covered and emptied at least once each shift. Also, most patient rooms now have a wall-mounted, puncture-resistant container into which used needles or other sharp objects are placed (Fig. 21-8).

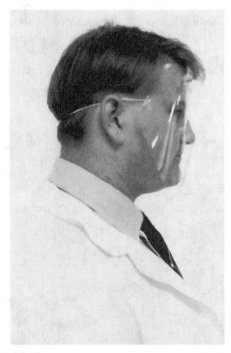

FIGURE 21-7
Face shield. (Courtesy of Ken Timby.)

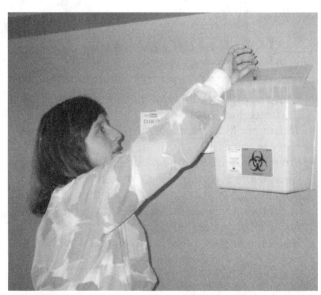

FIGURE 21-8
Sharps container. (Courtesy of Ken Timby.)

Keeping the Environment Clean

Health agencies employ laundry staff and housekeeping personnel to assist with cleaning tasks. For the most part, as long as soiled linen is bagged appropriately or handled with gloves, the detergents and heat from the water and dryers renders laundry sufficiently clean and free of pathogenic organisms.

Housekeeping personnel are responsible for collecting and disposing of accumulated refuse and for concurrent and terminal disinfection. **Concurrent disinfection** refers to those measures that keep the patient environment clean on a daily basis. Housekeepers are trained to carry out principles of medical asepsis in the following ways:

- Less soiled areas are cleaned before those that are grossly dirty.
- Floors are wet mopped and furniture is damp dusted to avoid distributing microorganisms on dust and air currents.
- Solutions used for mopping are discarded frequently in a flushable hopper.
- Clean items are never placed on the floor.

Terminal disinfection, on the other hand, refers to the more thorough cleaning of patient rooms, like scrubbing the mattress and insides of drawers and bedside stands, after patient discharge.

Nurses employed in home health care may teach the patient and family simple aseptic practices for cleaning contaminated articles.

Surgical Asepsis

Surgical asepsis, also known as *sterile technique*, refers to measures that prevent contaminating items that are totally free of microorganisms. Therefore, before surgical asepsis can be practiced, equipment and supplies must be sterilized.

STERILIZATION

Sterilization refers to techniques that destroy all microorganisms, including spores. Many disposable medical supplies are manufactured and delivered in sterile condition. However, reusable equipment is resterilized after each use. Sterilization is accomplished by physical or chemical means.

Physical Sterilization

Microorganisms and spores can be destroyed physically by using radiation or heat. Heat may be applied by using boiling water, free-flowing steam, dry heat, and steam under pressure.

Radiation. Ultraviolet radiation can kill bacteria. Sunlight has also been used in the past to eliminate microorganisms, especially the one that causes tuberculosis. Currently, radiation is combined with other methods of sterilization because many factors can affect its reliability (Boutotte, 1993).

Boiling Water. Boiling water is a convenient way to sterilize items used in the home. To be effective, contaminated equipment is boiled for 15 minutes at 212°F (100°C). The time may need to be lengthened in places that are above sea level because water begins boiling before it reaches 212°F at higher altitudes.

Free-Flowing Steam. Free-flowing steam is a method in which items are exposed to the heated vapor that escapes from boiling water. It requires the same temper-

---

 PATIENT TEACHING FOR CLEANING POTENTIALLY INFECTIOUS EQUIPMENT

Teach the patient and family to do the following:
- Wear waterproof gloves if items are heavily contaminated or if there are open skin areas on the hands.
- Designate one container for the sole purpose of cleaning contaminated articles.
- Disassemble and rinse reusable equipment as soon as possible after use.
- Rinse grossly contaminated items *first* under cool, running water because hot water causes protein substances in body fluids to thicken or congeal.
- Soak reusable items in a solution of water and detergent or disinfectant if a thorough cleaning is not immediately possible.

- Use a sponge, scrub brush, or cloth to create friction and loosen dirt, body fluids, and microorganisms from the surface of contaminated articles.
- Force sudsy water through the hollow channels of items to remove debris.
- Rinse washed items well under running water.
- Drain rinsed equipment and air dry.
- Perform handwashing after cleaning equipment.
- Store clean, dry items in covered containers or within a clean, folded towel.

ature and time requirements as the boiling method. Free-flowing steam is not as reliable as boiling because it may be difficult to expose all the surfaces of contaminated items to the steam.

Dry Heat. Dry heat, or hot air sterilization, is similar to baking items in an oven. To destroy microorganisms with dry heat, temperatures of 330°F to 340°F (165°C–170°C) must be maintained for at least 3 hours. Dry heat is a good technique for sterilizing sharp instruments and reusable syringes because moist heat damages cutting edges and the ground surfaces of glass. Dry heat prevents rust from forming on objects that are not made of stainless steel.

Steam Under Pressure. Steam under pressure is the most dependable method for destroying all forms of microorganisms and spores. The *autoclave* is a type of pressure steam sterilizer that most health agencies use (Fig. 21-9). Using pressure makes it possible to achieve much hotter temperatures than the boiling point of water or free-flowing steam. Heat-sensitive tape that changes color or displays a pattern when exposed to high temperatures is often used on sterilized packages as a visual indicator that the wrapped item is sterile.

Chemical Sterilization

Both gas and liquid chemicals are used for sterilizing invasive equipment. Two common substances include peracetic acid and ethylene oxide gas.

Peracetic Acid. Peracetic acid is a combination of acetic acid and hydrogen peroxide. Although early trials demonstrated that peracetic acid is highly corrosive, new methods of buffering it have eliminated this negative aspect. The major advantage of its use is the short time it takes to sterilize equipment—12 minutes at a temperature of 122°F to 131°F (50°C–55°C)—with the entire process taking approximately a half-hour from start to finish (Crow, 1993). Therefore the use of peracetic acid is

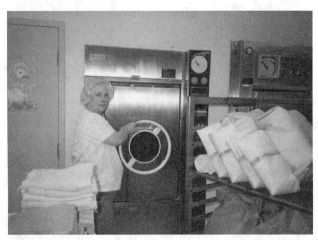

FIGURE 21-9
Autoclave. (Courtesy of Ken Timby.)

gaining popularity as a reliable method for sterilizing heat-sensitive instruments like endoscopes.

Ethylene Oxide Gas. Ethylene oxide gas is the chemical used for gas sterilization. It has the capacity to destroy a broad spectrum of microorganisms, including spores and viruses, when contaminated items are exposed for 3 hours at a temperature of 86°F (30°C). Gassed items, however, must be aired for 5 days at room temperature or 8 hours at 248°F (120°C) to remove traces of the gas, which can cause chemical burns.

Gas sterilization with ethylene oxide gas, however, continues to be used as a traditional method for destroying microorganisms. It is preferred if, and when, items are likely to be damaged by heat or moisture or when a better method is unavailable.

PRINCIPLES OF SURGICAL ASEPSIS

Surgical asepsis is based on the premise that once equipment and areas are free of microorganisms, they can remain in that state only if contamination is prevented. Consequently, health professionals observe the following principles:

- Sterility is preserved by touching one sterile item with another one that is sterile.
- Once a sterile item touches something that is not, it is considered contaminated.
- Any partially unwrapped sterile package is considered contaminated.
- If there is a question as to the sterility of an item, it is considered nonsterile.
- The longer the time since sterilization, the greater the probability that the item may no longer be sterile.
- A commercially packaged sterile item is not considered sterile past its recommended expiration date.
- Once a sterile item is opened or uncovered, it is only a short matter of time before it becomes contaminated.
- The outer 1-inch margin of a sterile area is considered a zone of contamination.
- A sterile wrapper, if it becomes wet, wicks microorganisms from its supporting surface, causing contamination.
- Any opened sterile item or sterile area is considered contaminated if it is left unattended.
- Coughing, sneezing, or excessive talking over a sterile field causes contamination.
- Reaching across an area that contains sterile equipment has a high potential for causing contamination, and is therefore avoided.
- Sterile items that are located or lowered below waist level are considered contaminated because they are not within critical view.

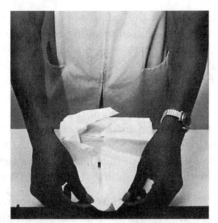

FIGURE 21-10
Unfolding away from the body.

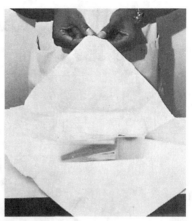

FIGURE 21-12
Unfolding toward the body.

The principles of surgical asepsis are observed during surgery, when performing invasive procedures such as inserting urinary catheters, and when caring for open wounds.

SURGICAL ASEPTIC PRACTICES

Examples of practices that involve surgical asepsis include creating a sterile field, adding sterile items to the sterile field, and donning sterile gloves.

Creating a Sterile Field

A **sterile field** is a work area that is free of microorganisms. The inner surface of a cloth or paper wrapper that holds sterile items is often used as a sterile field, much like a tablecloth is used. It enlarges the area where sterile equipment or supplies can be placed.

Therefore, the nurse opens sterile packages in such a way as to keep the inside of the wrapper and its contents sterile.

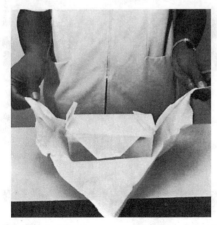

FIGURE 21-11
Unfolding the sides.

NURSING GUIDELINES FOR CREATING A STERILE FIELD

- Remove objects from the area where the field will be created.
  Rationale: Provides room for working without accidental contamination
- Perform handwashing.
  Rationale: Reduces the numbers of microorganisms on the hands
- Place the wrapped package on a surface that is at or above waist level.
  Rationale: Keeps sterile items within sight
- Position the package so that the outermost triangular edge of the wrapper can be moved away from the front of the body (Fig. 21-10).
  Rationale: Prevents reaching over the sterile area
- Unfold each side of the wrapper by touching the area that will be in direct contact with the table or stand, or touch no more than the outer 1-inch (2.5-cm) edge of the wrapper (Fig. 21-11).
  Rationale: Maintains a sterile zone
- Unfold the final corner of the wrapper by pulling it toward the body (Fig. 21-12).
  Rationale: Avoids reaching over a previously uncovered area

Adding Items to a Sterile Field

There are times when it may be necessary to add sterile items or sterile solutions to the sterile field.

Sterile Supplies. Agency-sterilized supplies or those that have been commercially prepared may be added to the sterile field. The former are usually wrapped in a cloth towel. The cloth wrapper is unwrapped in a way similar to the technique described for creating a

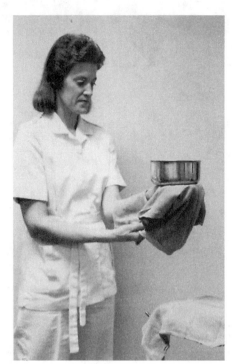

FIGURE 21-13
Adding a sterile basin. (Courtesy of Ken Timby.)

sterile field, except the nurse supports the wrapped item in one hand rather than laying it on a solid surface. Each of the four corners is held so they do not hang loosely (Fig. 21-13). Once the item is unwrapped, it is placed on the sterile field and the cloth cover is discarded.

Commercially prepared supplies, like sterile gauze squares, are enclosed in paper wrappers. The paper cover usually has two loose flaps that extend above the sealed edges. By separating the flaps, the sterile contents can be dropped onto the sterile field (Fig. 21-14).

Sterile Solutions. Sterile solutions, like normal saline, come in a variety of volumes. Some containers are sealed with a rubber cap or a screw top. Either may be replaced if the inside surface has not been contaminated. To avoid contamination, the cap is placed upside down on a flat surface or held by the fingers during pouring.

After a sterile solution has been uncapped, all subsequent uses from the same container are preceded by pouring and discarding a small amount of the container's contents. This practice, called *lipping* the container, washes any airborne contaminants from the mouth of the container.

When pouring the sterile solution, the container is held above and in front of the nurse. Care is taken to avoid touching any sterile areas on or within the field. Also, the solution is poured close to the container to avoid splashing the sterile field, causing an area of contamination (Fig. 21-15). Sterile solutions are re-

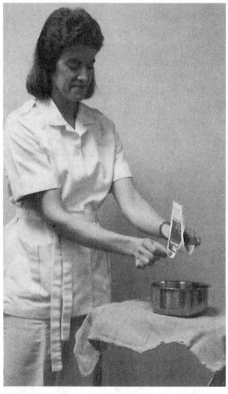

FIGURE 21-14
Adding sterile gauze. (Courtesy of Ken Timby.)

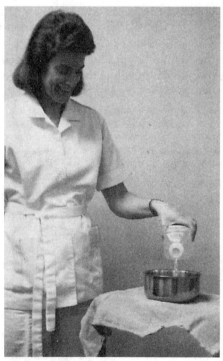

FIGURE 21-15
Adding sterile solution. (Courtesy of Ken Timby.)

placed on a daily basis, even if the entire volume has not been used.

Donning Sterile Gloves

When applied correctly (Skill 21-2), sterile gloves may be safely used to handle sterile equipment and supplies. They provide a barrier that prevents transferring microbes present on the hands. Sterile gloves are included in some packages of supplies. They may also be packaged separately in glove wrappers.

Donning a Sterile Gown

A sterile gown is used to protect the patient and sterile equipment from microorganisms that collect on the surface of uniforms, scrub suits, or scrub gowns. Sterile gowns are required during surgery and delivery of infants. They may be used during other sterile procedures as well.

Sterile gowns are made of cloth. They are laundered and sterilized after each use. Before wrapping a gown for sterilization, it is folded so that the inside surface of the gown can be touched during the process of donning it. To avoid contamination, the following guidelines are observed.

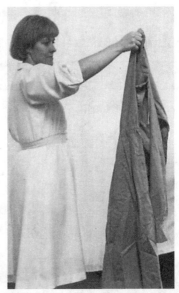

FIGURE 21-16
Unfolding a sterile gown. (Courtesy of Ken Timby.)

NURSING GUIDELINES FOR DONNING A STERILE GOWN

- Apply a mask and hair cover.
  Rationale: Prevents contamination of the hands after they are washed
- Perform a surgical scrub (see Table 21-3).
  Rationale: Removes resident as well as transient microorganisms

- Pick up the sterile gown at the inner neckline.
  Rationale: Preserves sterility of the outer gown
- Hold the gown away from your body and other nonsterile objects in the immediate area (Fig. 21-16).
  Rationale: Prevents contamination
- Allow the gown to unfold while suspending it high enough to avoid contact with the floor.
  Rationale: Prevents contamination
- Insert an arm within each sleeve without touching the outer surface of the gown.
  Rationale: Maintains sterility

(text continues on page 446)

SKILL 21-2
Donning Sterile Gloves

Suggested Action	Reason for Action
Assessment	
Determine if the procedure requires surgical asepsis.	Complies with infection control measures
Read the contents of prepackaged sterile equipment to determine if sterile gloves are enclosed.	Indicates whether extra supplies are needed
Discover how much the patient understands about the subsequent procedure.	Provides a basis for teaching
Planning	
Explain what is about to take place to the patient.	Promotes understanding and cooperation

SKILL 21-2
Donning Sterile Gloves *(Continued)*

Suggested Action	Reason for Action
Select a package of sterile gloves of the appropriate size.	Ensures ease when donning and using gloves
Remove unnecessary items from the overbed table or bedside stand.	Ensures an adequate, clean work space

Implementation

Perform handwashing.	Reduces the potential for transmitting micro-organisms
Open the outer wrapper of the gloves.	Provides access to inner wrapper

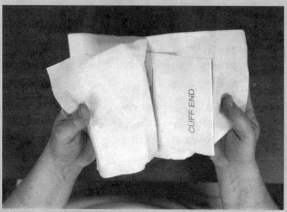

Opening glove wrapper. (Courtesy of Ken Timby.)

Place the inner wrapper so that the left glove is on your left side, and the same for the right.	Facilitates donning gloves

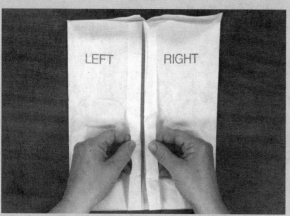

Positioning inner wrapper. (Courtesy of Ken Timby.)

(continued)

SKILL 21-2
Donning Sterile Gloves (Continued)

Suggested Action	Reason for Action
Pick up one glove at the folded edge of the cuff using your thumb and fingers.	Avoids contaminating the outer surface of the glove

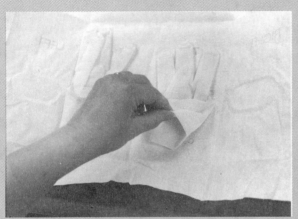

Picking up first glove. (Courtesy of Ken Timby.)

Insert your fingers while pulling and stretching the glove over your hand, taking care not to touch the outside of the glove to anything that is nonsterile.	Avoids contaminating the outer surface of the glove
Unfold the cuff so the glove extends above the wrist, but touch only the surface that will be in direct contact with the skin.	Extends the sterile area
Insert the gloved hand beneath the sterile folded edge of the remaining glove.	Maintains sterility of each glove

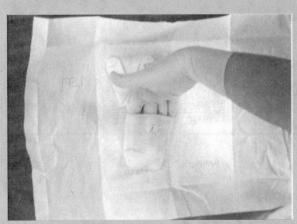

Picking up second glove. (Courtesy of Ken Timby.)

(continued)

SKILL 21-2
Donning Sterile Gloves (Continued)

Suggested Action	Reason for Action
Insert the fingers within the second glove while pulling and stretching it over the hand.	Facilitates donning the glove

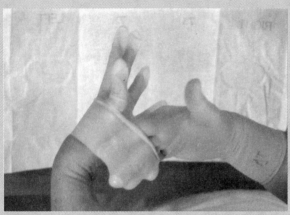

Pulling on second glove. (Courtesy of Ken Timby.)

Suggested Action	Reason for Action
Take care to avoid touching anything that is not sterile.	Maintains sterility
Maintain your gloved hands at or above waist level.	Prevents the potential for contamination
Repeat the procedure if contamination occurs.	Protects the patient from acquiring an infection

Evaluation
- Gloves are donned
- Sterility is maintained

Document
- The procedure that was performed
- Outcome of procedure

Sample Documentation

Date and Time   Sterile dressing changed over abdominal incision. Wound edges are approximated, with no evidence of redness or drainage. _____ **Signature, Title**

- Have an assistant pull at the inside of the gown to adjust the fit, expose the hands, and then tie it closed (Fig. 21-17).
  Rationale: Preserves the sterility of the front of the gown
- Proceed with donning sterile gloves.
  Rationale: Ensures sterile condition of the hands and cuff of the gown.

 APPLICABLE NURSING DIAGNOSES

- Risk for Infection
- Risk for Infection Transmission
- Altered Protection
- Knowledge Deficit

- Conscientious handwashing is necessary when caring for all patients, but it is especially important when patients are older adults because they are more susceptible to infections.
- Maintaining intact skin is an excellent first-line defense against acquiring nosocomial infections, but one that is often compromised among older adults.
- The aged and debilitated are at high risk for infections, especially those that are resistant to antibiotics.
- According to surveillance surveys conducted by the Centers for Disease Control and Prevention, many nursing home residents, older hospitalized patients, and health care personnel are colonized with antibiotic-resistant bacteria (Shoevin & Young, 1992).
- Older adults are more likely to experience life-threatening consequences of infections than younger adults.
- Nursing home residents tend to acquire infections involving the urinary tract, skin, and respiratory tract (Matteson & McConnell, 1988).
- Infections are often transmitted to vulnerable older adult patients via equipment reservoirs such as indwelling urinary catheters, humidifiers and oxygen equipment that are not maintained adequately, or intravenous sites that are not changed regularly.
- When caring for older patients, attention to perineal hygiene and handwashing is a priority because they may fall victim to opportunistic infections from organisms present in stool.
- Older adults and health care personnel who work closely with older patients should obtain immunizations against influenza and pneumococcal pneumonia, which may be life threatening when acquired by older adults.
- Visitors with respiratory infections should be tactfully advised to avoid visiting older adults until their symptoms have been relieved, or they may be provided with a mask.
- Health care workers who are ill should take sick leave rather than expose susceptible patients to infectious microorganisms.

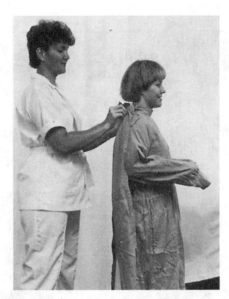

FIGURE 21-17
Assisting with donning a sterile gown. (Courtesy of Ken Timby.)

NURSING IMPLICATIONS

Everyone is susceptible to infections. However, pertinent nursing diagnoses such as those subsequently listed in Applicable Nursing Diagnoses usually are identified when caring for particularly susceptible patients.

The accompanying Nursing Care Plan has been developed to illustrate how aseptic principles are incorporated within a teaching plan for the nursing diagnosis of Knowledge Deficit. The NANDA taxonomy (1994) at present does not contain a definition for this category. Carpenito (1993), however, defines this nursing diagnosis as "the state in which an individual or group experiences a deficiency in cognitive knowledge or psychomotor skills regarding the condition or treatment plan." Some authorities would argue that the more correct nursing diagnosis would be the problem that is likely to occur as a consequence of the knowledge deficit in this case, Risk for Infection (Jenny, 1987).

KEY CONCEPTS

- Microorganisms are living animals or plants that are so small they cannot be seen except with a microscope.
- Nonpathogens are generally harmless microorganisms, whereas pathogens have a high potential for causing infections and contagious diseases. Resident microorganisms are generally nonpathogens that

NURSING CARE PLAN:
Knowledge Deficit

Assessment

Subjective Data

States, "The school nurse sent this note home saying there's been a case of hepatitis in my daughter's fifth-grade class. Isn't that what drug users get? Should I keep my daughter home from school? What will prevent her from catching it?" Daughter is not experiencing any anorexia or tenderness in right upper quadrant.

Objective Data

11-year-old girl in the fifth grade. Public health department confirms one case of hepatitis A at school. TPR is currently normal. Liver is not palpable. Denies nausea or diarrhea. Sclera of OU are white. Freshly voided urine is light yellow and tests negative for bilirubin with a chemstrip and Ictotest tablet. Will receive gamma globulin injection today.

Diagnosis

Knowledge Deficit: Cause and prevention of hepatitis A related to unfamiliarity with infectious disease transmission.

Plan

Goal

The child will satisfactorily return a demonstration of handwashing and mother will list at least three signs and symptoms of hepatitis at the end of this office visit.

Orders: 11/17

1. Explain that hepatitis A is spread primarily from stool of an infected person to the mouth of a susceptible person.
2. Provide the following information and ask mother to recall at least three signs and symptoms:
   a. Hepatitis B is usually associated with IV drug use and contaminated blood.
   b. The incubation period of hepatitis A is 25 to 30 days.
   c. Handwashing is an excellent preventive measure when performed before eating and after each use of the toilet; staying home from school is not necessary.
   d. Signs and symptoms include low-grade fever, reduced activity, loss of appetite, nausea, abdominal pain, dark urine, light-colored stool, and yellowing of the skin and white portion of the eyes.
3. Demonstrate handwashing and observe return demonstration, emphasizing the following:
   a. Turn handles of school faucet on using a paper towel and let water run.
   b. Wet hands and lather with liquid soap from a hand-pump dispenser.
   c. Rub lathered hands for at least 30 seconds to 1 minute.
   d. Rinse, letting water flow from wrists to fingers.
   e. Dry hands with paper towel.
   f. Use a paper towel to turn faucet handle off. _____ A. JOHANSON, RN

Implementation 11/7 1630 Differentiated between hepatitis A and B. States, "I'm so relieved that this case isn't caused by sharing drug needles." Provided with additional information on hepatitis as identified in care plan. Handwashing demonstration given.
(Documentation) _____ A. JOHANSON, RN

Evaluation 1645 Mother recalled the following signs and symptoms: fever, loss of appetite, nausea, and yellowing of eyes and skin. Child performed handwashing procedure as demonstrated. Given immune serum globulin injection in L. vastus lateralis muscle. _____ A. JOHANSON, RN
(Documentation)

permanently inhabit the skin. Transient microorganisms are generally pathogens that cling to the skin surface but can be more easily removed through handwashing. Aerobic microorganisms require oxygen for survival, whereas anaerobic microorganisms do not.

- The components of the infectious process cycle include: (1) an infectious agent, (2) a reservoir for growth and reproduction, (3) an exit route from the reservoir, (4) a method for transmission, (5) a port of entry, and (6) a susceptible host.
- Some microorganisms have ensured their survival by developing the capacity to form spores and resist antibiotic drug therapy.
- Nosocomial infections are those that are acquired by previously uninfected people while they are being cared for in a health care agency like a hospital or nursing home.
- "Asepsis" is a term that refers to practices that decrease the numbers of infectious agents, their reservoirs, and vehicles for transmission. Medical asepsis involves those practices that confine or reduce the presence of microorganisms; surgical asepsis refers to measures that prevent contaminating sterile items.
- Some principles of medical asepsis include: (1) frequent handwashing and maintaining intact skin are the best methods for reducing the transmission of microorganisms; (2) barriers like gloves, gown, mask, goggles, hair and shoe covers further interfere with the transmission of microorganisms; and (3) keeping the environment clean reduces the numbers of microorganisms.
- Examples of medically aseptic practices include using antimicrobial agents, handwashing, wearing hospital garments, confining soiled articles, and keeping the environment clean.
- Microorganisms may be totally destroyed by using ultraviolet radiation, heat, or chemicals.
- There are several principles of surgical asepsis. Three of them include: (1) sterility can be preserved by touching one sterile item with another; (2) once a sterile item touches something that is not, it is considered contaminated; and (3) any partially unwrapped sterile package is considered contaminated.
- Principles of surgical asepsis are applied when nurses create a sterile field, add supplies or liquids to a sterile field, and when sterile gloves are donned.

CRITICAL THINKING EXERCISES

- Use the infectious process cycle to trace the transmission of a common cold from one person to another.
- Describe methods of medical asepsis that would be helpful in controlling the infectious process cycle of the common cold.
- Discuss possible interventions that might be used should you observe that a nurse contaminates a pair of sterile gloves.

SUGGESTED READINGS

Boutotte J. Protecting yourself against T.B. Nursing October 1993;23:64.

Carpenito LJ. Nursing Diagnosis: Application to Clinical Practice. 5th ed. Philadelphia: JB Lippincott, 1993.

Centers for Disease Control and Prevention. Draft guidelines for isolation precautions in hospitals. Federal Register November 7, 1994;59:55552–55570.

Centers for Disease Control and Prevention. Guidelines for preventing the transmission of tuberculosis in health-care facilities. Morbidity and Mortality Weekly Report 1994;43(RR-13):7–132.

Crow S. Sterilization processes: meeting the demands of today's health care technology. Nursing Clinics of North America September 1993;28:687–695.

Fritsch DE, Pilat DMF. Exposing latex allergies. Nursing August 1993;23:46–48.

Handwashing. Mayo Clinic Health Letter. July 1993;11:4.

Jenny J. Knowledge deficit: not a nursing diagnosis. Image 1987;19: 184–185.

Korniewicz DM. Effectiveness of glove barriers used in clinical settings. MEDSURG Nursing September 1992;1:29–32.

Mallison MB. The staph that eats hospitals. American Journal of Nursing February 1992;92:7.

Matteson MA, McConnell ES. Gerontological Nursing: Concepts and Practice. Philadelphia: WB Saunders, 1988.

Miller CA. Infections, resistant microbes, and older adults. Geriatric Nursing January–February 1993;14:55–56.

Pritchard V. Infection control programs for long-term care. Journal of Gerontological Nursing July 1993;19:29–32.

Ralph IG. Infectious medical waste management: a home care responsibility. Home Healthcare Nurse May–June 1993;11:25–33.

Rice R, Jorden JU. Infection control education. Caring April 1992;11: 54–59.

Rodts B, Meister S. Infection control takes top priority. RN December 1990;53:59–62.

Shovein J, Young MS. MRSA: Pandora's box for hospitals . . . methicillin-resistant Staphylococcus aureus. American Journal of Nursing February 1992;92:48–52.

Tortora GJ, Funke BR, Case CL. Microbiology: An Introduction. 4th ed. Redwood City, CA: Benjamin Cummings, 1992.

CHAPTER 22

Infection Control

Key Terms

Acute Stage
Airborne Precautions
Colonization
Contact Precautions
Contagious Diseases
Convalescent Stage
Double-bagging
Droplet Precautions
Incubation Period

Infection
Infection Control
Prodromal Stage
Resolution
Standard Precautions
Transmission Barriers
Transmission-Based
Precautions

Learning Objectives

An understanding of the content within this chapter will be evidenced by the student's ability to:

- Explain the meaning of contagious diseases, and give two other terms that are commonly used when referring to contagious diseases
- Differentiate between infection and colonization
- List five stages in the course of an infectious disease
- Explain the meaning of infection control measures
- Name two major categories of infection control
- Discuss when Standard Precautions and Transmission-Based Precautions are used
- Name three types of Transmission-Based Precautions, and the basis for using them
- Describe Airborne, Droplet, and Contact Precautions
- Explain the purpose of transmission barriers
- Discuss one principle that is followed when removing barrier garments
- Explain how double-bagging is performed
- List two psychological problems that are common among patients with infectious diseases
- Provide at least three teaching suggestions for preventing infections
- Discuss one unique characteristic of older adults in relation to infectious diseases

At one time, **contagious diseases**, also called *infectious* or *communicable diseases* because they are are spread from one person to another, were the leading cause of death. But because of the development of vaccines, implementation of aggressive public health measures, and advances in drug therapy, that is no longer the case. Nevertheless, contagious diseases have not disappeared.

Timby BK: *Fundamental Skills and Concepts in Patient Care, Sixth Edition* © 1996 Lippincott-Raven Publishers

In fact, the microorganisms that cause tuberculosis, gonorrhea, and some forms of wound and respiratory infections have developed drug-resistant strains. Add to that the grim reality that there is an epidemic of acquired immune deficiency syndrome (AIDS), a contagious disease spread by blood and some body fluids (Display 22-1), and it is easy to see that the war against pathogens has not been won.

Therefore, this chapter addresses those precautions that confine the reservoir of infectious agents and block their transmission from one host to another. To understand the concepts of infection control, it is important to understand the infectious process cycle (see Chap. 21) and the course of an infection.

INFECTION

An **infection** is a condition that results when microorganisms cause injury to their host. **Colonization** refers to a condition in which microorganisms are present,

---

DISPLAY 22-1. *Methods of Contracting AIDS**

AIDS may be acquired by:
- Contact with the blood, semen, or vaginal secretions of a human immunodeficiency virus (HIV)-infected person during unprotected vaginal, anal, or oral sexual intercourse
- Contact with the blood, semen, or vaginal secretions of an HIV-infected person during medical, dental, and nursing procedures in which these fluids enter through an open cut or splash into a caregiver's eyes or nose
- Contact with the blood of an HIV-infected person by
    sharing intravenous needles or syringes
    receiving a transfusion of contaminated blood or blood cell components
    receiving plasma or clotting factors that have not been heat treated
    contaminated ear-piercing, tatooing, or dental equipment

The virus that causes AIDS also may be transmitted from infected mothers to their infants during pregnancy, birth, or breast-feeding

* Contact with saliva, tears, or sweat has never been shown to result in the transmission of HIV; nor has casual contact, closed-mouth kissing, being bitten by insects, or receiving immunoglobulin, albumin, plasma protein fraction, or hepatitis B vaccines.

Source: Centers for Disease Control and Prevention. Facts About the Human Immunodeficiency Virus and its Transmission. Washington, DC: United States Department of Health and Human Services, May, 1994.

---

but the host is not damaged nor shows any signs or symptoms. That does not mean, however, that a colonized person cannot transmit pathogens.

Infections progress through distinct stages (Table 22-1); however, the characteristics and lengths of each stage may differ depending on the infectious agent. For example, the incubation period for the common cold is approximately 2 to 4 days before symptoms appear, whereas it make take months or years before a person infected with the human immunodeficiency virus (HIV) demonstrates symptoms of AIDS.

Infection control depends on knowing the mechanisms by which an infectious disease is transmitted and the methods that will interfere with the infectious process cycle.

INFECTION CONTROL

Infection control refers to physical measures that attempt to curtail the spread of infectious or contagious diseases. The Centers for Disease Control and Prevention (CDC) (1994) has recently drafted a new proposal outlining two major categories for infection control. They include Standard Precautions and Transmission-Based Precautions.

Standard Precautions

Standard Precautions (Display 22-2) are used when caring for *all* patients regardless of their infection status. If adopted, Standard Precautions combine what was previously referred to as *Universal Precautions* and *Body Substance Isolation*. Standard Precautions reduce the potential for transmitting blood-borne pathogens and those from moist body substances like feces, urine, sputum, saliva, wound drainage and other body fluids. They are followed whenever there is the potential for contact with:

- Blood
- All body fluids, secretions and excretions, regardless of whether they contain visible blood
- Nonintact skin
- Mucous membranes

Transmission-Based Precautions

Transmission-Based Precautions, also called *isolation precautions*, are measures that are recommended for use *in addition to* Standard Precautions. Their purpose is to control the spread of infectious agents from patients known or suspected of being infected or colonized with highly transmissable or significant pathogens.

There are three types of Transmission-Based Precautions, namely, Airborne Precautions, Droplet Precau-

TABLE 22-1. *The Course of Infectious Diseases*

Stage	Characteristic
Incubation period	Infectious agent reproduces, but there are no recognizable symptoms. The infectious agent may, however, exit the host at this time and infect others.
Prodromal stage	Initial symptoms appear, which may be vague and nonspecific. They may include mild fever, headache, and loss of usual energy.
Acute stage	Symptoms become severe and specific to the tissue or organ that is affected. For example, tuberculosis is manifested by respiratory symptoms.
Convalescent stage	The symptoms subside as the host overcomes the infectious agent.
Resolution	The pathogen is destroyed. Health improves or is restored.

tions, and Contact Precautions (Table 22-2). These three Transmission-Based Precautions will replace the previous categories of Strict Isolation, Contact Isolation, Respiratory Isolation, Tuberculosis [Acid-Fast Bacillus (AFB)] Isolation, Enteric Precautions, and Drainage/ Secretion Precautions. The decision to use one or a combination of precautions is based on the mechanism for the transmission of the respective pathogen.

Transmission-Based Precautions may be required for various lengths of time depending on the nature of the infecting microorganisms. Some precautions, with the exception of Standard Precautions, may be discontinued when culture findings are negative, when a wound or lesion stops draining, or after the initiation of effective therapy. In some cases, they may be used throughout the duration of treatment and care.

DISPLAY 22-2. *Standard Precautions*

- Wear clean gloves when touching:
    blood, body fluids, secretions and excretions, and items containing these body substances
    mucous membranes
    nonintact skin
- Perform handwashing immediately
    when there is direct contact with blood, body fluids, secretions and excretions, and contaminated items
    after removing gloves
    between patient contacts
- Wear a mask, eye protection, face shield
    during procedures and patient care activities that are likely to generate splashes or sprays of blood, body fluids, secretions, and excretions
- Wear a cover gown
    during procedures and patient care activities that are likely to generate splashes or sprays of blood, body fluids, secretions, or excretions or cause soiling of clothing
- Remove soiled protective items promptly when the potential for contact with reservoirs of pathogens is no longer present.
- Clean and reprocess all equipment before reuse by another patient.
- Discard all single-use items promptly in appropriate containers that prevent contact with blood, body fluids, and secretions and excretions, contamination of clothing, and transfer of microorganisms to other patients and the environment.
- Handle, transport, and process linen soiled with blood, body fluids, and secretions and excretions in such a way as to prevent skin and mucous membrane exposures, contamination of clothing, or transfer to other patients and the environment.
- Prevent injuries with used needles, scalpels, and other sharp devices by
    never removing, recapping, bending, or breaking used needles
    never pointing the needle toward a body part
    using a one-handed "scoop" method, special syringes with a retractable protective guard or shield for enclosing a needle, or blunt-point needles (see Chaps. 34 and 35)
    depositing disposable and reusable syringes and needles in puncture-resistant containers
- Use a private room or consult with an infection control professional for the care of patients who contaminate the environment, or who cannot or do not assist with appropriate hygiene or environmental cleanliness measures.

TABLE 22-2. *Transmission-Based Precautions*

Type of Precaution	Patient Placement	Protection	Examples of Diseases
Airborne	Private room Negative air pressure* Discharge of room air to environment or filtered before being circulated	Follow Standard Precautions. Wear a mask for airborne pathogens or particulate air filter respirator in the case of tuberculosis. Place a mask on the patient if transport is required.	Tuberculosis Measles Chickenpox
Droplet	Private room, or in a room with a similarly infected patient(s) or one in which there is at least 3 feet between other patient(s) and visitors	Follow Standard Precautions. Wear a mask when entering the room, but especially when within 3 feet of the infected patient. Place a mask on the patient if a transport is required.	Influenza Rubella Streptococcal pneumonia Meningococcal meningitis
Contact	Private room, or in a room with similarly infected patient(s), or Consult with an infection control professional if the above options are not available.	Follow Standard Precautions. Don gloves before entering the room. Remove gloves before leaving the room. Change gloves after contact with infective material. Perform handwashing with an antimicrobial agent immediately after removing gloves. Wear a gown when entering the room if there is the possibility that your clothing will touch the patient or items in the room, or if the patient is incontinent, has diarrhea, an ileostomy, a colostomy, or wound drainage not contained by a dressing. Avoid transporting the patient, but, if required, use precautions that minimize transmission. Clean bedside equipment and patient care items daily. Use items such as a stethoscope, sphygmomanometer and other assessment tools exclusively for the infected patient and terminally disinfect them when precautions are no longer necessary.	Gastrointestinal, respiratory, skin, or wound infections that are drug resistant Acute diarrhea Draining abscess

*Negative air pressure pulls air from the hall into the room when the door is opened, as opposed to positive air pressure, which pulls room air into the hall.

Source: Centers for Disease Control and Prevention. Draft guideline for isolation precautions in hospitals; notice. Federal Register November 7, 1994;59:55552–55570.

AIRBORNE PRECAUTIONS

Airborne Precautions are measures used to block pathogens 5 microns or smaller that (1) are present within the residue of evaporated droplets that remain suspended in the air, and (2) are attached to dust particles.

DROPLET PRECAUTIONS

Droplet Precautions are measures used to block pathogens within moist droplets that are larger than 5 microns. These microorganisms commonly exit the body during coughing, sneezing, laughing, and talking.

CONTACT PRECAUTIONS

Contact Precautions are measures used to block the transmission of pathogens by (1) direct hand-to-skin or skin-to-skin contact, or (2) indirect contact with an intermediate object within the patient's environment.

INFECTION CONTROL MEASURES

Infection control measures involve the use of transmission barriers. **Transmission barriers** are garments or techniques that block the transfer of pathogens from infected patients, the environment, or contaminated substances to oneself or others (Fig. 22-1). Depending on the type of precautions being used, all or only some of the following measures may be used:

- Locating a patient and equipping a room so as to confine or restrict pathogens within one area
- Using barrier garments like cover gowns, face-protective devices, and gloves to prevent spreading microorganisms through direct and indirect contact
- Disposing of contaminated linen, equipment, and supplies in such a way that pathogens are not transferred to others
- Using infection control measures to keep pathogens from spreading when transporting laboratory specimens or patients themselves

Patient Care Environment

The patient care environment includes the actual room designated for the care of a patient with an infectious disease and the equipment and supplies that are essential to controlling its transmission.

INFECTION CONTROL ROOM

Except when Standard Precautions are used, most actual or potentially infectious patients are assigned to

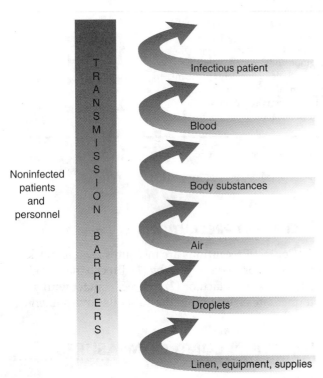

FIGURE 22-1
Blocking sources of infectious disease transmission.

a private room. Some alternatives may be used if this option is not feasible (see Table 22-2). The door to the room is kept closed to control air currents and the circulation of dust particles.

The room that is used has a private bathroom to facilitate flushing contaminated liquids and biodegradable solids. A sink with running water is also located within the room to enable handwashing.

An instruction card indicating the barrier methods that are required is posted on the door (Fig. 22-2). Nurses are responsible for teaching visitors how to implement the specified infection control measures.

Following principles of medical asepsis, housekeeping personnel clean the infectious patient's room last to avoid transferring organisms on the wet mop to other patient areas. The mop head, if not disposable, is deposited with the soiled linen. The mop handle is wiped with a disinfectant. Solutions used for cleaning are flushed down the toilet in most cases.

EQUIPMENT AND SUPPLIES

The isolation room contains essentially the same equipment and supplies as any other hospital room, with a few modifications. Items like a container for soiled laundry (Fig. 22-3), lined waste containers, and a liquid soap dispenser are placed within the room for concurrent disinfection. Equipment that would ordinarily be shared among noncontagious patients, such as a stethoscope and sphygmomanometer, is left in the room whenever possible for the patient's exclusive use. This prevents the added task of cleaning and disinfecting them each time they are removed.

For the same reason, disposable thermometers are usually preferred. If a glass thermometer is used, it is left at the patient's bedside in a container of disinfectant that is replaced on a regular basis. Electronic thermometers are disinfected to make them safe for the next patient.

Barrier Garments

All infection control measures involve using one or more barrier garments (Fig. 22-4) like a gown, mask or particulate respirator, goggles or face shield, and gloves (see Chap. 21). These items are located just outside the patient's room or within an anteroom (Fig. 22-5).

USING A COVER GOWN

Cover gowns are worn for two reasons. First, they prevent contamination of clothing and protect the skin from contact with blood and body fluids. Second, they reduce the possibility of transmitting pathogens to others following patient care.

Visitors—Report to Nurses' Station Before Entering Room

1. Masks are indicated for all persons entering room.
2. Gowns are indicated for all persons entering room.
3. Gloves are indicated for all persons entering room.
4. HANDS MUST BE WASHED AFTER TOUCHING THE PATIENT OR POTENTIALLY CONTAMINATED ARTICLES AND BEFORE TAKING CARE OF ANOTHER PATIENT.
5. Articles contaminated with infective material should be discarded or bagged and labeled before being sent for decontamination and reprocessing.

FIGURE 22-2
Door instructional card.

Many variations of cover gowns exist, but all have the following common characteristics:

- They open in the back to reduce inadvertent contact with the patient.
- They have close-fitting wristlets to help avoid contaminating the skin of the forearms.
- They fasten at the neck and waist to keep the gown securely closed, thus covering all the wearer's clothing (Fig. 22-6).

A cover gown is worn only once and then discarded. Discarded cloth gowns are placed within the patient's laundry hamper, removed with the soiled linen, and then washed before being used again. Disposable paper gowns are placed in a waste container and eventually incinerated.

WEARING FACE-PROTECTIVE DEVICES

Depending on the mode of transmission, a mask or particulate filter respirator, goggles, or a face shield may be worn (see Chap. 21). These items are always applied before entering the patient's room.

USING GLOVES

Gloves are required when an infectious disease is transmissable by direct contact or contact with blood and body substances. They are always donned before or immediately after entering the patient's room. After one use, they are discarded.

A word of caution: *gloves are not a total and complete barrier to microorganisms*. Gloves can be easily punctured, and occult leakage occurs approximately 2% of the time (Korniewicz, 1989). The percentage increases with the stress of their use.

Also, one must not be lulled into thinking that wearing gloves replaces the need to perform handwashing. It has been shown that the skin may become contaminated during the process of glove removal, and that microorganisms grow and multiply rapidly while within the warm, moist environment inside gloves.

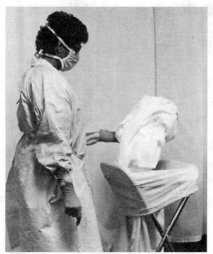

FIGURE 22-3
Containing soiled laundry. (Courtesy of Ken Timby.)

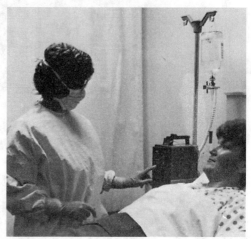

FIGURE 22-4
Barrier garments. (Courtesy of Ken Timby.)

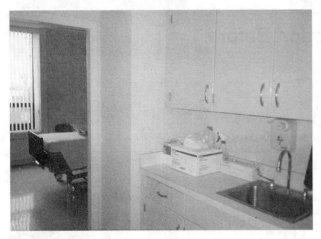

FIGURE 22-5
An anteroom outside the infection control room. (Courtesy of Ken Timby.)

REMOVING BARRIER GARMENTS

Regardless of which barrier garments are worn, there is an order that is followed when they are removed (Skill 22-1). The object is to remove the barrier garments in such a way as to leave the patient's room without contaminating oneself or one's uniform. To do so, garments are removed by always making contact between two contaminated surfaces or two clean surfaces.

Garments of greater contamination are removed first while preserving the clean uniform underneath. With this principle as a guide, the technique may be modified to accommodate the removal of any combination of barrier garments. The most important nursing action is to perform thorough handwashing before leaving the patient's room and before touching any other patient or personnel.

Disposing of Contaminated Linen, Equipment, and Supplies

Various receptacles within the patient's room are used to hold and collect contaminated items. Soiled waste containers are emptied at the end of each shift or more often if their contents accumulate. To avoid spreading pathogens, some items are double-bagged.

DOUBLE-BAGGING

Double-bagging is a measure in which one bag of contaminated items, like trash or laundry, is placed within another held by someone outside the patient's room. The person holding the second bag prevents contamination by manipulating the bag underneath a folded cuff (Fig. 22-7).

The CDC is now relaxing its recommendation concerning double-bagging. Its revised position is that a single bag probably provides adequate protection as long as it is strong enough to resist puncturing and care is taken to avoid touching the outside of the bag with articles that are placed within (CDC, 1983). When neither of these two criteria can be met, double-bagging is still appropriate. Even when linen is contaminated with blood or body fluids, double-bagging is unnecessary as long as the bags that are used prevent leakage (American Hospital Association, 1988). One study (Maki et al., 1986) at the University of Wisconsin Hospital and Clinics found that a single 2-mL polyethylene bag did not result in significantly greater surface contamination than that found on the outside of doubled

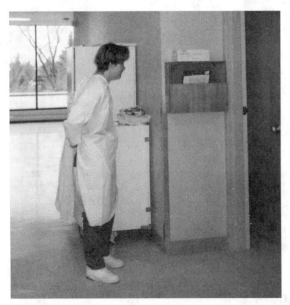

FIGURE 22-6
Donning a cover gown. (Courtesy of Ken Timby.)

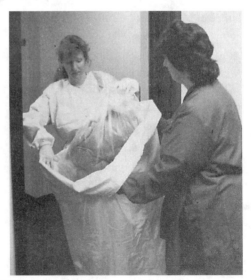

FIGURE 22-7
Double-bagging. (Courtesy of Ken Timby.)

SKILL 22-1
Removing Barrier Garments

Suggested Action	Reason for Action
Assessment	
Determine which type of infection control precautions are being used.	Indicates whether garments must be removed and discarded within or outside the room
Note if there is sufficient soap and paper towels, a laundry hamper, and a lined waste receptacle within the room.	Provides a means for washing and confining soiled garments
Planning	
Make sure that all direct care of the patient has been completed.	Avoids having to don barrier garments a second time
Implementation	
Untie the waist closure if it is fastened at the front of the cover gown before removing gloves.	Provides hand protection while touching a part of the gown that is considered grossly contaminated
Remove your gloves and discard them in a lined waste container.	Confines grossly contaminated items
Wash your hands (see Chap. 21).	Removes microorganisms
Remove your mask (see Chap. 21) and other disposable face-protective items and discard them in the waste container.	Confines contaminated items
Untie or unfasten the neck closure of the cover gown.	Prevents contaminating the back of the uniform and the hands
Remove the gown, but avoid touching the front, by either inserting your fingers at the shoulder or sliding a finger under the cuff and pulling the sleeve down.	Prevents gross contamination of the hands

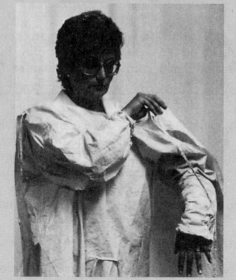

Removing a cover gown. (Courtesy of Ken Timby.)

(continued)

SKILL 22-1
Removing Barrier Garments (Continued)

Suggested Action	Reason for Action
Fold the soiled side of the gown to the inside while holding it away from your uniform.	Prevents contamination of the hands and uniform
Roll up the gown and discard it in the waste container, if it is constructed of paper. If the gown is made of cloth, discard it in the laundry hamper within the room.	Confines contaminated garments
Wash your hands.	Removes microorganisms that may have been inadvertently transferred during mask and gown removal
Use a clean paper towel to open the room door.	Protects clean hands from recontamination
Discard the paper towel within the waste container within the patient's room.	Confines contaminated material
Leave the room, taking care not to touch anything.	Prevents recontamination
Go directly to the utility room and wash your hands one final time.	Removes microorganisms; it is always safer to overdo than underdo any practice that controls the spread of pathogens

Evaluation
- Appropriate barrier garments were worn
- Garments were removed with the least contamination possible
- Handwashing was performed appropriately

Document
- Type of Transmission-Based Precautions being followed
- Care provided
- Response of patient

Sample Documentation

Date and Time   Contact Precautions followed. Assisted with bath while wearing gloves and gown. States, "I wish the door to my room could be left opened. It gets rather boring in here." Reinforced the purpose for keeping the door closed. _____ **Signature, Title**

bags. Despite these findings, some health agencies may continue to require double-bagging. Existing policies should be followed.

Discarding Biodegradable Trash

Biodegradable trash is that which will decompose naturally into less complex compounds. Some items like uneaten food, paper tissues, the contents of drainage collectors, urine, and stool may be flushed down the toilet within the patient's room. Chemicals and filtration methods in sewage treatment centers are sufficient for destroying pathogens in human wastes.

Bulkier items may be placed in a lined trash container and removed from the room by single- or dou-

ble-bagging. Moist items such as soiled dressings, however, are wrapped so that during their containment pathogens cannot be transferred by flying or crawling insects. Eventually, the bag and its contents are destroyed by incineration, or they are autoclaved. Autoclaved items may be safely disposed of in landfills.

Removing Reusable Items

To reduce the need for concurrent disinfection of reusable items, disposable equipment and supplies such as plastic bedpans, basins, eating utensils, and paper plates and cups are used as much as possible. However, if reusable items are necessary for care, they are cleaned, bagged, and sterilized by heat or chemicals.

Delivering Laboratory Specimens

Specimens are delivered to the laboratory in sealed containers. The agency's infection control guidelines are followed as to whether the sealed containers are additionally bagged. When the testing is complete, most specimens are flushed, incinerated, or sterilized.

Transporting Patients

Patients with infectious diseases may need to be transported elsewhere, such as to the x-ray department. During the time of transport, it is necessary to use practices that prevent the direct or indirect spread of pathogens from the patient. For example, to prevent contamination of transport equipment, the surface of the wheelchair or stretcher is protected from direct patient contact by lining it with a clean sheet or bath blanket. A second one is used to cover as much of the patient's body as possible during transport. A mask or particulate respirator is worn by the patient in cases where the pathogen is transmitted by the airborne or droplet route (Fig. 22-8). Any hospital personnel having direct contact with the patient dons and removes barrier garments similar to those used in patient care.

Furthermore, interdepartmental coordination is important. The department to which the patient will be transported is made aware that the patient has a contagious disease. This reduces unnecessary waiting in an area used by other patients.

When returning the patient, the nurse deposits the soiled linen in the linen hamper within the patient's room, taking care to touch only the outside surface of the protective covers. Some agencies also spray or wash the transport vehicle with disinfectant before reuse by another patient.

Although infection control measures are necessary, they often leave patients feeling as though they are being shunned or abandoned.

PSYCHOLOGICAL IMPLICATIONS

No matter how ill or well patients with infectious diseases may feel, they continue to need human contact and interaction. Both are often minimal because of the elaborate precautions that must be taken on entering and leaving the room. Added to this are the decreased socialization that occurs when fearful family and friends avoid visiting, and the fact that infectious patients are restricted from leaving their room. Therefore, conscientious nurses plan measures for relieving feelings of isolation by providing social interaction and sensory stimulation.

Promoting Social Interaction

While Transmission-Based Precautions are being used, it is important to plan frequent contact with the patient. Visitors are encouraged to come whenever and as often as the agency's policies and the patient's condition permit. Every opportunity is used to emphasize that as long as the infection control precautions are followed, visitors are not likely to acquire the disease.

Combating Sensory Deprivation

Sensory deprivation is a condition that results when a person experiences less-than-adequate amounts of sensory stimulation or is exposed to sensory stimulation that is continuous but monotonous. The goal is to provide a variety of sensory experiences at intermittent intervals.

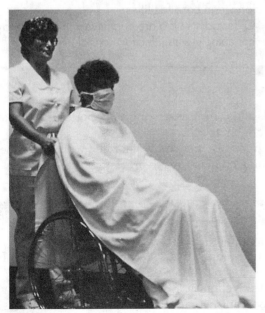

FIGURE 22-8
Transporting an infectious patient. (Courtesy of Ken Timby.)

NURSING GUIDELINES FOR PROVIDING SENSORY STIMULATION

- Move the bed to various places within the room or rearrange the furnishings within the room.
  Rationale: Provides a change in perspective
- Position the patient in such a way that he or she may look out windows.
  Rationale: Reduces boredom
- Encourage the use of the telephone.
  Rationale: Provides vicarious social interaction

- Communicate via the intercom system if it is inconvenient to enter the room.
  Rationale: Demonstrates concern for attention
- Engage in conversations about what is happening in current events on the community, state, federal, and global levels.
  Rationale: Stimulates a variety of thought processes
- Help the patient select television or radio programs.
  Rationale: Captivates attention
- Change the location of equipment that produces monotonous sounds.
  Rationale: Varies the volume or pitch of stimuli
- Encourage activity within the confines of the room.
  Rationale: Provides a means of self-stimulation
- Provide leisure activities that can be done independently like reading, working crossword puzzles, playing solitaire, putting together picture puzzles.
  Rationale: Offers diversion
- Offer a wide choice of foods that provide different flavors, temperatures, and textures.
  Rationale: Stimulates oral and olfactory sensations
- Use touch appropriately by giving a backrub or changing the patient's position.
  Rationale: Produces tactile stimulation

NURSING IMPLICATIONS

Caring for patients with contagious diseases requires skills for meeting both their physical as well as emotional needs. Some frequently identified nursing diagnoses include those listed in Applicable Nursing Diagnoses.

The accompanying Nursing Care Plan demonstrates how the nursing process is applied when providing care for a patient with the nursing diagnosis of Risk for Infection Transmission. Carpenito (1995) defines this diagnostic category as "The state in which an individual is at risk for transferring an opportunistic or pathogenic agent to others."

Nurses also play a pivotal role by providing health teaching on measures to prevent infections.

 FOCUS ON OLDER ADULTS

- Older adults are more susceptible to infectious diseases because they have decreased lymphocyte cells and a decreased antibody response.
- Chronic diseases reduce the older person's ability to resist infections.
- Symptoms of infections tend to be more subtle among older adults, but infections are more likely to have a rapid course once one becomes established.
- Recognizing an infectious process early may prevent the necessity for admitting older adults to an acute care setting.
- Confusion and changes in behavior are often signs of infection among older adults (Fraser, 1993).
- Infections are often the major reason for admitting nursing home residents to hospitals (Jackson & Schafer, 1993).
- Pneumonia is the fourth leading cause of death among older adults, whereas influenza is the fifth cause of death in people older than 65 years of age (Fraser, 1993).
- Inadequate nutrition predisposes the elderly to infections.
- All long-term care facilities are required to test each resident on admission and each new employee for tuberculosis.
- The limited number of private rooms and sinks for handwashing increases the risk for the transmission of pathogens among residents in long-term care facilities.
- Older adults who are cognitively impaired may not comply with infection control measures.

APPLICABLE NURSING DIAGNOSES

- Risk for Infection
- Altered Protection
- Risk for Infection Transmission
- Social Isolation
- Ineffective Individual Coping
- Diversional Activity Deficit
- Powerlessness
- Fear

KEY CONCEPTS

- Contagious diseases, also called infectious or communicable diseases, are those that are spread from one person to another.
- An infection is a condition that results when microorganisms cause injury to their host, whereas colonization refers to a condition in which microorganisms are present, but the host is not damaged nor shows any signs or symptoms.

NURSING CARE PLAN:
Risk for Infection Transmission

Assessment

Subjective Data

States "The health department informed me that my preemployment TB test was positive and my chest x-ray showed some suspicious cavities. The doctor put me in the hospital until my sputum tests are complete."

Objective Data

30-year-old man who is a recent immigrant from India presents with a nonproductive cough and an unexplained weight loss of 7 lbs in 1 month. No current fever.

Diagnosis

Risk for Infection Transmission related to airborne spread of pathogen causing tuberculosis.

Plan

Goal

Will comply with infection control measures and accurately describe postdischarge drug therapy and medical follow-up by time of discharge.

Orders: 5/11
1. Follow Airborne Transmission Precautions until sputum smear is negative; follow Standard Precautions throughout length of stay.
2. Post infection control measures on room door.
3. Wear a particulate filter respirator during patient care.
4. Teach patient to cover nose and mouth with a paper tissue when coughing, sneezing, or laughing, and dispose of it in a paper bag.
5. Directly observe patient taking prescribed drug therapy.
6. Explain the purpose of combination drug therapy and the need to continue uninterrupted administration to avoid treatment failure and development of drug-resistant strain.
7. Inform patient to provide a sputum specimen at the public health department within 2 to 3 weeks (5/28 to 6/1) if discharged earlier.
8. Recommend TB skin testing for close family members or friends.

_____ L. STRONG, RN

Implementation 5/11 1130 Placed in private infection control room. Instruction card posted. Explained
(Documentation) the purpose for wearing a respirator mask. Instructed on how to use tissues when coughing, sneezing, and laughing. Paper bag for tissue disposal taped to side rail of bed. _____ L. CUPP, LPN

Evaluation 2000 Spent 15 minutes talking with patient during the time of medication adminis-
(Documentation) tration. Using paper tissues as instructed. Concerned that immigration sponsor has not visited and how patient's illness will affect visa status. Left a message with social worker about contacting sponsor._____ L. STONER, LPN

- Infectious diseases usually follow five stages: the incubation period, the prodromal stage, the acute stage, the convalescent stage, and resolution.
- Infection control measures are physical measures that attempt to curtail the spread of infectious or contagious diseases.
- There are two major categories of infection control measures: Standard Precautions and Transmission-Based Precautions.
- Standard Precautions are used when caring for all patients, regardless of their infection status.

- Transmission-Based Precautions are used in addition to Standard Precautions to control the spread of infectious agents from patients known or suspected of being infected or colonized with highly transmissable or significant pathogens.
- There are three types of Transmission-Based Precautions: Airborne Precautions, Droplet Precautions, and Contact Precautions.
- Airborne Precautions are measures used to block very small pathogens that remain suspended in the air or are attached to dust particles. Droplet Precau-

PATIENT TEACHING FOR PREVENTING INFECTIONS

Teach the patient and family to do the following:
- Bathe daily and perform other forms of personal hygiene such as oral care.
- Keep the home environment clean and uncluttered.
- Use diluted household bleach (1:10 or 1:100) as a good disinfectant.
- Obtain appropriate immunizations; tetanus vaccine is recommended at 10-year intervals, the influenza vaccine must be repeated yearly, and a pneumococcal pneumonia immunization will last a lifetime.
- Investigate vaccines, water purification techniques, and foods to avoid when traveling outside the United States.
- Practice a healthy lifestyle such as eating the recommended servings from the food pyramid (see Chap. 14).

- Perform frequent handwashing, especially before eating and after contact with nasal secretions and use of the toilet.
- Use and immediately discard disposable tissues rather than reuse a cloth handkerchief.
- Avoid sharing personal care items like washcloths, towels, razors, and drinking cups.
- Stay home from work or school when ill rather than expose others to infectious pathogens.
- Relieve an ill family member from the responsibility of cooking meals.
- Keep food refrigerated and heat it thoroughly when preparing food for consumption.
- Avoid crowds and public places when there are local outbreaks of influenza.
- Follow infection control instructions when visiting hospitalized family members and friends.
- Comply with drug therapy when prescribed.

tions are measures used to block larger pathogens contained within moist droplets. Contact Precautions are used to block the transmission of pathogens by direct or indirect contact.
- Transmission barriers are a form of infection control in which garments or special techniques are used to block the transfer of pathogens from infected patients, the environment, or contaminated substances to oneself or others.
- When removing barrier garments, those with greater contamination are always removed first while preserving the clean uniform underneath.
- Double-bagging is a measure in which one bag of contaminated items like trash or laundry is placed within another held by someone outside the patient's room.
- Patients with infectious diseases often experience decreased social interaction and sensory deprivation as a result of being confined to their room.
- To prevent infections, the nurse can recommend that people (1) obtain appropriate immunizations, (2) practice a healthy lifestyle, and (3) avoid sharing personal care items.
- Unfortunately, symptoms of infectious disorders tend to be more subtle among older adults.

CRITICAL THINKING EXERCISES

- Discuss the similarities between the transmission and control of infections in day-care centers for young children and nursing home facilities that house older adults.

- Explain why the incidence of AIDS continues at such an alarming rate despite the fact that its mode of transmission is known.

SUGGESTED READINGS

American Hospital Association. Management of HIV Infection in the Hospital. 3rd ed. Chicago: Author, 1988.

Brinsko V. Infection control. Nursing Clinics of North America September 1993;28:597–598.

Carpenito LJ. Nursing Diagnosis: Application to Clinical Practice. 6th ed. Philadelphia: JB Lippincott, 1995.

Centers for Disease Control and Prevention (CDC). Aids Prevention Guide. Washington, DC: United States Department of Health and Human Services, August, 1994.

Centers for Disease Control and Prevention (CDC). Draft guidelines for isolation precautions in hospitals. Federal Register November 7, 1994;59:55552–55570.

Centers for Disease Control and Prevention (CDC). Guidelines for Isolation Precautions in Hospitals. 1983.

Fraser D. Patient assessment, infection in the elderly. Journal of Gerontological Nursing July 1993;19:5–11.

Jackson MM, Schafer K. Identifying clues to infections in nursing home residents. Journal of Gerontological Nursing July 1993;19: 33–42.

Korniewicz DM, Laughn BE, Butz A, et al. Integrity of vinyl and latex procedure gloves. Nursing Research May–June 1989;38:144–6.

Maki DG, Alvarado C, Hassemer C. Double-bagging of items from isolation rooms is unnecessary as an infection control measure: a comparative study of surface contamination with single and double-bagging. Infection Control 1986;7:535–537.

Miller CA. Infections, resistant microbes, and older adults. Geriatric Nursing January–February 1993;14:55–56.

Pritchard V. Infection control programs for long-term care. Journal of Gerontological Nursing July 1993;19:29–32.

Rice R, Jorden JU. Infection control education. Caring April 1992; 11:54–59.

UNIT VII

Assisting the Inactive Patient

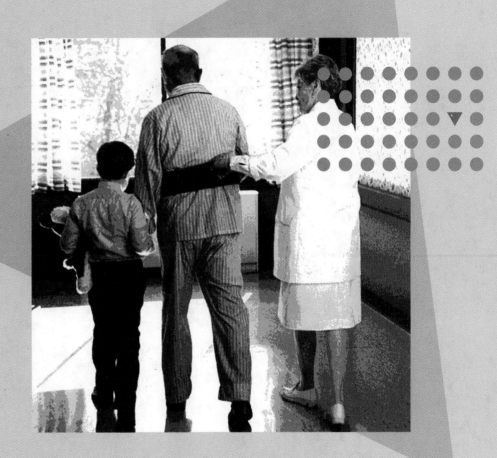

CHAPTER 23

Body Mechanics, Positioning, and Moving

NURSING GUIDELINES

Using Good Body Mechanics
Using a Trochanter Roll
Transferring Patients

SKILLS

Turning and Moving a Patient
Transferring Patients

NURSING CARE PLAN

Risk for Disuse Syndrome

Key Terms

Activity	Internal Rotation
Alignment	Lateral Position
Balance	Lateral Oblique Position
Base of Support	Line of Gravity
Bed Board	Muscle Spasms
Body Mechanics	Neutral Position
Center of Gravity	Oblique Position
Contracture	Plantar Flexion
Disuse Syndrome	Posture
Dorsiflexion	Prone Position
Extension	Rotation
External Rotation	Shearing
Flexion	Sims' Position
Foot Board	Supine Position
Foot Drop	Syndrome
Fowler's Position	Transfer
Functional Position	Trapeze
Gravity	

Learning Objectives

An understanding of the content within this chapter will be evidenced by the student's ability to:

- Identify characteristics of good posture in a standing, sitting, or lying position
- Describe a minimum of three principles of correct body mechanics
- Describe at least 10 signs or symptoms associated with the disuse syndrome
- List five positioning devices used for safety and comfort and explain the purpose of each
- List three pressure-relieving devices and one advantage for each
- Give at least five general guidelines that apply to transferring patients
- Name and describe six common patient positions
- List five suggested measures to prevent inactivity among older adults

Research has shown that activity is essential for health. Inactive patients require movement and positioning. This chapter describes principles for good posture, the use of body mechanics, and how to position and move patients to prevent complications associated with inactivity.

MAINTAINING GOOD POSTURE

Posture refers to the position of the body or the way in which it is held. Good posture, whether in a standing, sitting, or lying position, distributes gravity through the center of the body over a wide base of support (Fig. 23-1).

When a person performs work while using poor posture, muscle spasms often result. **Muscle spasms** are sudden, forceful, involuntary muscle contractions that occur when muscles are strained and forced to work beyond their capacity.

Standing

For good posture in a standing position (Fig. 23-2):

- Keep the feet parallel, at right angles to the lower legs, and about 4 to 8 inches (10–20 cm) apart. Distribute weight equally on both feet to provide a broad base of support.
- Bend the knees slightly to avoid straining the joints.

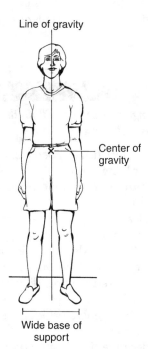

FIGURE 23-1
With good posture, gravity is aligned through the center of the body. A wide stance provides a stable base for support.

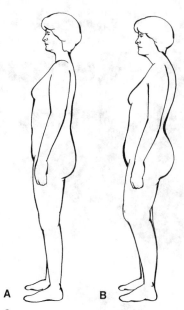

FIGURE 23-2
(*A*) Good standing posture. (*B*) Poor standing posture.

- Maintain the hips at an even level.
- Pull in the buttocks and hold the abdomen up and in to keep the spine properly aligned. This position supports the abdominal organs and reduces strain on both back and abdominal muscles.
- Hold the chest up and slightly forward and extend or stretch the waist to give internal organs more space and maintain good alignment of the spine.
- Keep the shoulders even and centered above the hips.
- Hold the head erect with the face forward and the chin slightly tucked.

Sitting

In a good sitting position (Fig. 23-3), the buttocks and upper thighs become the base of support. Both feet rest on the floor. The knees are bent and the popliteal area is free from the edge of the chair to avoid interfering with distal circulation.

Lying Down

Good posture in a lying position looks the same as a standing position, except the person is horizontal (Fig. 23-4). The head and neck muscles are in a neutral position centered between the shoulders. The shoulders are level, whereas the arms, hips, and knees are slightly flexed, with no compression of the arms or legs under the body. The trunk of the body is straight and the hips are level. The legs are parallel to each other with the feet at right angles to the leg.

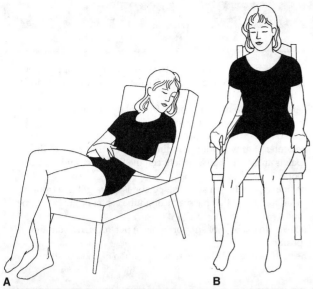

FIGURE 23-3
(*A*) Incorrect sitting posture. (*B*) Correct sitting posture. (Courtesy of Lowren West, New York, NY.)

Good posture is important for both nurses and patients. Furthermore, because nursing requires lifting, turning, and positioning of patients, it is also important to use proper body mechanics to avoid injury to oneself.

PRINCIPLES OF BODY MECHANICS

Body mechanics is defined as the efficient use of the body. Basic principles of body mechanics can be applied regardless of the worker or the task. Common terms used when speaking of body mechanics are defined in Table 23-1.

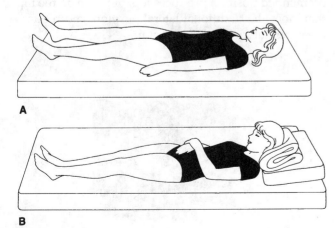

FIGURE 23-4
(*A*) Correct lying posture. (*B*) Incorrect lying posture. (Courtesy of Lowren West, New York, NY.)

NURSING GUIDELINES FOR USING GOOD BODY MECHANICS

- Use the longest and strongest muscles of the arms and legs.
  Rationale: Provides the greatest strength and potential for performing work
- Center a heavy load that is being lifted over the feet.
  Rationale: Creates a base of support
- Hold objects close to the body.
  Rationale: Facilitates balance
- Bend the knees.
  Rationale: Prepares the spine to accept the weight of the load
- Use the internal girdle and make a long midriff.
  Rationale: Protects the muscles of the abdomen and pelvis and prevents strain and injury to the abdominal wall
- Push, pull, or roll objects whenever possible, rather than lifting them.
  Rationale: Reduces work effort
- Use body weight as a lever to assist with pushing or pulling an object.
  Rationale: Reduces muscle strain
- Keep feet apart for a broad base of support.
  Rationale: Lowers the center of gravity
- Bend the knees and keep the back straight when lifting an object, rather than bending over from the waist with straight knees.
  Rationale: Makes best use of the longest and the strongest muscles in the body, and improves balance by keeping the weight of the object being lifted close to the center of gravity
- Avoid twisting and stretching muscles during work.
  Rationale: Prevents straining muscles from placing the line of gravity outside the body's base of support
- Rest between periods of exertion.
  Rationale: Promotes work endurance

If the principles of good posture and body mechanics are practiced, the result is an attractive appearance, good balance, increased muscle effectiveness, and less fatigue or injury to the musculoskeletal system—an important benefit when positioning and moving inactive patients.

COMMON POSITIONS

Proper body positioning is essential to promote comfort and provide for correct body alignment. An inactive patient's position is changed at least every 2 hours.

TABLE 23-1. *Basic Terminology of Body Mechanics*

Term	Definition	Example
Gravity	A force that pulls objects toward the center of the earth	The pull of gravity causes objects, such as an item dropped from the hand, to fall to the ground. It causes water to drain to its lowest level.
Energy	The capacity to do work	Energy is used to move the body from place to place. Energy is required to overcome the force of gravity.
Balance	Having a steady position with weight	A person falls when off balance.
Center of gravity	The point at which the mass of an object is centered	The center of gravity for a standing person is the center of the pelvis and about halfway between the umbilicus and the pubic bone.
Line of gravity	An imaginary, vertical line that passes through the center of gravity	The line of gravity in a standing person is a straight line from the head to the feet that passes through the center of gravity of the body.
Base of support	The area on which an object rests	The feet are the base of support when a person is in a standing position.
Alignment	Having parts of an object in proper relationship to one another	The body is in good alignment in a position of good posture.

There are six common body positions that may be used: the supine, lateral, lateral oblique, prone, Sims', and Fowler's positions. There are two additional terms that refer to body positioning. The term *neutral position* defines the position of a limb that is turned neither toward nor away from the body's midline. When a limb or body part is placed in *functional position*, it is in a position to perform an activity or to work properly and normally.

Supine Position

The **supine position** is one in which the person lies on his or her back (Fig. 23-5). There are two primary concerns when using the supine position. One is that pressure on the back, especially in the area at the end of the spine, may lead to skin breakdown. The second is the pressure exerted on the toes by the bed linens, which, when combined with gravity, forces the feet into a downward position known as **foot drop.** Foot drop may result in a permanent dysfunctional position caused by shortening of the calf muscles and lengthening of the opposing muscles on the anterior leg (Fig. 23-6).

Lateral Position

A **lateral position** is one in which a person lies on his or her side (Fig. 23-7). Foot drop is of less concern in this position because the feet are not being pulled down by gravity, as they are when the patient is supine. However, unless the upper shoulder and arm are supported, they may rotate forward and interfere with breathing.

Lateral Oblique Position

A **lateral oblique position** (Fig. 23-8) is one in which the patient lies on his or her side with the top leg placed in 30° of hip flexion and 35° of knee flexion. The calf of the top leg is placed behind the midline of the body on a support such as a pillow. The back is supported and the bottom leg is in neutral position. This newly recommended position produces less pressure on the hip than does the traditional lateral position, and reduces the potential for skin breakdown.

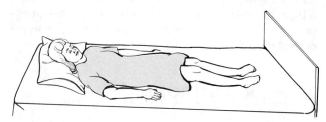

FIGURE 23-5
Supine position.

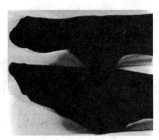

FIGURE 23-6
Position of foot drop.

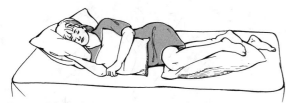

FIGURE 23-7
Lateral position.

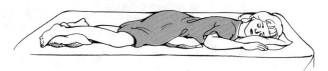

FIGURE 23-9
Prone position.

Prone Position

A **prone position** (Fig. 23-9) is one in which a person lies on his or her abdomen. Lying on the abdomen is a comfortable and relaxing position for many patients. It is an alternative position for the person with skin breakdown due to pressure sores. A prone position also provides for good drainage from bronchioles, stretches the trunk and extremities, and keeps the hips in an extended position. However, the prone position is often contraindicated when the patient has respiratory distress or heart disease because it interferes with chest expansion. It may also be uncomfortable for patients with recent abdominal surgery or those with back pain.

Sims' Position

Sims' position (Fig. 23-10) is a semiprone position in which the patient lies on his or her left side with the right knee drawn up toward the chest. The left arm is positioned along the patient's back, and the chest and abdomen are allowed to lean forward.

Fowler's Position

Fowler's position (Fig. 23-11) is a semisitting position. The hips and knees may or may not be elevated in this position; there are three variations commonly used. In the low-Fowler's position, the head and torso are elevated to 30°. A mid-Fowler's or semi-Fowler's position refers to an elevation of 45°. A 90° elevation is a high-Fowler's position. This position is especially helpful for patients with dyspnea because it causes the abdominal organs to drop away from the diaphragm, thereby relieving pressure on the chest cavity. This allows the lungs to fill efficiently. It also makes eating, conversing, and looking about easier than from a lying position.

POSITIONING DEVICES

There are many devices that help to maintain good body alignment in bed and prevent discomfort or pressure. Any position, however, no matter how comfortable or anatomically correct, must be changed frequently.

Adjustable Bed

The adjustable bed, described in Chapter 18, can be raised or lowered and allows the position of the head and knees to be changed. The high position facilitates nursing care. The low position enables the patient to get in and out of bed with greater ease. Raising the head of the bed helps bedridden patients see and look about without twisting and bending. It also promotes drainage of the upper lobes of the lungs and prepares the patient for the day when standing and walking will begin.

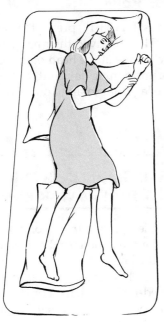

FIGURE 23-8
Lateral oblique position.

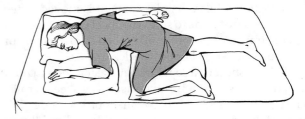

FIGURE 23-10
Sims' position.

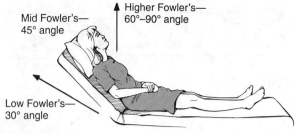

FIGURE 23-11
Fowler's position.

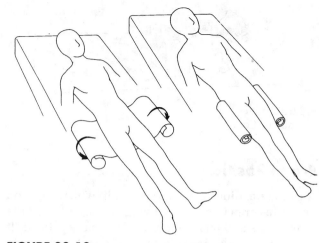

FIGURE 23-12
Placement of trochanter rolls.

Mattress

For a mattress to be comfortable and supportive, it must be firm but have sufficient flexibility to permit good body alignment. A nonsupportive mattress promotes an unnatural curvature of the spine.

Bed Board

A **bed board** is a rigid structure placed under a mattress to provide skeletal support. Bed boards usually are made of plywood or some other firm material. The size varies with the needs of the situation. If sections of the bed such as the head and foot can be raised, it may be necessary to have the board divided and held together with hinges. For home use, full bed boards can be purchased, or they can be made from sheets of plywood.

Pillows

The primary purposes of pillows are to provide support and elevate a body part. Small pillows, like contour pillows, triangular wedges, and bolsters, are ideal for support or elevation of the head, extremities, and shoulders. For home use, specially designed, heavy pillows are useful to elevate the upper part of the body when an adjustable bed is not available.

Turning Sheet

A turning sheet that extends from the upper back to thighs is a helpful positioning device. It is used to prevent friction while a helpless patient is moved, lifted, and turned from side to side. The sheet can also be used to help transfer a patient from the bed onto another surface such as a stretcher or wheelchair.

A draw sheet or a separate flat sheet folded in quarters can be used as a turning sheet. The sheet is rolled close to the patient's body by nurses on each side of the patient. Working as a team, they slide and roll the patient into an alternate position. Care is taken to keep the

sheet dry and free of wrinkles because it is usually left under the patient.

Sandbags

Sandbags, which are available in various sizes, are used when an extremity needs firm support. When properly filled, sandbags are pliable, not hard or rigid. For example, sandbags can be placed alongside the leg from the hip to the knee or ankle to promote proper alignment and positioning. Sandbags are covered with absorbent material, such as a sheet or bath blanket, to avoid accumulation of moisture next to the skin. These precautions help prevent skin breakdown.

Trochanter Rolls

Trochanter rolls (Fig. 23-12) prevent the legs from turning outward. They received their name from the bony ridges or trochanters at the head of the femur near the hip. Placing a positioning device at the trochanter helps to prevent the leg from rotating outward.

◄ NURSING GUIDELINES FOR USING A TROCHANTER ROLL

---

* Fold a sheet lengthwise in half or in thirds and place it under the patient so that it extends from the hips to the knees.
  Rationale: Anchors the body in position
* Place a rolled-up bath blanket or two bath towels under each end of the sheet that extends on either side of the patient.
  Rationale: Provides support to the leg

- Roll the sheet around the blanket so that the end of the roll is underneath.
  Rationale: Prevents unrolling
- Secure the rolls next to each hip and thigh.
  Rationale: Prevents external rotation of the hip
- Permit the leg to rest against the trochanter roll.
  Rationale: Allows normal alignment of the hips, preventing internal or external rotation

Hand Rolls

Hand rolls (Fig. 23-13) are devices that preserve the ability to grasp and pick up objects. To maintain this function and to prevent **contractures**, permanent stiffness of a joint, the thumb is positioned slightly away from the hand and at a moderate angle to the fingers. A rolled washcloth or a ball secured in the hand can be used as an alternative to commercial hand supports. Hand rolls are removed regularly to facilitate movement and exercise.

Foot Boards and Foot Splints

Foot boards and foot splints are devices that are used to keep the feet in the normal walking position, thus preventing foot drop. A foot board keeps the foot in a functional position that facilitates walking. On some commercial foot boards, there are supports that prevent outward rotation of the foot and lower leg (Fig. 23-14).

If the patient is short and cannot reach a foot board, a foot splint can be used (Fig. 23-15). A foot splint allows more variety of body positioning while still maintaining the foot in a neutral position. Some nurses have found that having the patient wear ankle-high tennis shoes in bed also helps prevent foot drop. The shoes are removed regularly, and proper foot care is given.

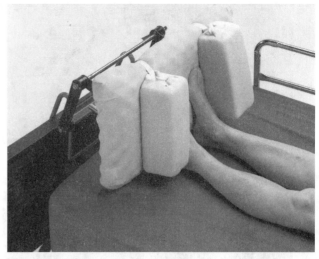

FIGURE 23-14
Foot board with lateral supports. (Courtesy of the J. T. Posey Company, Arcadia, CA.)

If a foot splint or foot board is not readily available, a temporary foot support can be made with a pillow and large sheet. The pillow is rolled in the sheet, and the ends of the sheet are twisted before being tucked under the foot of the mattress. A pillow support does not provide the firmness of a board or splint, and therefore it is replaced as soon as possible with a sturdier device.

Trapeze

A trapeze is a triangular piece of metal hung by a chain over the head of the bed (Fig. 23-16). The patient grasps

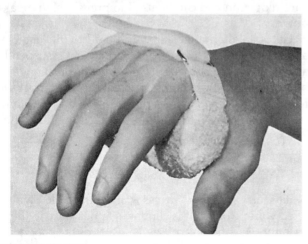

FIGURE 23-13
Hand roll. (Courtesy of the J. T. Posey Company, Arcadia, CA.)

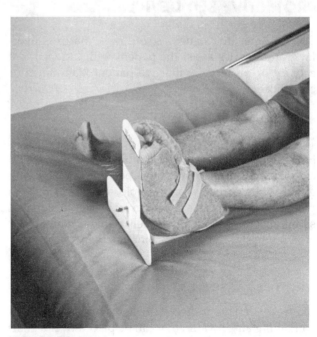

FIGURE 23-15
Foot splint (© 1994 Total Care, Gaithersburg, MD.)

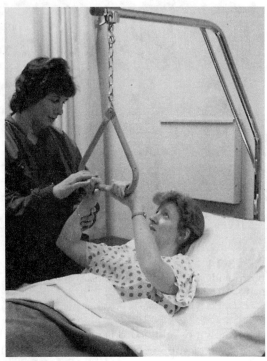

FIGURE 23-16
Using a trapeze to facilitate movement. (Courtesy of Ken Timby.)

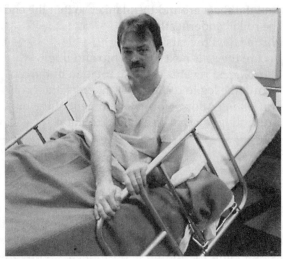

FIGURE 23-17
Using side rails to change position. (Courtesy of Ken Timby.)

a trapeze to lift his or her body and move about in bed. Unless arm movement or lifting is undesirable, a trapeze is an excellent device for helping a bedridden patient to be active.

PROTECTIVE BED DEVICES

Several other items such as side rails, mattress overlays, and cradles assist the patient with independent activity or protect the inactive patient from harm or complications.

Side Rails

Side rails (Fig. 23-17) are a valuable self-help device to aid patients in changing their position and moving about while in bed. For example, with side rails in place, the patient can safely turn from side to side and sit up in bed. These activities help patients maintain or regain muscle strength and joint flexibility.

Mattress Overlays

Mattress overlays are accessory items made of foam, or containing air or water, that can be placed over a standard hospital mattress. They are used to reduce pressure and restore the integrity of the skin (see Chap. 28).

FOAM MATTRESS

Several types of foam mattresses, made from latex or polyethylene, are available. Foam acts like a layer of subcutaneous tissue because it conforms to the patient's body shape and acts like a cushion. Consequently, it redistributes pressure over a greater area, thus reducing the compressive effect on skin and tissue. Foam also contains channels and cells filled with air, which allows for evaporation of moisture and escape of heat.

Some foam mattresses are convoluted or made with a series of elevations and depressions so as to resemble an egg crate (see Chap. 18) or waffle. The density of the foam and the manner in which the foam is formed determines the degree of pressure reduction.

Egg-crate foam mattresses that provide minimal pressure reduction are recommended for comfort only. Thicker, waffle-shaped foams offer much greater pressure reduction and can be used to prevent skin breakdown.

Gel is an alternative substance used to fill cushions and mattresses. It differs from foam in that it suspends and supports the body part. Gel and foam cushions can be placed in a wheelchair to prevent the "hammock effect." The hammock effect refers to the posterior and lateral compression that occurs when sitting in a sling-like seat.

STATIC AIR MATTRESS

A static air pressure mattress is one that is filled with a fixed volume of air. It is similar in appearance to those used for recreation purposes. It suspends the patient on a buoyant surface and distributes the pressure on the underlying tissue. However, if the mattress becomes underinflated, its effectiveness as a pressure-relieving

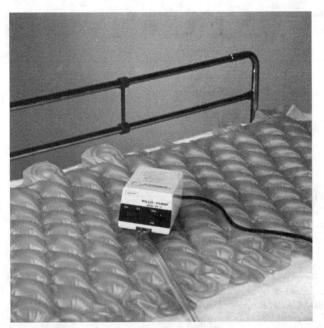

FIGURE 23-18
Alternating air mattress. (© 1994 Total Care, Gaithersburg, MD.)

device is lost. Air mattresses permit less evaporation of moisture than foam because of the nonabsorbent quality of plastic. Also, sharp objects can damage the integrity of the mattress.

ALTERNATING AIR MATTRESS

An alternating air mattress (Fig. 23-18) is similar to one that is static, with one exception: every other channel inflates as the next one deflates. The process is then reversed. Through the wave-like redistribution of air, pressure over bony prominences is cyclically changed. This repetitive process promotes blood flow and keeps the tissue supplied with oxygen.

It is important that the tubing connecting the mattress to its motor-driven compressor does not become kinked. Some patients also are disturbed by the noise.

WATER MATTRESS

A water mattress not only supports the body weight but equalizes the pressure per square inch over the body surface. This effect is maintained regardless of any shift in a patient's body position. Many claim that sleeping in a water bed produces a feeling of tranquility, which may provide beneficial emotional effects.

Water mattresses weigh a great deal; therefore, the structure of the floor and the frame of the bed must ensure that the weight can be supported. Puncturing leads to damage. Filling and emptying, although done infrequently, are nevertheless time consuming.

Cradle

A cradle is a frame that is made of metal and constructed so that it can be secured to the mattress or, in some instances, placed on top of the mattress. It forms a shell over the patient's lower legs and may be used to keep bed linen off the patient's feet or legs. A cradle is often used for patients with burns, painful joint disease, and fractures of the leg.

SPECIALTY BEDS

Specialty beds like low–air-loss beds, air-fluidized beds, oscillating support beds, and circular beds provide modified mattresses and frames with more functions than a standard hospital bed. They are used to relieve pressure as well as prevent other problems associated with inactivity and immobility (Table 23-2).

Low–Air-Loss Bed

A low–air-loss bed (Fig. 23-19) is one that contains inflated air sacs within its mattress. It maintains capillary pressure well below that which can interfere with blood flow. Regardless of changes in body position, the mattress selectively responds by redistributing the air to maintain low pressure to all skin areas.

Air-Fluidized Bed

An air-fluidized bed (Fig. 23-20) contains a collection of tiny beads within a mattress cover. The beads are blown upward on warm air. When suspended, the dry beads take on the characteristics of fluid, allowing the patient to float on the lifted beads. Excretions and secretions drain away from the body and through the beads, thereby preventing skin irritation and maceration from moisture. The pressure-relieving effects of this type of bed have been shown to speed the healing of severely impaired tissue.

An air-fluidized bed is better allocated for a patient who is likely to remain in bed for long periods of time. Fluid balance may become a patient care problem because of accelerated evaporation caused by the warm, blowing air. Puncturing or tearing the mattress is also a potential problem affecting function.

Oscillating Support Bed

An oscillating bed (Fig. 23-21) slowly and continuously rocks the patient from side to side in a 124° arc.

Oscillation relieves skin pressure and helps to mobilize respiratory secretions. Foam-covered supports applied to the head, arms, and legs prevent sliding and **shearing** of skin. **Shearing** is the force exerted against the surface and layers of the skin as tissues slide in opposite but parallel directions. Compartments within

TABLE 23-2. *Pressure-Relieving Devices*

Device	Examples	Indications for Use
Foam mattress or gel cushion	Egg crate Geo-Matt Spencegel pad	Intact skin and minimal risk for breakdown Changes in position occur spontaneously or require minimal assistance
Static air, alternating air, or water mattress	TENDER Cloud Sof-Care Pulsair Lotus	At some risk for skin breakdown OR The skin has a superficial or single deep break but pressure is easily relieved
Oscillating support bed	Roto Rest Tilt and Turn Paragon 9000	Need for prolonged bed rest with immobilization At high risk for systemic effects of immobility, such as pneumonia and skin breakdown
Low–air-loss bed	KinAir FLEXICAIR Mediscus	Combination of the following: Impaired skin Risk factors for further skin breakdown continue to exist Alternative positions are limited, less than adequate, or impossible Requires assistance for frequent transfers from bed
Air-fluidized bed	CLINITRON FluidAir	Combination of the following: Impaired skin Risk factors for further skin breakdown continue to exist Alternative positions are limited, less than adequate, or impossible Seldom transferred from bed
Circular bed	CircOlectric	Current or high risk for skin breakdown because of multiple trauma, especially if it involves the head, neck, or spine Burns that require frequent dressing changes or topical applications

the bed can be removed temporarily to facilitate assessment and care of the posterior body.

Circular Bed

A circular bed supports the patient on a 6- or 7-foot anterior or posterior platform suspended across the

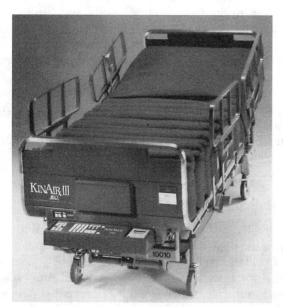

FIGURE 23-19
Low–air-loss bed. (Courtesy of Kinetic Concepts, Inc., San Antonio, TX.)

diameter of the frame (Fig. 23-22). This type of bed allows the patient to remain passively immobilized during a position change. The bed has the capacity to rotate the patient, who is sandwiched between the anterior and posterior frames, in a 180° arc. Turning facilitates access to the patient for nursing care. Instructed patients can learn how to operate the bed to make minor adjustments in their own position. This promotes a sense of control among otherwise dependent patients.

DANGERS OF INACTIVITY

Some patients are so inactive that their health deteriorates. Multiple complications can and do occur among people whose activity and movement are limited. These complications are collectively referred to as **disuse syndrome**.

The word **syndrome** means a set of signs and symptoms that occur together. The **disuse syndrome** refers to the collective signs and symptoms that develop as a result of inactivity. These signs and symptoms occur in many systems of the body, not just in the musculoskeletal system (Table 23-3). The dangers of inactivity illustrate the importance of a nursing care plan that includes turning and moving the patient. See Display 23-1 for a list of positioning principles.

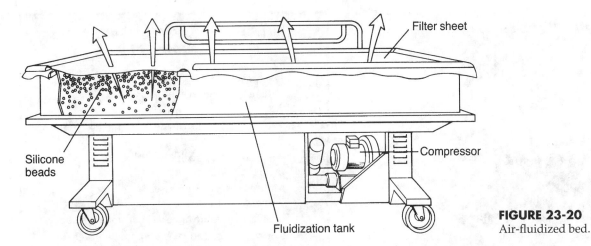

FIGURE 23-20
Air-fluidized bed.

TURNING AND MOVING PATIENTS

Turning and moving skills are important to prevent injury to the nurse and the patient, whose weight may equal or exceed that of the nurse. Skill 23-1 describes and illustrates the suggested actions when patients require repositioning and moving.

TRANSFERRING PATIENTS

The word **transfer** refers to moving a patient from place to place. For example, a patient is transferred when moved from a bed to a chair and back to bed, or to and from a stretcher. The patient assists in an *active* transfer. A transfer done entirely by others or by mechanical means is a *passive* transfer.

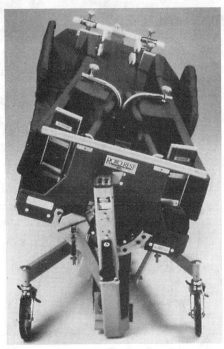

FIGURE 23-21
Oscillating bed. (Courtesy of Kinetic Concepts, Inc., San Antonio, TX.)

NURSING GUIDELINES FOR TRANSFERRING PATIENTS

- Be realistic about how much you can safely lift.
  Rationale: Demonstrates good judgment
- Always practice good body mechanics.
  Rationale: Reduces the potential for injury
- Put on braces and other supportive devices before getting a patient out of bed.
  Rationale: Provides maximum organization of time and work
- Dress the patient appropriately with shoes or non-skid slippers.
  Rationale: Provides support and prevents foot injuries
- Plan to transfer patients across the shortest distance.
  Rationale: Reduces the potential for injury
- Make sure that the patient's stronger leg, if there is one, is nearest the chair to which the patient is transferring.
  Rationale: Ensures safety
- Stand on the side of the bed to which the patient will be moving.
  Rationale: Facilitates assisting the patient
- Explain what will be done to the patient, step by step.
  Rationale: Informs the patient
- Solicit the patient's help as much as possible.
  Rationale: Encourages self-help and reduces the workload

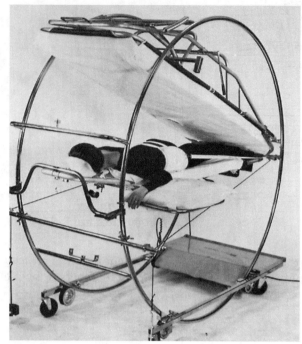

FIGURE 23-22
Circular bed.

If a patient cannot stand, it is best to have two people lift the patient from the bed into a chair (Fig. 23-23). Or, as an alternative, a mechanical lift is used (Fig. 23-24). When used correctly, a mechanical lift is safe and helps prevent injuries among personnel. For a single-person transfer and others that are more frequently re-

DISPLAY 23-1. *Positioning Principles*
• Positions are changed at least every 2 hours if patients are inactive.
• Adequate help is enlisted.
• The bed is raised to an appropriate height for the nurse.
• All pillows and positioning devices are removed before repositioning.
• Mattress overlays are used to relieve pressure points on bony prominences.
• Drainage tubes are unfastened from the bed linen.
• The patient is turned as a complete unit to avoid twisting the spine.
• The body is placed in good alignment.
• The joints are slightly flexed.
• Pillows and positioning devices are replaced after repositioning.
• Limbs are supported in a functional position.
• Elevation is used to relieve swelling or provide comfort.
• Proper alignment promotes good circulation to the extremities.
• Skin care is given after repositioning to maintain integrity.

quired in health care institutions, refer to the suggested actions in Skill 23-2.

NURSING IMPLICATIONS

Many nursing diagnoses, actual or potential, may apply to the care of inactive patients (see Applicable Nursing Diagnoses).

(text continues on page 488)

TABLE 23-3. *Dangers of Inactivity*	
Systems	**Effects**
Muscular	Weakness
	Decreased tone/strength
	Decreased size (atrophy)
Skeletal	Poor posture
	Contractures
	Foot drop
Cardiovascular	Impaired circulation
	Thrombus (clot) formation
	Dependent edema
Respiratory	Pooling of secretions
	Shallow respirations
	Atelectasis (collapsed alveoli)
Urinary	Oliguria (scanty urine)
	Urinary tract infections
	Calculi (stone) formation
	Incontinence (inability to control elimination)
Gastrointestinal	Anorexia (loss of appetite)
	Constipation
	Fecal impaction
Integumentary	Pressure sores
Endocrine	Decreased metabolic rate
	Decreased hormonal secretions
Central nervous	Sleep pattern disturbances
	Psychosocial changes

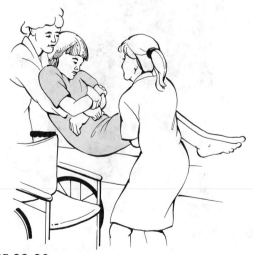

FIGURE 23-23
Passive transfer to a wheelchair.

SKILL 23-1
Turning and Moving a Patient

Suggested Action	Reason for Action
Assessment	
Assess for risk factors that may contribute to inactivity.	Indicates a need to reposition more frequently
Determine the time of the last position change.	Ensures following the plan for care
Assess physical ability to assist in turning, positioning, or moving.	Determines if additional help may be needed
Inspect for the presence of drainage tubes and equipment.	Ensures that they will not be displaced or cause discomfort to the patient
Planning	
Explain the procedure to the patient.	Increases cooperation and decreases anxiety
Remove all pillows and current positioning devices.	Reduces interference during repositioning
Raise the bed to a comfortable working height.	Prevents back strain by maintaining the center of gravity
Secure extra help if needed.	Ensures safety
Close the door or draw the bedside curtain.	Demonstrates respect for privacy
Implementation	
Turning the Patient From Supine to Lateral or Prone Position	
Wash hands.	Reduces the transmission of microorganisms
Lower the side rail and move the patient to one side of the bed	Provides room when turning
Raise the side rail.	Ensures safety
Move to the other side of the bed and lower the side rail on that side.	Facilitates assistance
Flex the patient's far knee over the near one with the arms across the chest.	Aids in turning and protects the patient's arms

![Positioning arms and legs.]

Positioning arms and legs.

(continued)

SKILL 23-1
Turning and Moving a Patient

Suggested Action	Reason for Action
Spread your feet, flex your knees, and place one foot behind the other.	Provides a broad base of support
Place one hand on the patient's shoulder and one on the hip on the far side.	Facilitates turning

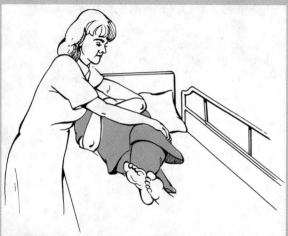

Turning the patient.

Roll the patient toward you.	Reduces effort
Replace pillows behind the back and between the legs and under the upper arm.	Aids in maintaining position and provides comfort
Raise the side rails and lower the height of the bed.	Ensures safety

For a Prone Position

Begin as described earlier for the lateral position.	Follows same principles
Have the patient turn his or her head opposite to the direction for rolling and leave the arms extended at each side.	Prevents pressure on the face and arms during and after repositioning

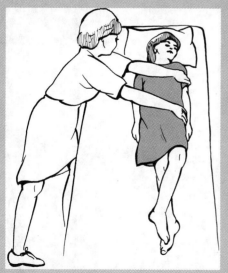

Preparing for prone positioning.

(continued)

SKILL 23-1
Turning and Moving a Patient

Suggested Action	Reason for Action
Shift your hands from the posterior of the shoulder and hip to the anterior as the patient rolls onto his or her abdomen.	Controls the speed with which the patient is repositioned

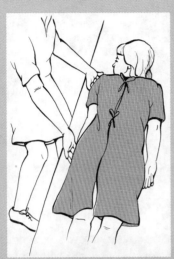

Bracing the patient during turning.

Suggested Action	Reason for Action
Center the patient in bed.	Prevents pressure on arms
Arrange pillows.	Provides for comfort and support
Raise the side rails and lower the height of the bed.	Ensures safety

Moving the Mobile Patient up in Bed (One-Nurse Technique)

Suggested Action	Reason for Action
Remove pillow from under the patient's head.	Prevents strain on the neck and head during moving
Place the pillow against the headboard.	Cushions the head from contact with the headboard
Instruct the patient to bend both knees while keeping the feet flat on the bed.	Aids in assisting by using the stronger muscles of the legs

(continued)

SKILL 23-1
Turning and Moving a Patient (Continued)

Suggested Action	Reason for Action
Place your arm under the patient's shoulders and the other under the hips.	Facilitates moving the heaviest section of the body

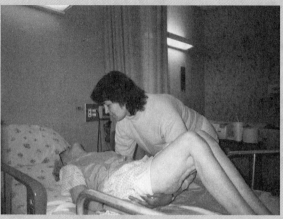

Supporting the upper and mid-sections of the body. (Courtesy of Ken Timby.)

Bend your hips and knees, spread your feet.	Provides a wide base of support and makes use of stronger muscles in the legs rather than the back
Rock toward the head of the bed while the patient pushes with his or her feet.	Creates momentum to facilitate moving

Alternate Technique

Stand facing the head of the bed.	Facilitates moving upward
Lock arms with the patient.	Uses combined strength of patient and nurse

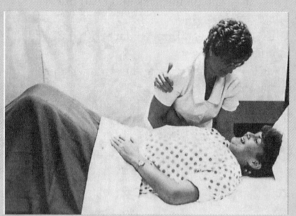

Locking arms. (Courtesy of Ken Timby.)

Bend from the hips and knees; spread your feet.	Follows principles of good body mechanics
Instruct the patient to push with his or her legs while pulling locked arms.	Coordinates momentum and effort to move upward

(continued)

SKILL 23-1
Turning and Moving a Patient *(Continued)*

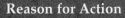

Suggested Action	Reason for Action
Two-Nurse Technique	
Protect the headboard with a pillow.	Ensures patient safety
Stand facing each other on opposite sides of the bed between the patient's hips and shoulders.	Distributes weight equally between nurses
Lock hands beneath the patient's buttocks and shoulders.	Doubles the muscular strength

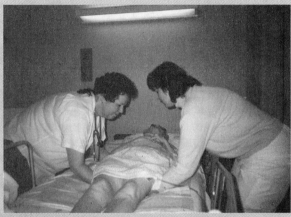

Locking hands. (Courtesy of Ken Timby.)

Bend hips and knees; spread feet; and rock toward the head of the bed.	Follows principles of good body mechanics
Move the patient up on reaching a previously agreed signal, such as the count of three.	Promotes coordination of effort
Using a Drawsheet	
Stand opposite one another on each side of the bed.	Facilitates distributing the patient's weight equally between nurses
Roll the drawsheet close to the patient.	Acts as a sling to slide the patient upward

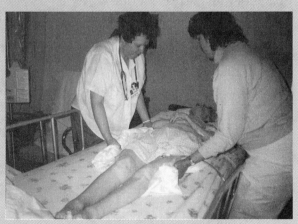

Rolling the drawsheet. (Courtesy of Ken Timby.)

Bend hips and knees; spread feet.	Follows principles of good body mechanics

(continued)

SKILL 23-1
Turning and Moving a Patient (Continued)

Suggested Action	Reason for Action
Rock back and forth in unison; move the patient up in bed on reaching an agreed signal.	Coordinates efforts

Evaluation
- Movement is achieved
- Patient is comfortable
- Pressure is relieved
- Joints and limbs are supported

Document
Frequency of turning and moving

- Positions used
- Use of positioning devices
- Assistance required
- Patient's response

Sample Documentation

Date and Time   Position changed q 2 h from supine to R and L lateral positions with assistance of patient. Pillows used to support limbs and maintain positions. Foot board in place. No shortness of breath noted. No evidence of discomfort during repositioning.
_____ **Signature, Title**

SKILL 23-2
Transferring Patients

Suggested Action	Reason for Action
Assessment	
Check the Kardex, nursing care plan, and medical orders for activity level.	Complies with the plan for care
Assess strength and mobility of the patient.	Determines the need for additional personnel or a mechanical lifting device.
Planning	
Consult with the patient on the preferred time for getting out of bed.	Helps patient participate in decision-making
Locate a straight-backed chair, wheelchair, or stretcher to which the patient will be transferred.	Facilitates efficient time management
Arrange the chair or stretcher next to or close to the bed on the patient's stronger side, if there is one.	Ensures safety
Lock the wheels of the bed, wheelchair, or stretcher.	Prevents rolling
Explain how the transfer will be accomplished.	Reduces anxiety and promotes cooperation

(continued)

SKILL 23-2
Transferring Patients (Continued)

Suggested Action	Reason for Action
Implementation	
From Bed to Chair	
Assist the patient to a sitting position on the side of the bed.	Reduces dizziness; enables the patient to stand
Help the patient to don a bathrobe and nonskid slippers.	Ensures warmth, modesty, and safety
Place the chair parallel to the bed on the patient's stronger side; raise the foot rests if a wheelchair is used.	Provides easy access
Apply a transfer belt or other assistive device, if needed.	Reduces the risk for falling

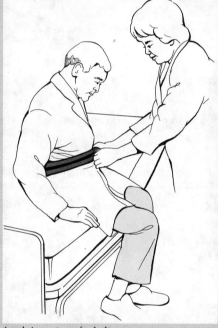

Applying a transfer belt.

Grasp the transfer belt or reach under the patient's arms.	Helps support the upper body
Instruct the patient to grasp your shoulders.	Gives the patient leverage for rising

(continued)

SKILL 23-2
Transferring Patients (Continued)

Suggested Action	Reason for Action
Bend the hips and knees; brace the patient's knees.	Stabilizes the patient and follows principles of good body mechanics

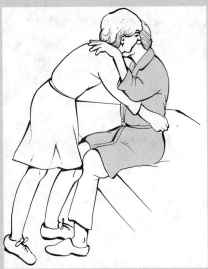

Bracing the patient's knees.

Suggested Action	Reason for Action
Rock the patient to a standing position at an agreed signal while encouraging the patient to straighten his or her knees and hips.	Provides momentum and reduces the need to lift the patient
Pivot the patient with his or her back toward the chair.	Positions the patient for sitting
Tell the patient to step back until he or she feels the chair at the back of the legs.	Places the patient in close proximity with the chair
Instruct the patient to grasp the arms of the chair while you stabilize his or her knees and lower the patient into the chair.	Promotes safety

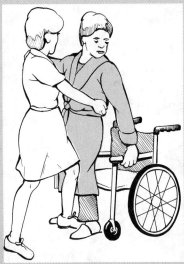

Backing into wheelchair.

(continued)

SKILL 23-2
Transferring Patients (Continued)

Suggested Action	Reason for Action
Support the feet on the footrests.	Facilitates good posture
Using a Transfer Board	
Remove an arm from the wheelchair.	Reduces interference with transfer
Slide the patient to the edge of the bed.	Maintains shortest distance for transfer
Angle the transfer board from the patient's buttocks and hips down toward the seat of the chair.	Places the board where there is maximum weight

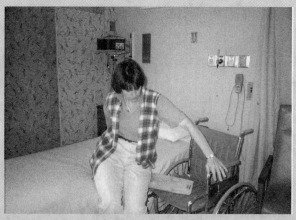

Using a transfer board. (Courtesy of Ken Timby.)

Raise the bed to a sitting position and grasp the patient under the axillae.	Supports upper body
Have an assistant support the lower legs at the knees.	Prevents injury
Slide the patient down the transfer board into the seat of the chair at an agreed on signal.	Reduces the need to lift patient
From Bed to a Stretcher Using a Sheet	
Place the patient in a supine position.	Maintains alignment
Loosen the bottom sheet or place a folded sheet beneath the patient's hips. Roll the sheet close to the patient's body.	Aids in sliding the patient without causing friction
Raise the bed to the same height as the stretcher.	Facilitates movement
Lower the side rail, position the stretcher parallel with the bed, and lock the wheels.	Maintains the shortest distance for transfer
Place the patient's arms over his or her chest.	Prevents injury
Have an assistant stand by the stretcher and grasp one side of the rolled sheet.	Facilitates pulling the patient
Climb onto the mattress next to the patient's buttocks and hips.	Enables use of stronger muscles in arms and thighs

(continued)

SKILL 23-2
Transferring Patients *(Continued)*

Suggested Action	Reason for Action
Have the assistant pull the sheet while lifting together at a prearranged signal.	Facilitates coordination and reduces workload

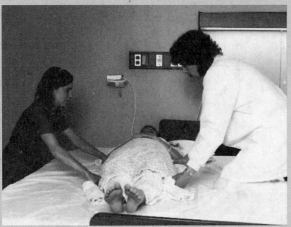

Using a lift sheet. (Craven RF, Hirnle CJ: Fundamentals of Nursing: Human Health and Function, p 736. Philadelphia, JB Lippincott, 1992)

Suggested Action	Reason for Action
From Bed to Stretcher Using a Three-Carrier Lift	
Place the stretcher at a right angle to the foot of the bed with the brakes locked.	Gives carriers room to pivot
Arrange three carriers according to height, with the tallest person at the patient's head and chest.	Uses the person with the longest arms for grasping the widest part of the patient
Bend hips and knees; spread feet.	Follows principles of good body mechanics
Slide arms beneath the patient so that one carrier supports the neck and chest, another the buttocks and hips, and the remaining carrier the thighs and lower legs.	Distributes burden of lifting among three carriers

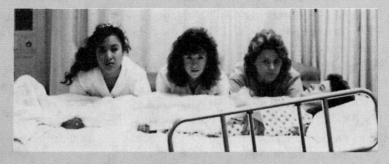

Positioning carriers and patient. (Courtesy of Ken Timby.)

(continued)

SKILL 23-2
Transferring Patients *(Continued)*

Suggested Action	Reason for Action
Logroll the patient toward the carriers' chests.	Facilitates placing the patient's mass over the carriers' center of gravity
Stand on a prearranged signal, thus lifting the patient in unison from the bed.	Uses stronger muscles of arms and legs and protects the back from injury

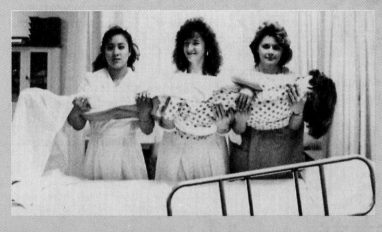

Lifting the patient. (Courtesy of Ken Timby.)

Suggested Action	Reason for Action
Pivot and move toward the stretcher; lower the patient to the stretcher in unison while bending the hips and knees.	Follows principles of good body mechanics
Secure safety belt and raise side rails on stretcher.	Prevents injury

Evaluation
- Patient is relocated
- No injury to patient or personnel

Document
- Method of transfer
- Response of patient

Sample Documentation

Date and Time Transferred from bed to wheelchair by standing and pivoting with weight bearing on right leg. Transient pain experienced in left hip during transfer. Refused pain medication. Up in chair approximately 1 hr. _____ **Signature, Title**

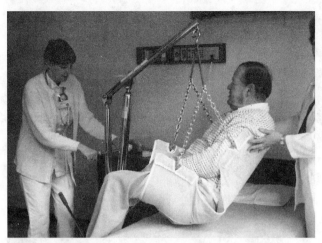

FIGURE 23-24
Using a mechanical lift. (Craven RF, Hirnle CJ: Fundamentals of Nursing: Human Health and Function, p 740. Philadelphia, JB Lippincott, 1992)

 FOCUS ON OLDER ADULTS

- The disuse syndrome is a serious threat to the older adult and aggressive efforts are made to prevent it.
- Muscle strength declines gradually by the seventh or eighth decade.
- Expect that older adults may require extra time during positioning and transferring.
- Older adults with short-term memory loss may be unable to follow directions regarding positioning and transferring.
- Some older adults have an increased susceptibility to fractures and fear of falling.
- Health care expenses for older adults reflect the economic impact of falls, fractures, and degenerative bone disease.

 PATIENT TEACHING FOR MOBILITY

Teach the patient or the family to do the following:
- Balance periods of activity with periods of rest.
- Become aware of the dangers of inactivity.
- Allow adequate time for performing activities.
- Join a senior citizens club for social activities.
- Develop hobbies or recreational interests.
- Volunteer services at hospitals, church, or city government.
- Investigate local support groups (eg, coffee clubs, needlework, football friends, or playing bingo and cards).
- Prevent injury by removing any objects that might pose a safety hazard (eg, throw rugs, electrical cords, chair legs, and water on the floor).
- Rent or purchase hospital equipment from a medical supply company.
- Investigate the loan of equipment for home-bound terminal patients from national companies (eg, American Cancer Society, American Heart Association, American Lung Association, and others).
- Investigate services in the community that aid in fostering independent living (eg, home-maker services, home-delivered meal services, social services, and religious organizations).

The accompanying Nursing Care Plan illustrates how the steps in the nursing process are applied when caring for a patient with the nursing diagnosis of Risk for Disuse Syndrome. The NANDA taxonomy (1994) describes this diagnostic category as "The state in which an individual is at risk for deterioration of body systems as the result of prescribed or unavoidable musculoskeletal inactivity."

 APPLICABLE NURSING DIAGNOSES

- Activity Intolerance
- Altered Tissue Perfusion
- Bathing/Hygiene Self-Care Deficit
- Body Image Disturbance
- Risk for Impaired Skin Integrity
- Risk for Infection
- Risk for Injury
- Impaired Physical Mobility
- Impaired Tissue Integrity
- Powerlessness
- Risk for Disuse Syndrome

NURSING CARE PLAN:
Risk for Disuse Syndrome

Assessment

Subjective Data
States, "Please don't move me; just let me alone."

Objective Data
82-year-old woman recuperating from the surgical repair of a fractured left femur. Weight approximately 95 pounds; occasional incontinence of bladder and bowel; skin translucent and dry; incision line clean and dry with good approximation; skin staples removed yesterday; reddened area on right hip approximately 2.5 × 3 cm; unable to turn self; non-weight bearing; regular mattress; overhead trapeze in place.

Diagnosis

Risk for Disuse Syndrome

Plan

Goal
The patient will demonstrate
- Intact skin/tissue integrity
- Full range of joint motion
- Negative Homans' sign
- Bowel, bladder, and renal functioning within normal limits by 1/22.

Orders: 1/20
1. Reposition q 2 h around the clock.
2. Provide clean, dry, and wrinkle-free bedding at all times
3. Use incontinence pads on bed continuously.
4. Assist to bedside commode q 4 h when awake.
5. Use foam mattress on bed.
6. Use trochanter rolls for supine positioning.
7. Use foot board.
8. Encourage active exercise with use of trapeze t.i.d.
9. Vary daily routine when possible.
10. Include the patient in planning the daily routine.
11. Teach family how to turn and position the patient. _____ J. SCALES, RN

Implementation 1/21 0745
(Documentation)

Right side-lying; incontinent of dark, foul-smelling urine. Reddened area approximately 2.5 × 3 cm over right trochanter. Skin cleansed; lotion applied to right hip. Incision line on left hip dry and pink. Repositioned to back; trochanter rolls in place. Served breakfast: consumed 50% of diet.
_____ J. SCALES, RN

Evaluation 1/21 1400
(Documentation)

Able to move about in bed with assistance of trapeze. Area on right trochanter 2 × 2.5 cm; skin translucent and dry. Incision line on left hip dry and pink. States appetite "getting better." Urine continues concentrated; cranberry juice encouraged._____ J. SCALES, RN

KEY CONCEPTS

- Characteristics of good posture include: (1) standing—keep the feet parallel; distribute weight equally on both feet to provide a broad base of support; (2) sitting—the buttocks and upper thighs are the base of support on the chair; both feet rest on the floor; and (3) lying—looks same as standing but in horizontal; body parts in neutral position.

- Three principles of correct body mechanics include: distribute gravity through the center of the body over a wide base of support; push, pull or roll objects rather than lift; and hold objects close to the body.

- Ten signs or symptoms associated with disuse syndrome include: weakness, atony, poor alignment, contractures, foot drop, impaired circulation, atelectasis, urinary tract infections, anorexia, and pressure sores.
- Five positioning devices and their purposes include: (1) adjustable bed—allows the position of the head and knees to be changed; (2) pillows—provide support and elevate a body part; (3) trochanter rolls—prevent legs from turning outward; (4) hand rolls—maintain functional use of the hand and prevent contractures; and (5) foot boards—keep the feet in normal walking position.
- Three pressure-relieving devices and one advantage of each include: (1) side rails—aid patients in changing their own positions; (2) mattress overlays—reduce pressure and restore skin integrity; and (3) cradle—keeps linen off patient's feet or legs.
- Five guidelines that apply to transferring patients include: (1) know the patient's diagnosis, capabilities, weaknesses, and activity level; (2) be realistic about how much you can safely lift; (3) transfer patients across the shortest distance possible; (4) solicit the patient's help; and (5) use smooth rather than jerky movements when transferring the patient.
- Six common patient positions include: (1) supine—person lies on the back; (2) lateral—person lies on the side; (3) lateral oblique—person lies on the side with slight hip and knee flexion; (4) prone—person lies on the abdomen; (5) Sims'—person lies semiprone on left side with the right knee drawn up to chest; and (6) Fowler's—person lies in semisitting position.
- Five measures to prevent inactivity in the older adult include: (1) balance periods of activity with periods of rest, (2) allow adequate time for performing activities, (3) develop hobbies or recreational interests, (4) investigate local support groups, and (5) prevent injury by removing any objects that pose a safety hazard.

CRITICAL THINKING EXERCISES

- You observe one of your coworkers using incorrect body mechanics while giving patient care. How would you approach this coworker? What suggestions would you give?
- The patient for whom you are caring is unable to assist with movement. How will you plan your care for this patient?

SUGGESTED READINGS

Basta S. Lateral positioning: new protocol. Nursing July 1991;21:69.

Booth B. Soft options . . . the range of products available to relieve pressure. Nursing Times August 1993;89:60, 62.

Brannon M. A hands-on rehab technique that really works. RN November 1989;52:65–66, 68.

Carnevali DL, Patrick M. Nursing Management for the Elderly. 3rd ed. Philadelphia: JB Lippincott, 1993.

Clark M, Cullum N. Matching patient need for pressure sore prevention with the supply of pressure redistributing mattresses. Journal of Advanced Nursing March 1992;17:310–316.

Conine TA, Choi AK, Lim R. The user-friendliness of protective support surfaces in prevention of pressure sores. Rehabilitation Nursing May 1989;14:261–263.

Eustace C. Back up and wait. RN June 1991;54(6):49–51.

Eustace C. Body mechanics: your aching back. Nursing June 1991; 21:71.

Fletcher J. Mattresses on trial. Nursing Times October 1993;89:70, 72.

Fink S. The mechanics of motion: mastering the physiology of footwork is a matter of keeping your whole body in line. Health September 1989;21:56.

Hempel S. Home truths . . . houses are far from safe when it comes to handling patients. Nursing Times April 14–20 1993;89:40–41.

Kane ME, et al. Knowledge and use of lifting techniques among a group of undergraduate student nurses. Journal of Clinical Nursing January 1994;3:35–42.

Love C. Rolling or lifting following hip replacement? Professional Nurse July 1994;9:456, 458, 460–462.

Matteson MA, Mc Connell ES. Gerontological Nursing: Concepts and Practice. Philadelphia: WB Saunders, 1988.

Miller CA. Nursing Care of Older Adults. Glenview, IL: Scott, Foresman and Company, 1990.

Munro BH, Brown L, Heitman BB. Pressure ulcers: one bed for another? Geriatric Nursing April 1989;10:190–192.

Owen BD, et al. Reducing risk for back pain in nursing personnel. American Association of Occupational Health Nursing Journal January 1991;39:24–33.

Owen BD, et al. Back stress isn't part of the job. American Journal of Nursing February 1993;93:48–51.

Rithalia S. Reducing the pressure. Nursing Times October 1993;89: 67–68.

Scopa M. Comparison of classroom instruction and independent study in body mechanics. Journal of Continuing Education for Nurses July–August 1993;24:170–173.

Tartling C. The right equipment. Nursing Times December 9–15 1992;88:38–40.

Walsh R. Human kinetics: good movement habits. Nursing Times 1988; 84:59–61.

Willey T. High-tech beds and mattress overlays: a decision guide. American Journal of Nursing September 1989;89:1142–1145.

Wilson RW, Patterson MA, Alford DM. Services for maintaining independence. Journal of Gerontological Nursing June 1989;15: 31–37, 43–44.

CHAPTER 24

Therapeutic Exercise

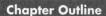

NURSING GUIDELINES

Performing Range-of-Motion Exercises

SKILLS

Performing Range-of-Motion (ROM) Exercises
Using a Continuous Passive Motion (CPM) Machine

NURSING CARE PLAN

Unilateral Neglect

Key Terms

Abduction	Inversion
Active Exercise	Isometric Exercise
Adduction	Isotonic Exercise
Aerobic Exercise	Metabolic Energy
Body Composition	Equivalent
Circumduction	Passive Exercise
Dorsiflexion	Plantar Flexion
Eversion	Pronation
Exercise	Range-of-motion Exercise

Extension	Recovery Index
External Rotation	Rotation
Fitness	Step Test
Fitness Exercise	Stress Electrocardiogram
Flexion	Supination
Goniometer	Therapeutic Exercise
Hyperextension	Walk-a-mile Test
Internal Rotation	

Learning Objectives

An understanding of the content within this chapter will be evidenced by the student's ability to:

- Give at least five benefits of regular exercise
- Define fitness and list seven factors that interfere with it
- Name three methods for assessing fitness
- Differentiate fitness exercises from therapeutic exercises.
- Explain the term "metabolic energy equivalent"
- Describe the difference between isotonic and isometric exercise, and give at least one example of each
- Explain how to calculate one's maximum heart rate and target heart rate
- Describe the difference between active and passive exercise
- Discuss how range-of-motion exercises are performed
- Give two reasons for performing range-of-motion exercises
- Provide at least two suggestions for helping older adults become more physically active

Exercise is a form of physical activity that provides benefits to all age groups. It has both preventive advantages as well as restorative potential (Display 24-1). Because the health risks among sedentary adults are well documented, this chapter addresses techniques for improving health and maintaining or restoring muscle and joint functions by promoting forms of exercise. Exercise, however, must always be individualized. Therefore, it is important to assess the fitness of each patient on a person-by-person basis.

ASSESSING FITNESS

Fitness refers to a person's capacity to perform physical activities. There are various factors that tend to interfere with fitness, such as chronic inactivity, concurrent health problems, impaired musculoskeletal function, obesity, advancing age, smoking, and high blood pressure.

Before someone with one or more of these health risks makes a rash decision to begin a regimen of strenuous exercise, it is wise to evaluate his or her fitness level. Some assessment techniques include measuring body composition, evaluating trends in vital signs, and conducting fitness tests.

Body Composition

Body composition refers to the amount of body tissue that is lean versus that which is fat (see section on Anthropometric Data, Chap. 14). Inactivity without adjustments in caloric intake tends to promote obesity. Therefore, one can conclude that overweight or obese people are less fit than their leaner counterparts and

may need to proceed gradually when initiating any exercise program.

Vital Signs

Vital signs, which include pulse rate, respiratory rate, and blood pressure, provide a window to a person's physical status (see Chap. 11). Elevated vital signs during rest are an ominous indication that the person may experience life-threatening cardiovascular symptoms during periods of exercise. After a period of modified exercise, however, it is possible that the vital signs will be lowered, thus reducing the potential for heart-related complications.

Fitness Tests

There are specific tests that may more objectively determine a person's potential to exercise safely. One is to undergo a stress electrocardiogram; two others that are less sophisticated self-tests include the step test and walk-a-mile test.

STRESS ELECTROCARDIOGRAM

A **stress electrocardiogram** is a test in which the electrical conduction through the heart is monitored during activity (Fig. 24-1). Vital signs and any symp-

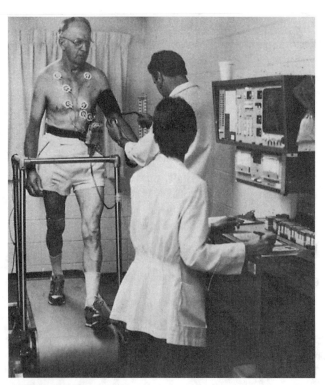

FIGURE 24-1
A stress electrocardiogram in progress. (Courtesy of Borgess Hospital, Kalamazoo, MI.)

DISPLAY 24-1. *Benefits of Physical Exercise*

- Improved cardiopulmonary function
- Reduction of blood pressure
- Increased muscle tone and strength
- Greater physical endurance
- Increased lean mass and weight loss
- Reduction of elevated blood sugar
- Decreased low-density blood lipids
- Improved physical appearance
- Increased bone density
- Regularity of bowel elimination
- Promotion of sleep
- Reduction in tension and depression

TABLE 24-1. *Step Test Recovery Index*

Cumulative Pulse Rate for Men	Cumulative Pulse Rate for Women	Fitness Level
≤132	≤135	Excellent
150–133	155–136	Good
165–149	170–154	Average
180–164	190–171	Fair
>180	>190	Poor

From Getchell B. Physical Fitness, A Way of Life. 3rd ed. New York: Macmillan, 1983. Reprinted with permission of Macmillan Publishing Company.

toms like chest pain are also noted. If an abnormal rhythm develops or the blood pressure becomes dangerously elevated, the test is stopped. People with cardiac risks may still exercise, but the level and length of time may require careful planning.

STEP TEST

The **step test** is a physical exercise test in which a person alternates going up and down two steps for a period of 3 minutes. The pace should average approximately 26 to 27 steps per minute. The pulse is counted at 1-minute intervals. The **recovery index** (Table 24-1), which is the cumulative rate for the three pulse rate measurements, indicates the person's state of fitness.

Despite its simplicity, life-threatening risks are still possible with this test. Consequently, the step test is used with caution and where medical assistance is available. If the subject experiences any discomfort or fatigue, the test is stopped.

WALK-A-MILE TEST

The **walk-a-mile test**, devised by the American College of Sports Medicine, uses walking time over a prescribed distance of a mile as a measure of fitness. When this test is used, a person is instructed to walk a mile as fast, yet as comfortably, as possible. The time from start to finish is then calculated and interpreted using established guidelines (Table 24-2).

TYPES OF EXERCISE

Basically, exercise is performed to promote fitness or to achieve therapeutic outcomes (Fig. 24-2).

Fitness Exercise

Fitness exercise, which may be isotonic or isometric, refers to those physical activities that develop and maintain cardiorespiratory function, muscular strength, and endurance in *healthy* adults (American College of Sports Medicine, 1989). To promote cardiorespiratory conditioning, exercise should be performed 3 or more days a week for 20 or more minutes (U.S. Department of Health and Human Services, 1992). Furthermore, the exercise should be sufficiently strenuous to maintain the heart rate at 60% of a person's maximum heart rate. Maximum heart rate is calculated by subtracting one's age from 220.

ISOTONIC EXERCISE

Isotonic exercise is that which involves movement and work. One of the best examples is aerobic exercise. **Aerobic exercise** involves rhythmically moving all parts of the body at a moderate to slow speed without impeding the ability to breathe. In other words, a person should be able to talk comfortably with another if the exercise is within his or her level of fitness.

Because there are variations in fitness levels, isotonic exercise may be prescribed in metabolic energy equiv-

TABLE 24-2. *Evaluation Criteria for the Walk-a-Mile Test*

Performance Time for Men	Performance Time for Women	Fitness Level
≥17.5 minutes	≥16.5 minutes	Needs work
≤15 minutes	≤14 minutes	Average
≤11.75 minutes	≤10.25 minutes	Good

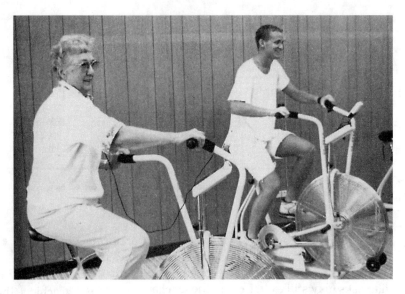

FIGURE 24-2
Stationary cycling. (Courtesy of Ken Timby.)

alents (METs) according to each person's activity tolerance. **Metabolic energy equivalent** is the measure of energy and oxygen consumption associated with particular activities. Some examples of low to vigorous physical activities and their approximate MET are listed in Table 24-3.

ISOMETRIC EXERCISE

Isometric exercise refers to stationary exercises that tend to be performed against a resistive force. Examples of isometric exercise include body building, weight lifting, and less intense activities like simply contracting and relaxing muscle groups while sitting or standing in place.

Isometric exercises tend to increase muscle mass, define muscle groups, and increase muscle strength and tone. Although isometric exercises do improve the circulation of blood, they do not promote cardiorespiratory function. In fact, strenuous isometric exercises tend to elevate the blood pressure while they are being performed.

Regardless of the form of exercise, certain information is provided to enhance safety.

Therapeutic Exercise

Therapeutic exercise is that which is performed to prevent health-related complications, or to restore lost functions (see sections on Performing Leg Exercises in

TABLE 24-3. *Levels of Physical Activity*

Metabolic Energy Equivalent (MET)	Examples of Activities
1 MET	Sewing Watching television Dressing
1–2 METs	Walking 1 mph on level ground Bowling
2–3 METs	Golfing with a cart Mowing lawn with a power mower
3–4 METs	Playing badminton (doubles) Raking leaves
4–5 METs	Slow swimming Lifting 50 lbs
5–6 METs	Square dancing Shoveling snow
6–7 METs	Water skiing Moving heavy furniture
7–8 METs	Playing basketball Playing noncompetitive handball
8–9 METs	Cross-country skiing Playing contact football
≥10 METs	Running 6 mph or faster

PATIENT TEACHING FOR A SAFE EXERCISE PROGRAM

Teach the patient or family to do the following:
- Seek a pre-exercise fitness evaluation.
- Identify activities within one's prescribed level of METs.
- Choose a form of exercise that seems pleasurable and involves as many muscle groups as possible.
- Plan 3 days of exercise per week at a convenient time of day.
- Exercise with a partner for safety and motivational purposes.
- Avoid exercising in extreme weather conditions such as when there is high humidity or when smog is evident.
- Dress in layers according to the temperature and weather conditions.
- Purchase supportive footwear.
- Wear reflective clothing when on the roadside.
- Walk or jog against traffic; cycle in the same direction as traffic.

- Eat complex carbohydrates (pasta, rice, cooked cereal) rather than fasting or eating simple sugars (cookies, chocolate, sweetened drinks).
- Avoid drinking alcohol, which dilates the blood vessels, promotes heat loss, and interferes with good judgment.
- Calculate the target heart rate (maximum heart rate × 60%).
- Warm up for 5 minutes by stretching muscle groups or doing light calisthenics.
- Monitor the heart rate two or three times while exercising.
- Slow the pace down if the heart rate exceeds the preestablished target.
- Try to sustain the target heart rate for at least 20 minutes.
- Never stop exercising abruptly.
- Cool down for at least 5 minutes in a manner similar to the warm-up

Chap. 27 and Strengthening Pelvic Floor Muscles in Chap. 30). Therapeutic exercise may be isotonic or isometric. Isotonic exercises may be actively or passively performed.

ACTIVE EXERCISE

Active exercise is that which is done independently. For example, after the removal of a breast, patients are taught to exercise the arm on the surgical side by combing their hair, squeezing a soft ball, climbing the wall with their fingers, and swinging a rope attached to a doorknob.

Active therapeutic exercise is often limited to one particular part of the body that is in a weakened condition. It can be assumed that patients thus affected will be using the remaining muscle groups during the performance of activities of daily living, such as bathing and dressing.

PASSIVE EXERCISE

Passive exercise is that which is performed with assistance. Passive exercise is used when patients are paralyzed after a stroke or spinal injury, or while in a comatose state. One form of passive therapeutic exercise that is frequently provided is range-of-motion exercises. Another is provided with a continuous passive motion machine.

Range-of-Motion Exercises

Range-of-motion (ROM) **exercises** are those in which joints are moved in the directions the normal joint permits (Table 24-4). In general, the patient actively exercises as many joints as possible while the nurse assists with those that are compromised in some way. ROM exercises are usually performed for the following reasons:

- To assess joint flexibility and evaluate the response to a therapeutic exercise program
- To maintain joint mobility and flexibility, especially among inactive patients.
- To prevent contracture deformities (restriction of joint flexibility)
- To stretch joints before performing more strenuous activities

NURSING GUIDELINES FOR PERFORMING RANGE-OF-MOTION EXERCISES

- Use good body mechanics (see Chap. 23).
  Rationale: Conserves energy and avoids muscle strain and injury
- Remove pillows and other positioning devices.
  Rationale: Prevents mechanical interference

- Position the patient so as to facilitate moving a joint through all its usual positions.
  Rationale: Facilitates a comprehensive system of exercise
- Follow a repetitive pattern, such as beginning from the head and moving downward.
  Rationale: Prevents overlooking a joint
- Perform similar movements with each extremity.
  Rationale: Exercises joints bilaterally
- Support the joint being exercised.
  Rationale: Reduces discomfort
- Move each joint until there is resistance, but not pain.
  Rationale: Exercises the joint to its point of limitation
- Watch for nonverbal communication.
  Rationale: Helps evaluate the patient's subjective response
- Avoid exercising a painful joint.
  Rationale: Contributes to injury
- Stop if spasticity develops, as manifested by sudden, continuous, muscle contraction.
  Rationale: Allows muscles time to relax and recover
- Apply gentle pressure to the muscle or move the joint more slowly.
  Rationale: Relieves spasticity
- Expect that the patient's respiratory and heart rates may increase during the exercises, but return to a resting rate later.
  Rationale: Demonstrates response to activity
- Teach the family to perform ROM with the patient.
  Rationale: Improves the potential for regaining function

TABLE 24-4. *Joint Positions*

Position	Description
Flexion	Bending so as to decrease the angle between two adjoining bones
Extension	Straightening so as to increase the angle between two adjoining bones up to 180°
Hyperextension	Increasing the angle between two adjoining bones more than 180°
Abduction	Moving away from the midline
Adduction	Moving toward the midline
Rotation	Turning from side to side as in an arc
External rotation	Turning outward, away from the midline of the body
Internal rotation	Turning inward, toward the midline of the body
Circumduction	Forming a circle
Pronation	Turning downward
Supination	Turning upward
Plantar flexion	Bending toward the sole of the foot
Dorsiflexion	Bending the foot toward the dorsum or anterior side
Inversion	Turning the sole of the foot toward the midline
Eversion	Turning the sole of the foot away from the midline

Manually assisted ROM is very therapeutic for most patients (Skill 24-1). However, a continuous passive motion machine may be more effective during the rehabilitation of burn patients and those who undergo knee or hip replacement surgery.

(text continues on page 508)

SKILL 24-1
Performing Range-of-Motion (ROM) Exercises

Suggested Action	Reason for Action
Assessment	
Review the medical record and nursing plan for care.	Determines if activity problems have been identified and the measures for treating those that exist
Assess the patient's level of activity and joint mobility.	Indicates whether, and the extent to which, joints should be passively exercised
Assess the patient's understanding of the hazards of inactivity and purposes for exercise.	Determines the type and amount of health teaching
Planning	
Explain the procedure for performing ROM.	Reduces anxiety and promotes cooperation

(continued)

SKILL 24-1
Performing Range-of-Motion (ROM) Exercises *(Continued)*

Suggested Action	Reason for Action
Consult with the patient on when ROM exercises may be best performed.	Shows respect for independent decision-making
Suggest performing ROM during a time that requires general activity, such as during bathing.	Demonstrates efficient time management
Perform ROM exercises at least twice a day.	Promotes recovery or maintains functional use
Exercise each joint at least two to five times during each exercise period.	Increases exercise benefits
Implementation Wash your hands.	Reduces the potential for transferring micro-organisms
Help the patient to a sitting or lying position.	Promotes relaxation and access to the body
Pull the privacy curtains.	Demonstrates respect for modesty
Drape the patient loosely or suggest loose-fitting underwear or shorts.	Avoids exposing the patient
Begin at the head.	Facilitates organization
Support the patient's neck and bring the chin toward the chest and then as far back in the opposite position as possible.	Flexes and hyperextends the neck

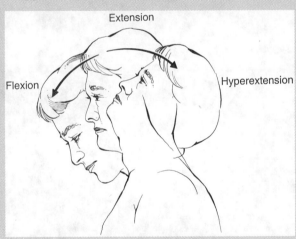

Neck flexion, extension, and hyperextension.

(continued)

SKILL 24-1
Performing Range-of-Motion (ROM) Exercises *(Continued)*

Suggested Action	Reason for Action
Place a hand on either side of the head and bend the neck from side to side.	Rotates the neck

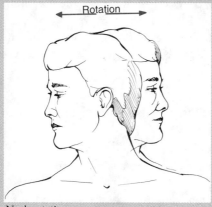

Neck rotation.

Turn the head in a circular fashion.	Puts the head and neck through circumduction

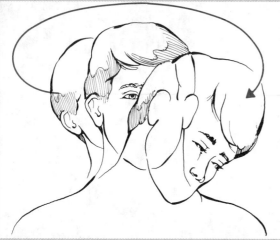

Circumduction of the neck.

(continued)

SKILL 24-1
Performing Range-of-Motion (ROM) Exercises *(Continued)*

Suggested Action	Reason for Action
Support the elbow and wrist while moving the straightened arm above the head and behind the body.	Flexes, extends, then hyperextends the shoulder

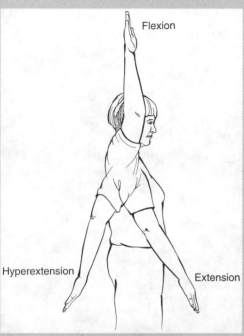

Flexion, extension, and hyperextension of the shoulder.

Suggested Action	Reason for Action
Move the straightened arm away from the body and then toward the midline.	Abducts and adducts the shoulder

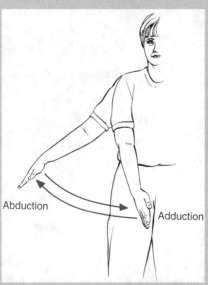

Abduction and adduction of the shoulder.

(continued)

SKILL 24-1
Performing Range-of-Motion (ROM) Exercises *(Continued)*

Suggested Action	Reason for Action
Bend the elbow and move the arm so that the palm is upward and then downward.	Produces internal and external rotation of the shoulder

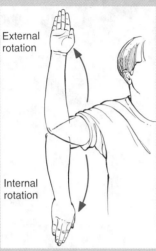

Internal and external rotation of the shoulder.

Move the arm in a full circle.	Circumducts the shoulder

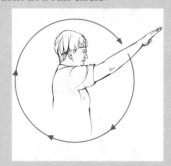

Circumduction of the shoulder.

Place the arm at the side of the patient and bend the forearm toward the shoulder, and then straighten it again.	Flexes and extends the elbow

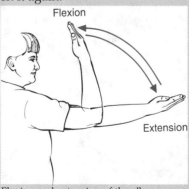

Flexion and extension of the elbow.

(continued)

SKILL 24-1
Performing Range-of-Motion (ROM) Exercises *(Continued)*

Suggested Action	Reason for Action
Bend the wrist backward and then forward.	Moves the wrist from extension to hyperextension and then flexion

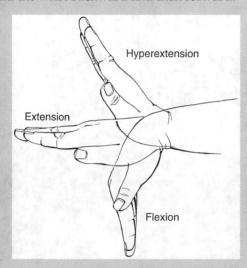

Twist the wrist to the right and then left.	Rotates the wrist joint

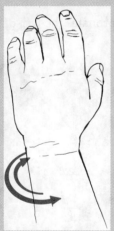

Rotation of the wrist.

(continued)

SKILL 24-1
Performing Range-of-Motion (ROM) Exercises *(Continued)*

Suggested Action	Reason for Action
Bend the thumb side of the hand toward the wrist and then away.	Provides abduction and then adduction of the wrist

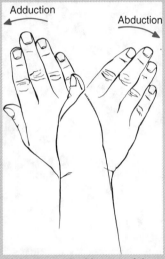

Abduction and adduction of the wrist.

Turn the palm upward and then downward.	Supinates and pronates the wrist.

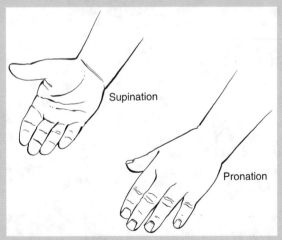

Supination and pronation of the wrist.

Open and close the fingers as though making a fist.	Flexes and extends fingers.

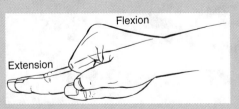

Flexion and extension of the fingers.

(continued)

SKILL 24-1
Performing Range-of-Motion (ROM) Exercises *(Continued)*

Suggested Action	Reason for Action
Bend the thumb toward the center of the palm and then back to its original position.	Flexes and extends the thumb

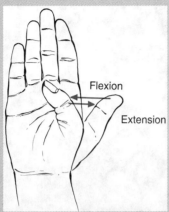

Flexion and extension of the thumb.

Suggested Action	Reason for Action
Spread the fingers and thumb as widely as possible and then bring them back together again.	Abducts and adducts the fingers and thumb

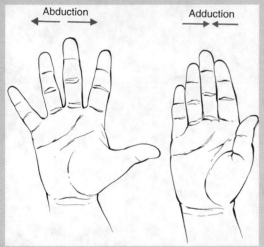

Abduction and adduction of the fingers and thumb.

(continued)

SKILL 24-1
Performing Range-of-Motion (ROM) Exercises (Continued)

Suggested Action	Reason for Action
Bring the straightened leg forward of the body and backward from the body.	Flexes, extends, and hyperextends the hip

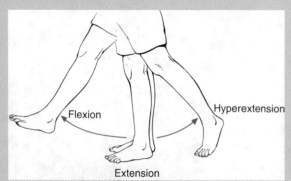

Flexion, extension, and hyperextension of the hip.

Suggested Action	Reason for Action
Move the straightened leg away from the body and back beyond the midline.	Abducts and then adducts the hip

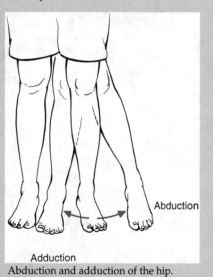

Abduction and adduction of the hip.

(continued)

SKILL 24-1
Performing Range-of-Motion (ROM) Exercises (Continued)

Suggested Action	Reason for Action
Turn the leg away from the other leg and then toward it.	Rotates the hip externally and then internally

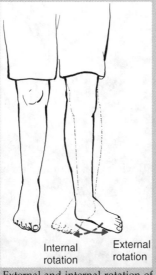

Internal rotation   External rotation

External and internal rotation of the hip.

Turn the leg in a circle.	Circumducts the hip

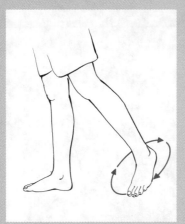

Circumduction of the hip.

(continued)

SKILL 24-1
Performing Range-of-Motion (ROM) Exercises *(Continued)*

Suggested Action	Reason for Action
Bend the knee and then straighten it again.	Flexes and extends the knee

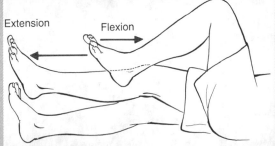

Flexion and extension of the knee.

Bend the foot toward the ankle and then away from the ankle.	Causes dorsiflexion and plantar flexion

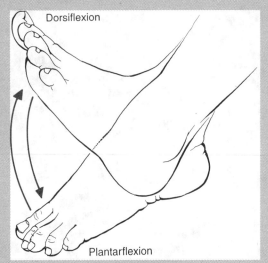

Dorsiflexion and plantar flexion of the foot.

(continued)

SKILL 24-1
Performing Range-of-Motion (ROM) Exercises *(Continued)*

Suggested Action	Reason for Action
Bend the sole of the foot toward the midline and then away from midline.	Inverts and everts the ankle

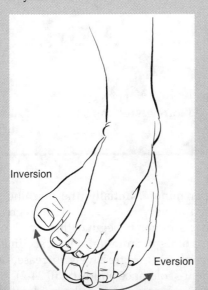

Inversion and eversion of the ankle.

Suggested Action	Reason for Action
Bend and then straighten the toes.	Flexes and extends the toes

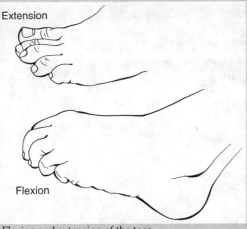

Flexion and extension of the toes.

(continued)

SKILL 24-1
Performing Range-of-Motion (ROM) Exercises (Continued)

Suggested Action	Reason for Action
Evaluation	
• All joints are exercised to the extent possible	
Document	
• Performance of exercise regimen	
• Response of the patient	
Sample Documentation	
Date and Time Assisted to perform ROM exercises during bath. Actively moves all joints on R side of body. Joints on L side passively exercised through full ranges. No resistance or pain experienced. _____ **Signature, Title**	

Continuous Passive Motion Machine

A **continuous passive motion** (CPM) **machine** (Fig. 24-3) is an electrical device that passively exercises joints for a set period of time. It can be used as a supplement or substitute for manually assisted exercise.

The machine can be adjusted for both the speed and the degree of desired joint flexion. Most machines can produce anywhere from 0° to 110° of motion 2 to 10 times per minute. Initially, the machine settings are regulated at very low speeds and degrees of movement. It is common to begin with 5° or 10° of flexion cycling two times per minute, at least six times a day. The adjustments are progressively increased each day as the patient's tolerance builds (Skill 24-2).

Several advantages have been identified with the use of a CPM machine. Besides restoring and increas-

SKILL 24-2
Using a Continuous Passive Motion (CPM) Machine

Suggested Action	Reason for Action
Assessment	
Review the medical record and nursing plan for care for the amount of joint flexion, cycles per minute, frequency, and duration of exercise.	Determines the exercise prescription for the individual patient
Explore how much the patient understands about CPM, especially if this is the first time it is being used.	Determines the level and type of health teaching to provide
Assess the quality of peripheral pulses, capillary refill, edema, temperature, sensation, and mobility of the affected extremity.	Provides a baseline of data for future comparisons
Compare assessments with the unaffected extremity.	Provides comparative data
Determine the patient's need for pain-relieving medication before the use of the CPM machine.	Controls pain before it intensifies with exercise
Planning	
Develop a schedule with the patient for when to use the machine.	Involves the patient in decision-making.

(continued)

SKILL 24-2
Using a Continuous Passive Motion (CPM) Machine (Continued)

Suggested Action	Reason for Action
Instruct the patient on techniques for muscle relaxation and pain control such as deep breathing, listening to audiotapes, watching television, or applying an ice bag.	Empowers the patient with techniques for controlling pain
Obtain the CPM machine and secure a length of sheepskin or soft flannel cloth to the horizontal bars to form a cradle (sling) for the calf.	Prepares the machine for supporting the leg
Don gloves and empty any wound drainage containers; change or reinforce the dressing (see Chap. 28).	Prevents leakage during exercise, when drainage is likely to increase
Wash hands.	Reduces the transmission of microorganisms
Implementation	
Explain the purpose, application, and use of the CPM machine.	Reduces anxiety and promotes cooperation
Position the patient flat or slightly elevate the head of the bed.	Promotes comfort during exercise
Place the CPM machine on the bed and position the patient's foot so that it rests against the foot cradle.	Prepares the patient for exercise

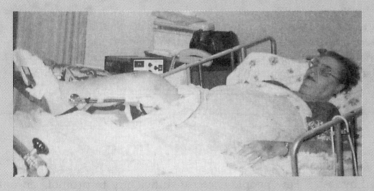

Positioned for continuous passive motion machine use. (Courtesy of Ken Timby.)

Suggested Action	Reason for Action
Check that the knee joint corresponds to the foot actuator knob and **goniometer**, a device for measuring range of motion (refer to Fig. 24-3 for location).	Positions the knee correctly
Use Velcro or canvas straps to secure the leg within the fabric cradle of the machine.	Supports and stabilizes leg
Adjust the machine to a lower than prescribed rate and degree of flexion.	Provides gradual progression to prescribed parameters
Turn on the machine and observe the patient's response.	Indicates level of tolerance
Readjust the alignment of the leg or position of the machine for optimum comfort.	Demonstrates concern for the patient's well-being

(continued)

SKILL 24-2
Using a Continuous Passive Motion (CPM) Machine (Continued)

Suggested Action	Reason for Action
Increase the degree of flexion and cycles per minute gradually until the prescribed levels are reached.	Facilitates adaptation
Turn off the machine with the leg in an extended position at the end of the prescribed period of exercise.	Facilitates lifting the leg from the machine
Release the straps and support the joints beneath the knee and ankle while lifting the leg.	Reduces discomfort
Remove the machine from the bed; encourage active range-of-motion exercises and isometric exercises.	Potentiates effects from CPM

Evaluation
- CPM used according to exercise prescription

Document
- Assessment data
- Use of machine
- Current amount of flexion, cycles per minute, and duration
- Tolerance of exercise

Sample Documentation

Date and Time   Knee incision is dry and intact. Toes on both feet are warm with capillary refill < 3 sec. Pedal pulses present and strong bilaterally. CPM machine used for 15 minutes with ROM at 30° of knee flexion for 5 cycles per minute. Discomfort increased from a level 4 before exercise to level 7 during exercise. Pain at a level of 5 after 15 minutes of rest following exercise. _____ **Signature, Title**

ing range of motion, the movement prevents pooling of venous blood, thus decreasing the risk of forming blood clots. Also, wound healing is accelerated by facilitating the circulation of synovial fluid about the joint.

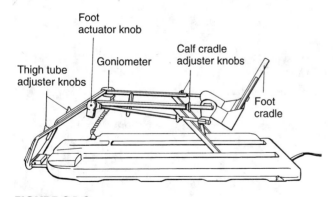

FIGURE 24-3
Continuous passive motion machine.

NURSING IMPLICATIONS

Few people exercise sufficiently to promote an optimum level of health. With this in mind, the United States Department of Health and Human Services (1992) established goals and strategies for improving the nation's health (Display 24-2). Nurses can set an example on a personal level by improving their own physical fitness and encouraging others to do likewise.

For those who have already acquired medical disorders, the nurse may identify one or more of the nurs-

 APPLICABLE NURSING DIAGNOSES

- Impaired Physical Mobility
- Risk for Disuse Syndrome
- Unilateral Neglect

DISPLAY 24-2. *National Strategies for Improving Physical Activity and Fitness*

- Increase daily participation in physical education in elementary and secondary schools
- Include more physical activity during physical education classes
- Involve children in physical activities that may be readily carried into adulthood
- Increase employer-sponsored physical activities and fitness programs
- Increase community availability and accessibility to physical activity and fitness facilities
- Increase counseling and the provision of exercise prescriptions for patients under the care of a physician

Adapted from United States Department of Health and Human Services. Healthy People 2000: National Health Promotion and Disease Prevention Objectives. Boston: Jones and Bartlett Publishers, 1992.

 FOCUS ON OLDER ADULTS

- Periods of activity are balanced with periods of rest when caring for older adults.
- Older adults can be encouraged to join organizations that promote activities for senior citizens such as the American Association of Retired Persons (AARP) and programs sponsored by the Commission on Aging (COA).
- Many shopping malls permit members of the community to use their indoor environment for walking before the stores open for business.
- Swimming or exercising in water creates less stress on the joints of older adults.
- Many physically challenging sports like bowling, golfing, walking in marathons, and even weight-lifting have competition categories for older adults.
- Precautions are taken to prevent falls, like wearing safe walking shoes with nonskid soles, when assisting older adults to exercise. Complications from falls contribute to the morbidity and mortality among people in this age group.
- Exercise in a rocking chair is a safe activity that can be carried out by most older adults.

ing diagnoses listed in Applicable Nursing Diagnoses. These diagnoses, if present, may be treated with various forms of activity and exercise.

The accompanying Nursing Care Plan illustrates how exercise is incorporated into the care of a stroke

NURSING CARE PLAN:
Unilateral Neglect

Assessment

Subjective Data
States, "Somebody's arm and leg are in my bed."

Objective Data
76-year-old man previously treated for hypertension. Admitted now for a stroke. Left side of face droops. Unable to fully smile or show teeth. Tongue deviates from midline. Not able to see objects placed on L. side of body. Does not eat food on left side of plate and tray. No movement of L. upper or lower extremities. No response to touch or pain stimuli on L. side. Cannot differentiate between warm or cold on the left, but can do so on right.

Diagnosis
Unilateral Neglect related to unawareness of objects in L. visual field secondary to stroke.

Plan

Goal
The patient will identify his own L. arm and leg and assist with bathing, exercising, and dressing the L. side of his body by 4/21.

(continued)

NURSING CARE PLAN:
Unilateral Neglect *(continued)*

Orders: 4/19

1. Each shift, show the patient three objects on the R. side of the patient's visual field.
2. Locate the same three objects on the L. side of the bed, wall, or room and instruct the patient to turn his head and identify where each is located.
3. Have the patient locate and touch his left arm and leg.
4. Instruct the patient to bathe his left arm in the A.M. and follow with inserting sleeve over left hand and arm; on remaining shifts have patient grasp his left arm and perform range of motion of shoulder, elbow, wrist, and fingers.

_____ S. LABADIE, RN

Implementation 4/19 1745 While standing on R. side of bed, patient was shown a pen, flashlight, and
(Documentation)   watch. Flashlight placed by left hand, watch buckled to left side rail, and pen
                                        placed on top sheet. Instructed to turn head to the left and identify relocated
                                        items, L. arm, and L. leg. _____ J. PERRY, LPN

Evaluation   1800 Able to scan left side and correctly identify objects and body parts. Able to
(Documentation)   grasp left hand and extend arm over head. Right elbow flexed and extended;
                                        arm adducted. Pronation, supination of hand, flexion and hyperextension of
                                        R. wrist and fingers performed by patient five times each. Assisted with abduc-
                                        tion of arm and circumduction of shoulder._____ J. PERRY, LPN

patient for whom the nursing diagnosis of Unilateral Neglect has been made. The NANDA taxonomy (1994) defines Unilateral Neglect as "A state in which an individual is perceptually unaware of and inattentive to one side of the body."

KEY CONCEPTS

- Regular exercise has many benefits, some of which include a reduction in blood pressure, blood sugar, and blood lipid levels, increased bone density, and reduction in tension and depression.
- Fitness refers to a person's capacity to perform physical activities. There are various factors that tend to interfere with fitness, such as chronic inactivity, concurrent health problems, impaired musculoskeletal function, obesity, advancing age, smoking, and high blood pressure.
- There are three ways to determine one's level of fitness. They include measuring body composition, monitoring vital signs, and undergoing fitness tests like a stress electrocardiogram or step test.
- Fitness exercises are physical activities that develop and maintain cardiorespiratory function, muscular strength, and endurance in healthy adults, whereas

therapeutic exercise involves physical activities that are designed to prevent health-related complications or restore lost physical functions.

- Metabolic energy equivalent (MET) is the measure of energy and oxygen consumption that a person's cardiovascular system can safely support. When an exercise prescription is given, exercises are correlated with the person's MET value.
- Isotonic exercise is that which involves movement and work. One of the best known examples is aerobic exercise. Isometric exercise refers to stationary activities that are performed against a resistive force. Examples of isometric exercise include body building and weight lifting.
- Exercise, regardless of the type, should be performed within one's target heart rate. Target heart rate is calculated by subtracting one's age from 220 (the maximum heart rate) and then multiplying that number by 60% (0.60).
- Active exercise is that which is done independently. Passive exercise is that which is performed with the assistance of another person.
- Range-of-motion (ROM) exercise is a form of therapeutic exercise in which joints are moved in the directions the normal joint permits.
- Two of the most common reasons for performing ROM exercises are to (1) maintain joint mobility and

flexibility, especially among inactive patients; and (2) prevent contracture deformities.

- Older adults may exercise more often if it is suggested that they use shopping malls as a location for walking or join social groups that promote physical exercise, such as line or ballroom dancing.

CRITICAL THINKING EXERCISES

- How might you remotivate a friend who began an exercise program and then gradually stopped?
- List at least five excuses people give for not exercising, and offer a counterargument.

SUGGESTED READINGS

American College of Sports Medicine. Guidelines for Exercise Testing and Prescription. 4th ed. Philadelphia: Lea & Febiger, 1989.

American Heart Association. Statement on exercise: a position statement for health professionals by the Committee on Exercise and Cardiac Rehabilitation of the Council on Clinical Cardiology. Circulation January 1990;81:396–398.

Birdsall C. How do you use the continuous passive motion device? American Journal of Nursing June 1986;86:657–658.

Blaylock B. Mobility and ambulation: not easy tasks for all older adults. Advancing Clinical Care November–December 1991;6:20–21, 41.

Edmunds MW. Strategies for promoting physical fitness. Nursing Clinics of North America December 1991;26:855–866.

Farrell J. Nursing Care of the Older Person. Philadelphia: JB Lippincott, 1990.

Gillett PA, Johnson M, Juretich M. The nurse as exercise leader. Geriatric Nursing May–June 1993;14:133–137.

Hays P. Exercise guidelines: an update. Clinical Management September–October 1992;12:54–55.

Making exercise a part of your life. Patient Care December 15 1991;25:129–130.

United States Department of Health and Human Services. Healthy People 2000: National Health Promotion and Disease Prevention Objectives. Boston: Jones and Bartlett Publishers, 1992.

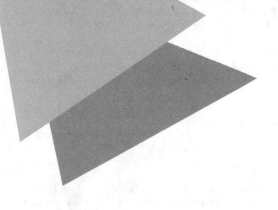

CHAPTER 25

Casts and Traction

Learning Objectives

An understanding of the content within this chapter will be evidenced by the student's ability to:

- List at least three purposes for immobilization
- Name four types of splints
- Discuss why slings and braces are used
- Explain the purpose of a cast and name two substances used to make casts
- Name three types of casts
- Describe at least five nursing actions that are appropriate when caring for patients with casts
- Discuss how casts are removed
- Explain what traction implies
- List three types of traction
- Name the seven principles that apply to maintaining effective traction

Some patients are inactive and physically immobile because of an overall debilitating condition. For others, becoming inactive or immobile is a consequence of treatment. Such is the case for patients who are temporarily restricted because of the application of a cast, traction, or other types of mechanical devices. Consequently, these types of situations require specialized skills if they are to accomplish their intended purpose. This chapter describes the techniques for caring for patients who require mechanical immobilization.

Timby BK: *Fundamental Skills and Concepts in Patient Care, Sixth Edition* © 1996 Lippincott-Raven Publishers

PURPOSES OF IMMOBILIZATION

Most patients for whom mechanical immobilization is used have sustained trauma to the musculoskeletal system. These injuries are painful and do not heal as rapidly as those of the skin or soft tissue. They require a period of inactivity during the time that new cells are restoring the integrity of the damaged structures.

Casts, traction, and similar immobilizing devices may be applied to accomplish any one or a combination of the following:

- Relieve pain and muscle spasm
- Support and align skeletal injuries
- Restrict movement while injuries heal
- Maintain functional positions until healing is complete
- Allow activity while restricting movement of an injured area
- Prevent further structural damage and deformity

Before the application of casts or traction, or in lieu of their use, some conditions may be treated with a splint.

SPLINTS

Splints are devices that immobilize and protect an injured part of the body. Splints are often applied as a first-aid measure. Doing so requires following principles to avoid contributing further to the pre-existing injury.

NURSING GUIDELINES FOR APPLYING AN EMERGENCY SPLINT

- Avoid changing the position of the injured part, even if it appears grossly deformed.
  Rationale: Prevents additional injuries
- Leave a high-top shoe or a ski boot in place if the injury involves an ankle.
  Rationale: Limits movement, reduces pain and swelling
- Cover any open wounds with clean material.
  Rationale: Absorbs blood and prevents the entrance of dirt and additional pathogens
- Select rigid splinting material like flat boards, broom handles, and rolled newspaper.
  Rationale: Provides support while restricting movement
- Pad bony prominences with soft material.
  Rationale: Relieves pressure and prevents friction on the skin

- Apply the splinting device so that it spans the injured area from the joint above the injury to the joint below the injury.
  Rationale: Immobilizes the injured tissue
- Use an uninjured area of the body adjacent to the injured part if no other sturdy material is available.
  Rationale: Substitutes for an external splint
- Use wide tape or wide strips of fabric to confine the injured part to the splint.
  Rationale: Prevents displacement and reduces the risk of compromising circulation
- Loosen the splint or the material used to attach it, if the fingers or toes are pale, blue, or cold.
  Rationale: Facilitates circulation
- Elevate the immobilized part, if that is possible, so that the lowest point is higher than the heart.
  Rationale: Reduces swelling
- Provide for the person's warmth and safety and seek assistance in transporting the injured person to a health agency.
  Rationale: Facilitates more sophisticated treatment

Commercial splints, which are more effective than those that are improvised, come in a variety of designs depending on the need for their use. Some examples include inflatable splints, traction splints, immobilizers, and molded splints.

Inflatable Splints

Inflatable splints, also called *pneumatic splints*, are soft devices that limit motion by becoming rigid when filled with air. Besides limiting motion, they also control bleeding and swelling by virtue of the pressure they exert.

To apply this type of device, the injured body part is inserted into the deflated splint. When air is infused, the splint molds to the contour of the injured part and prevents movement.

An inflatable splint is filled with air up to the point at which it can be indented ½ inch (1.3 cm) with the fingertips. Examination and treatment should take place within 30 to 45 minutes after the splint has been applied, or circulation may be affected.

Traction Splints

Traction splints, for example, a *Thomas splint*, are metal devices that are applied in such a way as to immobilize and pull on muscles that are in a state of contraction. They are not as easily applied as an inflatable splint and require special training to avoid causing additional injuries.

Both pneumatic and traction splints are intended for very brief periods of use. They are commonly applied immediately after an injury occurs and removed shortly after the injury has been assessed more thoroughly. Immobilizers and molded splints, on the other hand, are used for longer periods of time.

Immobilizers

Immobilizers are a type of splint made from cloth and foam (Fig. 25-1). They are held in place by adjustable Velcro straps. As their name implies, immobilizers are used to limit motion in the area of a painful, but healing injury, such as in the neck and knee. They can be removed for brief periods, allowing for dressing and hygiene.

Molded Splints

Molded splints (Fig. 25-2) are used by patients with chronic injuries or diseases. They provide prolonged support and limit movement so as to prevent further injury and pain. Because they are molded, they offer the advantage of maintaining the body part in a functional position to prevent contractures and muscle atrophy during the period of immobility.

Once an injury has been immobilized and examined, sometimes the only additional treatment is to provide some form of external support. In addition to splints,

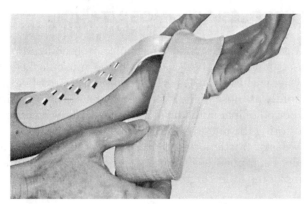

FIGURE 25-2
Molded splint.

there are other supporting devices like slings and braces that may be used in the concomitant treatment of an injury.

SLINGS

Slings are cloth devices that are used to elevate, cradle, and support parts of the body, like an arm (Fig. 25-3), leg, or the pelvis.

Although the commercial type of arm sling used by ambulatory patients is probably the type that comes to mind, it is still possible that a triangular piece of muslin cloth might be used to fashion a sling. To be effective, slings must be properly applied (Skill 25-1).

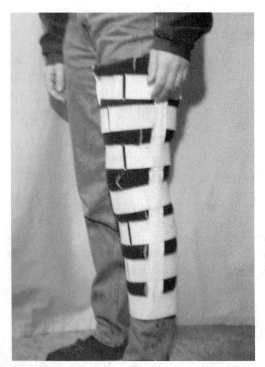

FIGURE 25-1
Leg immobilizer. (Scherer JC, Timby BK: Introductory Medical–Surgical Nursing, 6th ed, p 988. Philadelphia, JB Lippincott, 1995)

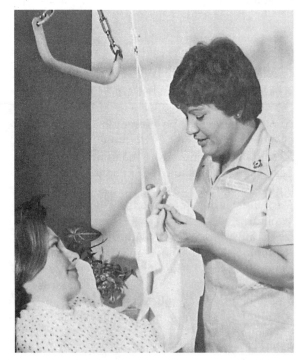

FIGURE 25-3
A sling used for arm suspension.

BRACES

Braces are usually custom-made or custom-fitted devices that are designed to support weakened structures during periods of activity. For this reason they are made of sturdy materials such as tough plastic, metal, and leather.

Leg braces may be incorporated into a shoe. Some back braces are cloth with metal staves, or strips, that are sewn within the fabric of the brace. Any improperly applied or ill-fitting brace can cause discomfort, deformity, and pressure sores.

Although slings and braces are frequently used, probably the most common devices used for treating musculoskeletal injures are casts and traction.

CASTS

A **cast** is a rigid mold that encircles a part of the body. Casts are used to immobilize an injured structure that has been restored to correct anatomic alignment. Casts are formed using either wetted rolls of plaster of paris or premoistened rolls of fiberglass (Table 25-1).

Types of Casts

There are three basic types of casts: cylinder casts, body casts, and spica casts.

CYLINDER CASTS

A **cylinder cast** is a rigid mold that surrounds an arm or leg, leaving the toes or fingers exposed. The same principle for immobilizing an injury with a splint applies to the application of a cast—namely, the cast extends to include the joints above and below the injury. This prevents movement, thereby maintaining the corrected alignment while healing takes place. As healing progresses, the cast may be trimmed or shortened.

(text continues on page 520)

SKILL 25-1
Applying an Arm Sling

Suggested Action	Reason for Action
Assessment	
Check the medical orders.	Collaborates nursing activities with medical treatment
Assess the color, skin temperature, capillary refill time, amount of edema, and verify the presence of peripheral pulses in the arm that has been injured (don gloves if there is a potential for contact with blood or nonintact skin).	Provides baseline objective data for future comparisons
Ask the patient to describe how the fingers or arm feel and to rate pain, if it is present, on a scale of 1 to 10.	Provides baseline subjective data for future comparisons
Determine if the patient has ever required an arm sling in the past.	Indicates the level and type of health teaching needed
Planning	
Explain the purpose for the sling.	Adds to the patient's understanding
Obtain a canvas or triangular sling, whichever is available or prescribed for use.	Complies with medical practice
Implementation	
Have the patient sit or lie down.	Promotes comfort and facilitates applying the sling
Position forearm across the patient's chest with the thumb pointing upward.	Flexes the elbow
Avoid more than 90° of flexion, especially if the elbow has been injured.	Facilitates circulation

(continued)

SKILL 25-1
Applying an Arm Sling (Continued)

Suggested Action	Reason for Action
Canvas Sling Slip the flexed arm into the canvas sling so that the elbow fits flush with the corner of the sling.	Encloses the forearm and wrist

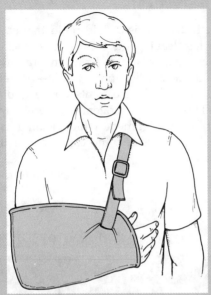

Commercial arm sling. (Scherer JC, Timby BK: Introductory Medical–Surgical Nursing, 6th ed, p 985. Philadelphia, JB Lippincott, 1995)

Bring the strap around the opposing shoulder and fasten it to the sling.	Provides the means for support
Tighten the strap sufficiently to keep the elbow flexed and the wrist elevated.	Promotes circulation

(continued)

SKILL 25-1
Applying an Arm Sling (Continued)

Suggested Action	Reason for Action
Triangular Sling Place the longer side of the sling from the shoulder opposite the injured arm to the waist.	Positions the sling where length is needed

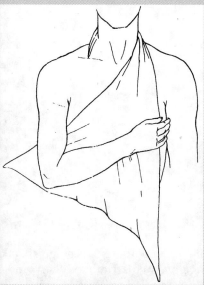

Positioning a triangular sling.

Suggested Action	Reason for Action
Position the apex or point of the triangle under the elbow.	Facilitates making a hammock for the arm
Bring the points at the neck and waist together and tie them.	Encloses the injured arm

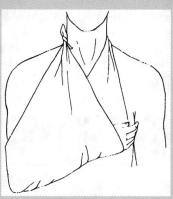

Completed sling.

Suggested Action	Reason for Action
Keep the knot to the side of the neck.	Avoids pressure on the vertebrae
Fold and secure excess fabric at the elbow; a safety pin may be necessary.	Keeps the elbow enclosed
Inspect the condition of the skin at the neck, and the circulation, mobility, and sensation of the fingers at least once per shift.	Provides comparative data

(continued)

SKILL 25-1
Applying an Arm Sling (Continued)

Suggested Action	Reason for Action
Pad the skin at the neck with soft gauze or towel material, if the skin becomes irritated.	Reduces pressure and friction
Tell the patient to report any changes in sensation, especially pain with limited movement or pressure.	Indicates developing complications

Evaluation
- Forearm is supported
- Wrist is elevated
- Pain and swelling are reduced
- Circulation, mobility, and sensation are maintained

Document
- Baseline and comparative assessment data
- Type of sling applied or used
- To whom significant, abnormal assessments were reported
- Outcomes of the verbal report

Sample Documentation

Date and Time	Fingers on R hand are pale, cool, and swollen. Capillary refill is sluggish, taking 4 sec for color to return. Able to move all fingers. Can discriminate sharp and dull stimuli. No tingling identified. Pain rated at 8 on a scale of 0–10. All above data reported to Dr. Stuckey. Orders received for pain medication and canvas sling. Demerol 75 mg given IM in vastus lateralis. Sling applied. _____ **Signature, Title**

BODY CASTS

A **body cast** is simply a larger form of a cylinder cast. Instead of encircling an extremity, a body cast encircles the trunk. It usually extends from the nipple line to the hips. For some people with spinal problems, the body cast may extend from the back of the head and chin areas to the hips, with modifications made for exposing the arms.

A body cast may be cut in two and worn like a clam shell. Bathing and skin care are provided by removing half of the cast shell.

TABLE 25-1. *Cast Materials*

Substance	Advantages	Disadvantages
Plaster of paris	Inexpensive Easy to apply	Takes 24–48 hours to dry Weight bearing must be delayed until thoroughly dried Heavy Prone to cracking or crumbling, especially at the edges Softens when wet
Fiberglass	Lightweight Porous Dries in 5–15 minutes Permits immediate weight bearing Durable Unaffected by water	Expensive Not recommended for severe injuries or those that are accompanied by excessive swelling Macerates skin if padding becomes wet Cast edges may be sharp and cause skin abrasions

SPICA CASTS

A **spica cast** encircles one or more extremities (arms or legs) and the chest or trunk. When applied to the upper body, they are referred to as a **shoulder spica**, whereas those on lower extremities are called **hip spicas**. A spica cast may be strengthened by attaching a reinforcement bar (Fig. 25-4). Spica casts, especially those on lower extremities, are very heavy, hot, and frustrating because they severely restrict activity.

When applied to a lower extremity, the cast is trimmed in the anal and genital areas to provide room for the elimination of urine and stool. Unfortunately, patients with a hip spica are unable to sit during elimination. Consequently, the nurse protects the cast from soiling using plastic wrap and provides a small type of bedpan known as a fracture pan.

Cast Application

The application of a cast usually requires more than one set of hands. The nurse prepares the patient, assembles the cast supplies, and helps the physician during the cast application (Skill 25-2).

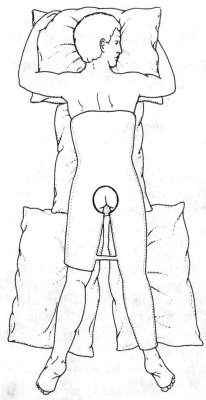

FIGURE 25-4
Hip spica cast. (Scherer JC, Timby BK: Introductory Medical–Surgical Nursing, 6th ed, p 975. Philadelphia, JB Lippincott, 1995)

SKILL 25-2
Assisting With a Cast Application

Suggested Action	Reason for Action
Assessment	
Check the medical orders.	Collaborates nursing activities with medical treatment
Assess the appearance of the skin that will be covered by the cast; also check circulation, mobility, and sensation.	Provides a baseline of data for future comparisons
Ask the patient to describe the location, type, and intensity of pain, if it is present.	Determines whether analgesic medication is needed
Determine what the patient understands about the application of a cast.	Indicates the need for and type of health teaching
Check with the physician as to whether a plaster of paris cast or fiberglass cast will be applied.	Facilitates assembling appropriate supplies
Planning	
Obtain a signature on a consent for treatment form, if that is required.	Ensures legal protection
Administer pain medication, if prescribed.	Relieves discomfort
Remove clothing that may not stretch over the cast once it is applied.	Avoids having to cut and destroy clothing

(continued)

SKILL 25-2
Assisting With a Cast Application

Suggested Action	Reason for Action
Provide a patient gown.	Preserves dignity and protects clothing
Assemble materials, which may include stockinette, felt padding, cotton batting, rolls of cast material, gloves, and aprons.	Facilitates organization and efficient time management
Anticipate that if the cast is being applied to a lower extremity, the patient may need crutches and instructions on their use (see Chap. 26).	Shows awareness of discharge planning
Have an arm sling available if the cast is being applied to an upper extremity.	Shows awareness of discharge planning

Implementation

Explain how the cast will be applied. If plaster of paris is used, be sure to tell the patient that it will feel warm for a period of time.	Reduces anxiety and promotes cooperation
Don gloves and an apron. Provide the physician with the same.	Protects the hands from contact with blood and cast materials
Wash the patient's skin with soap and water and dry well.	Removes dirt, body oil, and some microorganisms
Cover the skin with stockinette, stretchy fabric that comes knitted in a tube.	Protects the skin from direct contact with the cast material
Help the physician apply felt around bony prominences and cotton batting over the stockinette.	Provides a fabric cushion that protects the skin
Open rolls and strips of plaster gauze material. Dip them, one at a time, briefly in water and wring out the excess moisture.	Prepares the cast material for application to the patient
If fiberglass material is used, open the foil packets, one at a time.	Reduces the risk of rapidly drying and becoming unfit for use
Support the extremity while the physician wraps the cast material about the arm or leg.	Facilitates going around the injured area
Help to fold back the edges of the stockinette at each end of the cast just before the final layer of cast material is applied.	Forms a smooth, soft edge at the margins of the cast, which may protect the skin from becoming scraped and sore
Elevate the cast on pillows while it dries.	Prevents flattening due to compression on a hard surface
Dispose of the water in which plaster rolls were soaked in a special sink with a plaster trap.	Prevents clogging plumbing
Provide verbal and written instructions on cast care.	Facilitates independence and safe self-care

Evaluation

- Skin has been cleaned and protected
- Cast has been applied and is drying or dried
- Circulation and sensation are not severely impaired
- Patient can repeat discharge instructions

(continued)

SKILL 25-2
Assisting With a Cast Application (Continued)

Suggested Action	Reason for Action

Document
- Assessment data
- Type of cast
- Cast material
- Name of physician who applied the cast
- Discharge instructions

Sample Documentation

Date and Time   Wrist appears swollen but skin is warm, dry, and intact. Capillary refill <3 sec. X-ray Dept. reports a fracture of the wrist. Dr. Roberts notified. Cylinder fiberglass cast applied from middle of hand to above elbow by Dr. Roberts. Assessments remain unchanged after cast application. Casted arm supported in a canvas sling. Standard instructions for cast care provided (see copy attached). Instructed to call Dr. Roberts if pain or swelling increases and make an office appointment in 2 weeks.

_____ **Signature, Title**

Basic Cast Care

Some patients need extended care after the application of a cast. It then becomes the nurse's responsibility to care for the cast and make appropriate assessments to ensure that complications do not develop.

NURSING GUIDELINES FOR BASIC CAST CARE

- Leave the casted area uncovered.
  Rationale: Facilitates assessment and drying
- Assess the circulation and sensation in exposed fingers or toes at frequent intervals (Fig. 25-5).

Rationale: Provides comparative data for identifying neurovascular complications
- Monitor the mobility of the fingers (Fig. 25-6) or toes.
  Rationale: Provides data on neuromuscular function
- Report significant abnormal findings promptly, especially those that progressively get worse.
  Rationale: Ensures that complications are treated early
- Handle a wet cast with the palms of the hand, never the fingers (Fig. 25-7).
  Rationale: Prevents denting the plaster.
- Elevate the cast on pillows while it is wet.

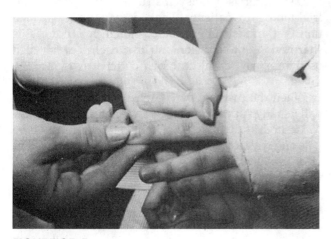

FIGURE 25-5
Assessing capillary refill.

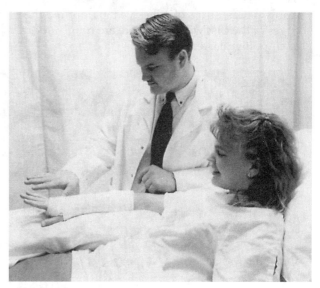

FIGURE 25-6
Checking mobility. (Courtesy of Ken Timby.)

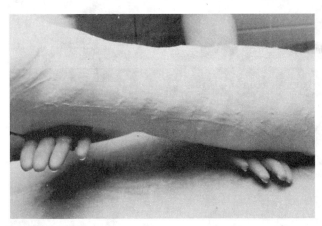

FIGURE 25-7
Support using the palms.

Rationale: Prevents changing the shape of the cast and interfering with the corrected alignment
- Remove residue of plaster from the skin with a wet washcloth.
Rationale: Prevents accumulation of plaster flakes inside the cast or bed.
- Swab fiberglass resin from the skin with alcohol or acetone.
Rationale: Acts as a chemical solvent
- Turn the patient frequently while a plaster cast is drying.
Rationale: Promotes drying of all surfaces and layers of the cast
- Apply ice packs to the cast where surgery has been performed.
Rationale: Reduces swelling and helps to control bleeding
- Circle areas where blood has seeped through the cast; note the time on the cast.
Rationale: Helps to evaluate the significance of blood loss
- Apply **petals**, strips of adhesive tape, around the edges of the cast wherever there are rough areas or chipping plaster (Fig. 25-8).

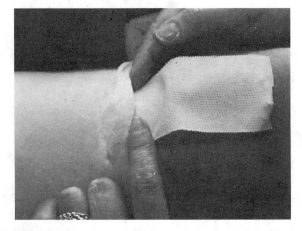

FIGURE 25-8
Applying petals.

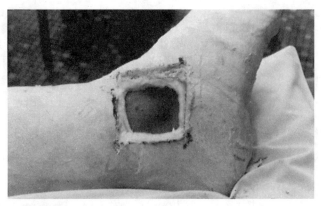

FIGURE 25-9
A cast with a window.

Rationale: Reinforces the edge of the cast
- Caution patients not to insert objects like straws, combs, eating utensils, and the like within the cast.
Rationale: Creates a risk for impairing the skin should they fall inside
- Replace cut squares, known as **windows** (Fig. 25-9), within their original site.
Rationale: Prevents bulging of tissue
- Ambulate patients as soon as possible or have them exercise in bed.
Rationale: Prevents complications from immobility

Cast Removal

Eventually casts are removed. This may happen earlier than anticipated, if complications like swelling develop. Otherwise, casts are removed when they need to be changed or when the injury has sufficiently healed that the cast is no longer necessary.

Most casts are removed with an electric cast cutter, an instrument that looks like a circular saw (Fig. 25-10). A cast cutter is a noisy instrument that can sound frightening to patients. There is a natural expectation that an instrument sharp enough to cut a cast is sharp enough to cut skin and tissue. However, when used properly, an electric cast cutter leaves the skin intact.

When the cast is removed, the unexercised muscle will usually appear smaller and weaker. The joints may be limited in their range of motion. The skin will be pale and waxy looking. It may contain scales or patches of dead skin. The skin may be washed as usual with warm, soapy water, but the semiattached areas of loose skin are not forcibly removed. Lotion applied to the skin may add moisture and prevent rough edges from catching on clothing.

The care of traction patients is often equally challenging.

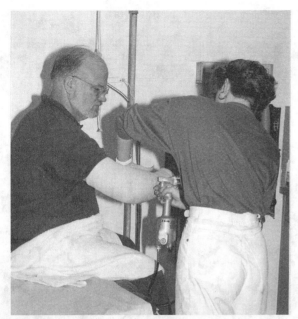

FIGURE 25-10
Cast removal. (Courtesy of Ken Timby.)

TRACTION

Traction is the application of a pulling effect on a particular part of the skeletal system. The pull of the traction is usually offset by the counterpull from the patients's own body weight. Traction is used for several purposes:

- To reduce muscle spasms
- To realign bones
- To relieve pain
- To prevent deformities

Types of Traction

There are three basic types of traction: manual, skin and skeletal traction. The categories reflect the manner in which traction is applied.

MANUAL TRACTION

Manual traction is achieved by pulling on the body using a person's hands and muscular strength (Fig. 25-11). This type of traction is most often used when realigning a broken bone. It may also be used when replacing a dislocated bone into its original position within a joint.

SKIN TRACTION

Skin traction produces a pulling effect indirectly on the skeletal system by applying devices such as a pelvic belt (Fig. 25-12) and cervical halter (Fig. 25-13) to the

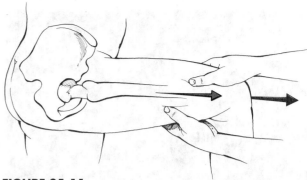

FIGURE 25-11
Manual traction.

skin. There are various names for commonly applied forms of skin traction, such as Buck's traction (Fig. 25-14) and Russell's traction (Fig. 25-15).

SKELETAL TRACTION

Skeletal traction pulls directly on the skeletal system by means of wires, pins, or tongs placed into or through bones (Fig. 25-16). Both skeletal and skin traction involve the use of weights that are connected in some fashion to the patient through a system of ropes, pulleys, slings, and other equipment.

Traction Care

Regardless of the type of traction that is used, its effectiveness depends on applying certain principles during patient care (Display 25-1).

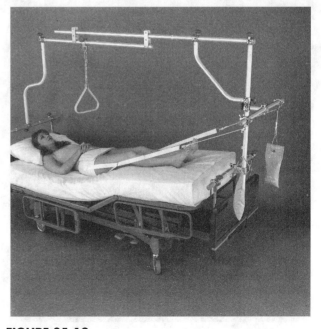

FIGURE 25-12
Pelvic belt. (Courtesy of Patient Care Division, Zimmer, Dover, OH.)

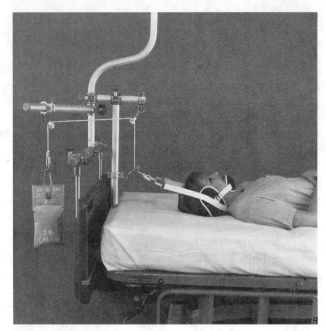

FIGURE 25-13
Cervical halter. (Courtesy of Patient Care Division, Zimmer, Dover, OH.)

NURSING GUIDELINES FOR CARE OF TRACTION PATIENTS

* Inspect the mechanical equipment used to apply traction.
  Rationale: Determines the status of existing equipment

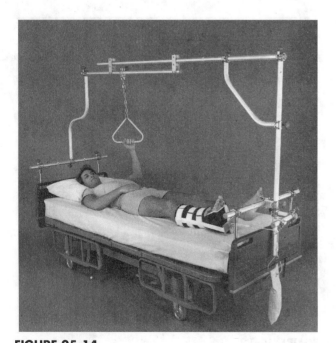

FIGURE 25-14
Buck's traction. (Courtesy of Patient Care Division, Zimmer, Dover, OH.)

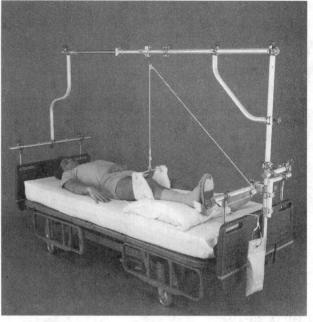

FIGURE 25-15
Russell's traction (Courtesy of Patient Care Division, Zimmer, Dover, OH.)

* Provide a trapeze and an overbed frame if none is present.
  Rationale: Facilitates mobility and self-care
* Position or reposition the patient so that the patient's body is in an opposite line to the pull of traction.
  Rationale: Supports one of the principles for maintaining effective traction
* Avoid tucking top sheets, blankets, or bedspreads beneath the mattress.
  Rationale: Interferes with the pull produced by traction equipment
* Keep the traction applied continuously unless there are medical orders to the contrary.
  Rationale: Fosters achieving desired outcomes
* Keep the weights from resting on the floor.
  Rationale: Maintains effective traction
* Ask the physician to replace fraying ropes or those

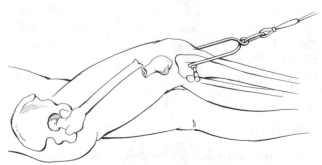

FIGURE 25-16
Skeletal traction.

DISPLAY 25-1. *Principles for Maintaining Effective Traction*

- Traction must produce a pulling effect on the body
- Countertraction (counterpull) must be maintained
- The pull of traction and the counterpull must be in exactly opposite directions
- Splints and slings must be suspended without interference
- Ropes must move freely through each pulley
- The prescribed amount of weight must be applied
- The weights must hang free

whose knots interfere with movement through pulleys.
Rationale: Maintains effective traction

- Limit the patient's positions to those indicated in the medical orders or standards for care.
Rationale: Avoids altering the pull and counterpull of effective traction

- Bathe the backs of patients who must remain in a supine or other back-lying position by depressing the mattress enough to insert a hand.
Rationale: Facilitates skin care and hygiene

- Make the bed by applying sheets from the bottom of the bed toward the top, rather than side to side.
Rationale: Maintains the patient in an opposite line to the traction

- Use a pressure-relieving device (see Chap. 28) or conscientious skin care if the patient is confined to bed for a prolonged time.
Rationale: Prevents skin breakdown

- Omit using a pillow if the patient's head or neck is in traction, unless medical orders indicate otherwise.
Rationale: Prevents disturbing the pull and counterpull

- Use a small bedpan, called a fracture pan, if elevating the hips alters the line of pull.
Rationale: Maintains effectiveness of traction

- Encourage isometric, isotonic, and active range-of-motion exercises.
Rationale: Maintains tone, strength, and flexibility of the musculoskeletal system

- Cleanse the skin around skeletal insertion sites using soap and water or an antimicrobial agent.
Rationale: Reduces the risk for infection

- Cover the tips of protruding metal pins or other

sharp traction devices with corks or other protective material.
Rationale: Prevents accidental injury

- Insert padding within slings if they tend to wrinkle.
Rationale: Helps cushion and distribute pressure, prevents interference with circulation, and reduces the risk for skin breakdown

- Provide diversional activities as often as possible.
Rationale: Relieves boredom and sensory deprivation

 FOCUS ON OLDER ADULTS

- Fractures of the hip are very common in older adults, especially women who lose bone density as a consequence of osteoporosis.
- Before having a fractured hip repaired, almost all patients are placed in Buck's or Russell's skin traction and remain so even while being transported to the operating room.
- The bones of older adults take longer to heal than those of younger age groups.
- Older adults are mobilized as soon as possible to avoid life-threatening complications.
- To promote healing of a musculoskeletal injury, older adults are encouraged to consume a diet rich in protein and calcium. Because their appetites may be reduced from inactivity, it may be beneficial to offer older adults a glass of liquid nourishment like Ensure, Sustacal, or Carnation Instant Breakfast several times a day.
- Although musculoskeletal injuries can be quite painful, it is important to exercise caution when administering narcotic analgesics to older adults. This category of drugs relieves pain, but they may also cause constipation, dizziness, confusion, depressed respirations, and inactivity.
- Older adults who are inactive and immobilized with casts or traction require aggressive skin care to maintain its integrity. The elbows, heels, coccyx, shoulder blades, and hips are especially vulnerable to skin breakdown.
- Older adults have diminished tactile sensation and may be unaware of developing problems associated with skin pressure.
- As adults live longer, many are forced to deal with the pain and limited mobility caused by arthritis. Consequently, more and more older adults are choosing to have joint replacement surgery that may involve rehabilitation with various types of mechanical devices.

NURSING IMPLICATIONS

Nurses who care for patients with casts, traction, or other immobilizing devices commonly identify one or more of the nursing diagnoses listed in the accompanying Applicable Nursing Diagnoses.

The accompanying Nursing Care Plan has been developed to illustrate the nursing process as it applies to a patient with Impaired Physical Mobility. NANDA (1994) defines this problem as "A state in which the individual experiences a limitation of ability for independent physical movement."

APPLICABLE NURSING DIAGNOSES

- Pain
- Impaired Physical Mobility
- Risk for Disuse Syndrome
- Risk for Peripheral Neurovascular Dysfunction
- Risk for Impaired Skin Integrity
- Altered Tissue Perfusion
- Bathing/Hygiene Self-Care Deficit

NURSING CARE PLAN:
Impaired Physical Mobility

Assessment

Subjective Data
States, "I wish I could just get up and move around. My hip hurts and I feel so scared about walking."

Objective Data
70-year-old man admitted for a L. total hip replacement done on 2/7. Must maintain limited flexion of operative hip and continuous abduction of operative leg. Schedule for physical therapy instruction on performing a three-point partial weight-bearing gait 2/10.

Diagnosis

Impaired Physical Mobility related to restricted positioning, limited weight bearing, pain, and fear.

Plan

Goal
The patient will ambulate 6 feet with the assistance of a walker by 2/10.

Orders: 2/9
1. Instruct and supervise dorsiflexion, plantar flexion, and quad-setting exercises of both legs q 1 h while awake.
2. Maintain abduction wedge between legs to keep knees apart at all times while in bed.
3. Keep bed flat or with slight elevation (30°–45°) of head.
4. Encourage use of patient-controlled analgesia (PCA) pump at frequent intervals to control pain.
5. Transfer from bed to standing position at the bedside, following these directions:
   a. Slide affected L. leg to edge of bed; remove abduction wedge.
   b. Have patient use trapeze or elbows and hands to slide buttocks and legs perpendicular to bed. Remind to avoid leaning forward and praise efforts at moving.
   c. Lower unaffected R. foot to floor and help with lowering affected L. foot, keeping knees apart.
   d. Apply safety belt around waist.
   e. Brace feet and pull forward on belt.
   f. Stand at bedside, putting only partial weight on L. leg.
   g. Reverse actions for returning to bed. _____ D. FENTON, RN

(continued)

NURSING CARE PLAN:
Impaired Physical Mobility (continued)

Implementation (Documentation)	2/9	0730	Positioned from back to R. side with abduction wedge between legs. _____ F. CLINTON, LPN
		0930	Positioned on back with head of bed raised 45° for breakfast. Active isotonic and isometric exercises done. Assisted with bathing legs and back. Having sharp, throbbing pain in L. hip. Encouraged to use PCA pump. Pain reduced after administration of morphine by PCA pump. _____ F. CLINTON, LPN
		1000	Assisted to transfer out of bed and stand at bedside following procedure outlined in written plan of care. _____ F. CLINTON, LPN
Evaluation (Documentation)		1030	Follows directions well when transferring from bed. Needs frequent reminding to lean backward. Alternated full weight bearing on R. leg with partial weight bearing on L. States, "That was easier than I imagined." Assisted back to bed keeping knees apart and hips slightly flexed. Abduction splint reapplied. _____ F. CLINTON, LPN

KEY CONCEPTS

- Purposes for immobilization include but are not limited to the following: relieving pain and muscle spasm, supporting and aligning skeletal injuries, and restricting movement while injuries heal.
- There are four types of splints: inflatable splints, traction splints, immobilizers, and molded splints.
- Slings are cloth devices that are used to elevate and support parts of the body. Braces are devices that support weakened structures during periods of activity.
- Casts are rigid molds that are used to immobilize an injury that has been restored to correct anatomic alignment. Casts are formed from plaster of paris or fiberglass.
- There are three basic types of casts: cylinder casts, body casts, and spica casts.
- Appropriate care of patients with casts includes: checking circulation, mobility, and sensation in the area of the cast; using the palms of the hands to handle a wet cast; elevating the casted extremity to reduce swelling; circling areas where blood has seeped through; and padding and reinforcing the cast edges to prevent skin breakdown.
- Most casts are removed with an electric cast cutter.
- Traction is the application of a pulling effect on a particular part of the skeletal system.
- There are three types of traction: manual traction, skin traction, and skeletal traction.
- To be effective, traction must produce a pulling effect on the body; countertraction must be maintained; the pull of traction and the counterpull must be in opposite directions; splints and slings must be suspended without interference; ropes must move freely through each pulley; the prescribed amount of weight must be applied; and the weights must hang free.

CRITICAL THINKING EXERCISES

- Discuss the differences and similarities between caring for patients with casts and those in traction.
- Discuss ways of providing diversion for cast and traction patients who are confined to bed while their injuries heal.
- Identify activities that provide exercise and can be performed in bed by patients with casts or in traction.

SUGGESTED READINGS

Bailey MM, Michalski J. Close-up on radial head fracture. Nursing September 1993;23:43.

Brady R, Chester FR, Pierce LL. Geriatric falls: prevention strategies for the staff. Journal of Gerontological Nursing September 1993; 19:26–32, 40–41.

Carnevali D, Patrick M. Nursing Management for the Elderly. 3rd ed. Philadelphia: JB Lippincott, 1993.

Farrell J. Nursing Care of the Older Person. Philadelphia: JB Lippincott, 1990.

Johnson PA, Stone MA, Larson A, Hromek CA. Applying nursing diagnosis and nursing process to activities of daily living and mobility. Geriatric Nursing January–February 1992;13:25–27.

Jones IH. Making sense of traction. Nursing Times June 6–12 1990;86 (23):39–41.

McConnell EA. Providing cast care. Nursing January 1993;23:19.

Morris L, Kraft S, Tessem S, Reinisch S. Nursing the patient in traction. RN January 1988;51:26–31.

Morris L, Kraft S, Tessem S, Reinisch S. Special care for skeletal traction. RN February 1988;51:24–29.

Redheffer GM, Bailey M. Assessing and splinting fractures. Nursing June 1989;19:51–59.

Sumner ED, Simpson WM Jr. Intervention in falls among the elderly. Journal of Practical Nursing June 1992;42:24–34.

Ambulatory Aids

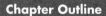

Learning Objectives

An understanding of the content within this chapter will be evidenced by the student's ability to:

- Name four activities that prepare patients for ambulation
- Give two examples of isometric exercises that tone and strengthen lower extremities
- Identify one technique for building upper arm strength
- Explain the reason for dangling patients or using a tilt table
- Name two devices that are used to assist patients with ambulation
- Give three examples of ambulatory aids
- Identify the ambulatory aid that is the most stable and that which is least stable
- Describe three characteristics of appropriately fitted crutches
- Name four types of crutch-walking gaits
- Discuss age-related changes that affect older adults' gait and ambulation

Patients with disorders or injuries affecting their musculoskeletal system and those who become weak or unsteady because of age-related or neurologic problems may have difficulty walking. This chapter provides information on the nursing activities and devices that are used to promote continued mobility.

PREPARING FOR AMBULATION

Debilitated patients, that is, those who are frail or weak from prolonged inactivity, may require physical conditioning before they are able to ambulate again. Some techniques for increasing muscular strength and the ability to bear weight include performing isometric exercises with the lower limbs, isotonic exercises for the upper arms, dangling at the bedside, and using a device called a tilt table.

Isometric Exercises

Isometric exercises (see Chap. 24) are used to promote muscle tone and strength. **Tone** refers to the ability of muscles to respond when stimulated. **Strength** is the power to perform. Muscle tone and strength are maintained or improved by frequently contracting muscle fibers. Active people maintain these two qualities through everyday activities, but inactive people and those who have been immobilized while in a cast or traction may require focused periods of exercise to reestablish their previous ability to walk.

Two types of isometric exercises that promote tone and strength in weight-bearing muscles are quadriceps setting and gluteal setting exercises.

QUADRICEPS SETTING

Quadriceps setting, sometimes shortened to *quad setting*, is a form of isometric exercise in which the quadriceps group of muscles are alternately tensed and relaxed. The quadriceps muscles, which include four muscles, the *rectus femoris, vastus intermedius, vastus medialis,* and *vastus lateralis,* cover the front and side of the thigh. Together they aid in extending the leg. Quadriceps exercise therefore enables patients to stand and support their body weight.

GLUTEAL SETTING

Gluteal setting is a form of isometric exercise that strengthens and tones the gluteal muscles. The gluteal muscles include the *gluteus maximus, gluteus medius,* and *gluteus minimus.* These three make up the muscles in the buttocks. As a group, they aid in extending, abducting, and rotating the leg, functions that are essential to walking.

Quadriceps and gluteal setting exercises are easily performed in bed or when seated in a chair; thus, they can be initiated long before ambulation takes place. Furthermore, most patients are capable of performing these exercises independently once they have been instructed.

Upper Arm Strengthening

Upper arm strength is needed by patients who will be ambulating with the assistance of a walker, cane, or crutches. Modified push-ups strengthen the upper arms.

There are several ways that modified push-ups can be performed, depending on the age and condition of the patient. While seated in bed, the patient may lift his or her hips off the bed by pushing down on the mattress with the hands. If the mattress is soft, a block or books are placed on the bed under the patient's hands. If there is a sturdy armchair available, the patient can raise his or her body from the seat while pushing on the arm rests.

If the patient can lie on his or her abdomen, push-ups may be performed by:

1. Flexing the elbows
2. Placing the hands, palms down, at approximately shoulder level, and then
3. Straightening the elbows so as to lift the head and chest off the bed.

To be effective, push-ups are performed three or four times a day.

Dangling

Dangling is a term that refers to having the patient sit on the edge of the bed (Fig. 26-1). This position is

---

 PATIENT TEACHING FOR PERFORMING QUADRICEPS AND GLUTEAL SETTING EXERCISES

Teach the patient to do the following:
- Tighten (contract) the quadriceps muscles of the thigh by flattening the back of the knees into the mattress, or, if that is not possible,
- Place a rolled towel under the knee or heel before attempting to tighten the quadriceps muscles.
- Check to see that the kneecaps move upward as an indication that the exercise is being performed correctly.

- Hold the contracted position for a count of five.
- Relax and repeat two or three times each hour.
- Tighten (contract) the gluteal muscles by pinching the cheeks of the buttocks together.
- Hold the contracted position for a count of five.
- Relax and repeat two or three times each hour.

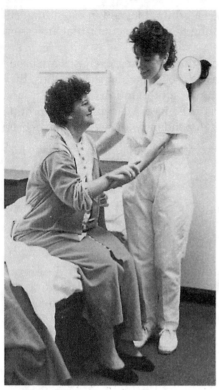

FIGURE 26-1
Dangling. (Courtesy of Ken Timby.)

used to help patients normalize their blood pressure, which may drop momentarily after rising from a reclining position (see section on Postural Hypotension, Chap. 11).

◄ NURSING GUIDELINES FOR DANGLING PATIENTS

- Use dangling before ambulating whenever a patient has been inactive for an extended period of time.
  Rationale: Demonstrates a concern for safety
- Place the patient in a Fowler's position for a few minutes.
  Rationale: Maintains safety in the event the patient becomes dizzy or faints
- Lower the height of the bed.
  Rationale: Facilitates using the floor for support
- Fold back the top linen.
  Rationale: Reduces interference with movement
- Provide the patient with a robe and slippers.
  Rationale: Maintains warmth and shows respect for modesty
- Help the patient pivot a quarter of a turn so as to swing his or her legs over the side and sit on the edge of the bed.

Rationale: Helps the patient become accustomed to sitting up
- Stay with the patient.
  Rationale: Ensures immediate assistance

Using a Tilt Table

A **tilt table**, which looks like a stretcher with a foot rest, is a device that is used to help patients get acclimated to being upright and bearing weight on their own feet. Although the tilt table is located in the physical therapy department, nurses often prepare the patient for this type of preambulation therapy and communicate with the therapists as to the response of the patient.

Just before using a tilt table, the nurse applies elastic stockings (see section on Using Antiembolism Stockings, Chap. 27). These stockings help to compress vein walls, thus preventing pooling of blood in the extremities, which may trigger fainting.

After being transferred from the bed or stretcher to the horizontal tilt table, the patient is strapped securely to avoid falling. Both feet are positioned against the foot rest. The entire table is then tilted in successive increments of 15° to 30° until the patient is in a vertical position, unless symptoms develop. If the patient experiences symptoms, the table is lowered somewhat or returned to the horizontal position.

ASSISTIVE DEVICES

Despite strengthening exercises, some patients may still need progressive assistance to achieve independent ambulation. Using parallel bars and a walking belt provide support and assistance with walking.

Parallel Bars

Parallel bars look like stationary bars separated by enough room to walk through. The bars are used as handrails while patients gain practice in ambulating. In some cases, the tilt table can be positioned immediately in front of the parallel bars so that patients can progress from being upright to actually walking again.

Walking Belt

A **walking belt** is a device worn about the waist that allows the nurse or physical therapist to assist a patient who is beginning to ambulate (Fig. 26-2). The walking belt is designed with handles at the sides and back so that if the patient loses his or her balance, the nurse can support the patient and prevent injuries from an uncontrolled fall.

When assisting a patient to ambulate, the nurse uses the following precautions:

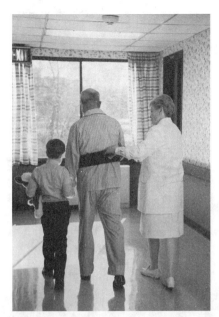

FIGURE 26-2
Using a walking belt. (©1994 Total Care, Gaithersburg, Maryland.)

- Walk alongside the patient.
- Hold onto the handles of the walking belt, or, if one is unavailable:
- Hold onto a belt securing the patient's robe or clothing.
- Support the patient's arm.

If fainting seems likely to occur, the patient may be supported by sliding an arm under the axilla and placing a foot to the side, forming a wide base of support. With the patient's weight braced, a fall can be averted either by balancing the patient on a hip until help arrives or by sliding the patient down the length of the nurse's leg to the floor.

AMBULATORY AIDS

There are three aids that may be used for assistive ambulation: canes, walkers, and crutches.

Canes

A **cane** is a hand-held ambulation device used by patients who have weakness on one side of their body. Canes may be made of wood or aluminum. Those made of aluminum are more commonly used. All canes have rubber tips at their base to reduce the potential for slipping.

There may be slight variations among canes depending on the physical deficits of patients. For instance, a *T-handle cane* has a handgrip with a slightly bent shaft that gives the user more stability. A *quad cane*

has four supports at the base and provides more stability than either of the other two types (Fig. 26-3).

For optimum use, a cane must be adjusted to an appropriate height for the patient. When fitted correctly, the cane's handle is parallel with the patient's hip and provides approximately a 15° angle of elbow flexion. Wooden canes can be shortened by removing a portion of their length from the lower end. Aluminum canes can be shortened or lengthened by depressing metal buttons within the shaft. This allows the shaft of the cane to telescope within itself to accommodate the patient's height.

When patients are beginning to use a cane, the nurse may assist by applying a walking belt and standing toward the back of the patient's stronger side.

Walkers

A **walker** is the most stable form of ambulatory aid. Walkers are used by patients who require considerable support and assistance with balance. Patients who are beginning to ambulate after prolonged bed rest or after hip surgery often use a walker initially.

Standard walkers are constructed of curved aluminum bars that form a three-sided enclosure with four legs for support. Some may be modified with front wheels (Fig. 26-4) or even a seat. Other adaptations can be made for patients who have compromised use of one or both arms or for those who must use stairs when they ambulate. The height of a walker can be adjusted similarly to the technique used for canes.

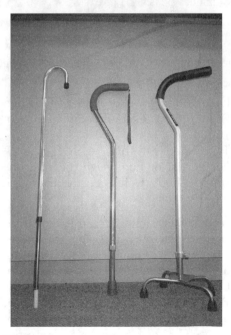

FIGURE 26-3
Straight, T-handle, and quad cane. (Courtesy of Ken Timby.)

PATIENT TEACHING FOR USE OF A CANE

Teach the patient to do the following:
- Place the cane on the stronger side of the body.
- Stand upright with the cane 4 to 6 inches (10–15 cm) to the side.
- Move the cane forward at the same time as the weaker extremity.
- Take the next step with the stronger extremity.

For stairs
- Use a stair rail rather than the cane when going up or down stairs, if that is possible.
- Take each step up with the stronger leg followed by the one that is weaker, but reverse the pattern for descending the stairs.
- If no stair rail is available, the cane is advanced just before rising or descending with the weaker leg.

To sit
- Back up to a chair until the seat is felt against the back of the legs.
- Rest the cane close by.
- Grip the armrests with both hands.
- Be seated.

To rise
- Grip the armrests while holding the cane in the stronger hand.
- Advance the stronger leg.
- Lean forward.
- Push with both arms against the armrests.
- Stand until balanced and any symptoms of dizziness pass.

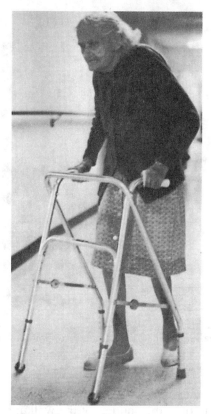

FIGURE 26-4
Using a wheeled walker.

When using a walker, patients are instructed to:

- Stand within the walker.
- Hold onto the walker at the padded handgrips.
- Pick up the walker and advance it 6 to 8 inches (15–20 cm).
- Take a step forward.
- For partial or non-weight bearing on one leg, support body weight on the hand grips when moving the weaker leg.

Using a walker to sit in a chair is similar to the technique used by patients with a cane, with one exception. When the legs are at the back of the chair, the patient grips an arm rest with one arm while still using the other hand on the walker and the stronger leg for support. Then the walker can be released as the patient uses the free hand to grasp the opposite arm rest and lower himself or herself into the chair. To rise, the patient moves to the edge of the chair and repositions the

walker. After pushing up with both arms until the body weight is centered, one hand is used to grasp the walker followed by the other.

Crutches

Crutches are a form of ambulatory aid usually used in pairs. They may be constructed of wood or aluminum, and most have an axillary bar and handgrips. Because the use of crutches requires a great deal of upper arm strength and balance, they are not commonly used by older adults or weak patients.

TYPES OF CRUTCHES

There are three basic types of crutches. **Axillary crutches** are the standard type of crutches with which most people are familiar. Patients who need brief, temporary assistance with ambulation most likely will use axillary crutches.

Lofstrand or **Canadian crutches** have no axillary support. Instead, they have a metal cuff that extends beyond the handgrip (Fig. 26-5). These crutches are used by patients who need permanent assistance with walking.

Another type of crutch is the **platform crutch**. Platform crutches are designed to support the forearm; they

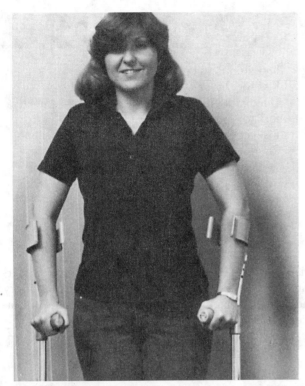

FIGURE 26-5
Lofstrand or Canadian crutches.

are especially useful for patients unable to bear weight with their hands and wrists. Many patients with arthritis use them. Sometimes a patient may use one axillary crutch and one platform crutch, for example when one arm has been disabled because of a fracture.

Once the type of crutches is selected, they are measured to fit each patient.

MEASURING FOR CRUTCHES

It is possible to obtain an approximate crutch measurement by subtracting 16 inches (40 cm) from the patient's height. However, actual measurements are more accurate. When measuring a patient, one of two techniques may be used. One method is used when patients are confined to bed; the other is used when patients can stand.

NURSING GUIDELINES FOR MEASURING CRUTCHES

For the Bedfast Patient
- Place the patient in a supine position with the shoes that will be used when crutch-walking.

Rationale: Simulates the patient's height in a standing position
- Measure the distance from the anterior skin fold of the axilla to the heel and add 2 inches (5 cm).
Rationale: Accommodates for the length that will be needed when standing with the crutches in place

For Patients Who Can Stand
- Assist the patient with supportive shoes.
Rationale: Affects the height of the patient and length of the crutches
- Measure from the anterior skin fold of the axilla to approximately 6 to 8 inches (15–20 cm) diagonally from the foot.
Rationale: Approximates the length required for appropriate use

Based on the patient's measurements, wooden crutches can be lengthened or shortened by removing wing nuts and replacing metal screws in an appropriate hole within the stem of the crutch (Fig. 26-6). Aluminum crutches usually telescope up or down.

Adjusting the length of the crutches may also affect the location of the handgrip. Therefore, before crutches are used, they should be evaluated for proper fit. Crutches that are of an appropriate height demonstrate the following characteristics—they:

- Allow the patient to stand upright with the shoulders relaxed
- Provide space for two fingers between the axilla and the axillary bar

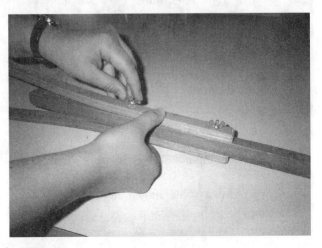

FIGURE 26-6
Adjusting crutch length. (Courtesy of Ken Timby.)

- Facilitate approximately 30° of elbow flexion and slight hyperextension of the wrist

Once crutches have undergone their final adjustment, the patient may be taught a specific crutch-walking gait (Skill 26-1).

CRUTCH-WALKING GAITS

The term *gait* refers to one's manner of walking. A crutch-walking gait is the walking pattern used when ambulating with crutches. However, some of the same gaits may be used with a walker or cane.

Basically, there are four types of crutch-walking gaits. They include the **four-point gait**; the **three-point gait**, which may be performed either in a non–weight-bearing (NWB) or partial weight-bearing (PWB) fashion; the **two-point gait**; and the **swing-through gait** (Table 26-1). The word *point* refers to the sum of the crutches and legs used when performing the gait.

APPLICABLE NURSING DIAGNOSES

- Impaired Physical Mobility
- Risk for Disuse Syndrome
- Unilateral Neglect
- Risk for Trauma
- Risk for Peripheral Neurovascular Dysfunction
- Risk for Activity Intolerance

NURSING IMPLICATIONS

Many nursing diagnoses may be identified when caring for patients who require the use of an ambulatory aid. Some are included in the accompanying Applicable Nursing Diagnoses.

(text continues on page 542)

SKILL 26-1
Assisting With Crutch-Walking

Suggested Action	Reason for Action
Assessment	
Review the medical orders for the type of activity and crutch-walking gait.	Reflects implementation of the medical treatment
Read any previous nursing documentation regarding the patient's efforts at crutch-walking.	Provides evaluative data and indicates need to simulate or modify nursing interventions
Observe the condition of the patient's axillae and palms.	Provides objective data concerning the weight-bearing effects on the upper body
Ask the patient if there is any muscle or joint pain, or tingling or numbness in the fingers.	Provides subjective data concerning the effects of crutch-walking and possible nerve irritation
Inspect the condition of the axillary pads and rubber crutch tips.	Demonstrates concern for safety
Planning	
Consult with the patient about the preferred time for ambulation.	Shows respect for individual decision-making
Assist the patient to don clothes or a robe and supportive shoes or slippers with nonskid soles.	Demonstrates concern for modesty and safety
Apply a walking belt if the patient is weak or inexperienced in the use of crutches.	Demonstrates concern for safety
Clear a pathway where the patient will ambulate.	Demonstrates concern for safety
Review the technique for performing the prescribed crutch-walking gait.	Reinforces prior learning

(continued)

Suggested Action	Reason for Action
Implementation	
Wash your hands.	Reduces the transmission of microorganisms
Help the patient to a standing position.	Prepares the patient for ambulation
Offer the crutches and observe that they are placed 4 to 8 inches (10–20 cm) to the side of the feet.	Forms a triangle for good balance

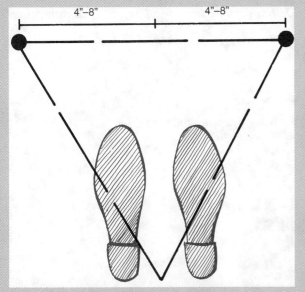

A tripod of support.

Suggested Action	Reason for Action
Remind the patient to stand straight with the shoulders relaxed.	Reduces muscle strain
Position yourself to the side and slightly behind the patient on the weaker side.	Facilitates assistance without causing interference

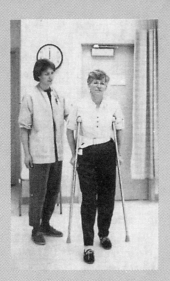

Positioning for assistance. (Courtesy of Ken Timby.)

(continued)

SKILL 26-1
Assisting With Crutch-Walking (Continued)

Suggested Action	Reason for Action
Take hold of the walking belt.	Helps steady or support the patient
Instruct the patient to advance the crutches, lean forward, put some weight on the handgrips, and move one or both feet, depending on the prescribed gait.	Promotes walking
Remind the patient to slow down if there is evidence of fatigue or intolerance to the activity.	Demonstrates concern for the patient's well-being

For Sitting

Recommend backing up to the seat of the chair.	Promotes a position for sitting
Place both crutches in the hand on the same side as the weaker leg.	Frees the opposite hand
While using the handgrips on the crutches for support, have the patient grasp one armrest with the free hand.	Reduces the potential for falling

Sitting down.

When balanced, tell the patient to lower himself or herself into the seat of the chair.	Facilitates sitting
To get up, help the patient to the edge of the chair.	Facilitates using the stronger muscles of the thighs
Instruct the patient to hold the crutches upright on the weaker side, balancing them with one hand.	Positions crutches for support

(continued)

SKILL 26-1
Assisting with Crutch-Walking (Continued)

Suggested Action	Reason for Action
Tell the patient to position the weaker leg forward of the body and the stronger leg toward the base of the chair.	Helps to distribute weight over the stronger leg.
Tell the patient to push on the handgrips and armrest, lean forward, and press down with the stronger leg.	Raises the patient from the chair

To Climb Stairs

Use a handrail that is on the stronger side of the body, if that is possible.	Balances needed support
Have the patient transfer both crutches to the hand opposite the handrail.	Frees one hand for grasping the handrail for support
Tell the patient to push down on the handrail and step up with the good leg.	Uses the stronger muscles for bearing weight

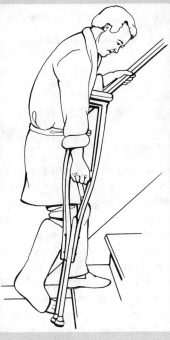

Climbing stairs.

Follow by raising the weaker leg.	Brings both legs to the same stair
Remind the patient that when going down the stairs, the weaker leg is advanced first with the support of the crutches or handrail; then the stronger leg is moved.	Enables safe descent

(continued)

SKILL 26-1
Assisting with Crutch-Walking *(Continued)*

Suggested Action	Reason for Action

Evaluation
- Crutches fit appropriately
- Patient performs crutch-walking gait correctly
- No fatigue or other symptoms develop
- Remains free of injury

Document
- Distance ambulated
- Gait used
- Response of the patient

Sample Documentation

Date and Time   Ambulated length of hospital corridor (approx. 100 feet) using crutches and a three-point non–weight-bearing gait. No breathlessness noted. States upper arms "ache" and attributes discomfort to "muscle strain" from previous day's ambulation efforts. Refuses medication for muscle discomfort. _____ **Signature, Title**

   FOCUS ON OLDER ADULTS

- Walking may be more difficult for older adults because of age-related postural changes. Older adults tend to acquire flexion of the spine as they get older, which may alter their center of gravity.
- Older adults may compensate for skeletal changes by flexing their hips and knees to accommodate for the shift in their center of gravity.
- Postural changes may result in a swaying or shuffling gait among older adults.
- If an unusual gait is noted, it is important to check the patient's feet because some problems may be caused by corns, calluses, bunions, and ingrown toenails.
- Older adults may refuse to use an ambulatory aid because, to them, it signifies dependence and loss of vitality.
- Before discharging an older adult who will be using an ambulatory aid, it is helpful to recommend that someone "fall-proof" their home by removing scatter rugs, extension cords, and the like.

- Older adults who may have difficulty climbing stairs may want to ask family members or friends to rearrange their homes so as to place all necessary furnishings on one level.
- A ramp may help older adults enter and leave their residence more conveniently and safely when using an ambulatory aid.
- Older adults sometimes use a "stop-stop" pattern when using an ambulatory aid—that is, they take one step, then stop, and repeat again. If that is the case, encourage them to ambulate at a smooth, progressive cadence.
- Another bad habit that some older adults develop is picking up and carrying a walker rather than having it make contact with the floor. Again, gentle, but frequent reminders may correct the problem.
- Instruct older adults to remove dust from the rubber tips on ambulatory aids or replace them when they are worn, because these conditions contribute to falls. Handgrips may also need replacing from time to time.

TABLE 26-1. *Crutch-Walking Gaits*

Gait	Indications for Use	Gait Pattern	Illustration
Four-point	Bilateral weakness or disability such as arthritis or cerebral palsy	One crutch, opposite foot, other crutch, remaining foot	
Two-point	Same as for four-point, but patients have more strength, coordination, and balance	One crutch and opposite foot moved in unison, followed by the remaining pair	
Three-point non–weight-bearing	One amputated, injured, or disabled extremity as in a fractured leg or severe ankle sprain	Both crutches move forward followed by the weight-bearing leg	
Three-point partial weight-bearing	Amputee learning to use prosthesis, minor injury to one leg, or previous injury showing signs of healing	Both crutches are advanced with weaker leg, stronger leg is placed parallel to weaker leg	
Swing-through	Injury or disorder affecting one or both legs, such as a paralyzed patient with leg braces or an amputee before being fitted with a prosthesis	Both crutches are moved forward, one or both legs are advanced beyond the crutches	

The Nursing Care Plan for this chapter has been developed to demonstrate how a plan of care is devised for a patient with the nursing diagnosis of Risk for Peripheral Neurovascular Dysfunction. In the NANDA Taxonomy (1994), this problem is defined as "A state in which an individual is at risk of experiencing a disruption in circulation, sensation, or motion of an extremity."

NURSING CARE PLAN:
Risk for Peripheral Neurovascular Dysfunction

Assessment

Subjective Data
States, "After using my crutches, my hands feel numb and like they're falling asleep, but they feel fine a few hours later."

Objective Data
68-year-old woman with a right knee replacement performed 3 days ago. Taught to perform a three-point non–weight-bearing (NWB) gait. Has been observed to rest weight on axillary bars.

Diagnosis

Risk for Peripheral Neurovascular Dysfunction related to compression of brachial nerve.

Plan

Goal
The patient will maintain normal sensation and mobility of fingers and hand.

Orders: 2/07
1. Explain the possible cause for symptoms.
2. Remeasure and fit crutches.
3. Check that there is room for two fingers between the axillae and axillary bars.
4. Reinforce that weight should be supported on handgrips and unoperative limb.
5. Observe performance of three-point NWB gait and monitor subjective symptoms each shift.
6. Substitute a walker for crutches if numbness and tingling reoccur. _____
    C. RUGGLES, RN

Implementation
(Documentation)   2/07   1430   Explained that symptoms may be caused by compressing the nerves in the axillae with the axillary bar of the crutches. Crutches shortened by one hole. Two fingers easily pass between axillae and axillary bar. _____ Y. GARCIA, LPN

Evaluation
(Documentation)   1500   Performs 3-point NWB gait correctly. Hands are warm. Capillary refill <3 sec. Able to move wrist through full range of motion independently. No tingling or numbness noted at this time. _____ Y. GARCIA, LPN

KEY CONCEPTS

- Four activities that help prepare patients for ambulation include performing isometric exercises with the lower limbs, strengthening upper arms, dangling at the bedside, and using a device called a tilt table.
- Two examples of isometric exercises that tone and strengthen lower extremities are quadriceps setting and gluteal setting.
- The upper arms can be strengthened by performing modified push-ups while in a bed or chair.
- Patients are dangled or placed on a tilt table to normalize their blood pressure and help them become acclimated to being upright.
- Two devices that may be used to assist patients with ambulation are parallel bars and walking belts.
- Three types of ambulatory aids are canes, walkers, and crutches.
- Walkers are the most stable form of ambulatory aid, whereas straight canes are the least stable.
- Three characteristics of appropriately fitted crutches are that they (1) permit the patient to stand upright with shoulders relaxed, (2) provide space for two fingers between the axilla and the axillary bar, and (3) facilitate approximately 30° of elbow flexion and slight hyperextension of the wrist.

- Older adults tend to acquire flexion of the spine as they age, which may alter their center of gravity. Consequently, older adults tend to compensate by flexing their hips and knees when walking, and may demonstrate a swaying or shuffling gait.

CRITICAL THINKING EXERCISES

- If you required the use of an ambulatory aid, which type would you prefer, and why? Which type would be least appealing to you, and why?
- Discuss stereotypes that are often applied to people who use an ambulatory aid.

SUGGESTED READINGS

Blaylock B. Mobility and ambulation: not easy tasks for all older adults. Advancing Clinical Care November–December 1991;6:20–21, 41.

Carnevali D, Patrick M. Nursing Management for the Elderly. 3rd ed. Philadelphia: JB Lippincott, 1993.

Farrell J. Nursing Care of the Older Person. Philadelphia: JB Lippincott, 1990.

Kanak MF. Interventions related to patient safety. Nursing Clinics of North America June 1992;27:371–395.

Nursing Procedures. Springhouse, PA: Springhouse Corporation, 1992.

Sumner ED, Simpson WM Jr. Intervention in falls among the elderly. Journal of Practical Nursing June 1992;42:24–34.

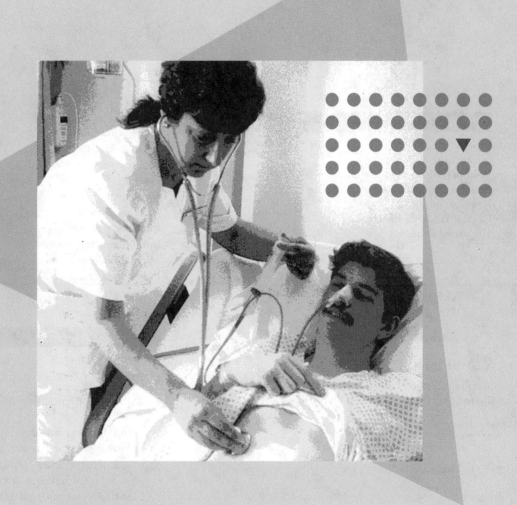

CHAPTER 27

Perioperative Care

NURSING GUIDELINES

Immediate Postoperative Care

SKILLS

Applying Antiembolism Stockings
Performing Presurgical Skin Preparation

NURSING CARE PLAN

Body Image Disturbance

Key Terms

Adynamic Ileus	Outpatient Surgery
Airway Occlusion	Perioperative Care
Anesthesiologist	Plume
Anesthetist	Pneumonia
Antiembolism Stockings	Postanesthesia Care Unit
Atelectasis	Postoperative Care
Autologous Transfusion	Postoperative Period
Depilatory Agent	Preoperative Checklist
Directed Donors	Preoperative Period
Discharge Instructions	Receiving Room

Emboli	Regional Anesthesia
Forced Coughing	Shock
General Anesthesia	Surgical Waiting Room
Hemorrhage	Thromboembolic Disorder
Homans' Sign	(TED) Hose
Hypoxemia	Thrombophlebitis
Inpatient Surgery	Thrombus
Informed Consent	Trendelenburg Position
Intraoperative Period	Urinary Retention
Microabrasions	Wound Infection
Pulmonary Embolus	

Learning Objectives

An understanding of the content within this chapter will be evidenced by the student's ability to:

- Explain the meaning of the term "perioperative care"
- Name three components of perioperative care
- Differentiate inpatient from outpatient surgery
- List at least four advantages of laser surgery
- Discuss two methods for predonating blood
- Identify five major nursing tasks that must be conducted during the immediate preoperative period
- Name three areas of preoperative teaching
- Explain the purpose for using antiembolism stockings
- Name three methods for removing hair when preparing the skin presurgically
- List at least three activities that are verified when completing a preoperative checklist
- Name three parts of a surgical department that are used during the intraoperative period
- Describe the focus of nursing care during the immediate postoperative period

Timby BK: *Fundamental Skills and Concepts in Patient Care, Sixth Edition* © 1996 Lippincott-Raven Publishers

- Give three examples of common postoperative complications
- Describe at least two items of information that are standard when providing discharge instructions for postsurgical patients
- Discuss at least two ways in which the surgical care of older adults differs from that of other age groups

Perioperative care refers to the nursing care that patients receive before, during, and after surgery. This chapter discusses the general responsibilities nurses assume when caring for patients during what are commonly referred to as the preoperative, intraoperative, and postoperative periods.

PREOPERATIVE PERIOD

The **preoperative period** begins when patients are informed that surgery is necessary and ends when they are transported to the operating room. One of the major factors that affects the length of the preoperative period is the urgency with which the surgery must be performed (Table 27-1). The trend today, however, is to keep the perioperative period as short as possible.

Inpatient Surgery

Inpatient surgery is that which is performed on patients who will remain in the hospital for a period of time. All except the sickest of patients are usually admitted the morning of their scheduled surgery. That does not mean, however, that a great deal of preparation has not already taken place.

Many people who have inpatient surgery have undergone prior laboratory and diagnostic tests. Some will have met with an **anesthesiologist**, a physician who administers chemical agents that temporarily eliminate sensation and pain (Table 27-2), or an **anesthetist**, a nurse who administers anesthesia under the direction of a physician. Most also will have received preoperative instructions from either the surgeon's office nurse or a hospital nurse.

The routine does not vary much for patients who are scheduled for surgery as outpatients.

Outpatient Surgery

Outpatient surgery, also called *ambulatory surgery* or *same-day surgery*, refers to those procedures from which patients recover and return home on the same day. Outpatient surgery is usually reserved for those patients who are in an optimum state of health and whose outcome is expected to remain uneventful. Despite its advantages, there are some disadvantages to outpatient surgery as well (Table 27-3).

One of the major factors that has increased outpatient surgery is the advances that have been made in laser surgery.

LASER SURGERY

"Laser" stands for *L*ight *A*mplification by the *S*timulated *E*mission of *R*adiation. To put it more simply, lasers convert a solid, gas, or liquid substance into light. When the light is focused, its energy is converted to heat, which allows it to vaporize tissue and coagulate bleeding vessels.

Laser surgery is being used as an alternative to many previously conventional surgical techniques. Besides its cost effectiveness, laser surgery offers many other advantages, including:

- Reduced need for general anesthesia
- Smaller incisions
- Minimal blood loss
- Reduced swelling
- Less pain
- Decreased wound infections
- Reduced scarring
- Less time recuperating

Laser technology, however, also creates a need for unique safety precautions when it is used.

Laser Safety
Laser safety involves protecting the eyes, preventing fires and reducing heat, and managing the risks from vaporized tissue.

TABLE 27-1. *Types of Surgery According to Their Urgency*		
Type	Description	Example
Optional	Surgery is performed at the request of the patient.	Surgery for cosmetic purposes
Elective	Surgery is planned at the convenience of the patient. Failure to have the surgery does not result in catastrophe.	Surgery for the removal of a superficial cyst
Required	Surgery is necessary and should be done relatively promptly.	Surgery for the removal of a cataract
Urgent	Surgery is required promptly, within a day or two if at all possible.	Surgery for the removal of a malignant tumor
Emergency	Surgery is required immediately for survival.	Surgery to relieve an intestinal obstruction

TABLE 27-2. *Types of Anesthesia*

Type	Description
General Anesthesia	Eliminates all sensation and consciousness or memory for the event
Inhalants	Gas or volatile liquids
Injectables	Given intravenously
Regional Anesthesia	Blocks sensation in an area, but consciousness is unaffected
Spinal (includes epidural)	Eliminates sensation in lower extremities, lower abdomen, pelvis
Local	Blocks sensation in a circumscribed area of skin and subcutaneous tissue
Topical	Inhibits sensation in epithelial tissues like skin and mucous membranes where directly applied

Eye Protection. Depending on the type of laser used, everyone—including the patient—wears goggles. In some cases, prescription glasses with side shields, but not contact lenses, may be allowed.

Fire and Heat Protection. Because lasers produce heat, fire and electrical safety are paramount. Therefore, volatile substances such as alcohol and acetone are not used around lasers. Surgical instruments may be coated black to avoid reflecting scattered light. Sometimes even the patient's teeth may be covered with plastic or a rubber mouth guard to shield metal fillings. For the same reason, no jewelry can be worn.

Vapor Protection. Vaporized tissue is referred to as **plume**. It contains carbon, water, and intact cells. Plume is accompanied by smoke, an offensive odor, and, for some, it causes burning and itching eyes. These effects, however, are nonhazardous and can usually be reduced with the use of smoke evacuators. The greater concern involves the consequences from inhaling plume that may not be totally evacuated.

The airborne cells in the inhaled plume may contain viruses; in theory, the human immunodeficiency virus (HIV) could be transmitted in this way. Although no cases of this have been documented, high-efficiency respirator masks (see Chap. 22) obviously provide more protection than conventional surgical masks.

Because there are potential hazards regardless of whether surgery is performed conventionally or with a laser, it is not unusual for patients to be fearful and anxious. In addition, because surgery is not an everyday event, many patients bring with them a multitude of questions and preconceived ideas about what surgery will involve. Some questions may be answered when the physician provides information for informed consent.

Informed Consent

Informed consent is the permission a person gives after having the risks, benefits, and alternatives explained (see section on Clarifying Explanations, Chap. 13). A signed form, which is usually witnessed by a nurse, is evidence that consent has been obtained (Fig. 27-1).

The rare, but potential, risk for acquiring HIV infection from a blood transfusion is sometimes discussed. Although publicly donated blood is tested for several pathogens, there is still a potential for acquiring a blood-borne disease. Therefore, some surgical patients may wish to arrange predonations of blood.

Predonating Blood

More and more patients are choosing to predonate their own blood. Predonated blood is held on reserve should the patient need a blood transfusion during or after surgery. Receiving one's own blood is called an **autologous transfusion**. Autologous transfusions may

TABLE 27-3. *Advantages and Disadvantages of Outpatient Surgery*

Advantages	Disadvantages
Lowers the surgical costs because of the reduced use of hospital services	Reduces the time for establishing a nurse–patient relationship
Reduces the time spent away from home, school, or place of employment	Requires intensive preoperative teaching in a short amount of time
Interferes less with the patient's usual daily routine	Reduces the opportunity for reinforcement of teaching and for answering questions
Provides the potential for more rest and sleep before and after surgery	Allows for fewer delays in assessing and preparing a patient once he or she arrives for surgery
Allows more opportunity for family contact and support	Requires that care of the patient after discharge be carried out by unskilled people

```
THREE RIVERS AREA HOSPITAL
THREE RIVERS, MICHIGAN   49093

AUTHORIZATION FOR MEDICAL
         AND/OR
  SURGICAL TREATMENT
```

Date **July 18** 19**88**   Time **2:30** a.m. **p.m.**

I, the undersigned, a patient in Three Rivers Area Hospital, hereby authorize Dr. **Robert Morrison, M.D.** (and whomever he may designate as his assistant) to administer such treatment as is necessary, and to perform the following operation **Exploratory Laparotomy and Appendectomy** .

(Name of operation and/or procedure)

and such additional operations or procedures as are considered therapeutically necessary on the basis of findings during the course of said operation, with the following exception, **None** .

I also consent to the administration of such anesthetics as are necessary, with the exception of **None** .

(None, spinal anesthesia, or other)

I hereby certify that I have read and fully understand the above AUTHORIZATION FOR MEDICAL and/or SURGICAL TREATMENT, the reasons why the above named surgery is considered necessary, its advantages and possible complications, if any, as well as possible alternative modes of treatments, which were explained to me by Dr. **Morrison** .

I also certify that no guarantee or assurance has been made as to the results that may be obtained.

Gary Holmes   _Judi Ebbert, RN_
(Patient or nearest relative)   (Witness)

_____
(Relationship)

I hereby certify that I have explained to **Gary Holmes** (a patient at Three Rivers Area Hospital), the reasons why the above named surgery is considered necessary, its advantages and possible complications, if any, as well as possible alternative modes of treatment.

Robert Morrison, M.D.   _7-18-88_
(Surgeon signature)   (Date)

FIGURE 27-1
Surgical consent form.

also be given by recycling blood that is suctioned from the patient during the surgical procedure.

Those who do not meet the criteria for self-donation may preselect their own blood donors from among relatives and friends. These people are known as **directed donors**. Some authorities believe that receiving blood from directed donors is not any safer than receiving blood from strangers. Although predonation of blood is common throughout the United States, criteria for autologous and directed donors (Table 27-4) may vary among regions and, in some cases, even hospitals.

Although some presurgical activities take place weeks in advance, there are others that cannot be performed until just before surgery.

Immediate Preoperative Care

During the immediate preoperative period, that is, the few hours before the actual procedure, several major tasks must be accomplished. They include conducting a nursing assessment, providing preoperative teaching, preparing the skin, and completing the surgical checklist.

TABLE 27-4. *Autologous and Directed Blood Donor Guidelines*	
Common Features	

Collected in blood centers, mobiles, hospitals
Require 72 hours from collection to delivery
Require donor appointment
Will be tested under routine protocol

Autologous Donation	Directed Donation
Donor must weigh 95 pounds.	Donor must weigh 110 pounds.
Donor must be at least 14 years old.	Donor must be at least 17 years old.
Exceptions made in medical history.	Must meet volunteer donor medical history criteria.
Requires physician order.	Patient's physician must be informed of directed donation.
Used only for transfusion to donor.	May be transfused to others if not needed by intended patient.
Blood type does not need to be known at time of donation.	Donors should know blood type of patient.
Units that test positive for disease (other than HIV) will be issued.	Units that test positive for HIV or hepatitis will not be used.
Donation frequency may be greater than 1 unit every 56 days; iron therapy may be necessary and is ordered by physician.	May donate 1 unit every 56 days.
Additional fee to hospital or recipient may be charged for holding blood on reserve.	Additional fees may be charged to the recipient, the donor, or hospital.

Information used with permission of Great Lakes Region, American Red Cross, 1990.

NURSING ASSESSMENT

Nurses share the responsibility for assessing preoperative patients with physicians. Experience has shown that certain risk factors (Display 27-1) increase the possibility that perioperative complications may occur. Some problems that nurses often detect, such as an unexplained elevation in temperature, abnormal laboratory data, current infectious disease, or significant deviations in vital signs, may be sufficient cause for postponing or canceling the surgical procedure.

PREOPERATIVE TEACHING

Before most patients are sent to surgery, they are given instructions on how to perform deep breathing, coughing, and leg exercises.

Deep Breathing

Deep breathing is a form of controlled ventilation that opens and fills small air passages within the lungs (see Chap. 20). It is especially advantageous for surgical patients who undergo general anesthesia or who breathe shallowly afterward because of pain. Breathing deeply reduces the postoperative risk for respiratory complications like **atelectasis**—airless, collapsed lung areas—and **pneumonia**, a lung infection, both of which can lead to hypoxemia.

It is beneficial to practice deep breathing exercises with patients before they actually go to the operating room (Fig. 27-2). Briefly, deep breathing involves inhaling deeply using the abdominal muscles, holding the breath for several seconds, and exhaling slowly. Pursing the lips may extend the period of exhalation.

Incentive spirometers (see Chap. 20) of one kind or another may be used to promote deep breathing.

DISPLAY 27-1. *Surgical Risk Factors*

- Extremes in age
- Dehydration
- Malnutrition
- Obesity
- Smoking
- Diabetes
- Cardiopulmonary disease
- Drug and alcohol abuse
- Bleeding tendencies
- Low hemoglobin and red cells
- Pregnancy
- Fear and foreboding

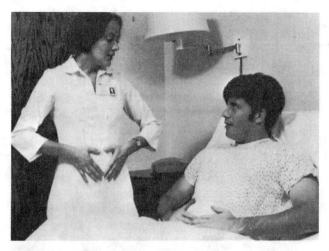

FIGURE 27-2
Teaching deep breathing.

 PATIENT TEACHING FOR PERFORMING FORCED COUGHING

Teach the patient to do the following:
- Sit upright.
- Take a slow, deep breath through the nose.
- Make the lower abdomen rise as much as possible.
- Lean slightly forward.
- Exhale slowly through the mouth.
- Pull the abdomen inward.
- Repeat, but this time cough three times in a row while exhaling.

Coughing

Less than optimal ventilation may be accompanied by the collection of thickened respiratory secretions. Coughing is an automatic method for clearing secretions from the airways. Deep breathing alone may be sufficient to produce a natural cough.

Although **forced coughing**, that which is purposely produced, may not be routinely necessary for all postoperative patients, it is important to prepare patients for the possibility. Forced coughing is most appropriate for those patients who have diminished or moist lung sounds or who raise thick sputum.

Postoperative patients with abdominal or chest incisions are less than enthusiastic about coughing. Expanding the chest and abdomen tends to intensify their pain. However, the discomfort may be reduced if coughing is performed after administering pain medication or if the the incision is splinted during coughing.

Splinting may be accomplished in three different ways: (1) by pressing on the incision with both hands, (2) by pressing on a pillow placed over the incision, and (3) by wrapping a bath blanket about the patient (Fig. 27-3).

Leg Exercises

Leg exercises are helpful for promoting circulation and reducing the possibility of forming a blood clot, or **thrombus**, in the veins. Blood clots form when venous circulation is sluggish and when the fluid component of blood becomes reduced. Both factors are to some degree unavoidable for surgical patients.

Surgical patients experience a reduction in their circulatory volume because of the preoperative restriction of food and fluids and as a consequence of blood loss during surgery. Also, blood tends to pool in the lower extremities as a result of the stationary position maintained during surgery and patients' reluctance to move

about afterward. By teaching patients to perform leg exercises, efforts to reduce circulatory complications can begin as soon as they recover from anesthesia.

Antiembolism Stockings. **Antiembolism stockings** are knee-high or thigh-high elastic stockings. They are sometimes called **TED** (thromboembolic disorder) **hose**. Wearing antiembolism stockings helps to prevent the development of thrombi, which are stationary clots, and **emboli**, which are moving clots. They do so by compressing superficial veins and capillaries, thus redirecting more blood to larger and deeper veins where it flows more effectively toward the heart.

To be effective, antiembolism stockings must fit patients appropriately and be applied correctly (Skill 27-1). Stockings that become soiled or dirty are laundered, during which time a second pair is used. If laundered by hand, the stockings are dried flat to prevent loss of elasticity.

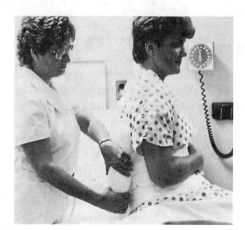

FIGURE 27-3
Using a bath blanket to splint. (Courtesy of Ken Timby.)

◈ PATIENT TEACHING FOR PERFORMING LEG EXERCISES

Teach the patient to do the following:
* Sit with the head slightly raised and the legs extended.
* Point the toes toward the head and then toward the mattress.
* Move both feet in clockwise and then counter-clockwise circles.

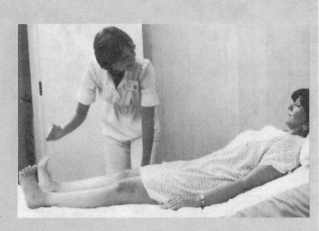

Exercising feet.

* Bend one knee and raise and hold the leg above the mattress for a few seconds.

* Lower the leg *gradually* back to the bed.
* Do the same with the other leg.

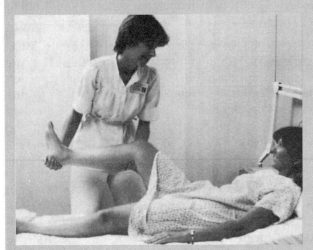

Leg raising.

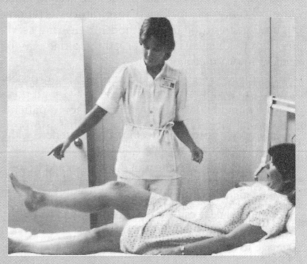

Leg lowering.

* Repeat the exercises five times every 2 hours while awake.

SKIN PREPARATION

Skin preparation involves removing hair and cleansing the skin (Skill 27-2), both of which are reservoirs of microorganisms. By reducing the presence of microorganisms, postoperative wound infections may be avoided.

In some cases, patients may have been instructed to shower with an antimicrobial soap or agent before coming for surgery. Some authorities believe that just washing the skin and hair is sufficient for preventing infections. Although the research is limited to statistically small numbers of patients, infection rates among those patients whose hair has been cleaned, yet re-

tained, do not differ significantly from those in patients from whom body hair was removed.

PREOPERATIVE CHECKLIST

A **preoperative checklist** is a form that identifies essential activities that must be carried out before it is safe to perform surgery. Some activities include verifying that:

* The history and physical examination have been documented.

(text continues on page 557)

SKILL 27-1
Applying Antiembolism Stockings

Suggested Action	Reason for Action
Assessment	
Review the medical orders and nursing plan for care.	Directs patient care
Assess the circulation of the toes and integrity of the skin.	Provides a baseline of data for future comparison
Check **Homans' sign** by dorsiflexing the foot and noting if pain is experienced in the calf, and report a positive finding.	Indicates the possibility of **thrombophlebitis**, inflammation of a vein due to the presence of a thrombus
Measure the patient's leg from the flat of the heel to the bend of the knee or to mid-thigh.	Determines the length needed for knee-high or thigh-high stockings
Measure the calf or thigh circumference.	Determines the size needed
Assess the patient's understanding of the purpose and use of elastic stockings.	Determines the type and amount of health teaching
Check the fit of stockings that are currently being worn.	Identifies the potential complications from tight, loose, or wrinkled stockings
Planning	
Obtain the correct size of stockings before surgery or as soon as possible after they are ordered.	Facilitates early preventive treatment
Plan to remove the stockings for 20 minutes once each shift or at least twice a day and then reapply them.	Facilitates assessment and hygiene
Elevate the legs for at least 15 minutes before applying the stockings, if the patient has been sitting or standing for a period of time.	Promotes venous circulation and avoids trapping venous blood in the lower extremities
Implementation	
Wash and dry the feet.	Removes dirt, skin oil, and some microorganisms
Apply corn starch or talcum powder if desired.	Reduces friction when applying the stockings
Avoid massaging the legs.	Prevents dislodging a thrombus if one is present
Turn the stockings inside out.	Facilitates threading the stockings over the foot and leg

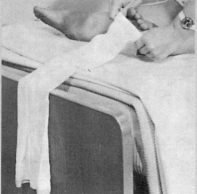

Antiembolism stocking turned inside out.

(continued)

SKILL 27-1
Applying Antiembolism Stockings *(Continued)*

Suggested Action	Reason for Action
Insert the toes and pull the stocking upward a few inches until it covers the foot.	Reduces bunching and bulkiness

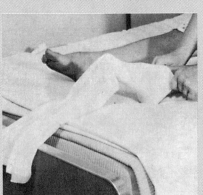

Inserting foot.

Suggested Action	Reason for Action
Gather the remaining length of stocking and pull it upward a few inches at a time.	Eases application and avoids forming wrinkles

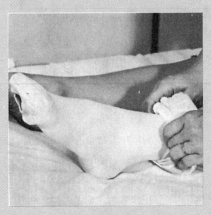

Pulling stocking upward.

Check - 3 times a day take off for 20 minutes

Evaluation
- Skin remains intact and circulation is adequate
- No calf pain on dorsiflexion of the foot
- Stockings are removed and reapplied at least b.i.d.

Document
- Assessment findings
- Removal and reapplication of elastic stockings
- To whom abnormal assessment findings have been reported, and the outcome of the communication

Sample Documentation
Date and Time   Toes are warm. Blood returns to nailbeds within 3 seconds of compression. Skin over legs is smooth and intact. Homans' sign is negative. TED hose applied after bathing. _____ **Signature, Title**

SKILL 27-2
Performing Presurgical Skin Preparation

Suggested Action	Reason for Action

Assessment

Consult the preoperative medical orders or a guide for surgical skin preparation.

Indicates the location and extent of skin preparation according to the planned surgical procedure

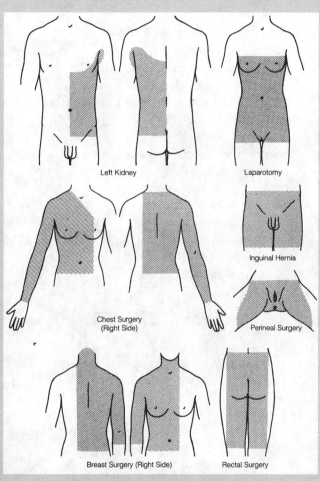

Left Kidney   Laparotomy

Chest Surgery (Right Side)   Inguinal Hernia

Perineal Surgery

Breast Surgery (Right Side)   Rectal Surgery

Guide for surgical skin preparation.

Assess the condition of the skin, looking especially for skin lesions.

Indicates areas that may bleed if irritated or present a reservoir of microorganisms

Explore how much the patient understands about the purpose and extent of skin preparation.

Helps identify the extent and level of health teaching

Planning

Arrange to perform the skin preparation shortly before the patient is scheduled for surgery.

Reduces the interim time during which microorganisms will recolonize the skin

Explain the procedure.

Reduces anxiety and promotes cooperation

Provide an opportunity for the patient to don a hospital gown.

Protects personal clothing and provides access for care

Obtain a skin preparation kit, towels, bath blanket, gloves, electric hair clippers, and source of water.

Provides essential supplies

(continued)

SKILL 27-2
Performing Presurgical Skin Preparation (Continued)

Suggested Action	Reason for Action
Implementation	
Wash your hands and don clean gloves.	Reduces the transmission of microorganisms
Provide privacy.	Shows respect for dignity
Position the patient so that the location for the skin preparation is accessible.	Facilitates performing the procedure
Drape the patient with a bath blanket.	Maintains dignity as well as warmth
Protect the bed with towels or an absorbent pad.	Collects moisture
Use electric hair clippers to remove hair from the designated area.	Prevents **microabrasions**, tiny cuts that may provide an entrance for microorganisms
If policy permits, use a **depilatory agent**, one that chemically removes hair, around bony prominences like the knuckles or ankle.	Removes hair where clippers or razors may be ineffective
Lather the designated skin area with soap or other antimicrobial agent like povidone iodine (Betadine)	Loosens dirt, debris, and microorganisms
Use a safety razor to remove hair, if that is agency policy.	Removes hair and epidermis
Pull the skin taut.	Stretches skin to produce a flatter surface
Move the razor in the direction of hair growth.	Increases effectiveness
Rinse the razor periodically.	Cleans the blade
Rinse the lather and loose hair from the skin.	Removes debris
Relather and scrub the skin from the center of the designated area outward toward the margins.	Follows principles of medical asepsis (see Chap. 21)

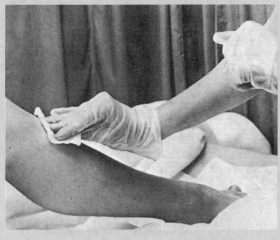

Scrubbing the skin.

Remove the soap, following a similar pattern.	Follows principles of medical asepsis
Dry the leg.	Eliminates moisture
Discard the razor, if one was used, in a biohazard container.	Reduces the potential for injury and transmission of blood-borne viruses

(continued)

SKILL 27-2
Performing Presurgical Skin Preparation (Continued)

Suggested Action	Reason for Action
Deposit the wet towels and bath blanket in a laundry hamper.	Restores comfort and orderliness
Place the used supplies in a waste receptacle.	Confines sources of infectious disease transmission
Remove gloves and wash hands.	Reduces the transmission of microorganisms

Evaluation
- Skin has been prepared according to policy and medical orders
- Skin remains essentially intact

Document
- Assessment findings
- Technique used
- Area prepared

Sample Documentation

Date and Time   Skin areas for laparotomy procedure cleansed with Betadine and shaved. Skin is intact. No evidence of bleeding. _____ **Signature, Title**

- The name of the procedure on the surgical consent form matches that which has been scheduled in the operating room.
- The surgical consent form has been signed and witnessed.
- All laboratory test results have been returned and reported if abnormal.
- The patient is wearing an identification bracelet.
- Allergies have been identified.
- The patient has had nothing by mouth (NPO—*nil per os*) since midnight.
- The skin preparation has been completed.
- Vital signs have been assessed and recorded.
- Nail polish, glasses, contact lenses, and hair pins have been removed.
- Jewelry has been removed or wedding rings have been secured.
- Dentures, if worn, have been removed or not.
- The patient is wearing only a hospital gown and hair cover.
- The patient has urinated.
- The prescribed preoperative medication has been given.

The nurse assigned to the patient is responsible for completing and signing the checklist. It is reviewed by operating room personnel when they arrive to trans-

port the patient. Surgery may be delayed if the checklist is incomplete (Fig. 27-4).

INTRAOPERATIVE PERIOD

The **intraoperative period** is the time during which the patient undergoes surgery. However, before that happens, patients may spend a brief period of time in an area called the receiving room.

Receiving Room

The **receiving room** (Fig. 27-5) is a holding area within the surgery department where patients are observed until the operating room has been cleaned and prepared for surgery.

It may be the practice in some hospitals to administer the preoperative medication when patients reach the receiving room. This practice coordinates the patient's sedation more closely with the actual time that surgery will take place.

Skin preparation may be delayed until this time as well. There is a direct relationship between the time after the skin preparation is performed and the rate of microbial proliferation, especially when skin preparation has involved shaving with a razor. The basis for

PREOPERATIVE CHECK LIST

DATE

NURSING UNIT CHECK LIST	YES	NO
1. DIAL BATH GIVEN	✓	
2. ORAL HYGIENE	✓	
3. MAKE-UP REMOVED	✓	
4. BOBBY PINS, COMBS, HAIR PIECES REMOVED	✓	
5. CARDIAC CATHETERIZATION FORM GIVEN TO PATIENT AND/OR FAMILY	✓	
6. VOIDED	✓	
7. RINGS, JEWELRY, RELIGIOUS MEDALS, OR OTHER ITEMS REMOVED (MAY BE WORN DURING CARDIAC CATHETERIZATION) WHEN REMOVED, DISPOSITION IS: *IN HOSPITAL SAFE. WEDDING RING TIED TO FINGER*		
8. ALLERGIES NOTED ON FRONT OF CHART	✓	
9. PREOPERATIVE MEDICINE GIVEN AS ORDERED	✓	
10. WHERE FAMILY CAN BE LOCATED DURING AND IMMEDIATELY AFTER SURGERY *WAITING ROOM AT RECOVERY ROOM*		

NURSING UNIT AND OPERATING ROOM NURSES CHECK LIST	YES	NO
11. GROIN PREP DONE (WHEN ORDERED) — CARDIAC CATHETERIZATION	✓	
12. CONSENTS: SURGERY	✓	
OB CONSULTATION OR SPECIAL		
13. URINALYSIS	✓	
14. HEMATOLOGY	✓	
15. HISTORY AND PHYSICAL	✓	
16. RETENTION CATHETER		✓
17. DENTURES (BRIDGES, PLATES, PARTIALS) (MAY BE WORN DURING CARDIAC CATHETERIZATION)		
REMOVED	✓	
PERMANENT		
CAPS	✓	
LOOSE TEETH		
18. PROSTHESIS		
ARTIFICIAL EYE	*NONE*	OUT
CONTACT LENS		OUT
PACEMAKER		
OTHER		

B. H. Becker, R.N.
R.N. OR TEAM LEADER SIGNATURE
R. Green R.N
CIRCULATING NURSE SIGNATURE

PATIENT IDENTIFICATION ON UNIT

A. PERSON FROM SURGERY CALLING FOR PATIENT
1. ASK FOR PATIENT BY NAME
2. CHECK PATIENT'S CHART
3. CHECK PATIENT'S CHART WITH CALL SLIP (NOT NECESSARY WITH CARDIAC CATHETERIZATION)

B. PERSON FROM UNIT MUST ACCOMPANY
1. ASK PATIENT HIS/HER NAME
   ASK PATIENT HIS/HER DOCTOR'S NAME
2. CHECK CHART FACE SHEET FOR PATIENT'S NAME NAME, AND HOSPITAL NUMBER WITH PATIENT IDENTIBAND
3. CHECK CALL SLIP WITH IDENTIBAND (NOT NECESSARY FOR CARDIAC CATHETERIZATION)

SIGNATURES: *B. H. Becker, R.N.*
NURSING UNIT PERSONNEL
C.R. Johnson
SURGERY PERSONNEL

SPECIAL COMMENTS TO OPERATING ROOM AND RECOVERY ROOM NURSES FROM NURSING UNIT: (PLEASE SIGN YOUR COMMENT)

Pt. very worried that she will need a radical mastectomy B.H. Becker, R.N.

PREOPERATIVE CHECK LIST

FIGURE 27-4
Preoperative checklist.

this lies in the fact that microbes tend to grow even more vigorously in the plasma-rich environment of abraded skin.

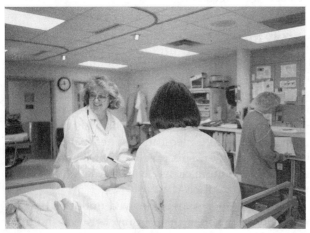

FIGURE 27-5
Receiving room. (Courtesy of Ken Timby.)

Operating Room

Eventually patients are taken to the operating room, where their care and safety are in the hands of a team of experts that includes physicians and nurses. Meanwhile, the family or friends of surgical patients may be directed to a surgical waiting area.

Surgical Waiting Area

The **surgical waiting area** is a special room where visitors who have accompanied the surgical patient may find comfort, support, and information about how surgery is progressing. Many agencies provide access to food and beverages, coffee, public telephones, television, and magazines in this area. Quite often, the surgeon comes here immediately after the procedure to communicate directly with those who are concerned about the welfare of the patient.

POSTOPERATIVE PERIOD

The **postoperative period** begins when the patient is transported from the operating room to the postanesthesia care unit (Fig. 27-6). The **postanesthesia care unit (PACU)**, also known as *postanesthesia reacting* (PAR) room or the *recovery room*, is an area within the surgical department where patients are intensively monitored to ensure their safe recovery from anesthesia. During this time, nurses on the general patient unit prepare for the patient's extended postoperative care.

Postoperative Care

Postoperative care, in general, refers to the care after surgery until the patient is discharged. However, the focus tends to be somewhat different during the immediate postoperative period than it is later, when patients are more stable.

Immediate Postoperative Care

The immediate postoperative period refers to the first 24 hours after the patient's surgery. During this period of time, nurses are involved in preparing the room for the return of the patient from surgery and monitoring the patient for potential complications.

PREPARING THE ROOM

While patients are in surgery, their beds are made with fresh linen. The top linen is folded toward the foot or side of the bed and left in high position to facilitate transferring the patient from the stretcher. Additional blankets often are provided because some patients feel quite cold as a result of being quiet and inactive.

Supplies and equipment that facilitate patient care may be assembled ahead of time. Some items that may

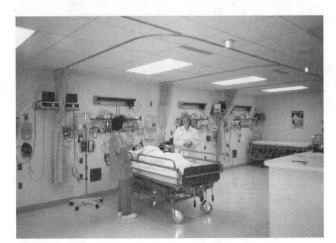

FIGURE 27-6
Postanesthesia care unit. (Courtesy of Ken Timby.)

be needed include oxygen equipment (see Chap. 20), a pole or infusion device for intravenous fluids (see Chap. 15), an emesis basin in case the patient feels nauseous, paper tissues, and a device for collecting and measuring urine (see Chap. 30). Suction canisters may also be necessary for patients who have gastric tubes (see Chap. 29).

MONITORING FOR COMPLICATIONS

Postoperative patients are at risk for many complications (Table 27-5), some of which are more likely to occur soon after surgery. Therefore, a safe postoperative recovery is facilitated by making frequent, focused assessments of the patient and equipment.

NURSING GUIDELINES FOR IMMEDIATE POSTOPERATIVE CARE

- Obtain a summary report from a PACU nurse.
  Rationale: Provides current assessment data concerning the progress of the patient
- Check the postoperative medical orders on the chart.
  Rationale: Provides instructions for individualized care
- Assist PACU personnel transfer the patient to bed.
  Rationale: Provides for continuous observation and care
- Observe the patient's respiratory pattern and auscultate the lungs.
  Rationale: Ensures breathing is maintained, a priority for care
- Check oxygen saturation using a pulse oximeter if the patient seems hypoxic (see Chap. 20).
  Rationale: Indicates the quality of internal respiration
- Administer oxygen if the oxygen saturation is less than 90%, or if prescribed by the physician.
  Rationale: Increases the oxygen that is available for binding with hemoglobin and becoming dissolved in the plasma
- Note the patient's level of consciousness and response to stimulation.
  Rationale: Indicates neurologic status
- Orient the patient and instruct him or her to take several deep breaths, as taught before surgery.
  Rationale: Improves ventilation and gas exchange
- Check vital signs.
  Rationale: Provides data for assessing the patient's current general condition
- Repeat vital sign assessment at least every 15 minutes until they are stable; then take them every hour to every 4 hours depending on the condition of the patient or on the medical orders.
  Rationale: Provides comparative assessment data

- Check the incisional area and the dressing for drainage.
  Rationale: Provides data concerning the status of blood loss
- Inspect all tubes, insertion sites, and connections.
  Rationale: Ensures that equipment is functioning appropriately
- Check the type of intravenous fluid, rate of administration, and volume that remains.
  Rationale: Provides data regarding fluid therapy
- Monitor urination; report a failure to void within 8 hours of surgery.
  Rationale: Indicates urinary retention
- Auscultate bowel sounds.
  Rationale: Provides data concerning bowel motility

- Assess the patient's level of pain and its location and characteristics.
  Rationale: Indicates the need for analgesia
- Administer analgesic drugs according to prescribed medical orders if it is safe to do so.
  Rationale: Relieves pain
- Remind the patient to perform leg exercises or apply antiembolism stockings.
  Rationale: Promotes circulation
- Use a side-lying position if the patient is lethargic or unresponsive.
  Rationale: Facilitates maintaining an open airway
- Raise the side rails unless providing direct care.
  Rationale: Ensures safety
- Fasten the signal device within the patient's reach.
  Rationale: Facilitates a means for communication and obtaining assistance

TABLE 27-5. *Postoperative Complications*

Complication	Description	Treatment
Airway occlusion	Obstruction of throat	Tilt head and lift chin Insert an artificial airway (see Chap. 36)
Hemorrhage	Severe, rapid blood loss	Control bleeding Administer intravenous fluid Replace blood
Shock	Inadequate blood flow	Place in **Trendelenburg** position

Trendelenburg position.

		Replace fluids Administer oxygen Give emergency drugs
Pulmonary embolus	Obstruction of circulation through the lung due to a wedged blood clot that began as a thrombus	Give oxygen Administer anticoagulant drugs
Hypoxemia	Inadequate oxygenation of blood	Give oxygen
Adynamic ileus	Lack of bowel motility	Treat cause Give nothing by mouth Insert a nasogastric tube and connect to suction Administer intravenous fluid
Urinary retention	Inability to void	Insert a catheter
Wound infection	Proliferation of pathogens at or beneath the incision	Cleanse with antimicrobial agents Open and drain incision Administer antibiotics
Dehiscence	Separation of incision	Reinforce wound edges Apply a binder (see Chap. 28)
Evisceration	Protrusion of abdominal organs through separated wound	Cover with wet dressing Reapproximate wound

Facilitating Recovery

All surgical patients are ambulated as soon as possible. Most are assisted from bed the evening of surgery.

Food and oral fluids are withheld until patients are awake, free of nausea and vomiting, and their bowel sounds are active. It is also essential to monitor fluid intake and output to make sure patients are adequately hydrated.

The condition of the wound and characteristics of drainage are assessed each shift. Dressings are reinforced or changed if they become saturated. Eventually, sutures or staples are removed (see Chap. 28). Most inpatients are discharged within 3 to 5 days of surgery to continue their recuperation at home.

Discharge Instructions

Discharge instructions are the directions the nurse provides patients for managing their self-care and medical follow-up. Common areas that are addressed when discharging surgical patients include:

- How to care for the incision site
- Signs of complications to report
- What drugs to use for relieving pain
- How to self-administer prescribed drugs
- When presurgical activity can be resumed
- If and how much weight can be lifted
- Which foods to consume or avoid
- When and where to return for a medical appointment

NURSING IMPLICATIONS

When caring for surgical patients, nurses are faced with unique patient care problems. Some nursing diagnoses that are commonly identified during the perioperative period include those in the accompanying Applicable Nursing Diagnoses.

APPLICABLE NURSING DIAGNOSES

- Knowledge Deficit
- Fear
- Pain
- Impaired Skin Integrity
- Risk for Infection
- Risk for Fluid Volume Deficit
- Ineffective Breathing Pattern
- Ineffective Airway Clearance
- Impaired Gas Exchange
- Body Image Disturbance
- Ineffective Management of Therapeutic Regimen: Individual

FOCUS ON OLDER ADULTS

- Older adult patients who undergo surgery are likely to have several chronic medical problems as well. According to the U.S. Senate Special Committee on Aging (1991), older adults averaged four diagnoses at the time of their discharge.
- Adults older than the age of 65 years are hospitalized three times as often, stay 50% longer, and use twice as many prescription drugs as adults younger than 65 years (U.S. Senate Special Committee on Aging, 1991).
- The average length of hospital stay was 8.2 days for patients between the ages of 65 and 74 years, and 9.5 days for those who are older (U.S. Senate Special Committee on Aging, 1991).
- Older adults are likely to be extremely self-conscious or sensory deprived if glasses, hearing aids, and dentures are removed before surgery. It may be helpful to collaborate with operating room personnel regarding their removal shortly before or during the administration of anesthesia.
- The period of fluid restriction before surgery may be shortened for older adults to reduce their risk for dehydration and hypotension.
- The cardiac status of older adults must be monitored carefully after surgery because they may not be able to circulate or eliminate intravenous fluids that are given at standard rates.
- Chronic use of aspirin by patients who have inflammatory conditions, like arthritis, makes them prone to postoperative bleeding. Aspirin use should be discontinued at least a week before elective surgery.
- Older adults may not demonstrate significant postoperative signs of an infection. Even a slight elevation in temperature may be cause for concern.
- Older adults may require extended or home care at the time of a surgical discharge if they are unable to manage their recuperation independently.
- Well before discharge, it is important to assess the extent of the older adult's support system regarding the ability to provide assistance after the patient's discharge.
- Five percent of patients older than 70 years of age experience dehiscence after abdominal surgery (Carnevali & Patrick, 1993).
- Wound healing is much slower in older adults because of impaired circulation, oxygenation, hydration, and nutrition.

NURSING CARE PLAN:
Body Image Disturbance

Assessment	**Subjective Data** States, "I hate myself for agreeing to this operation. This 'thing' fills up, it bulges, and smells. No one will ever want to come near me again." **Objective Data** 31-year-old woman with prior history of ulcerative colitis admitted 4 days ago for colectomy with ileostomy. Asks that room freshener be sprayed frequently. Applies perfume heavily. Positions herself more than 5 feet from visitors.
Diagnosis	Body Image Disturbance related to fear of rejection based on altered elimination.
Plan	**Goal** The patient will demonstrate acceptance and less self-consciousness about ostomy by interacting with a visitor within 3 feet by 10/9.

Orders: 10/5
1. Spend at least 15 minutes with patient midmorning, midafternoon, and early evening without performing direct care to communicate acceptance. During interaction:
   a. Sit within 3 feet to show by example that closeness is not a problem.
   b. Empathize with the patient; agree that this change is difficult to accept.
   c. Offer to contact another person with an ostomy through the United Ostomy Association to share mutual feelings and experiences while still in the hospital.
   d. Offer referral to an enterostomal nurse therapist for suggestions on odor-control techniques.
2. During ostomy teaching sessions and care of the stoma, implement the following:
   a. Avoid facial expressions that may communicate disgust or repulsion with the care of the ileostomy.
   b. Use terminology such as "your stoma" (avoiding any depersonalized or pet names) to promote the concept that the stoma is not a separate entity but rather part of her natural body. _____ N. NUNN, RN

Implementation *(Documentation)*	10/5	1330	Interacted socially for approx. 15 min. Sat within 3 feet. Patient moved her own chair away to provide more distance. Reinforced that adjusting to an ostomy is difficult. Explained the purpose of the United Ostomy Association and gave booklet, "So You Have. . .Or Will Have An Ostomy." Offered to contact another person with an ostomy or the enterostomal therapist. _____ G. ORSINI, LPN
Evaluation *(Documentation)*	10/6	1030	Demonstrated stoma care. Used the term "your ostomy" and "your appliance" during teaching session. Pt. used the term "Mt. Vesuvius" when referring to stoma. Page mark noted in ostomy booklet indicating that reading has begun. States "I don't know if talking with someone else will help. Not everyone has friends like mine." _____ G. ORSINI, LPN

The accompanying Nursing Care Plan has been developed to show how the nursing process is used to identify and resolve a diagnosis of Body Image Disturbance. NANDA defines this problem in its 1994 taxonomy as, "A disruption in the way one perceives one's body image." This diagnosis is especially pertinent to surgical patients who have in some way had their appearance altered.

KEY CONCEPTS

- Perioperative care refers to the nursing care that patients receive before, during, and after surgery.
- Perioperative care spans the preoperative, intraoperative, and postoperative periods.
- Inpatient surgery is that which is performed on patients who will remain in the hospital for a period of time. Outpatient surgery refers to those procedures from which patients recover and return home on the same day.
- Laser surgery, which can be performed on an outpatient basis, has several advantages, some of which are that it is cost effective; requires smaller incisions; results in minimal blood loss; and is accompanied by less pain.
- Some patients choose to reserve blood, if it is needed during or after surgery, by predonating their own blood or asking specific donors to do so.
- Five major tasks that must be completed during the immediate preoperative period include: conducting a nursing assessment, providing preoperative teaching, preparing the skin, and completing the surgical checklist.
- All preoperative patients are taught how to perform deep breathing, coughing, and leg exercises.
- Antiembolism stockings are worn by surgical patients to prevent the development of thrombi, which are stationary clots, and emboli, which are moving clots.
- During preoperative skin preparation, hair can be removed with electric clippers, depilatory agents, or a safety razor.
- Three examples of information verified on a preoperative checklist are (1) that the surgical consent form has been signed and witnessed, (2) that the patient is wearing an identification bracelet, and (3) that all laboratory test results have been returned and reported if abnormal.
- The receiving room, the operating room, and the surgical waiting room are three areas in the surgical department that are used during the intraoperative period.
- During the immediate postoperative care period, nurses focus on preparing the patient's room and monitoring for complications.

- Three common postoperative complications include airway obstruction, hemorrhage, and shock.
- When surgical patients are discharged, among other things, they are instructed on how to care for their incisional site, signs of complications to report, and how to self-administer prescription drugs.
- Older adults have unique surgical needs and problems. For example, the period of fluid restriction before surgery may be shortened for older adults to reduce their risk for dehydration and hypotension. Also, the cardiac status of older adults must be monitored carefully after surgery because they may not be able to circulate or eliminate intravenous fluids given at standard rates.

CRITICAL THINKING EXERCISES

- You assess a postoperative patient and obtain the following data: blood pressure 102/64, pulse rate 90, respirations 32 and shallow, responds when shaken, experiencing nausea. What finding is most serious at this time, and what nursing action(s) would be appropriate?
- A preoperative patient who is a Native American wants you to attach a dream catcher, a circular object with a woven web, to the intravenous pole. Discuss how you would respond to the patient's request.

SUGGESTED READINGS

Allison S, Latham G. Same day admission surgery. Canadian Nurse December 1991;87:25.

Brockopp DY, Warden S, Colclough G. Nursing knowledge: acute postoperative pain management in the elderly. Journal of Gerontological Nursing November 1993;19:31–37.

Cahill-Wright C. Managing postoperative pain. Nursing December 1991;21:42–45.

Carnevali D, Patrick M. Nursing Management for the Elderly. 3rd ed. Philadelphia: JB Lippincott, 1993.

Cushing M. Back to (PACU) basics . . . the legal side. American Journal of Nursing July 1992;92:21–22.

Kemmett V. Fit to consent? . . . caring for patients with mental illness who have to undergo surgery can be difficult. Nursing Times June 16–22, 1993;89:40–42

Kirkpatrick L, Kleinbeck SVM. Surgery trends change nursing care: operating room nurses share new procedures that will affect home healthcare. Home Healthcare Nurse November–December 1991;9:13–20.

Lawler M. Preventing postop complications: managing other complications. Nursing November 1991;21:33, 40–46.

McConnell EA. Preventing postop complications: minimizing respiratory problems. Nursing November 1991;21:33–39.

Metzler DJ, Fromm CG. Laying out a care plan for the elderly postoperative patient. Nursing April 1993;23:66–68, 71, 73–74.

United States Senate Special Committee on Aging. Aging Americans: Trends and Projections. Publication No. (FCoA) 91-28001. Washington, DC: U.S. Department of Health and Human Services, 1991.

CHAPTER 28

Wound Care

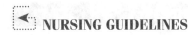
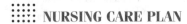
Learning Objectives

An understanding of the content within this chapter will be evidenced by the student's ability to:

- Explain the meaning of the term "wound"
- Discuss the purpose of the inflammatory response
- Name five signs and symptoms that are classically associated with the inflammatory response
- Discuss the purpose of phagocytosis and two cells that perform this activity
- Name three types of wound repair processes
- Explain first, second, and third intention healing
- Name two types of wounds
- List at least five risk factors for developing pressure sores
- Discuss three techniques for preventing pressure sores
- Give at least three purposes for using a dressing
- Discuss an advantage in keeping wounds moist
- Explain the purpose of a drain and name two types
- Name two ways that surgical wounds are held together until they heal

- Explain one reason for using a bandage and binder
- Name one type of binder and the purpose for its use
- Explain the purpose for administering an irrigation
- List four structures that are commonly irrigated
- Give two reasons to apply heat and two for cold
- List at least five methods for providing heat or cold applications

The body has remarkable ability to recover when tissue is injured. This chapter discusses several methods through which the body repairs damaged tissue. It also describes nursing actions that can be taken to prevent tissue injury from occurring and those that support the healing process.

WOUNDS

A **wound** is damaged skin or soft tissue. It occurs as a result of **trauma**, a general term referring to injury. Tissue trauma may occur, for example, from cuts, blows, poor circulation, strong chemicals, and excessive heat or cold. The trauma produces two basic types of wounds: open and closed (Table 28-1).

Open Wounds

An **open wound** is one in which the surface of the skin or mucous membrane is no longer intact. Such a wound may be caused accidentally, or it may be intentional, such as an incision made by a surgeon.

Closed Wounds

A **closed wound** is one in which there is no opening in the skin or mucous membrane. Closed wounds occur more often from blunt trauma or pressure.

Regardless of the type of wound, the body immediately responds first by initiating the inflammatory response and then by repairing the damage.

THE INFLAMMATORY RESPONSE

The **inflammatory response** (Fig. 28-1) is a physiologic defense that occurs when tissue is injured. Its purpose is to limit tissue damage, remove injured cells and debris, and prepare the wound for healing.

The inflammatory response progresses in several phases. During the first phase, local changes occur.

Local Changes

When an injury occurs, the damaged cells' membranes immediately become more permeable, allowing them to release chemical substances contained within. These chemicals trigger multiple responses to limit the effects of the injury. As a result of their actions, the characteristic signs and symptoms of inflammation, *swelling, redness, warmth, pain*, and *decreased function* are produced.

The second wave of defense occurs when white cells, known as **leukocytes** or **macrophages**, migrate to the site of injury as the body produces more and more to take their place in blood and tissue.

Leukocytosis and Phagocytosis

Leukocytosis is a term that describes a state in which there is an increased production of white blood cells. Leukocytosis is confirmed and monitored by counting the number and type of white blood cells in a sample of the patient's blood. The laboratory test is called a WBC (white blood cell) count and differential. A rise in white

TABLE 28-1. *Types of Wounds*	
	Description
Open Wounds	
Incision	A clean separation of skin and tissue with smooth, even edges
Laceration	A separation of skin and tissue in which the edges are torn and irregular
Abrasion	A wound in which the surface layers of skin are scraped away
Avulsion	Stripping away of large areas of skin and underlying tissue, leaving cartilage and bone exposed
Ulceration	A shallow crater in which skin or mucous membrane is missing
Puncture	An opening of skin, underlying tissue, or mucous membrane caused by a narrow, sharp, pointed object
Closed Wounds	
Contusion	Injury to soft tissue underlying the skin from the force of contact with a hard object; sometimes called a bruise

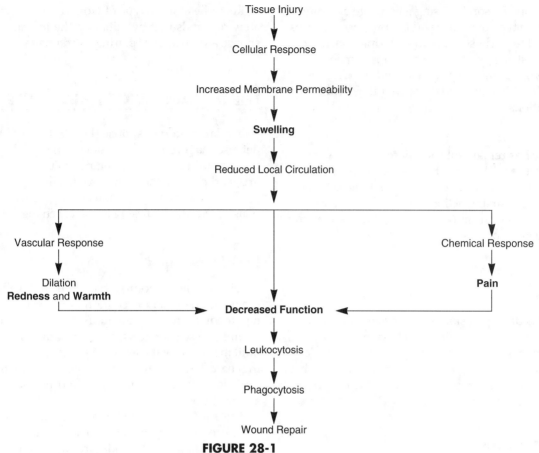

FIGURE 28-1
The inflammatory response.

blood cells, particularly neutrophils and monocytes, suggests that an inflammatory and, in some cases, an infectious process is occurring.

Neutrophils and monocytes, specific kinds of white blood cells, are primarily responsible for engulfing pathogens, coagulated blood, and cellular debris, a process called **phagocytosis**. They clean the area of injury and prepare the site for wound repair.

WOUND REPAIR

Wound repair depends on the magnitude of tissue damage. In general, the integrity of the skin and damaged tissue is restored by either resolution, regeneration, or scar formation.

Resolution is a reparative process in which cells that are slightly injured recover and reestablish their normal function. **Regeneration** occurs when some cells are destroyed and duplicates are produced to take their place. However, when cells are extensively destroyed and there is no potential for regeneration, the integrity of the area is restored by replacing it with scar tissue, a process referred to as **scar formation**.

Scar Tissue

Scar tissue, in its early stage, is highly vascularized connective tissue that contains **collagen**, a protein substance that is tough and inelastic. The initial scar tissue is referred to as **granulation tissue**. Granulation tissue can be recognized by the bright pink to red color produced by the extensive projections of capillaries into the area. The color gradually fades when the network of capillaries regresses.

The amount of scar tissue that is formed depends on whether the wound heals by first, second, or third intention (Fig. 28-2).

FIRST INTENTION HEALING

First intention healing, also called *primary intention*, occurs when wound edges are directly next to one another. Because the space is narrow, only a small amount of scar tissue forms. Most surgical wounds that are closely approximated heal by first intention.

SECOND INTENTION HEALING

Second intention healing occurs when the wound edges are widely separated. Because the margins of the

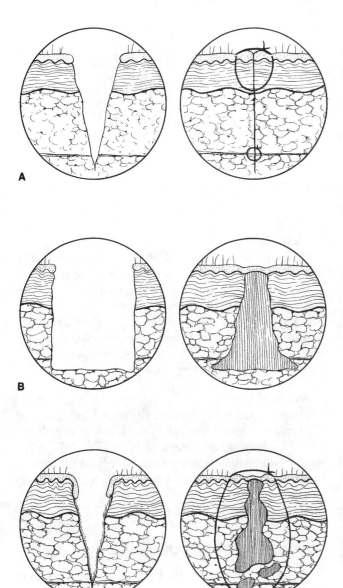

FIGURE 28-2
(*A*) First intention healing (*B*) Second intention healing (*C*) Third intention healing.

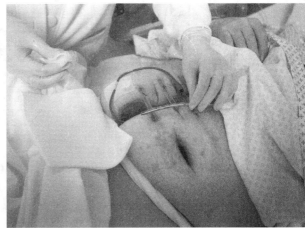

FIGURE 28-3
Example of third intention healing. (Courtesy of Ken Timby.)

ally is fairly deep and likely to contain extensive drainage and tissue debris. To speed healing, drainage devices may be placed in the wound, or it may be packed with absorbent gauze.

Healing, whether by first, second, or third intention, is further affected by a number of factors that may complicate wound care. These factors may include:

- Extent of injury
- Quality of circulation
- Type of injury
- Amount of foreign debris
- Infection
- Health of the patient

WOUND CARE

Wound care involves those techniques that promote healing. The approach may be somewhat different for tissue damaged by pressure as opposed to wounds that are surgically created.

Pressure Sores

The term **pressure sore**, or *decubitus ulcer*, refers to a specific tissue injury caused by an impairment in blood supply. Pressure sores usually appear over bony prominences of the lower spine, posterior pelvis, and hips, as well as the heels, elbows, shoulder blades, ears, and back of the head.

The tissues in these areas are particularly vulnerable because they often have less body fat to act as a pressure-absorbing cushion. Consequently, the tissue is particularly vulnerable to being compressed between the bony mass and a rigid surface like a chair or bed. Should the compression reduce the blood pressure in local capillaries below 32 mm Hg for a prolonged period of time, the cells die from lack of oxygen.

wound are not in direct contact with one another, granulation tissue must extend from the edges toward the center, resulting in a broader and deeper scar.

Healing by second intention is a slow process that may be prolonged by the presence of drainage from an infection or other wound debris. Furthermore, because granulation tissue is fragile while it is being formed, wound care must be performed cautiously to avoid disrupting the healing wound.

THIRD INTENTION HEALING

Third intention healing occurs when a widely separated wound is later brought together with some type of closure material (Fig. 28-3). This type of wound usu-

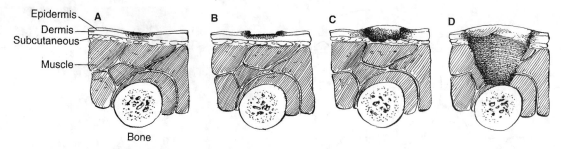

Epidermis
Dermis
Subcutaneous

Muscle

Bone

FIGURE 28-4
Pressure sore stages (A) Stage I (B) Stage II (C) Stage III (D) Stage IV.

The care and healing of pressure sores depend on the stage of injury that has occurred.

STAGES OF PRESSURE SORES

Pressure sores are categorized into four stages according to the extent of tissue injury that has occurred (Fig. 28-4). Without aggressive nursing care, incipient pressure sores may easily progress to stages that are much more serious.

Stage I

Stage I pressure sores are characterized by redness. Cellular damage has occurred if the skin fails to resume its normal color when the pressure is relieved.

Stage II

A Stage II pressure sore is red and is accompanied by blistering or a shallow break in the skin, sometimes described as a **skin tear**. Impairment of the skin may lead to colonization and infection of the wound.

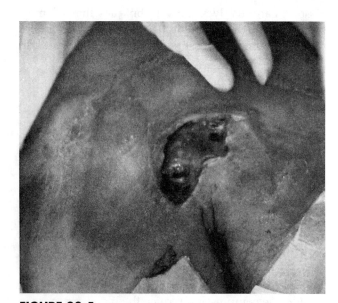

FIGURE 28-5
Example of stage IV pressure sore. (Courtesy of E. R. Squibb & Sons, Inc., Princeton, NJ.)

Stage III

Pressure sores classified as stage III are those in which the superficial skin impairment progresses to a shallow crater that extends to the subcutaneous tissue. Stage III pressure sores may be accompanied by **serous drainage** from leaking plasma or **purulent drainage**, white- or green-tinged fluid, caused by a wound infection. Although a stage III pressure sore is a significant injury, the area is relatively painless.

Stage IV

Stage IV pressure sores are the most traumatic and life threatening. At this stage, the tissue is deeply ulcerated, exposing muscle and bone (Fig. 28-5). The dead tissue may produce a rank odor. Local infection, which is the rule rather than the exception, easily spreads throughout the body, causing a potentially fatal condition referred to as **sepsis**.

PREVENTING PRESSURE SORES

Optimally, it would be best to prevent pressure sores rather than aggressively treat the wound once it has occurred. Prevention first involves identifying patients who are at greatest risk for pressure sores (Display 28-1), and, second, implementing measures that reduce conditions under which they are likely to form.

NURSING GUIDELINES FOR PREVENTING PRESSURE SORES

- Change the at-risk patient's position as frequently as every hour or two.
  Rationale: Relieves pressure and restores circulation
- Avoid using plastic-covered pillows when positioning patients.
  Rationale: Raises skin temperature and prevents evaporation of perspiration, both of which contribute to the growth of microorganisms

- Use a lateral oblique position (see Chap. 23) rather than the conventional lateral position when using a side-lying position.
  Rationale: Reduces the potential for pressure on vulnerable bony prominences
- Massage bony prominences *if the skin blanches with pressure relief.*
  Rationale: Improves circulation to normal tissue; but will further damage pressure sores that are already established
- Keep the skin clean, especially when patients are unable to control their bladder or bowel function.
  Rationale: Removes substances that may injure the skin chemically
- Use a moisturizing skin cleanser rather than soap, if possible.
  Rationale: Maintains skin hydration and avoids altering the skin's natural acidity, which serves to protect it from bacterial colonization
- Rinse and dry the skin well.
  Rationale: Removes chemical residues and surface moisture
- Use pressure-relieving mattresses like an alternating air mattress, or a specialized bed like the Clinitron bed (see Chap. 23).
  Rationale: Maintains capillary blood flow
- Pad body areas such as the heels, ankles, and elbows that are vulnerable to friction and pressure (Fig. 28-6).
  Rationale: Prevents friction and adds a cushioning layer over the bony prominence.
- Use seat-cushioning devices like a gel-filled pad when patients sit for extended periods of time.
  Rationale: Distributes pressure over a wider area; relieves direct pressure on the coccyx
- Keep the head at ≤ 30° of elevation when in bed.
  Rationale: Prevents **shearing force**, which is an effect that moves layers of tissue in opposite directions from each other—a situation that occurs when patients slide downward

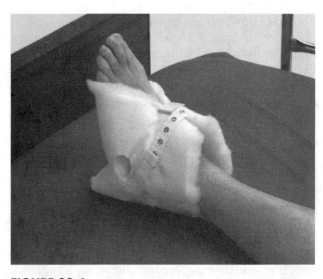

FIGURE 28-6
Heel and ankle protection. (Courtesy of J.T. Posey Company, Arcadia, CA.)

Surgical Wounds

Surgical wounds result from incising tissue with a laser (see Chap. 27) or an instrument called a scalpel. Surgical wound care involves the use of dressings, caring for drains, removing sutures or staples, applying bandages and binders, and administering irrigations.

DRESSINGS

A **dressing** is a substance that covers a wound. When used, a dressing may serve one or more purposes, such as:

- Keeping the wound clean
- Absorbing drainage
- Controlling bleeding
- Protecting the wound from injury
- Holding medication in place
- Maintaining a moist environment

There are several different types of dressings, depending on the purpose for their use.

Types of Dressings

The most common wound coverings include gauze, transparent, and hydrocolloid dressings. All dressing materials come in a variety of sizes that allow for customizing their application.

Gauze Dressings. Gauze dressings are made of woven cloth fibers. Their highly absorbent nature makes them ideal for covering fresh wounds that are likely to bleed or those that exude drainage.

Unfortunately, gauze dressings interfere with wound assessment. In addition, unless ointment is used on the wound, or the gauze is lubricated with an ointment like petroleum jelly, granulation tissue may adhere to the gauze fibers.

DISPLAY 28-1. *Risk Factors for Developing Pressure Sores*	
• Inactivity	• Incontinence
• Immobility	• Vascular disease
• Malnutrition	• Localized edema
• Emaciation	• Dehydration
• Diaphoresis	• Sedation

Gauze dressings are usually secured with tape. If gauze dressings need frequent changing, **Montgomery straps**, strips of tape with eyelets, may be used (Fig. 28-7). Some other method may be necessary if patients are allergic to tape (see the section on Bandages and Binders later in this chapter).

Transparent Dressings. Transparent dressings are clear wound coverings. One of their chief advantages is that they facilitate wound assessment without removing the dressing itself. In addition, they are less bulky than gauze and do not require tape because they consist of a single sheet of adhesive material (Fig. 28-8). They are commonly used to cover peripheral and central intravenous insertion sites.

Unfortunately, transparent dressings are not absorbent. If wound drainage accumulates, it has a tendency to loosen the dressing. Once the dressing is no longer intact, many of its original purposes are defeated.

Hydrocolloid Dressings. Hydrocolloid dressings are self-adhesive, opaque, air- and water-occlusive wound coverings (Fig. 28-9). Their best feature is that they keep wounds moist. A moist wound undergoes accelerated healing because new cells grow more rapidly in a wet environment. In addition, if they remain intact, they can be left in place for up to a week (Motta, 1993). Furthermore, their occlusive nature repels the entrance of pathogens from other body substances like stool.

Changing a Dressing

Dressings are changed when the wound requires assessment or care, and when they become loose or saturated with drainage. In some cases, the physician may choose to assume total responsibility for changing the dressing, at least for the first time. However, dressings can and should be *reinforced*, that is, additional absorbent layers applied, if the present dressing becomes moist. Reinforcing a dressing prevents "wicking" microorganisms toward the wound (see section on Surgical Asepsis, Chap. 21).

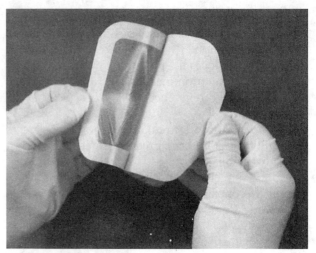

FIGURE 28-8
Transparent dressing. (Courtesy of Ken Timby.)

Because most surgical wounds are covered with gauze dressings, this example is used when describing the technique for changing a dressing in Skill 28-1. When other types of dressings are used, nurses can modify the dressing technique by following the manufacturer's directions.

DRAINS

Drains are tubes that provide a means for removing blood and drainage from a wound. Although some drains are placed directly within a wound, there is a trend to insert them so that they exit from a separate location beside the wound. This approach keeps the wound margins approximated and avoids creating a direct entry site for pathogens.

If drainage is needed, the physician may elect to use an open or closed drain.

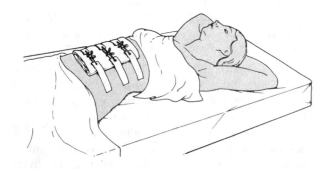

FIGURE 28-7
Montgomery straps.

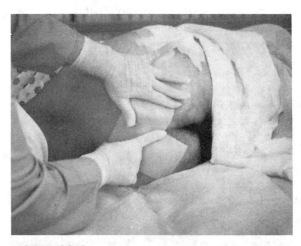

FIGURE 28-9
Hydrocolloid dressing. (Courtesy of E. R. Squibb & Sons, Inc., Princeton, NJ.)

Open Drains

Open drains are flat, flexible tubes. They provide a pathway for drainage toward the dressing. The drainage takes place passively by gravity and capillary action. **Capillary action** is the movement of a liquid at the point of contact with a solid.

Sometimes a safety pin or long clip is attached to the drain as it extends from the wound. This prevents the drain from slipping within the tissue. Occasionally, as the drainage decreases, the physician may instruct the nurse to shorten the drain. If so, the drain is pulled out from the wound for the specified length. The safety pin or clip is then repositioned near the wound.

Closed Drains

Closed drains are tubes that terminate in a receptacle. Some examples of closed drainage systems include a Hemovac and Jackson-Pratt (JP) drain (Fig. 28-10).

Closed drains are more efficient than open drains because they pull fluid by creating a vacuum or negative pressure. This is done by opening the vent on the receptacle, squeezing the drainage collection chamber, and capping the vent.

When caring for a wound with a drain, the insertion site is cleansed in a circular manner. After cleansing, a

(text continues on page 576)

SKILL 28-1
Changing a Gauze Dressing

Suggested Action	Reason for Action
Assessment	
Inspect the current dressing for the presence of drainage, integrity, and type of gauze dressing supplies that appear to have been used.	Provides assessments indicating a need to change the dressing and supplies that may be needed
Check the medical orders for a directive to change the dressing.	Shows collaboration with the prescribed medical treatment
Determine if the patient has any allergies to tape or antimicrobial wound agents.	Helps determine dressing supplies that may or may not be used
Assess the patient's level and characteristics of pain.	Determines if analgesia will be beneficial before changing the dressing
Planning	
Explain the need and technique for changing the dressing.	Relieves anxiety and promotes cooperation
Consult the patient on a preferred time for the dressing change if there is no immediate need for it.	Empowers the patient to participate in decision-making
Give pain medication, if it is needed, 15 to 30 minutes before the dressing will be changed.	Allows time for absorption and effectiveness
Gather the necessary supplies, which are likely to include a paper bag for the soiled dressing, clean and sterile gloves, individually packaged gauze dressings, tape, and, in some cases, an antimicrobial agent like povidone-iodine swabs, for wound cleansing.	Facilitates organization and efficient time management
Implementation	
Wash your hands.	Reduces the transmission of microorganisms
Pull the privacy curtain.	Shows respect for the patient's dignity
Position the patient in such a way as to allow access to the dressing.	Facilitates comfort and dexterity
Drape the patient so as to expose the area of the wound.	Ensures modesty, but facilitates care

(continued)

SKILL 28-1
Changing a Gauze Dressing *(Continued)*

Suggested Action	Reason for Action
Loosen the tape securing the dressing; pull the tape toward the wound.	Facilitates removal without separating the healing wound

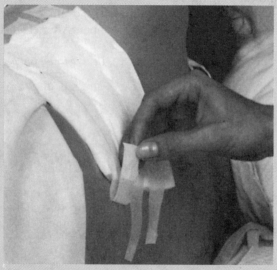

Loosening tape.

Suggested Action	Reason for Action
Don at least one glove and lift the dressing from the wound.	Provides a barrier against contact with blood and body substances

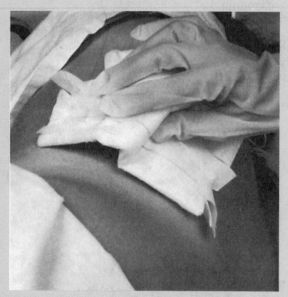

Removing dressing.

Suggested Action	Reason for Action
Moisten the gauze with sterile normal saline, if it adheres to the wound.	Prevents disrupting granulation tissue

(continued)

SKILL 28-1
Changing a Gauze Dressing *(Continued)*

Suggested Action	Reason for Action
Discard the soiled dressing in a paper bag or other receptacle along with the glove(s)	Confines sources of pathogens

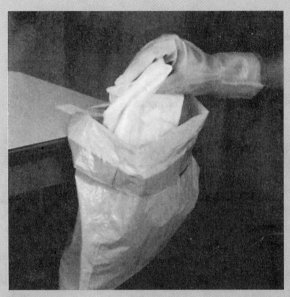

Dressing disposal.

Suggested Action	Reason for Action
Wash your hands again.	Removes transient microorganisms
Tear several long strips of tape and fold the ends over, forming tabs.	Facilitates handling tape later when wearing gloves and eases tape removal during the next dressing change

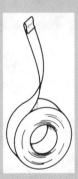

Forming tabs
on tape.

Suggested Action	Reason for Action
Open sterile supplies, using the inside wrapper of one of the gauze dressings as a sterile field, if needed.	Ensures sterile technique
Don sterile gloves.	Ensures sterility
Inspect the wound.	Provides data for description and comparison

(continued)

Suggested Action	Reason for Action
Cleanse the wound with the antimicrobial agent.	Removes drainage and microorganisms

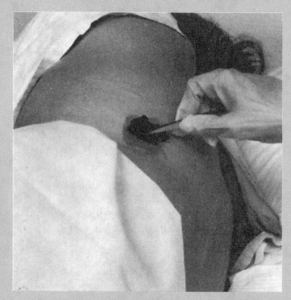

Cleansing wound.

| Use a technique that prevents transferring microorganisms back to a cleaned area. | Supports principles of medical asepsis |

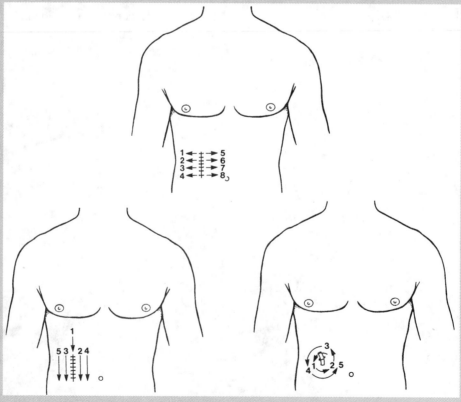

Wound cleansing techniques.

(continued)

Suggested Action	Reason for Action
Use a single swab or small gauze square for each stroke.	Prevents transferring microorganisms to clean areas
Allow the antimicrobial agent to dry.	Ensures that the tape will stay secured when applied
Cover the wound with the gauze dressing.	Protects the wound

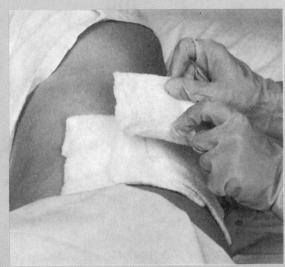

Applying the dressing.

Secure the dressing with tape.	Holds the dressing in place

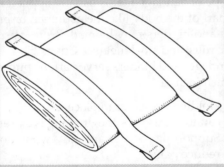

Securing the dressing.

Remove and discard gloves.	Confines sources of microorganisms

Evaluation
- Dressing covers the entire wound
- Dressing is secure, dry, and intact

Document
- Type of dressing
- Antimicrobial agent used for cleansing
- Assessment data

Sample Documentation

Date and Time   Gauze dressing changed over abdominal wound. Wound cleansed with povidone-iodine. Incision is well approximated with sutures. No drainage, swelling, or tenderness observed. _____ **Signature, Title**

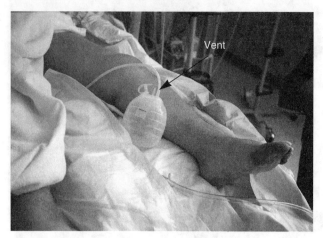

FIGURE 28-10
Jackson-Pratt (closed) drain. (Courtesy of Ken Timby.)

precut drain gauze, which is open to its center, is placed around the base of the drain. An open drain may require additional layers of gauze material because its drainage does not collect within a receptacle.

SUTURES AND STAPLES

Sutures are knotted ties that hold an incision together. They are usually constructed from silk or synthetic materials like nylon. **Staples** are wide metal clips that perform a similar function. Staples do not encircle a wound like sutures; instead, they form a bridge that holds the two wound margins together. An advantage of staples is that they do not compress the tissue should the wound swell.

Sutures and staples are left in place until the wound has healed sufficiently to prevent reopening. Depending on the location of the incision, this may be a few days to as long as 2 weeks.

The nurse may be directed by the physician to remove sutures (Fig. 28-11) and staples (Fig. 28-12)—sometimes half on one day, and the remaining half on another. A weak incision may be temporarily held together afterward with adhesive *Steri-strips* (3M Health Care, St. Paul, MN), also known as *butterflies* because of their winged appearance.

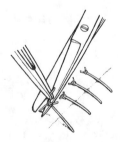

FIGURE 28-11
Technique for suture removal.

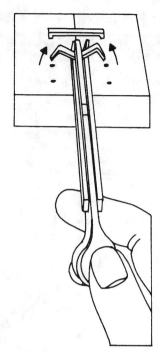

FIGURE 28-12
Technique for staple removal.

BANDAGES AND BINDERS

A **bandage** is a covering that is wrapped around a body part; one example is the Ace bandage. A **binder** is a type of bandage that is usually applied to a particular part of the body like the abdomen or breast. Bandages and binders may be made from gauze, muslin, elastic rolls, and stockinet (see Chap. 25).

Bandages and binders serve various purposes, some of which include:

- Holding dressings in place, especially when tape cannot be used or the dressing is extremely large
- Supporting the area around a wound or injury to reduce pain
- Limiting movement in the wound area to promote healing

Applying a Roller Bandage

Most bandages are prepared in rolls of varying widths. The end is held in one hand while the roll is passed repeatedly around the part being bandaged.

Several principles are followed when applying a roller bandage:

- Elevate and support the limb.
- Wrap from a distal to proximal direction.
- Avoid gaps between each turn of the bandage.
- Exert equal, but not excessive, tension with each turn.
- Keep the bandage free of wrinkles.
- Secure the end of the roller bandage with metal clips.

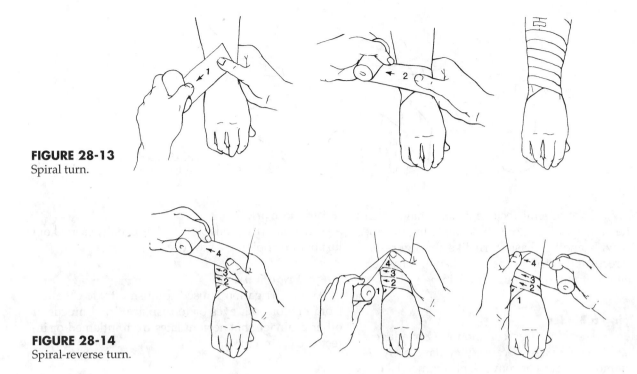

FIGURE 28-13
Spiral turn.

FIGURE 28-14
Spiral-reverse turn.

- Check the color and sensation of exposed fingers or toes often.
- Remove the bandage for hygiene, and replace it at least twice a day.

There are six basic techniques for wrapping a roller bandage. They include using a circular turn, spiral turn, spiral-reverse turn, figure-of-eight-turn, spica turn, and recurrent turn.

Circular Turn. A circular turn is used to anchor and secure a bandage when it is started and ended. It simply involves holding the free end of the rolled material in one hand and wrapping it about the area, bringing it back to the starting point.

Spiral Turn. A spiral turn partly overlaps a previous turn (Fig. 28-13). The overlapping varies from one-half to three-fourths of the width of the bandage. Spiral turns are used when wrapping a cylindrical part of the body like the arms and legs.

Spiral-Reverse Turn. A spiral-reverse turn is a modification of a spiral turn. When used, the roll is reversed halfway through the turn (Fig. 28-14).

Figure-of-Eight Turn. A figure-of-eight turn is best used when an area spanning a joint, like the elbow or knee, requires bandaging. This turn is made by making oblique turns that alternately ascend and descend, simulating the number "8" (Fig. 28-15).

Spica Turn. A spica turn (Fig. 28-16) is a variation of the figure-of-eight turn. It differs in that the wrap includes a portion of the trunk or chest (see section on Spica Cast, Chap. 25).

Recurrent Turn. The recurrent turn is made by passing the roll back and forth over the tip of a body part

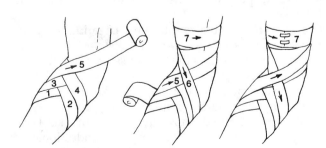

FIGURE 28-15
Figure-of-eight turn.

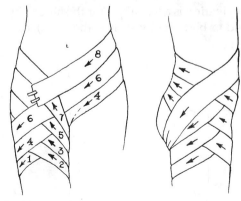

FIGURE 28-16
Spica turn.

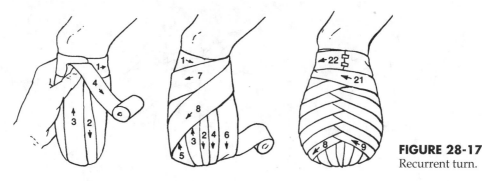

FIGURE 28-17
Recurrent turn.

(Fig. 28-17). Once several recurrent turns have been made, the bandage is anchored by completing the application with another basic turn like the figure-of-eight. A recurrent turn is especially beneficial when wrapping the stump of an amputated limb.

Applying a Binder

Binders are not used as commonly as bandages. Many have become passé because they have been replaced by more modern or convenient commercial devices. For example, brassieres have, for the most part, replaced breast binders. On rare occasions, nurses may be required to apply a T-binder.

T-Binder. As the name implies, a T-binder looks like the letter "T" (Fig. 28-18). T-binders are used for securing a dressing to the anus, perineum, or within the groin. To apply a T-binder, the crossbar of the T is fastened about the waist. Then the single or double tails are passed between the legs and pinned to the belt. Elastic sanitary belts serve the same purpose and may be preferred by women.

For the most part, wounds heal rapidly with conventional care. However, there are situations in which wounds and other areas of the body require irrigations.

IRRIGATIONS

An **irrigation** is a technique for flushing debris from a wound or body cavity such as the eye(s), ear(s), and vagina.

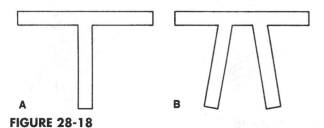

FIGURE 28-18
(*A*) Single T-binder. (*B*) Double T-binder.

Wound Irrigation

A wound irrigation (Skill 28-2) is usually carried out just before applying a new dressing

Eye Irrigation

An eye irrigation is used to flush a toxic chemical from one or both eyes or to displace dried mucus or other drainage that accumulates from inflamed or infected eye structures.

NURSING GUIDELINES FOR AN EYE IRRIGATION

- Assemble supplies, which include bulb syringe, irrigating solution, gauze squares, gloves and other Standard Precautions apparel, absorbent pads, and at least one towel.
  Rationale: Ensures organization and efficient time management
- Warm the solution to approximately body temperature by placing the container of solution in warm water, except when administering emergency first aid.
  Rationale: Promotes comfort
- Position the patient with the head tilted slightly toward the side.
  Rationale: Facilitates drainage
- Place absorbent material in the area of the shoulder.
  Rationale: Prevents saturating the patient's gown and bed linen
- Give the patient a kidney basin to hold beneath the cheek.
  Rationale: Facilitates collecting irrigating solution
- Wash hands and don gloves.
  Rationale: Reduces the transmission of micro-organisms
- Open and prepare supplies.
  Rationale: Facilitates implementing procedure
- Wipe a moistened gauze square from the nasal corner of the eye toward the temple; use additional gauze squares, one at a time, as needed.

(text continues on page 581)

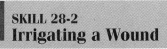

SKILL 28-2
Irrigating a Wound

Suggested Action	Reason for Action
Assessment	
Check the medical orders for a directive to irrigate the wound.	Shows collaboration with the prescribed medical treatment
Determine how much the patient understands about the procedure.	Indicates the need for and level of health teaching
Planning	
Plan to irrigate the wound at the same time that the dressing requires changing.	Makes efficient use of time
Gather the equipment required, which is likely to include a container of solution, basin, bulb or Asepto syringe, gloves, and absorbent material, including a towel to dry the skin.	Facilitates organization
Bring supplies for changing the dressing.	Makes efficient use of time
Consider additional items for standard precautions such as goggles or face shield, and cover apron or gown.	Follows infection control guidelines when there is a potential for being splashed with blood or body substances
Implementation	
Wash your hands.	Reduces the transmission of microorganisms
Pull the privacy curtain.	Shows respect for the patient's dignity
Drape the patient so as to expose the area of the wound.	Ensures modesty, but facilitates care
Follow earlier directions for removing the dressing.	Provides access to the wound
Wash your hands.	Reduces the transmission of microorganisms.
Position the patient in such a way as to facilitate filling the cavity with solution.	Ensures contact between the solution and all areas of the wound
Pad the bed with absorbent material and place a kidney basin adjacent to and below the wound.	Reduces the potential for saturating the bed linen
Open and prepare supplies following principles of surgical asepsis.	Confines and controls the transmission of microorganisms
Don gloves and other Standard Precautions apparel.	Reduces the potential for contact with blood and body substances

(continued)

SKILL 28-2
Irrigating a Wound

Suggested Action	Reason for Action
Fill the syringe with solution and instill it into the wound without touching the wound directly.	Dilutes and loosens debris

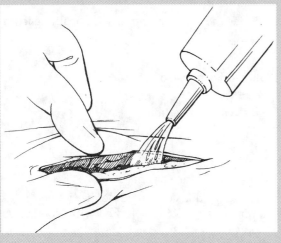

Instilling irrigant.

Suggested Action	Reason for Action
Hold the kidney basin close to the patient's body so as to catch the solution as it drains from the wound.	Collects irrigating solution
Repeat the process until the draining solution seems clear.	Indicates that debris has been evacuated

Draining irrigant.

Suggested Action	Reason for Action
Tilt the patient toward the basin.	Drains remaining solution from the wound
Dry the skin.	Facilitates applying a dressing
Dispose of the drained solution, soiled equipment, and linen.	Reduces the potential for transmitting microorganisms
Remove gloves, wash hands, and prepare to change the dressing.	Provides for absorption of residual solution and coverage of the wound

(continued)

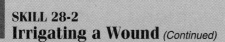

SKILL 28-2
Irrigating a Wound (Continued)

Suggested Action	Reason for Action
Evaluation • Irrigation caused removal of debris • Wound shows evidence of healing *Document* • Assessment data • Type and amount of solution • Outcome of procedure *Sample Documentation* **Date and Time** Dressing removed. Moderate amount of purulent drainage on soiled dressing. Wound is separated 3″. Approximately 300 mL of sterile NSS instilled within wound. Drained solution is cloudy with particles of debris. _____ **Signature, Title**	

Rationale: Removes gross debris
• Separate the eyelids widely with the fingers of one hand.
Rationale: Widens the exposed surface area
• Direct the solution onto the conjunctiva, holding the syringe or irrigating device approximately 1 inch (2.5 cm) above the eye (Fig. 28-19).
Rationale: Prevents injury to the cornea
• Instruct the patient to blink periodically.
Rationale: Distributes solution under the eyelids and about the eye
• Continue irrigating until debris is removed.
Rationale: Accomplishes purpose
• Dry the face and replace wet gown or linen.
Rationale: Restores comfort

• Dispose of soiled materials and gloves; wash hands.
Rationale: Reduces the transmission of micro-organisms
• Record assessment data, specifics of procedure, and outcome.
Rationale: Documents nursing care and patient response

Ear Irrigation
An ear irrigation removes debris from the ear. However, an ear irrigation is contraindicated if the tympanic membrane (eardrum) is perforated. Also, it is wise to perform a gross inspection of the ear if a foreign body is suspected. A bean, pea, or other dehydrated substance may swell if the ear is irrigated, causing it to

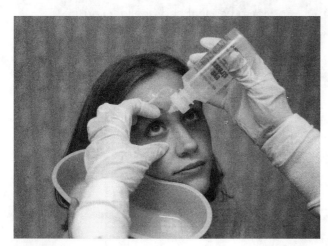

FIGURE 28-19
Eye irrigation. (Courtesy of Ken Timby.)

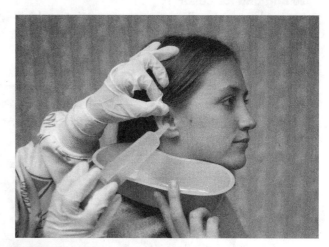

FIGURE 28-20
Ear irrigation. (Courtesy of Ken Timby.)

become tightly wedged. Solid objects may require removal with an instrument.

If an irrigation is not contraindicated, it is performed similarly to an eye irrigation except that the solution is directed toward the roof of the auditory canal (Fig. 28-20). Also, care is taken to avoid occluding the ear canal with the tip of the syringe because the pressure of the trapped solution could rupture the eardrum. After the irrigation, a cotton ball may be placed *loosely* within the ear.

Vaginal Irrigation

A vaginal irrigation is the same as a **douche**. Occasionally it may be necessary to irrigate the vagina to treat an infection or to instruct a patient on how to perform this procedure.

HEAT AND COLD APPLICATIONS

There are various therapeutic uses for heat and cold (Display 28-2). The terms "hot" and "cold," however, are subject to wide interpretation, and because the skin can be injured by extremes in temperature, certain guidelines must be followed to ensure safety (Table 28-2). Another safety precaution involves protecting the skin in some way to avoid direct contact with the heating or cooling device.

Not only are there many therapeutic uses for heat and cold, there are multiple ways in which each can be applied. Common methods for applying cold include the use of an ice bag, collar, or chemical pack, and cool compresses. An aquathermia pad serves a dual purpose; it may be used either for cooling or warming. Heat may be applied with a hot water bottle, electric heating pad, soaks and moist packs, and therapeutic baths.

Ice Bag and Ice Collar

An ice bag and collar are containers into which crushed or small cubes of ice are placed. Ice collars are usually applied after surgery when the tonsils have

PATIENT TEACHING ABOUT DOUCHING

Teach the patient to do the following:
- Refrain from douching as a routine practice because it removes helpful microbes called *Döderlein bacilli* that help to prevent vaginal infections.
- Avoid douching 24 to 48 hours before a Pap test (see Chap. 13) to ensure the presence of diagnostic cells.
- Consult with a physician about symptoms such as itching, burning, or drainage, rather than attempting self-diagnosis.
- Find out from a physician if one's sexual partner(s) also need to be treated with medications to avoid reinfection.
- Purchase douching equipment from a drug store or check about using a prefilled disposable container of solution.
- Warm the solution to a comfortable temperature (no more than 110°F [43.3°C]).
- Clamp the tubing, if using other than a disposable container, and fill the reservoir bag.
- Undress and recline in a bath tub.
- Suspend the douche bag approximately 18 to 24 inches (45–60 cm) above the hips.
- Insert the lubricated tip of the nozzle or prefilled container downward and backward within the vagina about the distance of a tampon.
- Unclamp the tubing and rotate the nozzle as the fluid is instilled.
- Contract the perineal muscles as though trying to stop urinating and then relax the muscles; repeat the exercise four or five times while douching.
- Sit up to facilitate drainage or shower afterward.
- Position a perineal pad (sanitary napkin) to absorb residual solution.

DISPLAY 28-2. *Common Uses for Heat and Cold Applications*

Uses for Heat	Uses for Cold
• Provides warmth	• Reduces fevers
• Promotes circulation	• Prevents swelling
• Speeds healing	• Controls bleeding
• Relieves muscle spasm	• Relieves pain
• Reduces pain	• Numbs sensation

TABLE 28-2. *Temperature Ranges for Applications of Heat and Cold*

	Temperature Range
Level of Heat	
Very hot	40.5°C to 46.1°C (105°F–115°F)
Hot	36.6°C to 40.5°C (98°F–105°F)
Warm and neutral	33.8°C to 36.6°C (93°F–98°F)
Level of Cold	
Tepid	26.6°C to 33.8°C (80°F–93°F)
Cool	18.3°C to 26.6°C (65°F–80°F)
Cold	10°C to 18.3°C (50°F–65°F)
Very cold	Below 10°C (below 50°F)

been removed. Ice bags are applied to any small injury that is in the process of swelling. Although some people own an ice bag, there are various ways that they can be improvised.

Chemical Packs

Commercially made cold packs become cool after having been struck or crushed to activate the chemicals that are stored inside. This type is usually included in most first aid kits. Unfortunately, once they are used, they must be discarded. However, there are some gel packs, designed for cold or hot applications, that are reusable (Fig. 28-21). They may be stored in a freezer until needed or heated in a microwave.

Compresses

Compresses are moist, warm or cool cloths that are applied to the skin. Before application, the compress material is soaked in a solution of warmed tap water or one containing medication. The excess moisture is then wrung from the cloth and it is applied to the skin. To maintain the moisture and temperature, plastic wrap may be used to cover the compress. The area is then secured within a towel.

If the skin is not intact, as in the case of a draining wound, gloves are worn. There also may be certain circumstances, such as when caring for an open wound, that call for sterile technique when applying compresses.

Aquathermia Pad

An **aquathermia pad**, sometimes called a *K-pad*, is an electrical heating or cooling device. It resembles a mat, but it contains hollow channels through which heated or cooled *distilled* water circulates (Fig. 28-22). An aquathermia pad may be used alone or to cover a compress.

A key-controlled thermostat on the pad automatically keeps the temperature of the water at the specified setting. The pad is covered before placing the patient on the pad or wrapping it about a part of the body. A roller bandage may help hold the pad in place. The electrical unit is positioned slightly higher than the patient to promote gravity circulation of the fluid.

Larger styles may be used to warm hypothermic pa-

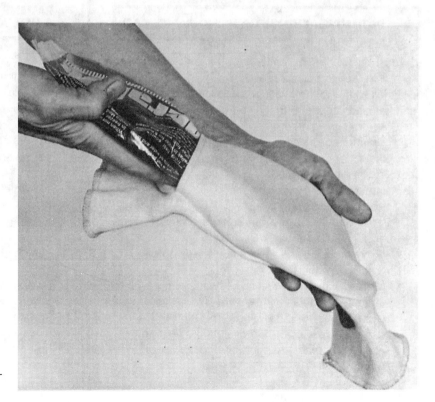

FIGURE 28-21
Commercial cold pack. (Courtesy of Hydro-Med Products, Inc., Dallas, TX.)

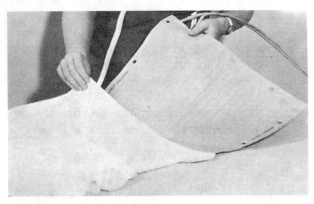

FIGURE 28-22
Aquathermia pad (K-pad).

Electric Heating Pad

An electric heating pad provides a mechanism for applying dry heat. The heating element consists of a web of wires that converts electric current into heat. Most pads have a heat selector for regulating the temperature; however, after people adapt to the heat, they often increase the temperature setting. Consequently, many people, especially older adults, have been burned in this manner.

In addition, electric heating pads have the potential for overheating, causing fires and electrical shocks. So, despite the fact that they are easy to use, many health agencies have a policy that prohibits them. If patients insist on their use, they may be required to sign a release from responsibility form.

Soaks and Moist Packs

A **soak** is a procedure in which a part of the body is submerged in warm water or medicated solution for a period of time. A **pack** is a commercial device for applying moist heat to a large area of the body (Fig. 28-23). Both offer the advantage of providing moist heat. Applications of moist heat seem to be more comforting and therapeutic than those that provide dry heat.

A soak usually lasts 15 to 20 minutes, during which time the temperature of the fluid is kept as constant as possible. This may mean that the basin is emptied and

tients or cool those who experience heat stroke. Because these applications involve treating patients with dangerously altered body temperature, it is essential to monitor their vital signs continuously.

Hot Water Bottle

A hot water bottle is not really a bottle at all. It is a flexible bag made of rubber-like material that is designed to hold warm water. Health agencies rarely use a hot water bottle, but they are common in many households. Because burns may occur during their use, home care patients are taught how to use them safely.

⚛ PATIENT TEACHING FOR USING AN ICE BAG

Teach the patient or family to do the following:
- Test the ice bag for leaks.
- Fill it one-half to two-thirds full of crushed ice or small cubes so that it can be easily molded to the injured area.
- Eliminate as much air from the bag as possible.
- Pour water over the ice to provide slight melting. This tends to smooth the sharp edges from frozen ice crystals.
- Cover the ice bag with a layer of cloth before placing it on the body.
- Leave the ice bag in place no more than one-half to one hour.
- Mottled skin and a feeling of numbness are indicators that the temperature is too severe.
- Use a rubber or plastic glove, plastic bag with a zipper closure, or bag of small frozen vegetables like peas, as substitutes for an ice bag.

⚛ PATIENT TEACHING FOR USING A HOT WATER BOTTLE

Teach the patient or family to do the following:
- Check the bag and cap for leaks.
- Avoid using extremely hot water.
- Warm the water between 105°F to 110°F (40.5°C–43.3°C) for children younger than 2 years of age, older adults, diabetics, or those who may be comatose to avoid burns.
- Use water at 115°F to 125°F (46.1°C–51.6°C) for older children and all but older adults.
- Fill the bag only two-thirds full to reduce its weight.
- Remove trapped air from the bag to facilitate molding it about the body.
- Cover the bag with a towel or cloth pouch.
- Remove the hot water bottle at least every 2 hours.
- Replace it, if necessary, after allowing the skin to recover.

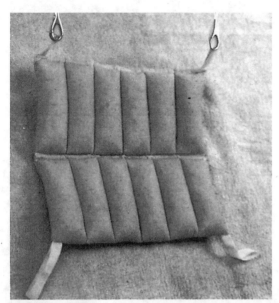

FIGURE 28-23
Hot pack. (Courtesy of Ken Timby.)

refilled frequently. Care is taken that the newly added water is not so hot that it causes discomfort or tissue damage.

Packs differ from soaks in two major ways: the duration of the application is usually longer, and the initial application of heat is usually more intense. Packs are usually applied at temperatures as hot as patients can tolerate. Because of the potential for causing burns, a pack is never used on an unresponsive patient or one who is paralyzed and cannot perceive temperatures. The nurse is ultimately accountable for the patient's safety. Therefore, it is essential that nurses conduct frequent assessments and remove a pack if there is any likelihood that it is producing thermal injury.

Therapeutic Baths

Therapeutic baths are those that are given other than for strictly hygiene purposes. For example, a *sponge bath*, or *alcohol bath*, is given to reduce a high

(text continues on page 590)

SKILL 28-3
Providing a Sitz Bath

Suggested Action	Reason for Action
Assessment	
Check the medical orders for a directive to administer a sitz bath.	Shows collaboration with the prescribed medical treatment
Determine how much the patient understands about the procedure.	Indicates the need for and level of health teaching
Assess the condition of the rectal or perineal wound and the patient's level of pain.	Provides baseline data for future comparisons; indicates if pain medication is needed
Planning	
Explain the procedure.	Relieves anxiety and promotes cooperation
Collaborate with the patient on whether the sitz bath is preferred before or after routine hygiene.	Involves the patient in the decision-making process
Obtain disposable equipment unless specially installed tubs are available.	Facilitates organization and efficient time management
Assemble other supplies such as a bath blanket and towels.	Prepares for maintaining warmth and provides a means for drying the skin
Inspect and clean the bathroom area or the tub room.	Supports principles of medical asepsis

(continued)

Suggested Action	Reason for Action
Place the basin inside the rim of the raised toilet seat.	Facilitates a means for submerging the rectum and perineum

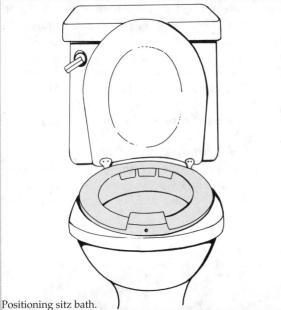

Positioning sitz bath.

Implementation

Suggested Action	Reason for Action
Wash your hands.	Reduces the transmission of microorganisms
Assist the patient with a robe and slippers.	Maintains warmth, safety, and comfort
Help the patient ambulate to the location where the sitz bath will be administered.	Demonstrates concern for safety
Shut the door to the bathroom or tub room.	Provides privacy
Clamp the tubing attached to the water bag.	Prevents loss of fluid
Fill the container with warm water, no hotter than 110°F (43.3°C).	Provides comfort without danger of burning the skin

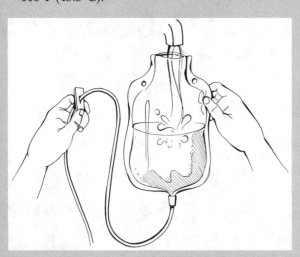

Filling solution container.

(continued)

SKILL 28-3
Providing a Sitz Bath (Continued)

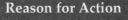

Suggested Action	Reason for Action
Hang the bag above the toilet seat.	Facilitates gravity flow
Insert the tubing from the bag into the front of the basin.	Provides a means for filling the basin

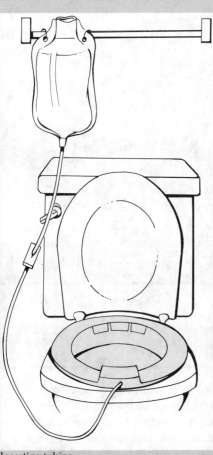

Inserting tubing.

Suggested Action	Reason for Action
Help the patient sit on the basin and unclamp the tubing.	Facilitates filling the basin
Cover the patient's shoulders with a bath blanket if the patient feels chilled.	Promotes comfort
Instruct the patient on how to signal for assistance.	Ensures safety
Leave the patient alone, but recheck at frequent intervals to add more warm water to the reservoir bag.	Provides sustained application of warm water
Help the patient pat his or her skin dry after soaking for 20 to 30 minutes.	Restores comfort
Assist the patient back to bed.	Ensures safety in case the patient feels dizzy from hypotension caused by peripheral vasodilation.

(continued)

SKILL 28-3
Providing a Sitz Bath (Continued)

Suggested Action	Reason for Action
Don gloves and clean the disposable equipment and bath area.	Supports principles of medical asepsis and infection control
Replace the sitz bath equipment within the patient's bedside cabinet or leave it in the patient's private bathroom.	Reduces hospital costs by reusing disposable equipment

Evaluation
- Sitz bath administered according to policy or standards of care
- Safety maintained
- Symptoms relieved

Document
- Procedure
- Response of the patient
- Assessment data

Sample Documentation
Date and Time   Sitz bath provided over 30 minutes. States "I always feel so good after this treatment." Perineum is slightly swollen. Margins of episiotomy are approximated. Continues to have moderate, bloody, vaginal drainage. _____ **Signature, Title**

 FOCUS ON OLDER ADULTS

- Skin cells are renewed at a much slower rate among older adults. The full cycle averages 30 days, compared to 20 days in younger adults, which explains why it takes older adults' wounds longer to heal (Ebersole & Hess, 1990).
- The amount of collagen also decreases with age, which indicates that healing wounds may be more fragile than those of younger people.
- A lifetime of exposure to sun hastens collagen fiber alterations (Ebersole & Hess, 1990).
- Because older adults have a thinner dermal layer to their skin and the amount of subcutaneous tissue decreases with age, they are much more susceptible to development of pressure sores.
- Diminished immune response due to a reduction in T cells predisposes older adults to wound infections.
- The rate at which neutrophils are released from the bone marrow may be reduced (Ebersole & Hess, 1990).
- A higher incidence of diabetes and its associated vascular changes among older adults contributes to slower rates of healing and a higher incidence of infection.
- Older adults are often insensitive to hot and cold applications. Consequently, they are at greater risk for sustaining thermal injuries.
- Compliance with a medical treatment regimen may be a problem for older adults who are economically limited, although there are many other reasons for this phenomenon. Another possibility is that health beliefs conflict with discharge instructions.
- Healing may be affected by nutritional deficits that are common among older adults who lose their motivation to prepare meals or cannot afford a well balanced diet.
- Signs of inflammation may be subdued among older adults.
- Placing absorbent undergarments on in-continent older adults may contribute to skin breakdown because the garments may not be changed as frequently as saturated bed linen.

NURSING CARE PLAN:
Impaired Tissue Integrity

Assessment

Subjective Data
States, "I have no feeling below my upper back and chest."

Objective Data
18-year-old man with spinal cord injury at the C7 (7th cervical vertebrae) level 2 years ago after an auto accident in which he was not wearing a seat belt and was thrown from the car. Admitted for treatment of a pressure sore over the coccyx that has not responded to home treatment. The skin over the coccyx is open and measures 2 in × 3 in × ½ in. Approximately 2 in of intact skin around the sore remain red and warm even after pressure is relieved. Tissue within the ulcer is gray with a yellow base. Elbows and heels are reddened but skin is intact. Wears an external catheter. Bowel elimination is regulated with the use of a suppository q 2 days.

Diagnosis

Impaired Tissue Integrity: Stage III pressure sore over coccyx and Stage I over bilateral heels and elbows related to unrelieved pressure secondary to immobility.

Plan

Goal
The coccygeal pressure sore will develop a ⅛ inch margin of granulation tissue around the circumference of the wound by 8/30. The elbows and heels will blanch with pressure relief by 8/18.

Orders: 8/15
1. Reposition q 2 h until an air-fluidized bed can be obtained.
2. Avoid the supine and Fowler's position as much as possible.
3. After bathing, spray heels and elbows with Bard Barrier Film.
4. Until results of wound culture are obtained, care for the open wound as follows:
   • Mix Shur Clens with water and cleanse wound.
   • Rinse with normal saline.
   • Pack the wound loosely with a continuous strip of gauze moistened with normal saline.
   • Cover with an ABD pad.
   • Repeat above routine q 4 h as the packing becomes dry.
5. If wound culture is negative for pathogens:
   • Eliminate wet to dry dressing.
   • Clean, dry, and cover wound with Op-Site and leave in place for 5 days.
   • If drainage collects, pierce Op-Site and aspirate fluid from underneath. Seal opened area with a small reinforcement of Op-Site over punctured area.
6. Measure open pressure sore q 3 days (8/18, 8/21, etc.) during day shift.
_____ R. ROSEN, RN

Implementation (Documentation) 8/16

1700 Turned q 2 h alternating side to side using a 30° lateral position with slight elevation of the upper body. _____ A. FOX, LPN

1900 Transferred from hospital bed to Clinitron bed. Explained principle for use and discontinuation of turning schedule. _____ A. FOX, LPN

2000 Dressing and packing removed. Wound cleansed with Shur Clens and rinsed with saline. Repacked with saline-moistened gauze and covered with ABD secured with paper tape. _____ A. FOX, LPN

Evaluation (Documentation)

2045 Removed packing contains white debris. Tissue within wound looks pink with slight bleeding. Wet to dry dressing drying more rapidly with Clinitron bed therapy. Will change in 3 h and evaluate again. Evidence of skin coating on elbows and heels. These areas still appear red over bony prominences. States, "I really like this bed, I wasn't sleeping much at night with all that turning going on." Advised that fluid intake must be increased to compensate for increased evaporation from skin due to blowing air from bed. Placed on I & O. _____ A. FOX, LPN

fever. Other types are used to apply medicated substances to the skin to treat skin disorders or discomfort. Examples include baths to which sodium bicarbonate (baking soda), corn starch, or oatmeal paste are added.

In health agencies, the most common type of therapeutic bath is called a sitz bath. A **sitz bath** is used to reduce swelling and inflammation and promote healing of wounds in the rectum or perineum like those after a hemorrhoidectomy (surgical removal of hemorrhoids) or episiotomy (an incision that facilitates a vaginal birth).

Although the term "bath" is used, a sitz bath involves soaking only the perineal area in water. The legs and feet usually remain dry. Some health agencies have special tubs for administering sitz baths, but most patients are provided with disposable equipment (Skill 28-3).

NURSING IMPLICATIONS

Patients with surgical wounds and other types of tissue injury are likely to have one or more nursing diagnoses from among the accompanying Applicable Nursing Diagnoses.

The Nursing Care Plan for this chapter has been developed for a patient diagnosed with Impaired Tissue Integrity. NANDA defines this diagnostic category in its 1994 taxonomy as "A state in which an individual experiences damage to mucous membrane, corneal, integumentary, or subcutaneous tissue."

KEY CONCEPTS

- A wound is damaged skin or soft tissue.
- The purpose of the inflammatory response is to limit tissue damage, remove injured cells and debris, and prepare the wound for healing.
- Five signs and symptoms that are classically associated with the inflammatory response are swelling, redness, warmth, pain, and decreased function.

- Phagocytosis is a process in which white blood cells, namely neutrophils and monocytes, engulf pathogens, coagulated blood, and cellular debris.
- The integrity of damaged skin and tissue is restored by either resolution, regeneration, or scar formation.
- Two common types of wounds that require special care include pressure sores and surgical wounds.
- Five factors that place patients at risk for development of pressure sores are inactivity, immobility, malnutrition, dehydration, and incontinence.
- Some techniques for preventing pressure sores include changing patients' positions every 1 to 2 hours, keeping the skin clean and dry, and preventing friction and shearing forces on the skin.
- Some, but not all, of the purposes for covering a wound with a dressing include keeping it clean, absorbing drainage, and controlling bleeding.
- One method for promoting wound healing is to keep wounds moist. A moist wound undergoes accelerated healing because new cells grow more rapidly in a wet environment.
- Open or closed drains may be placed within or near a wound to provide a means for removing blood and drainage.
- The edges of an incision are usually held together with either sutures or staples.
- One reason a bandage or binder may be used is to hold a dressing in place, especially when tape cannot be used or the dressing is extremely large.
- One type of binder that may be used is a T-binder. It is used for securing a dressing to the anus, perineum, or groin.
- An irrigation is used to flush debris from a wound or body cavity such as the eye(s), ear(s), and vagina.
- Heat may be applied to promote circulation and speed healing; cold applications are used to prevent swelling and control bleeding.
- Heat or cold may be applied with ice bags, hot water bottles, compresses, soaks, and therapeutic baths.

CRITICAL THINKING EXERCISES

- You are assigned to care for a patient with a stage III pressure sore, one with an abdominal incision, and one with a peripheral intravenous infusion site. Describe the wound care that would be appropriate for each.
- A 75-year-old patient is admitted from a nursing home to have hip surgery to repair a fracture. Discuss the potential problems that threaten this patient's wound healing.

SUGGESTED READINGS

Carr P. Choosing wound care products. Home Healthcare Nurse May–June 1993;11:53–55.

Carr P. Wound care. Home Healthcare Nurse January–February 1993;11:51–53.

Ebersole P, Hess P. Toward Healthy Aging: Human Needs and Nursing Response. 3rd ed. St. Louis: CV Mosby, 1990.

Krasner D. The 12 commandments of wound care. Nursing December 1992;22:34–42.

Krasner D. Wound measurements: some tools of the trade. American Journal of Nursing May 1992;92:89–90.

McConnell EA. Clinical do's and don'ts: how to irrigate the ear. Nursing January 1992;22:66.

McConnell EA. How to apply an ice bag, ice collar, or ice glove. Nursing July 1992;22:18.

Motta GJ. Dressed for success: how moisture-retentive dressings promote healing. Nursing December 1993;23:26–34.

Payne RL, Martin MC. Defining and classifying skin tears: need for a common language. Ostomy Wound Management June 1993;39:16–20, 22–24, 26.

Saltus R. How we heal. Health February 1989;21:82–83.

Willey T. Use a decision tree to choose wound dressings. American Journal of Nursing February 1992;92:43–46.

Gastrointestinal Intubation

NURSING GUIDELINES

SKILLS

NURSING CARE PLAN

Key Terms

Learning Objectives

An understanding of the content within this chapter will be evidenced by the student's ability to:

- Define the term "intubation"
- List six purposes for gastrointestinal intubation
- Identify four general types of gastrointestinal tubes
- Name at least four assessments that are appropriate before inserting a tube nasally
- Explain the purpose for and how to obtain an NEX measurement
- Describe three techniques for checking stomach placement
- Discuss three ways that nasointestinal feeding tubes or their insertion differ from their gastric counterparts
- Name two problems that are common among patients with transabdominal tubes
- Explain the meaning of enteral nutrition

Timby BK: *Fundamental Skills and Concepts in Patient Care, Sixth Edition* © 1996 Lippincott-Raven Publishers

- Name four schedules for administering tube feedings
- Explain the purpose for assessing gastric residual
- Name five nursing activities that are involved in managing the care of patients who are being tube-fed
- List four items of information that are included in the written instructions for patients who will administer their own tube feedings
- Name two responsibilities nurses assume when assisting with the insertion of a mercury-weighted tube

Patients, especially those having abdominal or gastrointestinal surgery, may require some type of tube placed within their stomach or intestine. This chapter discusses the uses for such tubes and the nursing guidelines and skills for managing patient care.

INTUBATION

Intubation is the term for placing a tube into a structure of the body. When the tube is inserted into the stomach by way of the mouth or nose, it is referred to as *nasogastric intubation* (Fig. 29-1); if the distal end of the tube is located within the digestive tract, but further than the stomach, it is referred to as *intestinal intubation*.

A tube may also be inserted within a surgically created opening, called an **ostomy**. The location of the opening is identified by a prefix indicating the anatomic site of the ostomy (eg, a gastrostomy is an artificial opening into the stomach).

Gastric or intestinal tubes are used for a variety of reasons.

Purposes for Intubation

Tubes may be inserted to:

- Provide nourishment, a process known as **gavage**
- Administer oral medications that cannot be swallowed
- Obtain a sample of secretions for diagnostic testing
- Remove poisonous substances, a process known as **lavage**
- Remove gas and secretions from the stomach or bowel, a process called **decompression**
- Control gastric bleeding, a process called **compression** or **tamponade**

TYPES OF TUBES

Although all gastric and intestinal tubes have a proximal and distal end, their size, construction, and composition vary somewhat according to their use (Table 29-1). The outside diameter of most tubes is measured using the French scale, indicated by a number followed by the letter "F." Each number on the French scale is the approximate equivalent of 0.33 millimeters (mm). The larger the number, the larger the diameter of the tube.

A common way to describe the various tubes is to identify them according to the location of their insertion, which may be the mouth, nose, or abdomen.

Orogastric Tube

An **orogastric tube**, such as the Ewald tube, is one that is inserted at the mouth into the stomach. This type of tube is used in an emergency to remove toxic substances that have been ingested. The diameter of the tube is large so as to remove pill fragments and stomach debris. Because of its size, the tube is introduced through the mouth rather than the nose.

Nasogastric Tubes

A **nasogastric tube** is one placed in the nose and advanced to the stomach. Nasogastric tubes are smaller in diameter than orogastric tubes, but larger and shorter than nasointestinal tubes. Some have more than one channel, or **lumen**, within the tube.

A Levin tube (Fig. 29-2) is a common, single-lumen gastric tube that has multiple uses, one of which is decompression. Gastric **sump tubes** (Fig. 29-3) are double-lumen tubes that are used almost exclusively to re-

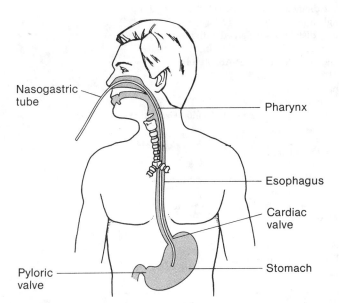

FIGURE 29-1
Nasogastric intubation pathway.

Labels: Nasogastric tube, Pharynx, Esophagus, Cardiac valve, Stomach, Pyloric valve

TABLE 29-1. *Types of Gastrointestinal Tubes*

Tube	Purpose	Characteristics
Orogastric		
Ewald	Lavage	• Large diameter: 36–40 F • Single lumen • Multiple distal openings for drainage
Nasogastric		
Levin	Lavage Gavage Decompression Diagnostics	• Usual adult size: 14–18 F • Single lumen • 42″–50″ (107–127 cm) long • Multiple drain openings
Salem sump	Decompression	• Same diameter as Levin • Double lumen • Pig-tail vent • 48″ (122 cm) length • Marked at increments to indicate depth of insertion • Radiopaque
Sengstaken- Blakemore	Compression Drainage	• Usual diameter: 20 F • 36″ (90 cm) long • Triple lumen; two lead to balloons in the esophagus and stomach, the third is for removing gastric drainage; a fourth lumen may be used to remove pharyngeal secretions
Nasointestinal		
Keofeed	Gavage	• Small diameter: 8 F • 36″ (90 cm) long • Polyurethane or silicone • Weighted tip • Extremely flexible and may require the use of a stylet during insertion • Radiopaque • Bonded lubricant that becomes activated with moisture
Miller-Abbott	Intestinal decompression	• Usual size: 16 F • 10′ (3 m) in length • Double lumen • Mercury is instilled into distal tip after the tube is beyond the pylorus
Cantor	Intestinal decompression	• Same diameter and length as Miller-Abbott tube • Single lumen • Bag at distal tip is weighted with mercury before tube insertion
Harris	Intestinal decompression	• Same diameter as Miller-Abbott tube • 6′ (1.8 m) • Single lumen • Weighted with mercury • Y-tube is usually attached to facilitate irrigation
Transabdominal		
Gastrostomy	Gavage; may be used for decompression while the patient is fed through a jejunostomy tube	• Sizes 12–24 F for adults • Rubber or silicone • Some may have additional side ports for balloon inflation to maintain placement • May be capped or plugged between feedings • Radiopaque
Jejunostomy	Gavage	• Sizes 5–14 F for adults • Silicone or polyurethane • Radiopaque

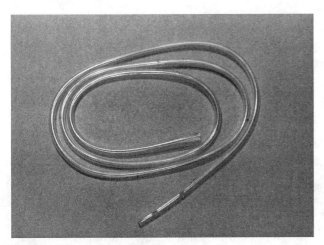

FIGURE 29-2
Levin tube. (Courtesy of Ken Timby.)

move fluid and gas from the stomach. Their second lumen serves as a vent. This feature allows a small amount of air to be drawn in when the tube is connected to suction. Sump tubes decrease the possibility of the stomach's wall adhering to and obstructing the drainage openings when suction is applied.

Because nasogastric tubes remain in place for several days or more, many patients complain of nose and throat discomfort. If the tube's diameter is inappropriately large or pressure from its placement is prolonged, tissue irritation or breakdown may occur. Furthermore, the gastric tube tends to dilate the esophageal sphincter, a circular muscle between the esophagus and the stomach. The stretched opening may allow **gastric reflux**, the reverse flow of gastric contents, especially when the tubes are used to administer liquid formula. If or when gastric reflux occurs, the liquid could potentially enter the airway and interfere with respiratory function.

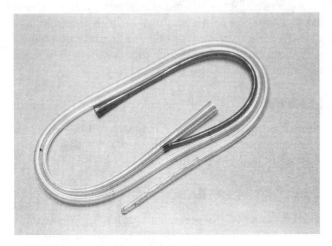

FIGURE 29-3
Vented Salem sump tube. (Courtesy of Ken Timby.)

Nasointestinal Tubes

Nasointestinal tubes are longer than their gastric counterparts, which permits them to be placed in the small bowel. They are used primarily for two reasons: to provide nourishment or to remove gas and liquid drainage from the small intestine.

FEEDING TUBES

Those tubes that are used for nutrition, like a Keofeed tube, are usually small in diameter and made of flexible substances like polyurethane or Silicone. Their narrow width and softer composition allow them to remain in the same nostril for up to 4 weeks. In addition, gastric reflux is less likely because they deliver liquid nutrition beyond the stomach.

Narrow tubes, however, are not free of disadvantages. They tend to curl during insertion because they are so flexible. Therefore, some are supplied with a **stylet**, a metal wire, that helps straighten and support the tube during its insertion. Almost all have a weighted tip that helps them descend past the stomach. Checking the placement of the distal end is also more difficult, and these tubes become obstructed more easily.

Despite the problems associated with maintenance, however, small-diameter tubes are preferred for their comfort. They are ideal for providing a continuous infusion of nourishment.

MERCURY-WEIGHTED TUBES

Nasointestinal tubes, like the Miller-Abbott, Cantor, and Harris tubes (Fig. 29-4), range in length from 6 to 10 feet and are weighted at their tip with a flexible bag containing mercury, a heavy liquid metal. The weight of the mercury propels the tip of the tube beyond the stomach by gravity and peristalsis. Mercury weighted tubes are used for intestinal decompression.

Transabdominal Tubes

Transabdominal tubes are placed through the abdominal wall into the stomach. A **gastrostomy tube** (G-tube) remains located within the stomach, whereas a **jejunostomy tube** (J-tube) leads to the jejunum of the small intestine.

A gastrostomy tube may be placed surgically or with the use of an endoscope. A surgically inserted G-tube looks like a long rubber catheter that is sutured to the abdomen. A G-tube inserted under endoscopic guidance, known as a **percutaneous endoscopic gastrostomy** (PEG) **tube**, contains internal and external crossbars, called bumpers (Fig. 29-5), that anchor the tube. A **percutaneous endoscopic jejunostomy** (PEJ) **tube** (Fig. 29-6) is actually a smaller tube that is passed through the PEG tube into the small intestine.

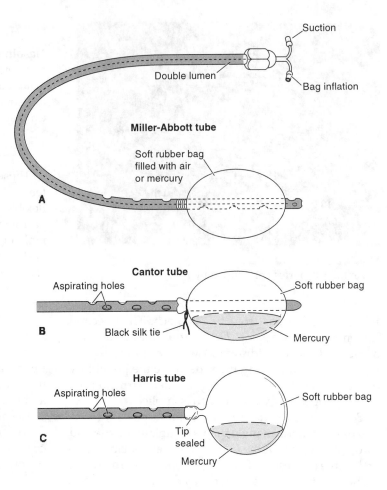

FIGURE 29-4
Mercury-weighted tubes for intestinal decompression. (Scherer JC, Timby BK: Introductory Medical-Surgical Nursing, 6th ed, p 705. Philadelphia, JB Lippincott, 1995)

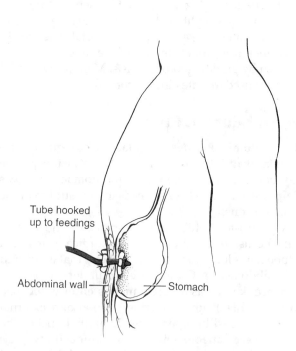

FIGURE 29-5
Percutaneous endoscopic gastrostomy (PEG) tube.

Transabdominal tubes are used in lieu of nasogastric or nasointestinal tubes when patients require an alternative to oral feeding for longer than a month.

Regardless of the type of gastrointestinal tube, nurses are responsible for managing safe patient care.

MANAGING NASOGASTRIC TUBES

Nasogastric tubes are usually inserted by nurses. When in place, nursing responsibilities include keeping them patent, or unobstructed, implementing their prescribed use, and removing them when they have accomplished their therapeutic purpose.

Insertion

The task of inserting a nasogastric tube involves preparing the patient, conducting preintubation assessments, and placing the tube.

PATIENT PREPARATION

Most patients are anxious about having to swallow a tube. Suggesting that the diameter of the tube is smaller than most pieces of food may psychologically foster a positive outcome.

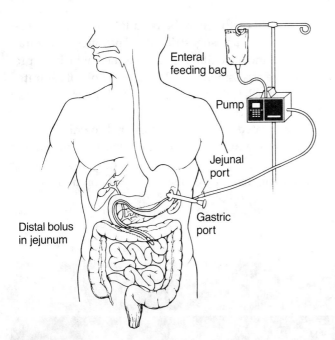

FIGURE 29-6
Percutaneous endoscopic jejunostomy (PEJ) tube. (Courtesy of Ivac Corporation, San Diego, CA, 1990.)

Patients' insecurity may further be reduced by providing a brief explanation of the procedure and instructions as to how they may assist while the tube is being passed. One of the most important mechanisms for supporting patients is to provide them with some means for control. This can be done by establishing a signal like raising the hand, whereby the patient can indicate that a pause is needed during the tube's passage.

ASSESSMENT

Before actually inserting a nasogastric tube, the nurse conducts a focused assessment (Display 29-1). Besides serving as a baseline for future comparisons, the focus assessment findings may suggest modifications in the manner in which a patient is intubated or the equipment that is used.

DISPLAY 29-1. *Preintubation Assessment Data*

- Level of consciousness
- Weight
- Characteristics of bowel sounds
- Extent of abdominal distention
- Integrity of nasal and oral mucosa
- Ability to swallow, cough, and gag
- Presence of nausea or vomiting

More to the point, however, patients are assessed to determine which nostril is best to use when inserting the tube, and the length to which the tube will be inserted.

Nasal Inspection
The nose is inspected after having the patient clear nasal debris by blowing into a paper tissue. Then the size, shape, and patency of each nostril is determined. The assessment can be facilitated by having the patient exhale while one and then the other nostril is occluded. The presence of *nasal polyps*, small growths of tissue, a *deviated septum*, displaced nasal cartilage in the midline of the nose, or a narrow nasal passage excludes one or the other nostril for placement.

Tube Measurement
Some tubes are premarked to indicate the approximate length at which the distal tip will be located within the stomach. However, these markings, if they are present—and, in some cases, they are not—may not correlate exactly with each patient's anatomy. Therefore, before a tube is inserted, the nurse obtains the patient's **NEX** (**n**ose, **e**arlobe, **x**iphoid) **measurement** (Fig. 29-7) and marks the tube appropriately.

The first mark on the tube is placed at the measured distance from the nose to the earlobe. It indicates the distance to the nasal pharynx, a location that places the tip at the back of the throat but above where the gag reflex is stimulated. A second mark is made at the point where the tube reaches the *xiphoid process*, the tip of the breastbone, indicating the depth required to reach the stomach.

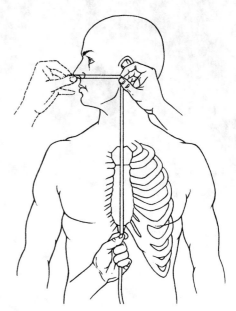

FIGURE 29-7
Obtaining the NEX measurement.

PLACEMENT

When placing, or inserting, a nasogastric tube (Skill 29-1), the nurse's primary concerns are that the tube is inserted with as little discomfort as possible, that the integrity of the nasal tissue is preserved, and that the tube is not inadvertently passed into the respiratory passages.

Checking Placement

Once the tube has been advanced to its final mark, it is checked to verify that it has, indeed, been placed within the stomach. There are three physical assess-

ment methods that may be used to determine the distal location of a nasogastric tube. They include aspirating fluid and auscultating the abdomen, which are presumptive assessments, and testing the pH of aspirated liquid, which is the most accurate technique other than x-ray.

If aspirated fluid appears clear, brownish-yellow, or green, the nurse can presume that its source is the stomach. Using the auscultation method for testing placement, the nurse instills 10 mL or more of air

(text continues on page 603)

SKILL 29-1
Inserting a Nasogastric Tube

Suggested Action	Reason for Action
Assessment	
Check that a medical order has been written.	Ensures that care is within the legal scope of practice
Determine the purpose for the nasogastric tube.	Facilitates evaluation of outcomes
Identify the patient.	Ensures that the procedure will be performed on the correct patient
Assess how much the patient understands about the procedure.	Indicates the need for and level of health teaching
Inspect the nose after the patient blows into a paper tissue.	Provides data that will determine which naris to use
Unwrap and stretch the tube.	Straightens tube and releases bends from product packaging

Clearing nose. (Courtesy of Ken Timby.)

(continued)

SKILL 29-1
Inserting a Nasogastric Tube (Continued)

Suggested Action	Reason for Action
Obtain the NEX measurements.	Determines length for insertion

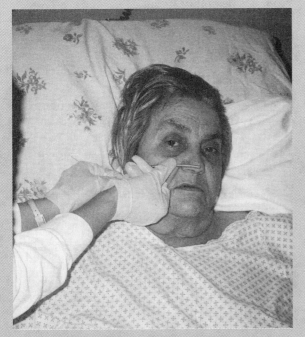

Measuring the tube. (Courtesy of Ken Timby.)

Suggested Action	Reason for Action
Mark the tube at the NE (nose-to-ear) and NX (nose-to-xiphoid) measurements.	Provides a guide during insertion

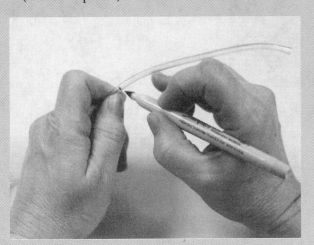

Marking the tube. (Courtesy of Ken Timby.)

(continued)

SKILL 29-1
Inserting a Nasogastric Tube *(Continued)*

Suggested Action	Reason for Action
Planning	
If a plastic tube feels quite rigid, place it in warm water or flush the tube with warm water.	Promotes flexibility
Assemble the following equipment, in addition to the tube: water, straw, towel, lubricant, tissues, tape, emesis basin, flashlight, stethoscope, clean gloves, 50-mL syringe.	Contributes to organization and efficient time management
Place a suction machine at the bedside if the patient is unresponsive or has difficulty swallowing.	Provides a method for clearing the patient's airway of vomitus
Remove dentures.	Avoids choking should they become loose or displaced
Establish a hand signal for pausing.	Relieves anxiety by providing the patient with some locus for control
Implementation	
Wash your hands.	Reduces the transmission of microorganisms
Pull the privacy curtain.	Demonstrates respect for dignity
Assist the patient to sit and hyperextend the neck as if in a sniffing position.	Facilitates inserting the tube
Protect the patient, bedclothing, and linen with a towel.	Avoids linen changes
Don gloves.	Reduces the transmission of microorganisms
Lubricate the tube with water-soluble gel over 6 to 8 inches (15–20 cm) at the distal tip.	Reduces friction and tissue trauma
Insert the tube into the nostril while pointing the tip backward and downward.	Follows the normal contour of the nasal passage

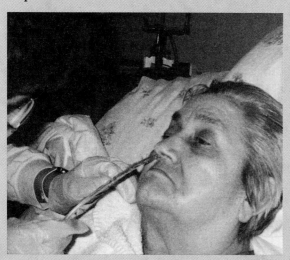

Inserting the tube. (Courtesy of Ken Timby.)

(continued)

SKILL 29-1
Inserting a Nasogastric Tube *(Continued)*

Suggested Action	Reason for Action
Do not force the tube. Relubricate the tube or rotate it if there is some resistance.	Prevents trauma
Stop when the first mark on the tube is at the tip of the nose.	Places the tip above the area where the gag reflex may be stimulated
Use a flashlight to inspect the back of the throat.	Confirms that the tube has been maneuvered around the nasal curve
Instruct the patient to lower his or her chin to the chest and swallow sips of water.	Narrows the trachea and opens the esophagus; helps advance the tube
Advance the tube 3 to 5 inches (7.5–12.5 cm) each time the patient swallows.	Coordinates insertion; reduces the potential for gagging or vomiting
Pause if the patient gives the preestablished signal.	Demonstrates respect and cooperation
Discontinue the procedure and raise the tube to the first mark if there are signs of distress such as gasping, coughing, a bluish skin color, or the inability to speak or hum.	Indicates that the tube is possibly in the airway
Assess placement when the second mark is reached.	Provides data on distal placement

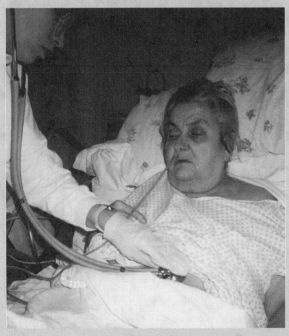

Assessing placement. (Courtesy of Ken Timby.)

Withdraw the tube to the first mark and reattempt insertion if the assessment findings are inconclusive, or consult with the physician about obtaining an x-ray.	Ensures safety

(continued)

SKILL 29-1
Inserting a Nasogastric Tube (Continued)

Suggested Action	Reason for Action
Proceed to secure the tube if data indicate the tube is in the stomach.	Prevents tube migration

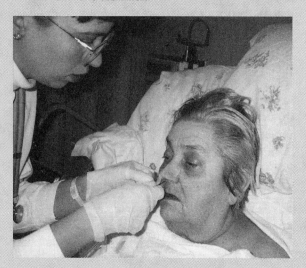

Securing the tube. (Courtesy of Ken Timby.)

Suggested Action	Reason for Action
Connect the tube to suction or clamp it while awaiting further orders.	Promotes gastric decompression or potential use
Remove gloves and wash your hands.	Reduces the transmission of microorganisms
Position the patient with a minimum head elevation of 30°.	Prevents gastric reflux
Remove equipment from the bedside.	Restores orderliness and supports principles of medical asepsis
Measure and record the volume of drainage at least every 8 hours.	Provides data for evaluating fluid balance

Evaluation
- Distal placement within the stomach is confirmed
- No evidence of respiratory distress
- Patient can speak or hum
- Lung sounds are present and clear bilaterally
- No bleeding or pain in area of nasal mucosa

Document
- Type of tube
- Outcomes of the procedure
- Method for determining placement
- A description of drainage
- The type and amount of suction, if the tube is used for decompression

Sample Documentation

Date and Time   16 F Levin tube inserted without difficulty. Placement verified by aspirating gastric secretions, which are yellowish-green and reveal a pH of 3 when tested. Levin tube secured to nose and connected to low, intermittent wall suction. Positioned with head of bed elevated 30°. _____ **Signature, Title**

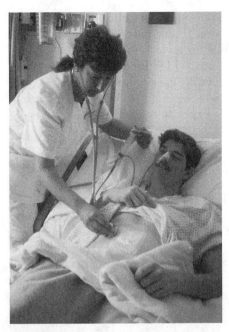

FIGURE 29-8
Checking distal placement. (Courtesy of Ken Timby.)

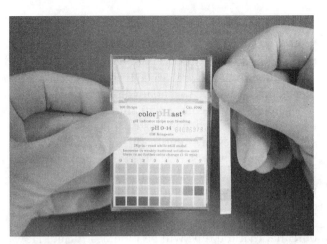

FIGURE 29-9
Checking pH. (Courtesy of Ken Timby.)

while listening with a stethoscope over the abdomen (Fig. 29-8).

If a swooshing sound is heard, the nurse can infer that it was caused by the air entering the stomach. Belching often indicates that the tip is still in the esophagus.

The most definitive assessment, however, involves testing the pH of aspirated fluid. Stomach fluid is acid and usually measures between 1 to 3 on the pH scale. If the pH measures 5 or greater, the fluid may be from the duodenum of the small intestine. A pH of 7 or greater is indicative of a respiratory location. Once stomach placement is confirmed, the tube is secured to avoid its upward or downward migration (Fig. 29-10). The tube may then be used for its intended purpose.

Use and Maintenance

Nasogastric tubes may be connected to suction for gastric decompression or used for tube feeding.

◄
⸽⸽⸽⸽**NURSING GUIDELINES FOR**
     ASSESSING THE PH
     OF ASPIRATED FLUID

- Wear gloves.
  Rationale: Reduces the transmission of microorganisms
- Aspirate a small volume of fluid from the tube with a clean syringe.
  Rationale: Ensures valid test results
- Drop a sample of gastric fluid onto an indicator strip.
  Rationale: Initiates a chemical reaction on contact and saturation
- Compare the color on the test strip with the color guide on the supplied container of reagent strips (Fig. 29-9).
  Rationale: Indicates results according to the color change

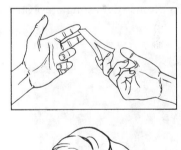

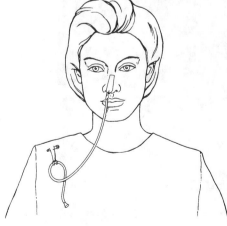

FIGURE 29-10
Technique for securing a nasal tube.

GASTRIC DECOMPRESSION

The suction for gastric decompression may come from either a wall outlet or portable suction machine. The suction setting is prescribed by the physician or indicated in the agency's standards for care.

Usually low (40–60 mm Hg), intermittent suction is used with unvented nasogastric tubes. Intermittent suction provides an interim during which stomach mucosa that adheres to the tip can be temporarily released. Because a vented tube prevents adherence, the prescribed amount of suction is likely to be maintained continuously.

Even with suction applied, there is always the potential that the tube will become obstructed. However, there are some techniques that may promote its patency.

Promoting Patency

Patency can be promoted by giving a patient who is otherwise NPO ice chips or occasional sips of water. The fluid helps to dilute the gastric secretions. However, both must be given sparingly because water is hypotonic and draws electrolytes into the gastric fluid. Because the diluted fluid is ultimately removed, giving the patient liberal amounts can deplete serum electrolytes (see Chap. 15).

Restoring Patency

The nurse frequently assesses whether the tube is remaining patent by monitoring the volume and characteristics of drainage (Fig. 29-11), as well as observing for signs and symptoms suggesting an obstruction. These

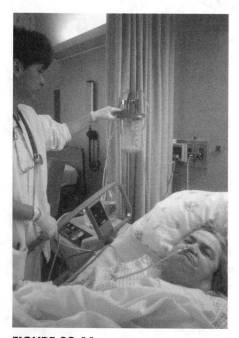

FIGURE 29-11
Monitoring drainage characteristics. (Courtesy of Ken Timby.)

include nausea, vomiting, and abdominal distention. An overall inspection of the equipment may help identify possible causes for the assessment findings (Table 29-2). Once the cause is identified, it may be resolved with a variety of simple nursing interventions.

However, in some cases, it may be necessary to irrigate the nasogastric tube to maintain or restore its patency (Skill 29-2).

PROVIDING ENTERAL NUTRITION

Enteral nutrition refers to nourishing patients via the stomach or small intestine rather than the oral route. Although enteral nourishment can be provided through a nasogastric tube, it is more likely that liquid formula will be administered through a nasointestinal or transabdominal tube (see section on Tube Feedings, later in this chapter).

Removal

A nasogastric tube may be removed when the patient's condition improves, the tube becomes hopelessly obstructed, or standards for care indicate that it must be changed to maintain the integrity of the nasal mucosa (Skill 29-3).

Before removal, some physicians may prescribe a trial period during which the nasogastric tube is clamped and the patient is allowed to resume drinking oral fluids. Remaining asymptomatic is a good indication that the patient no longer requires gastric intubation. If symptoms develop, the tube is already in place and the patient does not have to experience the discomfort of having it replaced.

MANAGING NASOINTESTINAL TUBES

Nasointestinal tubes, used for enteral feeding, are also inserted by nurses.

Insertion

The techniques for tube measurement, placement, and checking placement differ slightly from those described for nasogastric tubes.

TUBE MEASUREMENT

To estimate the length of tube required for intestinal placement, the nurse determines the NEX measurement and adds 9 inches (23 cm). The additional measurement is also marked on the tubing.

(text continues on page 610)

TABLE 29-2. *Troubleshooting a Poorly Draining Nasogastric Tube*

Possible Causes	Solutions
Drainage holes are adhering to the gastric mucosal wall	Turn the suction off momentarily. Change the patient's position.
Tube is displaced above the cardiac sphincter	If measured mark is not at the tip of the nose, remove tape, advance the tube, check placement, and resecure.
Portable suction machine is disconnected or turned off	Replace plug into electrical outlet or turn on power.
Drainage container is filled beyond capacity	Empty and record amount of drainage in suction container.
The vent is acting as a siphon	Instill a bolus of air into the vent to restore patency.
The vent is capped or plugged	Remove cap and restore port to atmospheric pressure.
The tubing is kinked or disconnected	Straighten tubing or reconnect to suction machine.
Inadequate suction	Check that pressure is between 40 to 60 mm Hg.
Loose cover on suction container	Resecure the lid to the container.
Solid particles or thick mucus obstructs lumen	Increase suction pressure momentarily.
	Obtain and implement a medical order for an irrigation.

SKILL 29-2
Irrigating a Nasogastric Tube

Suggested Action	Reason for Action
Assessment	
Monitor the patient's subjective symptoms, volume and rate of drainage, and evidence of abdominal distention.	Provides data for future comparisons
Check that a medical order has been written.	Complies with the legal scope of nursing practice
Identify the patient.	Ensures that the procedure will be performed on the correct patient
Assess how much the patient understands about the procedure.	Provides an opportunity for patient teaching
Planning	
Assemble the following equipment: Asepto or irrigating syringe, irrigating fluid, container, clean towel or pad, clean gloves, cover or plug for end of tube.	Contributes to organization and efficient time management
Turn off the suction.	Facilitates implementation
Implementation	
Pull the privacy curtain.	Demonstrates respect for dignity
Wash your hands.	Reduces the transmission of microorganisms
Place a clean pad or towel beneath where the tube will be separated.	Avoids changing bed linen
Don clean gloves.	Complies with standard precautions
Disconnect the nasogastric tube from the suction tubing and apply cover or insert plug.	Keeps connection area clean
Check the distal placement of the tube.	Ensures safety
Fill irrigating syringe with 30 to 60 mL of normal saline solution.	Provides an adequate quantity of isotonic solution to clear tubing

(continued)

SKILL 29-2
Irrigating a Nasogastric Tube (Continued)

Suggested Action	Reason for Action
Insert the tip of the syringe within the proximal end of the tube and allow the solution to flow in by gravity, or apply gentle pressure.	Dilutes and mobilizes debris

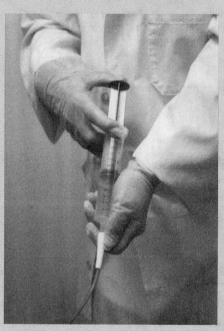

Instilling irrigation solution. (Courtesy of Ken Timby.)

Suggested Action	Reason for Action
Aspirate after the fluid has been instilled.	Removes substances that may impair future drainage
Reconnect the tube to the source of suction.	Resumes therapeutic management
Observe the characteristics of the aspirated solution; measure and discard.	Provides data for evaluating the effectiveness of the procedure

(continued)

SKILL 29-2
Irrigating a Nasogastric Tube (Continued)

Suggested Action	Reason for Action
Monitor for the flow of drainage through the suction tubing.	Provides evidence that patency is being maintained

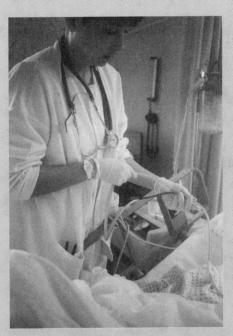

Monitoring drainage. (Courtesy of Ken Timby.)

Remove gloves and wash hands.	Reduces the transmission of microorganisms
Record the volume of instilled and drained fluid on the bedside intake and output sheet.	Provides accurate data for determining fluid balance

Evaluation
- Drainage is restored
- Nausea and vomiting are relieved
- Abdominal distention is reduced

Document
- Volume and type of fluid instilled
- Appearance and volume of returned drainage
- Response of patient

Sample Documentation
Date and Time   Levin tube irrigated with 60 mL of normal saline. Solution instilled with slight pressure. 100 mL of solution returned with several large mucus particles. Reconnected to low, intermittent suction. Draining well at the present time. Abdomen is soft. No vomiting. _____ **Signature, Title**

SKILL 29-3
Removing a Nasogastric Tube

Suggested Action	Reason for Action
Assessment	
Assess bowel sounds, condition of mouth and nasal mucosa, level of consciousness, and gag reflex.	Provides data for future comparisons and may affect the manner in which the procedure is performed
Check that a medical order has been written.	Complies with the legal scope of nursing practice
Identify the patient.	Ensures that the procedure will be performed on the correct patient
Assess how much the patient understands about the procedure.	Provides an opportunity for patient teaching
Planning	
Assemble the following equipment: towel, emesis basin, applicator sticks, oral hygiene equipment, clean gloves.	Contributes to organization and efficient time management
Implementation	
Pull the privacy curtain.	Demonstrates respect for dignity
Wash your hands.	Reduces the transmission of microorganisms
Place the patient in a sitting position, if alert, or in a lateral position if not.	Prevents aspiration of stomach contents
Cover the chest with a clean towel and place the emesis basin and tissues within easy reach.	Prepares for possible vomiting
Remove the tape securing the tube to the patient's nose.	Facilitates pulling the tube from the stomach
Don clean gloves.	Complies with Standard Precautions
Turn off the suction.	Prepares for removal
Clamp, plug, or pinch the tube.	Prevents fluid from leaking as the tube is withdrawn

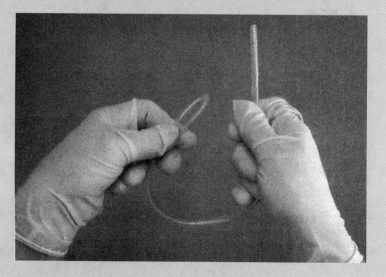

Occluding the tube. (Courtesy of Ken Timby.)

(continued)

SKILL 29-3
Removing a Nasogastric Tube *(Continued)*

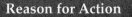

Suggested Action	Reason for Action
Enclose the tube within the towel or glove and discard the tube in a covered container.	Provides a transmission barrier against microorganisms

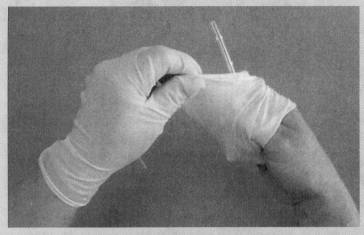

Enclosing the tube. (Courtesy of Ken Timby.)

Suggested Action	Reason for Action
Empty, measure, and record the drainage in the suction container.	Provides data for evaluating the patient's fluid status
Remove gloves and wash hands.	Reduces the transmission of microorganisms
Offer an opportunity for oral hygiene.	Removes disagreeable tastes from the patient's mouth
Encourage the patient to clear the nose of mucus and debris with paper tissues or cotton applicators.	Promotes integrity of nasal tissue
Discard disposable equipment; rinse and return portable suction equipment.	Preserves cleanliness and orderliness in the patient's unit; demonstrates accountability for equipment

Evaluation
* Tube is removed
* Resumes eating and taking fluids
* No nausea or vomiting experienced
* Airway remains clear
* Nasal mucosa is moist and intact

Document
* Type of tube removed
* Response of patient
* Appearance and volume of drainage
* Appearance of nose and nasopharynx

Sample Documentation

Date and Time   Levin tube removed. Brief period of retching during removal. Total of 75 mL clear green drainage emptied from suction container. Oral care provided. L. naris swabbed with applicator lubricated with petroleum jelly. Mucosa is red, but intact.

_____ **Signature, Title**

PLACEMENT

For the most part, the techniques for patient preparation, positioning, and advancement of a nasointestinal tube are similar to those for nasogastric tubes. However, some modifications are necessary because nasointestinal tubes are constructed somewhat differently.

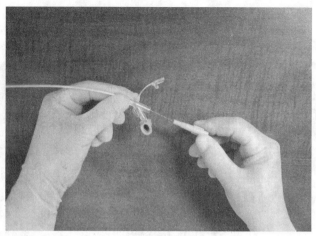

FIGURE 29-13
Removing stylet. (Courtesy of Ken Timby.)

◄ NURSING GUIDELINES FOR INSERTING A NASOINTESTINAL FEEDING TUBE

- Follow the manufacturer's suggestions for activating the lubricant that is bonded to the tube. A common technique is to instill water through the tube.
  Rationale: Transforms the dry bond to a gelatinous consistency
- Secure the stylet within the tube.
  Rationale: Stiffens the tube and facilitates insertion
- Insert the tube to the second mark.
  Rationale: Places the tube in the presumed area of the stomach
- Aspirate fluid using a *50-mL syringe* (Fig. 29-12) and test its pH.
  Rationale: Provides data for determining gastric placement
- Loop the tubing and tape it temporarily to the cheek, if the test for placement suggests that the tip is in the stomach.
  Rationale: Provides a bit of slack so the tube can descend into the small intestine
- Ambulate or position the patient on his or her right side for at least an hour, or the time specified in agency policy.
  Rationale: Provides time and gravity for moving the tube through the pyloric valve of the stomach

- Secure the tube at the nose when the third measured mark is at the nasal tip.
  Rationale: Prevents the tube from migrating further than the desired distance
- Verify placement by x-ray, especially in unconscious patients or those with a depressed gag reflex.
  Rationale: Provides reliable confirmation of the distal location
- Remove the stylet using gentle traction (Fig. 29-13), or follow the manufacturer's suggestions.
  Rationale: Opens the lumen to allow instillation of water and liquid nourishment
- Store the stylet in a clean wrapper at the patient's bedside.
  Rationale: Avoids charging the patient for a new tube should the current one need to be removed and reintroduced
- Never reinsert the stylet while the tube is within the patient.
  Rationale: Prevents trauma to the patient and damage to the tube
- Measure and record the length of tubing extending from the nose.
  Rationale: Provides data for reassessing distal placement

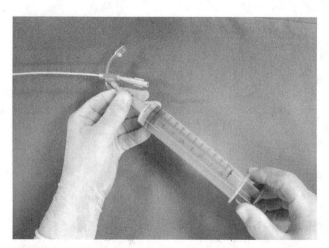

FIGURE 29-12
Aspirating to assess pH. (Courtesy of Ken Timby.)

Checking Tube Placement

Tube placement is always initially verified with an x-ray because checking placement by auscultating air may be inconclusive. Because of the small diameter of the tube, there may be a less pronounced escape of air from its tip. The literature also suggests that aspiration of stomach contents from small-diameter tubes is not always possible because the negative pressure that is created causes the tube to collapse on itself.

Nevertheless, checking placement throughout the period of patient care is essential. Repeated x-rays just

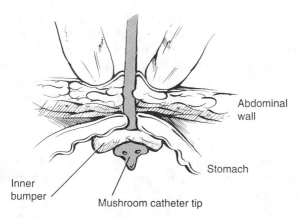

FIGURE 29-14
Inspecting for drainage.

to assess tube placement, however, are expensive, impractical, and potentially harmful. Pulling (1992) reports that by modifying the aspiration technique, it is possible to verify the tube's distal placement. The modification involves using a large-volume (50 mL) rather than a small-volume (3–5 mL) syringe to obtain a sample of fluid. The larger syringe creates less negative pressure during aspiration, and therefore usually provides enough fluid to test the pH 90% of the time.

MANAGING TRANSABDOMINAL TUBES

Transabdominal tubes, like gastrostomy and jejunostomy tubes, are inserted by the physician. However, nurses have a responsibility for assessing and caring

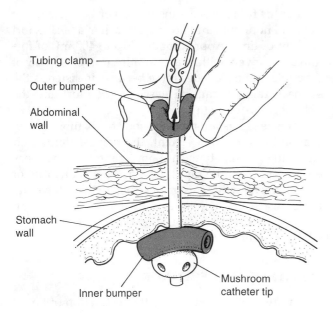

FIGURE 29-15
Inspecting the skin.

for the tube and its insertion site. Conscientious care is required because gastrostomy tubes may leak and cause skin breakdown.

▶ NURSING GUIDELINES FOR MANAGING A GASTROSTOMY

- Wash hands and don gloves.
  Rationale: Reduces the transmission of microorganisms
- Assess and replace the gauze dressing covering the gastrostomy if it becomes moist; expect that there may be slight bleeding or clear serum draining from the wound immediately after the procedure.
  Rationale: Reduces the conditions that support growth of microorganisms and maceration of the skin
- Remove and discontinue the dressing after the first 24 hours unless the physician orders otherwise.
  Rationale: Facilitates assessment
- Inspect the skin around the tube daily.
  Rationale: Provides assessment data about the status of wound repair
- Make sure that the sutures holding a surgically placed tube are intact.
  Rationale: Prevents tube migration
- Report any redness or tissue maceration.
  Rationale: Indicates evidence of early skin impairment
- Apply a skin barrier ointment, like zinc oxide, karaya gum wafer, hydrocolloid dressing, or ostomy pouch if the skin appears irritated (see section on Ostomy Care, Chap. 31).
  Rationale: Protects the skin and promotes healing
- Press down on the skin at the base of the tube (Fig. 29-14).
  Rationale: Aids in assessing for drainage, which normally disappears by the end of the first week
- Compress the arms of the external bumper together and lift them about 1 inch (2.5 cm) if the patient has a PEG tube (Fig. 29-15).
  Rationale: Facilitates inspection
- Clean the skin with half-strength hydrogen peroxide or whatever is the preferred antimicrobial solution. After a week's time, soap and water is sufficient.
  Rationale: Removes secretions and reduces the presence of microorganisms
- Rotate the direction of the external bumper 90° every 4 hours.
  Rationale: Relieves pressure; maintains skin integrity

- Slide the external bumper downward so it is again flush with the skin.
  Rationale: Restabilizes the tube
- Avoid placing any type of dressing material under the arms of the external bumper.
  Rationale: Creates pressure on the internal bumper and may cause damage to the tissue
- Tape the gastrostomy tube to the abdomen.
  Rationale: Maintains the tube's position
- Take care that the tube is not kinked nor the skin stretched.
  Rationale: Ensures patency of the tube and the integrity of the skin
- Insert a Foley catheter (see Chap. 30) 2 to 5 inches (5–10 cm) within the opening and inflate the balloon if the tube comes out.
  Rationale: Maintains temporary access to the stomach and, if done within 3 hours of accidental extubation, prevents the site from closing
- Use the gastrostomy tube in a manner similar to the way in which a nasogastric tube is used for administering feedings.
  Rationale: Serves as a method for providing nourishment

TUBE FEEDINGS

It is always best if nutrition can be provided by the oral route. If oral feedings are impossible or jeopardize the patient's safety, however, nourishment can be provided enterally or parenterally (see section on Total Parenteral Nutrition, Chap. 15).

Tube feedings are used when patients have intact stomach or intestinal function, but are unconscious or have extensive mouth surgery, difficulty swallowing, or esophageal or gastric disorders.

Benefits and Risks

Tube feedings can be delivered through a nasogastric, nasointestinal, or transabdominal tube. Each has its advantages and disadvantages (see Table 29-3).

Instilling nutritional formulas into the stomach uses the natural reservoir for food. It may also reduce the potential for *enteritis*, inflammation of the intestine, because the chemicals in the stomach tend to destroy microorganisms. However, gastric feedings create a greater potential for gastric reflux because of their volume and temporary retention within the stomach.

Although tubes placed within the intestine reduce the risk of gastric reflux, they do not totally eliminate

it. There are additional problems that are associated with intestinal tube feedings. For example, dumping syndrome may occur with an intestinally placed tube. **Dumping syndrome** is a cluster of symptoms that occurs when a concentrated solution, especially one containing glucose, is rapidly placed in the small intestine. The symptoms, which include weakness, dizziness, sweating, and nausea, are produced as a result of fluid shifts from the circulating blood to the intestine and low blood sugar caused by a surge of insulin. Diarrhea may also result from administering hypertonic formula solutions.

Formula Considerations

Selecting the type of tube and access site is only one factor that must be considered before implementing a regimen of tube feedings. The type of formula is also personalized according to the nutritional needs of the patient. Some factors that are considered include weight, present nutritional status, concurrent medical conditions, and projected length of therapy. The feeding schedule may also affect the choice of formula because calories may need to be concentrated if the patient is being fed several times a day rather than on a continuous basis. Most formulas provide 0.5 to 2.0 kcal/mL of formula (Young & White, 1992).

Tube Feeding Schedules

Tube feedings may be administered according to bolus, intermittent, cyclic, or continuous schedules (Skill 29-4).

BOLUS FEEDINGS

A **bolus feeding** is the instillation of a large volume of liquid nourishment into the stomach in a fairly short amount of time. Approximately 250 to 400 mL of formula are given within a few minutes. This type of schedule is the least desirable because it distends the stomach rapidly, causing gastric discomfort and the risk for reflux to occur.

Bolus feedings are repeated four to six times a day. This mimics, to some extent, the natural filling and emptying of the stomach. Some patients experience discomfort from the rapid delivery of this quantity of fluid. Patients who are unconscious or who have delayed gastric emptying are at greater risk for regurgitation, vomiting, and aspiration when this method of administration is used.

INTERMITTENT FEEDINGS

An **intermittent feeding** is the instillation of liquid nourishment into the stomach in the time most people

TABLE 29-3. *Comparison of Feeding Tubes*

Tube	Advantages	Disadvantages
Nasogastric	Low incidence of obstruction Accommodates crushed medications Facilitates bolus or intermittent feedings Easy to check distal placement and gastric residual	Can damage nasal and pharyngeal mucosa from pressure or friction Dilates esophageal sphincter, potentiating gastric reflux Potential for aspiration Requires frequent replacement to ensure integrity of nasal tissue
Nasointestinal	Easy to insert Comfortable Only slight dilation of esophageal sphincter Reduced danger for aspiration Can remain in place for up to 4 weeks	Requires x-ray to verify placement Becomes obstructed easily Best used for continuous feeding
Gastrostomy	No nasal tube Easily concealed Accommodates long-term use Infrequent tube replacement Patient can be taught self-care	Must wait 24 hours to use after initial placement May leak and cause skin breakdown Increased incidence for infection Requires skin care at tube site Can migrate or become dislodged if tube is not secured Gastric overfill and aspiration is possible
Jejunostomy	Same as gastrostomy Reduced potential for reflux and aspiration	Same as gastrostomy

would spend eating a meal. Usually the volume is 250 to 400 mL. Intermittent feedings are usually given by gravity drip from a suspended container over a period of 30 to 60 minutes. Feedings are scheduled four to six times a day. Gradual filling of the stomach at a slower rate reduces the bloated feeling experienced with bolus feedings.

CYCLIC FEEDINGS

A **cyclic feeding** is one that is given continuously for 8 to 12 hours followed by a 16- to 12-hour pause. This routine is often used to wean patients while continuing to maintain an adequate amount of nutrition. The tube feeding is given during the late evening hours and during sleep. During the day, patients eat some food orally. As the patient's oral intake increases, the volume and duration of tube feeding are gradually decreased.

CONTINUOUS FEEDINGS

A **continuous feeding** is the instillation of a small volume of liquid nourishment without any interruption. Approximately 1.5 mL/minute is administered. An electric feeding pump is used to regulate the infusion. Because there is only a small amount of fluid at any one time, the formula does not need to be held in the reservoir of the stomach; it can be delivered directly into the small intestine. Instilling small amounts of fluid beyond the stomach reduces the danger for vomiting and aspiration. Continuous feeding does, however, create some inconvenience. The pump must go wherever the patient goes.

Patient Assessment

The following daily assessments are standard for almost every patient who receives tube feedings: weight, fluid intake and output, bowel sounds, lung sounds, temperature, condition of the nasal and oral mucous membranes, breathing pattern, gastric complaints, abdominal distention, vomiting, bowel elimination patterns, skin condition at the site of a transabdominal tube. Once tube feedings have been initiated, it is also necessary to assess the patient's gastric residual on a routine basis.

GASTRIC RESIDUAL

Gastric residual is the volume of liquid remaining within the stomach after allowing a compensatory time for stomach emptying. The purpose for checking gastric residual is to determine if the rate or volume of feeding exceeds the patient's physiologic capacity. Overfilling the stomach can cause esophageal reflux, regurgitation, vomiting, aspiration, and pneumonia. As a rule of thumb, the gastric residual should be no more than 100 mL or no more than 20% of the previous hour's tube feeding volume (Bockus, 1993).

(text continues on page 622)

SKILL 29-4
Administering Tube Feedings

Suggested Action	Reason for Action
Bolus Feeding	
Assessment	
Check the medical order for the type of nourishment, volume, and schedule to follow.	Complies with the legal scope of nursing practice
Check the date and identifying information on the container of tube-feeding formula.	Ensures accurate administration and avoids using formula that may be outdated
Identify the patient.	Ensures that the procedure will be performed on the correct patient
Assess bowel sounds and measure gastric residual.	Provides data indicating safety for instilling liquids through the tube

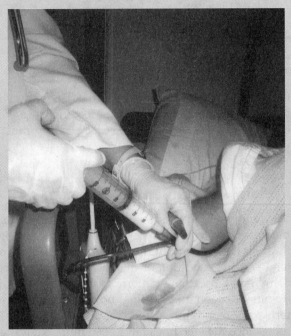

Measuring gastric residual. (Courtesy of Ken Timby.)

Measure capillary blood glucose or glucose in the urine.	Provides data indicating response to caloric intake
Assess how much the patient understands about the procedure.	Provides an opportunity for patient teaching
Planning	
Replace unused formula every 24 hours.	Reduces the potential for bacterial growth
Wait and recheck gastric residual in 1/2 hour if it exceeds 100 mL.	Avoids overfilling the stomach
Assemble the following equipment: Asepto syringe, formula, tap water.	Contributes to organization and efficient time management.
Warm refrigerated nourishment to room temperature in a basin of warm water.	Prevents chilling and abdominal cramping

(continued)

SKILL 29-4
Administering Tube Feedings (Continued)

Suggested Action	Reason for Action
Implementation	
Wash your hands.	Reduces the transmission of microorganisms
Place the patient in a 30° to 90° sitting position.	Prevents regurgitation
Refeed gastric residual by gravity flow.	Returns predigested nutrients without excessive pressure
Pinch the tube just before all the residual has instilled.	Prevents air from entering the tube
Add fresh formula to the syringe and adjust the height to allow a slow, but gradual instillation.	Provides nourishment

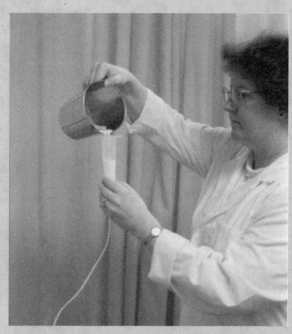

Administering a bolus feeding. (Courtesy of Ken Timby.)

Suggested Action	Reason for Action
Continue filling the syringe before it becomes empty.	Prevents air from entering the tube
If a gastrostomy tube is being used, tilt the barrel of the syringe during the feeding.	Permits air displacement from the stomach

(continued)

SKILL 29-4
Administering Tube Feedings (Continued)

Suggested Action	Reason for Action
Flush the tubing with at least 30 to 60 mL of water after each feeding or follow agency policy for suggested amounts.	Ensures that all of nourishment has entered the stomach; prevents fermentation and coagulation of formula in the tube; provides water for fluid balance

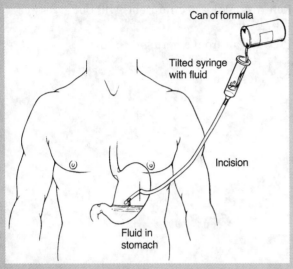

Bolus feeding through a gastrostomy tube.

Plug or clamp the tube as the water leaves the syringe.	Prevents air from entering the tubing; maintains patency
Keep the head of the bed elevated for at least 30 to 60 minutes after a feeding.	Prevents esophageal reflux
Wash and dry the feeding equipment. Return items to the bedside.	Supports principles of medical asepsis
Record the volume of formula and water administered on the bedside intake and output record.	Provides accurate data for assessing fluid balance and caloric value of nourishment
Provide oral hygiene at least twice daily.	Removes microorganisms and promotes comfort and hygiene of patient

Intermittent Feeding

Assessment

Follow the previous sequence for assessment.	Principles remain the same

Planning

In addition to those activities listed for bolus feeding:

Replace unused formula, feeding containers, and tubing every 24 hours.	Reduces the potential for bacterial growth

Implementation

Fill the feeding container with room-temperature formula.	Cold formula can cause cramping; room-temperature formula will be instilled before supporting bacterial growth
Purge the air from the tubing by gradually opening the clamp on the tubing.	Prevents instilling air

(continued)

SKILL 29-4
Administering Tube Feedings *(Continued)*

Suggested Action	Reason for Action
Connect the tubing to the nasogastric or naso-enteral tube.	Provides access to formula

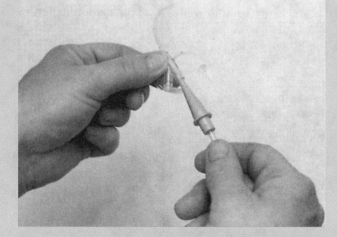

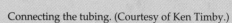

Connecting the tubing. (Courtesy of Ken Timby.)

Suggested Action	Reason for Action
Open the clamp and regulate the drip rate according to the physician's order or agency policy.	Supports safe administration of liquid nourishment
Check at 10-minute intervals.	Ensures early identification of infusion problems

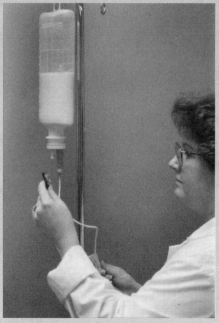

Checking the rate of flow. (Courtesy of Ken Timby.)

Suggested Action	Reason for Action
Flush the tubing with water after the formula has infused.	Clears the tubing of formula, prevents obstruction, and provides water for fluid balance.

(continued)

SKILL 29-4
Administering Tube Feedings (Continued)

Suggested Action	Reason for Action
Pinch the nasal tube just as the last volume of water is administered.	Prevents air from entering the tube
Clamp or plug the nasal tube.	Prevents leaking
Record the volume of formula and water instilled.	Provides accurate data for assessing fluid balance and caloric value of nourishment
Follow recommendations for postprocedural care as described with bolus feeding.	Principles for care remain the same

Continuous Feeding

Assessment

In addition to previously described assessments:	Principles remain the same
Check the gastric residual every 4 hours.	Ensures a routine pattern for assessment to accommodate the schedule of continuous feedings.

Planning

In addition to previously described planning activities:	
Obtain equipment for regulating continuous infusion, such as a tube-feeding pump.	Aids accurate administration and sounds an alarm if the infusion is interrupted
Replace unused formula, feeding containers, and tubing every 24 hours.	Reduces the potential for bacterial growth
Attach a time tape to a feeding container.	Facilitates periodic assessment

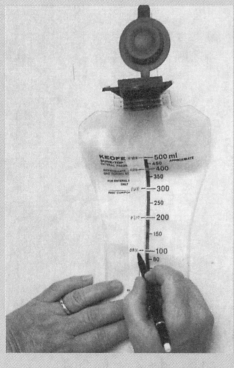

Attaching a time strip. (Courtesy of Ken Timby.)

(continued)

SKILL 29-4
Administering Tube Feedings (Continued)

Suggested Action	Reason for Action
Implementation	
Flush the new feeding container with water.	Reduces surface tension within the tube and enhances the passage of large protein molecules.
Fill the feeding container with no more than 4 hours' worth of refrigerated formula. *Exception:* commercially prepared, sterilized containers of formula or formula that is kept iced while infusing may hang for longer periods.	Prevents growth of bacteria Cold formula will be warmed by body heat when infused at a slow rate
Purge the tubing of air.	Prevents distention of the stomach or intestine
Thread the tubing within the feeding pump according to the manufacturer's directions.	Ensures correct mechanical operation of equipment and accurate administration to the patient

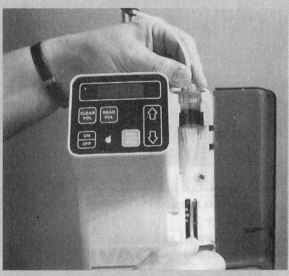

Preparing the pump. (Courtesy of Ken Timby.)

Suggested Action	Reason for Action
Connect the tubing from the feeding pump to the patient's feeding tube.	Provides access to formula

(continued)

SKILL 29-4
Administering Tube Feedings (Continued)

Suggested Action	Reason for Action
Set the prescribed rate on the feeding pump.	Complies with medical order

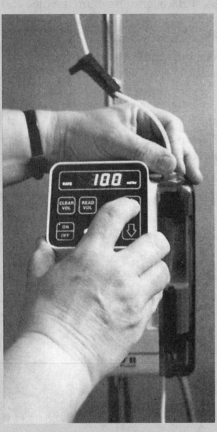

Programming the pump. (Courtesy of Ken Timby.)

(continued)

SKILL 29-4
Administering Tube Feedings (Continued)

Suggested Action	Reason for Action
Open the clamp on the feeding tube and start the pump.	Initiates infusion

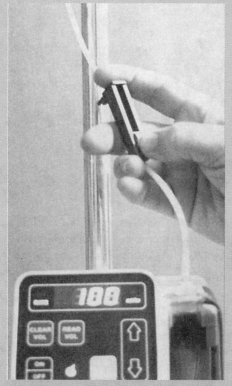

Releasing the clamp. (Courtesy of Ken Timby.)

Suggested Action	Reason for Action
Keep the patient's head elevated at all times.	Prevents reflux and aspiration
Flush the tubing with 30 to 60 mL of water, or more, every 4 hours after checking and refeeding gastric residual, and after administering medications.	Promotes patency and contributes to the patient's fluid balance
Record the volume of formula and water instilled.	Provides accurate data for assessing fluid balance and caloric value of nourishment
Follow recommendations for postprocedural care as described with bolus feeding.	Principles for care remain the same

(continued)

SKILL 29-4
Administering Tube Feedings (Continued)

Suggested Action	Reason for Action

Evaluation

• Receives prescribed volume of formula according to established feeding schedule
• Weight remains stable or reaches target weight
• Lungs remain clear
• Bowel elimination is normal
• Has a daily fluid intake between 2,000 and 3,000 mL, unless intake is otherwise restricted

Document

• Volume of gastric residual and actions taken if excessive
• Type and volume of formula
• Rate of infusion, if continuous
• Volume of water used for flushes
• Response of patient; if symptomatic, describe actions taken and results

Sample Documentation

Date and Time   50 mL of gastric residual. Residual reinstilled and tube flushed with 60 mL of tap water. 480 mL of Enrich with Fiber placed in tube feeding bag. Formula infusing at 120 mL/hr. No diarrhea or gastric complaints at this time. _____ **Signature, Title**

NURSING GUIDELINES FOR CHECKING GASTRIC RESIDUAL

• Stop the infusion of tube feeding formula.
  Rationale: Facilitates assessment
• Aspirate fluid from the feeding tube using a 50-mL syringe.
  Rationale: Allows collection of a large volume of fluid
• Continue aspirating until no more fluid is obtained.
  Rationale: Ensures an accurate assessment
• Measure the aspirated fluid and record the amount.
  Rationale: Provides objective data for evaluation
• Reinstill the aspirated fluid.
  Rationale: Returns partially digested nutrients and electrolytes to the patient
• Postpone tube feeding and report residual amounts that exceed agency guidelines or those established by the physician.
  Rationale: Reduces the risk of aspiration
• Recheck gastric residual again in 1/2 hour.
  Rationale: Allows time for a portion of the stomach contents to empty into the small intestine
• Provide or resume tube feeding, if gastric residual is within an acceptable range.
  Rationale: Prevents overfeeding the patient

Nursing Management

Caring for patients with feeding tubes generally involves maintaining tube patency, clearing obstructions should they occur, providing adequate hydration, dealing with common formula-related problems, and preparing patients for home care.

MAINTAINING TUBE PATENCY

Feeding tubes, especially those that are smaller than 12 French, are prone to becoming obstructed (Display 29-2). To maintain patency, it is best to flush feeding tubes with 30 to 60 mL of water:

DISPLAY 29-2. *Common Causes of Feeding Tube Obstructions*

• Introducing formulas with nutrients of large molecular size
• Refeeding partially digested gastric residual
• Administering formula at rates less than 50 mL/hour
• Instilling crushed or hydrophilic (water-absorbing) medications into the tube

- Immediately before and after administering a feeding or medications
- Every 4 hours if the patient is being continuously fed
- After refeeding the gastric residual

Although tap water is effective as a flush solution, cranberry juice and carbonated beverages may be used. Formula tends to curdle when coming in contact with cranberry juice, which detracts from the efficacy of this approach.

CLEARING AN OBSTRUCTION

If an obstruction occurs, the physician is consulted. Occasionally it may be possible to clear the tube with a solution of meat tenderizer or pancreatic enzyme. However, both require written medical orders.

Webber-Jones and colleagues (1992) suggest the following actions for unclogging a feeding tube:

◄ NURSING GUIDELINES FOR CLEARING AN OBSTRUCTED FEEDING TUBE

- Select a syringe with a minimum 50-mL capacity.
  Rationale: Reduces negative pressure during aspiration, which could lead to collapse of the tube walls
- Aspirate as much as possible from the feeding tube.
  Rationale: Clears the path above the obstructing debris
- Instill 5 mL of the selected solution.
  Rationale: Allows direct contact between the irrigating solution and the debris
- Clamp the tube and wait 15 minutes.
  Rationale: Ensures time for the substance in solution to have a physical effect on the obstructing debris
- Aspirate or flush the tube with water.
  Rationale: Uses negative pressure or positive pressure to restore patency
- Repeat if necessary.
  Rationale: Promotes patency

When an obstruction cannot be cleared, it is in the patient's best interest to remove the tube and insert another rather than compromise nutrition by the delay.

PROVIDING ADEQUATE HYDRATION

Despite the fact that tube feedings are approximately 80% water (Young & White, 1992), patients usu-

ally require more. Adults require 30 mL of water/kg of weight or 1 mL/kcal on a daily basis (Bockus, 1993).

To determine if a patient's hydration needs are being met, the listed amounts of moisture are identified on formula labels. This plus the total volume of flush solution can be added and compared with the recommended amount. If there is a significant deficit, the plan for care is revised to provide either an increase in the volume or, preferably, the frequency for flushing the tube. If the fluid volume is excessive, the urine output and lung sounds are monitored to determine if the patient is able to excrete comparable amounts (see Chap. 15).

DEALING WITH MISCELLANEOUS PROBLEMS

There are several common or potential problems that are experienced by patients who require enteral feeding. Many are associated with tube feeding formulas or the mechanical effects of the tubes themselves (Table 29-4). When problems occur, they are reported promptly, and changes are made in the patient's plan for care.

PREPARING FOR HOME CARE

Because of shortened lengths of stay in hospitals, some patients who continue to need tube feedings are being discharged to care for themselves at home. Before the procedure is demonstrated, a written instruction sheet is provided that includes:

- Resources for obtaining equipment and formula
- The amount and schedule for each feeding and flush, using household measurements
- Guidelines for delaying a feeding
- Special instructions for skin or nose care, including frequency and types of products to use
- Types of problems to report, such as weight loss, reduction in urination, weakness, diarrhea, nausea and vomiting, and breathing difficulties
- A list of phone numbers to call and names to ask for if questions arise during home care
- The date, time, and place for continued medical follow-up.

Most nasogastric, nasointestinal, and transabdominal tubes are used for enteral feeding or gastric decompression. However, there are occasions when nurses must assist with and manage the care of patients who require intestinal decompression.

INTESTINAL DECOMPRESSION

Intestinal decompression refers to the removal of gas and fluids from the small bowel. The procedure is done with unique nasointestinal tubes.

TABLE 29-4. Common Tube-Feeding Problems

Problem	Common Causes	Solutions
Diarrhea	Highly concentrated formula	Dilute initial tube feeding to 1/4 to 1/2 strength.
	Rapid administration	Start at 25 mL/hour and increase rate by 25 mL q12 h.
	Bacterial contamination	Wash hands.
		Change formula bag and tubing q 24 h.
		Hang no more than 4 hours' worth of formula.
		Refrigerate unused formula.
	Lactose intolerance	Consult with the physician on using a milk-free formula.
	Inadequate protein content	Raise serum albumin levels with total parenteral nutrition solutions containing supplemental protein or administer albumin intravenously.
	Medication side effects	Consult with the physician about adjusting drug therapy or administering an antidiarrheal.
Nausea and vomiting	Rapid feeding	Instill bolus and intermittent feedings by gravity.
	Overfeeding	Delay feeding until gastric residual is less than 100 mL or less than 20% of hourly volume.
		Maintain sitting position for at least 30 minutes after feeding.
		Consult with the physician about ordering medication that facilitates gastric emptying.
		Administer continuous feedings.
		Instill feedings within the small intestine.
	Air in stomach	Keep tubing filled with formula or water.
	Medication side effects	Consult with the physician about adjusting drug therapy or administering drugs to control symptoms.
Aspiration	Incorrect tube placement	Check placement before instilling liquids.
	Vomiting	Keep head elevated at least 30° during feedings and for 1/2 hour afterwards.
		Keep cuffed tracheostomy and endotracheal tubes inflated.
		Refer to measures for controlling vomiting.
Constipation	Lack of fiber	Change formula.
	Dehydration	Increase supplemental water.
		Consult with the physician on giving a laxative, enema, or suppository.
Elevated blood sugar	Calorie concentrated formula	Instill diluted formula and gradually increase concentration.
		Administer insulin according to medical orders.
Weight loss	Inadequate calories	Increase calories in formula.
		Increase rate or frequency of feedings.
Elevated electrolytes	Dehydration	Increase supplemental water.
Dry oral and nasal mucous membranes	Mouth breathing	Frequent oral and nasal hygiene.
	Dried nasal mucus	
Middle ear inflammation	Narrowing or obstruction of eustachian tube from presence of tube in pharynx	Turn from side to side q 2 h.
		Insert a small-diameter feeding tube.
Sore throat	Pressure and irritation from tube	Use a small-diameter feeding tube.
Plugged feeding tube	Instilling crushed or powdered medications through the tube	Use liquid medications.
		Dilute crushed drugs.
		Flush the tubing liberally after drug administration.
	Formula coagulation from drug–food interactions	Flush tubing with water before and after drug administration.
		Follow agency policy for alternative flush solutions such as carbonated beverages or solutions of meat tenderizer.
	Kinked tube	Maintain neck in neutral position or change position frequently.
	Large molecules in formula	Dilute formula.
		Flush tubing at least q 4 h.
		Use a larger-diameter feeding tube.
Dumping syndrome	Rapid and large instillation of highly concentrated formula into the intestine	Administer small, continuous volume.
		Adjust glucose content of formula.

Tube Insertion

Nasointestinal tubes like the Miller-Abbott, Cantor, and Harris tubes are inserted into the stomach by the physician in much the same manner as a nasogastric tube, but the nurse is responsible for promoting and monitoring their movement into the intestine.

Each type of intestinal tube contains a bag at the distal end for mercury. In the absence of peristalsis, the weight of the mercury-filled bag propels the tip of the tube beyond the stomach by gravity. If the Miller-Abbott tube is used, the mercury is instilled *after* the tube has passed into the stomach. The mercury is instilled in the balloon of the Cantor and Harris tubes with a needle *before* insertion. Leakage does not occur because the needle does not make an opening large enough to permit the escape of the mercury. The bag is elongated when the tube is inserted, so that it can be passed more easily and with less discomfort to the patient.

Openings throughout the distal end provide channels through which intestinal contents can be suctioned. These tubes are left in place until the intestinal lumen is patent and peristalsis resumes or some other form of treatment is instituted.

◄ NURSING GUIDELINES FOR ASSISTING WITH THE INSERTION OF MERCURY-WEIGHTED TUBES

- Assemble all the necessary equipment. In addition to the equipment needed for gastric intubation, the following should be available: the specified tube, long cotton-tipped applicators that will help to insert the balloon within the patient's nostril, mercury, and a 5-mL syringe with a 21-gauge needle.
  Rationale: Ensures organization and efficient time management
- Label the adapter on a Miller-Abbott tube through which mercury will be instilled.
  Rationale: Prevents confusion over which lumen is to be used for suction
- Test the balloon by inflating it with air and submerging it in water to observe for air bubbles.
  Rationale: Helps identify leaks in the balloon
- Replace the tube if it is defective.
  Rationale: Ensures patient safety
- Place the patient in a high-Fowler's position with the neck hyperextended.
  Rationale: Facilitates passage of the tube
- Generously lubricate the balloon and distal 6 inches of the tube.
  Rationale: Reduces friction
- Hand the physician a long cotton applicator.

  Rationale: Helps advance the tube through the nose and into the nasopharynx
- Instruct the patient to flex his or her chin to the chest when the tube is at the back of the throat.
  Rationale: Reduces the possibility that the tube will enter the airway
- Coach the patient to drink water or swallow when instructed.
  Rationale: Helps advance the tube
- Provide emotional support to the patient.
  Rationale: Acknowledges that this procedure can be stressful
- Thread the excess tubing through a sling of folded gauze taped to the forehead (Fig. 29-16).
  Rationale: Supports the tube as it advances
- Ambulate the patient.
  Rationale: Helps the tube move downward
- *When a radiograph indicates that the intestinal tube has advanced beyond the stomach, position the patient:*
  - On the right side for 2 hours, then
  - On the back in a Fowler's position for 2 hours, then
  - On the left side for 2 hours.
  Rationale: Uses gravity and positioning to promote movement through anatomic curves
- Follow the policy manual or physician's instructions for manually advancing the tube several inches each hour.
  Rationale: Supplements natural peristaltic advancement
- Observe the lines or numbers on the tube.
  Rationale: Provides a means for monitoring the tube's progression and approximate anatomic location
- Request x-ray confirmation when the tube has reached the prescribed distance.
  Rationale: Provides objective evidence verifying the terminal location of the distal tip
- Secure the tube once its distal location has been confirmed.

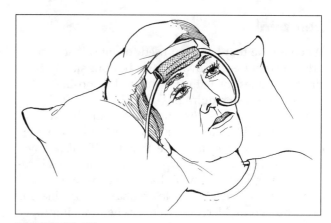

FIGURE 29-16
Fashioning a gauze sling.

PATIENT TEACHING FOR HOME TUBE FEEDING

Teach the patient or the family to do the following:
- Monitor weight on a weekly basis.
- Report a loss of 2 or more pounds in 1 week.
- Observe that a sufficient quantity of urine is passed five to six times a day and that the urine appears light yellow.
- Inspect and clean the skin area where the tube is located.
- Purchase two sets of formula containers with tubing.
- Change the feeding container and tubing daily if it is used for continuous feedings.
- Wash the feeding container, tubing, and all utensils for mixing and storing formula between uses with hot soapy water, rinse well, and drain dry.
- Wash your hands before mixing formula and equipment.
- Mix or open only enough formula for one feeding at a time.
- Keep opened or mixed formula refrigerated; store unopened, commercial formula at room temperature.

- Postpone the feeding if nausea and vomiting are experienced; reevaluate in 1 hour.
- Hang or hold the formula container approximately 24 to 36 inches above the stomach.
- Regulate the rate of infusion by tightening the roller clamp on the tubing or varying the height of the container—the lower the container, the slower the instillation.
- Consult someone in authority if you feel there is reason to delay a feeding beyond 1 hour.
- Flush the tube with the specified volume of water before and after each administration of formula, after the instillation of medications, or on a regularly scheduled basis if continuous feedings are being administered.
- Clamp or plug the tubing before the entire volume of flush solution has instilled.
- Remain in a sitting position during the instillation of formula and for at least a half-hour afterward.

Rationale: Stabilizes the tube and prevents further migration
- Coil the excess tubing and attach it to the patient's hospital gown.
Rationale: Prevents accidental extubation
- Connect the proximal end to wall or portable suction.
Rationale: Produces negative pressure to pull substances from their source

Once the tube has served its usefulness, the nurse is often instructed to begin the process of removing it.

Removal

When a tube that has been used for intestinal decompression requires removal, it must be done slowly. Special techniques for withdrawing and disposing of the mercury are also required.

First the tube is disconnected from the suction source. If a Miller-Abbott tube has been used, the mercury is withdrawn by aspirating it with a 10-mL syringe. The mercury in the other types of intestinal tubes is removed after the tube is withdrawn. Whenever the mercury is removed, it is placed in a biohazard container for proper disposal. Mercury is a toxic chemical; improper disposal contributes to environmental pollution.

To remove the tube, the tape securing it to the face is removed and the tube is withdrawn 6 to 10 inches (15–25 cm) at 10-minute intervals. When the last 18 inches (45 cm) of a Miller-Abbott tube remains, it is removed from the nose. If a Cantor or Harris tube has been used, however, the bag of mercury is grasped with a forceps when it reaches the pharynx, and the bag is withdrawn from the patient's mouth. Once the mercury is removed from the bag, the tube is withdrawn from the nose. Afterward, it is considerate to provide nasal and oral hygiene.

NURSING IMPLICATIONS

Depending on the data collected during the process of patient care, one or more of the nursing diagnoses listed in the Applicable Nursing Diagnoses may be identified.

The accompanying Nursing Care Plan, Risk for Aspiration, is offered as a model for managing the care of a patient with a large gastric residual. This particular diagnostic problem is defined by NANDA (1994) as "The state in which an individual is at risk for entry of gastro-intestinal secretions, oropharyngeal secretions, or solids or fluids into tracheo-bronchial passages."

FOCUS ON OLDER ADULTS

- In older adults, the gag reflex may become depressed because of repeated insertion and removal of dentures (Meehan, 1992).
- In older adults, who are at risk for dehydration, hyperglycemia (elevated blood glucose levels) may develop more quickly than in other adults who receive tube feedings.
- It is best to check an older patient's capillary blood glucose every 4 hours until the patient's blood sugar is within normal range for 48 hours while receiving full-strength concentrations of tube-feeding formula.
- Monitor older adults for agitation or confusion, which may cause them to remove the tube being used to provide nourishment.
- Older adults tend to tolerate small, but continuous feedings better.
- When teaching an older adult or older caregiver how to manage a gastrostomy tube or administer tube feedings at home, plan the teaching schedule to allow more time for processing the information, and several practice sessions.
- For older adults living on a very fixed income, the dietitian may suggest ways of preparing home-blenderized formulas that meet the nutritional needs of the patient.
- In 1992, the American Nurses Association published a position statement indicating that advance directives indicating a wish to avoid artificial nutrition and hydration should be followed (see Chap. 3).

 APPLICABLE NURSING DIAGNOSES

- Altered Nutrition: Less than body requirements
- Feeding Self-Care Deficit
- Impaired Swallowing
- Risk for Aspiration
- Altered Oral Mucous Membrane
- Diarrhea
- Constipation

KEY CONCEPTS

- "Intubation" refers to the insertion of a tube into a structure of the body.
- Gastrointestinal intubation is used for providing nourishment; administering medications; obtaining diagnostic samples; removing poisons, gas, and secretions; and controlling bleeding.
- Four types of tubes that may be used for intubating the gastrointestinal system include orogastric, nasogastric, nasointestinal, and transabdominal tubes.
- Some common assessments before inserting a tube nasally include determining the patient's level of consciousness, characteristics and location of bowel sounds, structure and integrity of the nose, and ability to swallow, cough, and gag.
- An NEX measurement, which helps to determine how far to insert a tube for stomach placement, is the distance from the nose to the earlobe and nose to the xiphoid process.
- Stomach placement is checked by aspirating gastric fluid, auscultating the abdomen as a bolus of air is instilled, and testing the pH of aspirated fluid.
- Nasointestinal feeding tubes differ from their nasogastric counterparts in that they are longer, narrower, and more flexible; their lubricant is bonded to the tube; they are frequently inserted with a stylet; and an x-ray is used to confirm their placement.
- Although transabdominal feeding tubes can be used for long periods of time, they are prone to leaking and causing skin impairment.
- "Enteral nutrition" refers to nourishing patients via the stomach or small intestine rather than the oral route.
- There are four common schedules for administering tube feedings: bolus, intermittent, cyclic, and continuous.
- The purpose for checking gastric residual is to determine if the rate or volume of feeding exceeds the patient's physiologic capacity.
- Caring for patients with feeding tubes generally involves maintaining tube patency, clearing obstructions should they occur, providing adequate hydration, dealing with common formula-related problems, and preparing patients for home care.
- Before discharging patients who will administer their own tube feedings, they are provided with written instructions that include, among other information, resources for obtaining equipment and formula, the amount and schedule for each feeding, guidelines for delaying a feeding, and instructions for skin or nose care.
- When assisting with the insertion of a mercury-weighted tube, nurses assume responsibility for promoting and monitoring its movement into the intestine.

NURSING CARE PLAN:
Risk for Aspiration

Assessment

Subjective Data
None obtained; patient is unresponsive.

Objective Data
35-year-old with head trauma after motor vehicle accident. Opens eyes, but makes no verbal response. Moves away when painful stimulus is applied. #16 nasogastric tube in L. naris. Tube placement verified by instilling air and auscultating over stomach. Gastric residual measures 150 mL 4 hours after previous bolus feeding of 400 mL.

Diagnosis

Risk for Aspiration related to slow gastric emptying.

Plan

Goal
Gastric residual will be less than 100 mL within 1 hour of feeding schedule.

Orders: 8/22
1. Keep cuff of endotracheal tube inflated.
2. Maintain head elevation at no less than 30° at all times.
3. Monitor bowel sounds; report if absent or less than five sounds per minute.
4. Measure gastric residual before all tube feedings.
5. Refeed gastric residual and follow with 30 mL tap water flush.
6. Postpone tube feeding for 1 hour if gastric residual measures ≥100 mL.
7. Report gastric residual volume to physician if ≥100 mL after delaying feeding for 1 hour and reassess.
8. Maintain suction machine at the bedside. _____ J. RHAMES, RN

Implementation
(Documentation)

8/23   0800   Bowel sounds present and active in all quadrants. Endotracheal tube cuff remains inflated. Head is elevated 30°. Gastric residual measures 150 mL. Residual reinstilled followed with 30 mL flush with tap water. Tube feeding postponed. _____ A. PETRY, LPN

0900   Gastric residual measures 100 mL after 1 hour delay of tube feeding. Volume of gastric residual reported to Dr. Burns. Orders received for metaclopramide and replacement of nasogastric tube with a small nasointestinal tube when residual measures 50 mL, and resume tube feeding on a continuous basis once tube is in intestine (see physician's orders). Head maintained in elevated position at 60°. _____ A. PETRY, LPN

Evaluation
(Documentation)

1030   Gastric residual measures 50 mL. Nasogastric tube replaced with 8 F Keofeed tube. Placement verified by x-ray. Tube feeding resumed at 100 mL/hr with feeding pump as ordered. _____ A. PETRY, LPN

CRITICAL THINKING EXERCISES

- Describe the similarities and differences between inserting a tube for gastric decompression and one for intestinal decompression.
- What questions would be important to ask a discharged tube-fed patient who calls to report the onset of diarrhea?

SUGGESTED READINGS

Ahern HL, Rice KT. How do you measure gastric pH. American Journal of Nursing May 1991;91:70.

Bockus S. When your patient needs tube feedings: making the right decisions. Nursing July 1993;23:34–43.

Eisenberg PG. Nasoenteral tubes: a nurse's guide to tube feeding. RN October 1994;57:62–66, 68–69.

Faller N, Lawrence KG. Comparing low-profile gastrostomy tubes. Nursing December 1993;23:46–48.

Faller NA, Lawrence KG. How to stabilize a percutaneous tube. Nursing July 1992;22:52–54.

Galindo-Ciocon DJ. Tube-feeding: complications among the elderly. Journal of Gerontological Nursing June 1993;19:17–22.

Gruver J. Selecting an enteral feeding pump. American Journal of Nursing June 1993;93:66–68.

Lehmann S, Barber JR. Giving medications by feeding tube: how to avoid problems. Nursing November 1991;21:58–61.

Martyn-Nemeth P, Fitzgerald K. Clinical considerations: tube feeding in the elderly. Journal of Gerontological Nursing February 1992;18:30–38.

Meehan M. Nursing Dx: potential for aspiration. RN January 1992; 55:30–35.

Metheny N, Reed L, Worseck M. How to aspirate fluid from a small-bore feeding tube. American Journal of Nursing May 1993;93:86–88.

Pulling R. The right place . . . feeding tubes . . . do nurses accurately assess their correct placement? Canadian Nurse February 1992; 88:29–30.

Shuster M. Preparing patients for tube feeding at home. American Journal of Nursing November 1992;92:21.

Surratt S, Ryan AB, Hallenbeck P. Troubleshooting a sump tube. American Journal of Nursing January 1993;93:42–47.

Webber-Jones J, Sweeney K, Winterbottom A. How to declog a feeding tube. Nursing April 1992;22:62–64.

Weiler K. Artificial nutrition and hydration . . . nurse's role in withholding and withdrawing food and fluids from patients. Journal of Gerontological Nursing July 1992;18:45.

Young CK, White S. Preparing patients for tube feeding at home. American Journal of Nursing April 1992; 92:46–53.

UNIT IX
Promoting Elimination

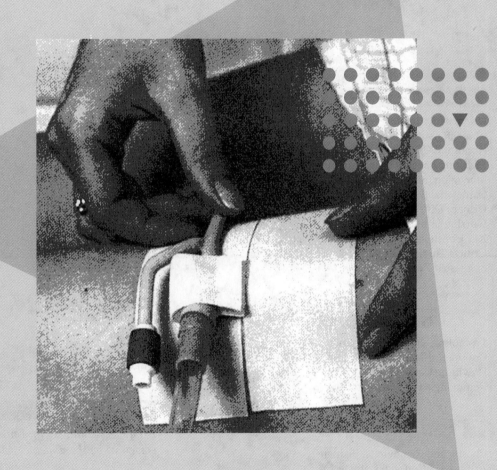

CHAPTER 30
Urinary Elimination

Learning Objectives

An understanding of the content within this chapter will be evidenced by the student's ability to:

- Name four urinary structures and their collective functions
- Name at least five factors that affect urination
- List four physical characteristics of urine
- Name four types of urine specimens that nurses frequently collect
- List six abnormal urinary elimination patterns
- Identify three devices that may be used for urinary elimination as alternatives to a conventional toilet
- Explain the meaning of continence training
- Name three types of urinary catheters
- Describe two principles that apply to using a closed drainage system

Timby BK: *Fundamental Skills and Concepts in Patient Care, Sixth Edition* © 1996 Lippincott-Raven Publishers

- Explain why catheter care is important in the nursing management of patients with retention catheters
- Discuss the purpose for irrigating a catheter and identify three ways in which this is done
- Explain the meaning of a urinary diversion
- Discuss some factors that contribute to skin impairment among patients with a urostomy
- Describe two incontinence aids that may promote older adults' self-esteem and decrease their social isolation

In this chapter the process of urinary elimination is briefly reviewed. In addition, nursing skills for assessing and maintaining urinary elimination are described.

URINARY ELIMINATION

Urinary elimination is the release of fluid and chemical substances in a waste solution called **urine**. When urinary elimination becomes impaired, the consequences can be life threatening.

Urinary Structures and Function

The urinary system (Fig. 30-1) consists of the kidneys, ureters, bladder, and urethra. These major components, along with some accessory structures, like the ring-shaped muscles called the internal and external sphincters, coordinate to produce urine, collect it, and excrete it from the body.

Urination

Urination is the process by which urine is released. Urination takes place several times each day. The need to urinate, or **void**, becomes apparent when the bladder distends with approximately 250 to 400 mL of urine (Sherwood, 1995). The increase in fluid pressure stimulates stretch receptors within the bladder wall, creating a desire to empty it of urine.

FACTORS AFFECTING URINATION

The patterns of urinary elimination vary depending on physiologic, emotional, and social factors. Some examples include:

- Neuromuscular development
- Integrity of the spinal cord
- Volume of fluid intake
- Fluid losses from other sources
- Amount and type of food consumed
- Circadian rhythm
- Opportunity for urination
- Personal habits
- Anxiety

PROMOTING NORMAL URINARY ELIMINATION

Normal urination can be promoted in several ways.

⟶ **NURSING GUIDELINES FOR PROMOTING URINARY ELIMINATION**

- Provide privacy.
  Rationale: Eliminates tension and worry about being publicly observed during what most consider a very personal activity
- Help women to assume a sitting position and men to stand.
  Rationale: Facilitates the most anatomically correct urinating position for each gender
- Maintain an adequate fluid intake.
  Rationale: Ensures an adequate circulatory volume from which urine is formed
- Use the power of imagery and suggestion to initiate voiding, like running water from the tap.
  Rationale: Provides the brain with sensory and psychological stimuli that trigger physiologic mechanisms for releasing urine

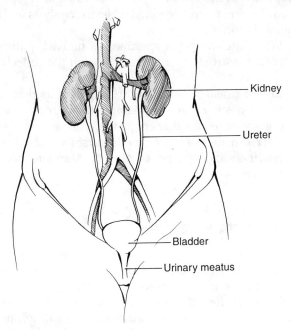

FIGURE 30-1
Major structures of the urinary system.

Kidney

Ureter

Bladder

Urinary meatus

TABLE 30-1. *Characteristics of Urine*

Characteristic	Normal	Abnormal	Common Causes of Variations
Volume	500–2,500 mL/day 1,200 mL average	<400 mL/day	Low fluid intake Excess fluid loss Kidney dysfunction
		>2,500 mL/day	High fluid intake Diuretic medication Endocrine diseases
Color	Light yellow	Dark amber Brown Reddish-brown Orange, green, blue	Dehydration Liver/gallbladder disease Blood Water-soluble dyes
Clarity	Transparent	Cloudy	Infection Stasis
Odor	Faintly aromatic	Foul Strong Pungent	Infection Dehydration Certain foods

CHARACTERISTICS OF URINE

The physical characteristics of urine include its volume, color, clarity, and odor. Nevertheless, despite specific quantitative and descriptive criteria, there can be wide variations within what is considered normal (Table 30-1).

Collecting Urine Specimens

Urine specimens, or samples of urine, may be collected to identify the microscopic or chemical constituents of urine. Common urine specimens that nurses collect include voided specimens, clean-catch specimens, catheter specimens, and 24-hour specimens.

VOIDED SPECIMENS

A **voided specimen** is a sample of urine that has been freshly urinated into a clean, dry collection container. The first voided specimen of the day is preferred, the rationale being that a morning specimen is most likely to contain a substantial accumulation of urinary substances.

In some cases, nurses perform tests on voided specimens with chemical reagent strips (Fig. 30-2). More often than not, however, the sample of urine is transferred into a specimen container and delivered to the laboratory for testing and analysis. If the specimen cannot be examined in less than 1 hour after its collection, the urine sample is labeled and refrigerated.

CLEAN-CATCH SPECIMENS

A **clean-catch specimen**, sometimes called a *midstream specimen*, is collected in such a way as to avoid contaminating the voided sample with microorganisms or substances other than those present in the urine. To do this, the urinary meatus, the opening to the urethra, and tissue surrounding it are cleaned and the urine is collected after the initial stream of urine has been released—hence the name, "midstream specimen."

If at all possible clean-catch specimens are preferred to randomly voided specimens. This method of collection is also preferrable whenever a urine specimen is needed during the menstruating cycle of a female patient. As soon as the specimen is collected, it is labeled and taken to the laboratory. A clean-catch urine specimen also must be refrigerated when the analysis will be delayed more than 1 hour.

When a clean-catch specimen is needed, patients are often instructed on how to perform the collection technique.

Recent research (Winslow, 1993) suggests that collecting a specimen in midstream without prior cleansing provides results that are just as reliable as those in which cleansing was performed. Nurses are advised to follow their agency's policy until the standard procedure is revised.

CATHETER SPECIMENS

It is possible to collect a urine specimen under sterile conditions using a catheter (see Skill 30-3). However, this is usually done only when patients are catheterized for other reasons. Another technique for patients who are already catheterized is to aspirate a sample of urine through the lumen of a latex catheter or from a self-sealing port (Fig. 30-3).

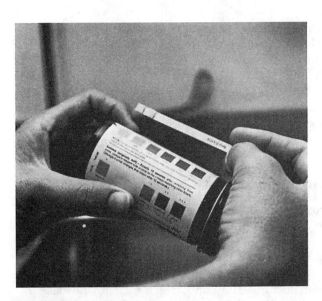

FIGURE 30-2
Chemical reagent strips for testing urine.

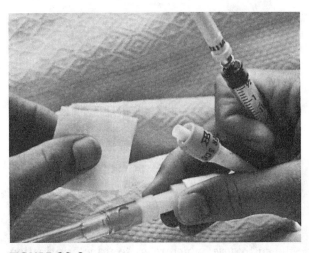

FIGURE 30-3
Location for collecting a catheter specimen.

TWENTY-FOUR–HOUR SPECIMENS

A **24-hour specimen** is one in which *all* the urine produced in a full 24-hour period is collected, labeled, and delivered to the laboratory for analysis. Because the urine may decompose over this period of time, the collected urine is placed in a container with a chemical preservative, or the container is placed in a basin of ice or a refrigerator.

To establish the 24-hour collection period accurately, the patient is instructed to urinate just before starting the test. This essentially empties the bladder. All urine voided at intervals thereafter becomes a part of the collected specimen. The final contribution to the specimen takes place the next day. Exactly 24 hours after the test was initiated, the patient is asked to void once again. After the final urination, the specimen is labeled and taken to the laboratory.

Laboratory analysis is a valuable diagnostic tool for identifying abnormal characteristics of urine.

Abnormal Urine Characteristics

There are specific terms that describe particular abnormal characteristics of urine and urination. Many terms

---

 PATIENT TEACHING FOR COLLECTING A CLEAN-CATCH SPECIMEN

Teach the *female* patient to do the following:
- Wash your hands.
- Remove the lid from the specimen container.
- Rest the lid upside down on its outer surface, taking care not to touch the inside areas.
- Sit on the toilet and spread your legs.
- Separate your labia with your fingers.
- Cleanse each side of the urinary meatus with a separate antiseptic swab, wiping toward the vagina.
- Use the final clean, moistened swab to wipe directly down the center of the separated tissue.
- Begin to urinate.
- After a small amount of urine has been released into the toilet, catch a sample of urine in the specimen container.
- Take care not to touch the mouth of the specimen container to your skin.

- Place the specimen container nearby.
- Release your fingers and continue voiding normally.
- Complete handwashing.
- Cover the specimen container with the lid.

Teach the *male* patient to do the following:
- Follow all of the steps for collecting the specimen as described for a woman, *except* follow this cleansing routine:
- Retract your foreskin, if you are uncircumcised; otherwise
- Cleanse in a circular direction around the tip of the penis toward its base using a premoistened antiseptic swab.
- Repeat with another swab.
- Continue retracting the foreskin while initiating the first release of urine and until the midstream specimen has been collected.

DISPLAY 30-1. *Abnormal Urine Characteristics*

Hematuria	Urine that contains blood
Pyuria	Urine that contains pus
Proteinuria	Urine that contains plasma proteins
Albuminuria	Urine that contains albumin, a plasma protein
Glycosuria	Urine that contains glucose
Ketonuria	Urine that contains ketones

use the suffix *uria*, which refers to urine or urination (Display 30-1).

ABNORMAL URINARY ELIMINATION PATTERNS

Analyzing assessment data may indicate that some patients have abnormal urinary elimination patterns. Some common problems include anuria, oliguria, polyuria, nocturia, dysuria, and incontinence.

Anuria

Anuria refers to the absence of urine or up to a 100-mL output in 24 hours. If the kidneys are not forming urine, the term **urinary suppression** may be used. The most distinguishing characteristic of urinary suppression is that the bladder is empty, and therefore there is no urge to urinate. This distinguishes anuria from urinary retention. **Urinary retention** refers to a condition in which urine is produced but is not released from the bladder. Urinary retention is identified by a progressively distending bladder.

Oliguria

Oliguria is a term meaning that the volume of voided urine is quite small. The term is used when the urine output falls below 400 mL over 24 hours.

Sometimes oliguria is a sign that the bladder is being partially emptied at the time of voiding. The unvoided volume of urine is referred to as **residual urine**. Retained urine can support the growth of microorganisms, leading to an infection. Also, when there is urinary **stasis** (lack of movement), dissolved substances like calcium can precipitate, causing stones to form.

Polyuria

Polyuria describes a condition in which a large volume of urine is eliminated without any reasonable explana-

tion. Ordinarily, urine output is nearly equal to fluid intake. When this is not the case, there is cause to believe that the excessive urination results from a pathologic disorder.

Common disorders associated with polyuria include *diabetes mellitus*, an endocrine disorder caused by insufficient insulin, and *diabetes insipidus*, an endocrine disease caused by insufficient antidiuretic hormone.

Nocturia

Nocturia is characterized by being awakened at night to urinate. Because the rate of urine production is normally reduced at night, nocturia may indicate an underlying medical problem.

An enlarging prostate gland is commonly associated with nocturia. The gland, which encircles the male urethra, may interfere with complete bladder emptying as it increases in size.

Dysuria

Dysuria refers to difficult or uncomfortable voiding. It is a common symptom of trauma to the urethra or a bladder infection. Dysuria is often accompanied by **frequency**, a need to urinate often, and **urgency**, a strong feeling that urine must be eliminated quickly.

Incontinence

Incontinence is the inability to control elimination. In the case of urine, the term is prefaced as *urinary* incontinence. However, the label is not to be used indiscriminately—any person may be incontinent if their need for assistance goes unnoticed. Spontaneous urination once the bladder has become extremely distended may be more of a personnel problem than a patient problem.

ASSISTING PATIENTS WITH URINARY ELIMINATION

Stable patients who can ambulate can be assisted to the bathroom to use the toilet. Others may need to use a commode.

Using a Commode

A **commode** is a chair with an opening in the seat under which a receptacle is placed. A commode is placed beside or a short distance from the bedside. It may be used for eliminating urine or stool. Immediately afterward, the waste container is removed, emptied, cleaned, and replaced.

Patients who are confined to bed must use a urinal and bedpan for their elimination needs.

Using a Urinal

A **urinal** is a container for collecting urine. Because of anatomic differences, urinals are more easily used by male patients.

When providing a urinal, make sure it is empty; otherwise, the bed linen may become wet and soiled. Some patients, however, may need assistance with placing the urinal. To do this:

- Pull the privacy curtain
- Don gloves
- Ask the patient to spread his legs
- Hold the urinal by its handle
- Direct the urinal at an angle between the patient's legs so that the bottom rests on the bed (Fig. 30-4)
- Lift the penis and place it well within the urinal

After use of a urinal, it is promptly emptied. The volume of urine is measured and recorded, if the patient's intake and output are being monitored (see Chap. 15). Patients are always offered an opportunity for handwashing after elimination.

Using a Bedpan

A **bedpan** is a plastic or metal container for elimination that is placed under the buttocks (Skill 30-1). It is designed for collecting either urine or stool. Most are several inches deep to provide a sufficient area for collecting the products of elimination. A *fracture pan*, on the other hand, is a modified version of a conventional bedpan. It is quite flat on the sitting end (Fig. 30-5). This

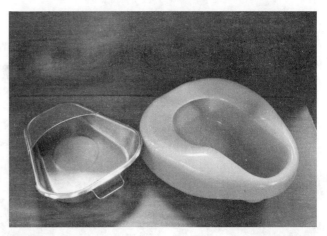

FIGURE 30-5
Two types of bedpans: fracture pan (*left*) and conventional bedpan (*right*). (Courtesy of Ken Timby.)

feature enables it to be used by patients with musculoskeletal disorders who may not be able to elevate their hips or sit on a bedpan in the usual manner.

MANAGING INCONTINENCE

There are six recognized types of urinary incontinence. They include stress, urge, reflex, functional, overflow, and total incontinence (Table 30-2). Urinary incontinence, depending on the type, may be either permanent or temporary.

The management of incontinence is complex because there are so many variations. Treatment is further complicated by the fact that some patients may have more than one type of incontinence. For example, stress incontinence is often combined with urge incontinence as well.

Some forms of incontinence respond to simple measures like modifying clothing so that elimination is more easily facilitated. Others may improve with a more regimented approach like continence training.

Continence Training

Continence training is the process of restoring the ability to empty the bladder at an appropriate time and place. Continence training is sometimes referred to as *bladder retraining*, but this term is somewhat inaccurate because various techniques involve mechanisms other than those that are unique to the bladder.

SELECTING APPROPRIATE CANDIDATES

Continence training is most beneficial for patients who have the cognitive ability and desire to participate in a rehabilitation program. This may include, but is

(*text continues on page 640*)

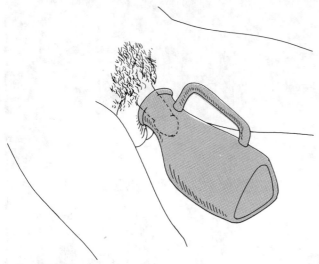

FIGURE 30-4
Placement of urinal. (Earnest VV: Clinical Skills in Nursing, 2nd ed, p 585. Philadelphia, JB Lippincott, 1992)

SKILL 30-1
Placing and Removing a Bedpan

Suggested Action	Reason for Action
Assessment	
Ask the patient if he or she feels the need to void.	Anticipates elimination needs
Palpate the lower abdomen for signs of bladder distention.	Indicates bladder fullness
Determine if there is a need to use a fracture pan or if there are any restrictions in turning or lifting.	Prevents further injury
Planning	
Gather needed supplies such as clean gloves, the bedpan, toilet tissue, and a disposable pad.	Promotes organization and efficient time management
Warm the bedpan by running warm water over it, especially if it is made of metal.	Demonstrates a concern for the patient's comfort
Implementation	
Wash your hands and don clean gloves.	Reduces the transmission of microorganisms
Place the adjustable bed in high position.	Promotes good use of body mechanics
Close the door and pull the privacy curtains.	Demonstrates the patient's right to privacy and dignity
Raise the top linen enough to determine the location of the patient's hips and buttocks.	Prevents unnecessary exposure
Instruct the patient to bend his or her knees and press down with the feet.	Helps in elevating the hips
Place a disposable pad over the bottom sheets, if it seems necessary.	Protects bed linen from becoming wet and soiled
Slip the bedpan beneath the patient's buttocks.	Ensures proper placement

Placing a bedpan from a sitting position. (Craven RF, Hirnle CJ: Fundamentals of Nursing: Human Health and Function, p 679. Philadelphia, JB Lippincott, 1992)

(continued)

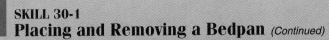

SKILL 30-1
Placing and Removing a Bedpan (Continued)

Suggested Action	Reason for Action
Or, roll the patient to the side and position the bedpan.	Reduces work effort and the potential for a work-related injury

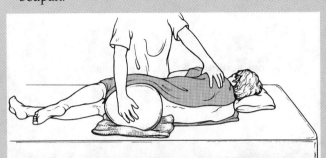

Placing a bedpan from a side-lying position. (Craven RF, Hirnle CJ: Fundamentals of Nursing: Human Health and Function, p 679. Philadelphia, JB Lippincott, 1992)

Suggested Action	Reason for Action
Raise the head of the bed.	Simulates the natural position for elimination

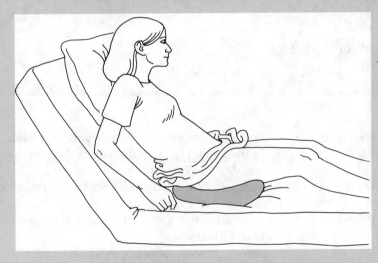

Position for elimination. (Earnest, VV: Clinical Skills in Nursing, 2nd ed, p 584. Philadelphia, JB Lippincott, 1992)

Suggested Action	Reason for Action
Ensure that the toilet tissue is within the patient's reach.	Provides supplies for hygiene
Identify the location of the signal device and leave the patient, if it is safe to do so.	Respects privacy yet provides a mechanism for communicating a need for assistance
Return and remove the bedpan.	Prevents discomfort
Assist with removing residue of urine from the skin, if that is necessary.	Prevents offensive odors and skin irritation
Wrap the gloved hand with toilet tissue and wipe from the meatus toward the anal area.	Supports principles of medical asepsis
Place soiled tissue in the bedpan.	Contains soiled tissue until the time of disposal
Help the patient to a position of comfort.	Ensures the patient's well-being
Provide supplies for handwashing.	Removes residue of urine and colonizing micro-organisms
Measure the volume of urine if the patient's intake and output are being monitored.	Ensures accurate data collection

(continued)

SKILL 30-1
Placing and Removing a Bedpan (Continued)

Suggested Action	Reason for Action
Save a sample of urine if it appears abnormal in any way.	Facilitates laboratory examination or further assessment
Empty the urine into a toilet and flush.	Facilitates disposal
Clean the bedpan and replace it in a place that is separate from clean supplies.	Supports principles of asepsis
Remove your gloves and wash your hands.	Removes colonizing microorganisms

Evaluation
- Bedpan is positioned without injury
- Urine (and stool) are eliminated
- Hygiene measures are accurately performed

Document
- Volume of urine eliminated for purposes of monitoring intake and output
- Appearance and other characteristics of the urine

Sample Documentation

Date and Time   Assisted to use the bedpan. Voided 300 mL of clear, amber urine without difficulty.

_____ **Signature, Title**

not limited to, patients with lower body paralysis who wish to facilitate urination without the use of urinary drainage devices such as a catheter.

Whomever the candidate, everyone involved must understand that continence training is often a slow process that requires the combined effort and dedication of the nursing team, patient, and family.

NURSING GUIDELINES FOR CONTINENCE TRAINING

- Compile a log of the patient's elimination patterns.
  Rationale: Aids in analyzing the patient's unique type of incontinence and how best to plan rehabilitation
- Set realistic, specific, short-term goals with the patient.
  Rationale: Prevents self-defeating consequences
- Discourage strict limitation of liquid intake.
  Rationale: Maintains fluid balance and ensures an adequate volume of urine
- Plan a trial schedule for voiding that correlates with the times when the patient is usually incontinent or experiences bladder distention.
  Rationale: Reduces the potential for accidental voiding or sustained urinary retention
- In the absence of any identifiable pattern, plan to assist the patient with voiding every 2 hours during the day and every 4 hours at night.
  Rationale: Accommodates for the time it takes to form a sufficient volume of urine
- Communicate the plan with nursing personnel, the patient, and family.
  Rationale: Promotes continuity of care and dedication to reaching goals
- Assist the patient to a toilet or commode; position the patient on a bedpan; or place a urinal before the scheduled time for trial voiding.
  Rationale: Readies the patient for releasing urine
- Simulate the sound of urination, such as running water from the faucet.
  Rationale: Stimulates relaxation of the sphincter muscles, allowing for the release of urine
- Suggest bending forward and applying hand pressure over the bladder, a technique referred to as **Credé's maneuver** (Fig. 30-6).
  Rationale: Increases abdominal pressure so as to overcome the resistance of the internal sphincter muscle
- Instruct paralyzed patients to identify any sensation that precedes voiding, like a chill, muscular spasm, restlessness, or spontaneous erection.
  Rationale: Provides a cue for anticipating urination

TABLE 30-2. Types of Incontinence

Type	Description	Example	Common Causes	Nursing Approach
Stress	The loss of small amounts of urine during situations when intra-abdominal pressure rises	Dribbling is associated with sneezing, coughing, lifting, laughing, or rising from a bed or chair	Loss of perineal and sphincter muscle tone secondary to childbirth, menopausal atrophy, prolapsed uterus, or obesity	Pelvic floor muscle strengthening Weight reduction
Urge	The need to void is perceived frequently, with short-lived ability to sustain control of the flow	Voiding commences when there is a delay in accessing a restroom	Bladder irritation secondary to infection; loss of bladder tone due to recent continuous drainage with an indwelling catheter	Maintain fluid intake of at least 2,000 mL/day Omit bladder irritants, such as caffeine or alcohol Administer diuretics in the morning
Reflex	Spontaneous loss of urine when the bladder is stretched with urine, but without prior perception of a need to void	Automatic release of urine that cannot be controlled by the person	Damage to motor and sensory tracts in the lower spinal cord secondary to trauma, tumor, or other neurologic conditions	Cutaneous triggering Straight intermittent catheterization
Functional	Control over urination is lost because of inaccessibility of a toilet or a compromised ability to use one	Voiding occurs while attempting to overcome barriers such as doorways, transferring from a wheelchair, manipulating clothing, acquiring assistance, or making needs known	Impaired mobility, impaired cognition, physical restraints, inability to communicate	Modify clothing Facilitate access to a toilet, commode, or urinal Assist to a toilet according to a pre-planned schedule Absorbent undergarments External catheter Indwelling catheter
Total	Loss of urine without any identifiable pattern or warning	A person passes urine without any ability or effort to control	Altered consciousness secondary to a head injury, loss of sphincter tone secondary to prostatectomy, anatomic leak through a urethral/vaginal fistula	
Overflow	Urine leaks because the bladder is not completely emptied and remains distended with retained urine	The person voids small amount frequently or urine leaks around a catheter	Overstretched bladder or weakened muscle tone secondary to obstruction of the urethra by debris within a catheter, an enlarged prostate, distended bowel, or postoperative bladder spasms	Hydration Adequate bowel elimination Maintain patency of catheter Perform Credé's maneuver

641

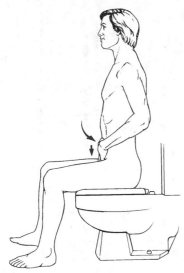

FIGURE 30-6
Credé's maneuver.

• Propose that paralyzed patients with *reflex* incontinence lightly massage or tap the skin above their pubic area, a method known as **cutaneous triggering**. *Rationale:* Initiates urination among patients who have retained a **voiding reflex**, a spontaneous sphincter response to physical stimulation

• Teach patients with *stress* incontinence to perform **Kegel exercises** (Display 30-2). *Rationale:* Strengthens and tones *pubococcygeal* and *levator ani* muscles used voluntarily to hold back urine as well as intestinal gas or stool

• Assist patients with *urge* incontinence to walk slowly and concentrate on holding their urine when nearing the area of the toilet. *Rationale:* Reverses previous mental conditioning wherein the urge to urinate becomes stronger and more overpowering the closer to the toilet

---

In cases that are not amenable to rehabilitation, use of absorbent undergarments or catheterization may be necessary alternatives.

CATHETERIZATION

Catheterization refers to the act of applying or inserting a device called a catheter. A **urinary catheter** may be used for various reasons, some of which include:

• Keeping incontinent patients dry
• Relieving bladder distention when patients are unable to void
• Assessing fluid balance accurately
• Keeping the bladder from becoming distended during procedures such as surgery
• Measuring the residual urine left in the bladder after voiding

---

DISPLAY 30-2. *Technique for Performing Kegel Exercises*

• Tighten the internal muscles used to prevent urination or interrupt urination once it has begun
• Keep the muscles contracted for at least 10 seconds
• Relax the muscles for the same period of time
• Repeat the pattern of contraction and relaxation 10 to 25 times each day
• Perform the exercise regimen three to four times a day for at least 2 weeks to 1 month

---

• Obtaining sterile urine specimens
• Instilling medication within the bladder

Types of Catheters

There are three common types of catheters: external catheters, straight catheters, and retention catheters.

EXTERNAL CATHETERS

An **external catheter** is a device that is applied to the skin so as to cover the urinary meatus. One type of external catheter is called a *condom catheter*; another is a *urinary bag* or *U-bag* (Fig. 30-7). Because of the differ-

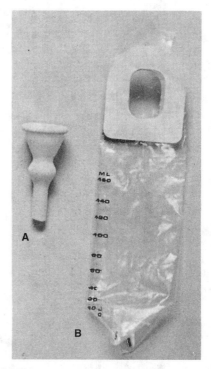

FIGURE 30-7
External urine collection devices: (*A*) Condom catheter, (*B*) "U" or urinary bag. (Courtesy of Ken Timby.)

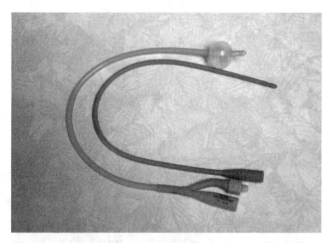

FIGURE 30-8
Types of urinary catheters: retention (Foley) catheter with balloon and straight catheter. (Courtesy of Ken Timby.)

ences in male and female anatomy, external catheters are more effective for men.

Condom catheters are helpful for managing incontinent patients being cared for at home because they are quite easy to apply. A condom catheter has a flexible sheath that is unrolled over the penis. The narrow end is connected to tubing that serves as a channel for draining urine. It can be attached to a leg bag or connected to a larger urine collection device.

A urinary bag is more often used for collecting urine specimens from infants. It is attached to the skin surrounding the genitals by removing an adhesive backing. Urine collects in the self-contained bag. Once a sufficient quantity of urine has been collected, the urinary bag is removed.

Applying a Condom Catheter

Despite the simplicity of condom catheters, there are three potential problems involved in their use. First, and perhaps the most hazardous, is that the sheath may be applied too tightly and may restrict blood flow to the skin and tissues of the penis. Second, moisture tends to accumulate beneath the sheath and can lead to skin breakdown. Third, condom catheters frequently leak. These problems, however, can be avoided by applying the catheter correctly and managing the patient's care appropriately (Skill 30-2).

STRAIGHT CATHETERS

A **straight catheter** (Fig. 30-8) is a narrow tube that is placed in the bladder until it is temporarily drained or a sufficient volume for a urine specimen is obtained.

RETENTION CATHETERS

A **retention catheter** (see Fig. 30-8) is also called an *indwelling catheter*, because it is placed within the bladder and secured there for a period of time. The most common type of retention catheter is called a *Foley* catheter.

Retention catheters differ from straight catheters in that they are held in place by a balloon that is inflated once the distal tip is within the bladder. Both straight and retention catheters are available in various diameters. They are sized according to the French scale (see Chap. 29). For adults, catheters of sizes 14, 16, and 18 French are usually used.

Inserting a Catheter

The technique for inserting a catheter is similar whether a straight or Foley retention catheter is used. The main difference is that the steps for inflating the retention balloon do not apply if a straight catheter is being inserted.

Because the anatomy, and consequently the techniques for insertion, are different for each gender, the skills are also described separately (Skills 30-3 and 30-4).

CONNECTING A CLOSED DRAINAGE SYSTEM

A **closed drainage system** is a device used to collect urine from a catheter. It consists of a calibrated bag, which can be opened at the bottom, tubing of sufficient length to accommodate for turning and positioning patients, and a hanger from which to suspend the bag from the bed (Fig. 30-9).

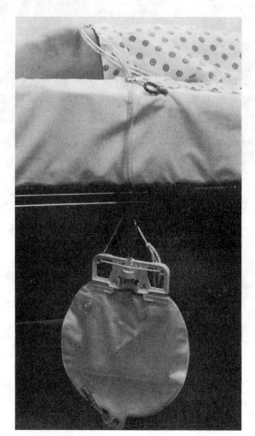

FIGURE 30-9
Closed urine drainage system.

NURSING GUIDELINES FOR PROVIDING CATHETER CARE

- Plan to cleanse the meatus and a nearby section of catheter at least once a day.
  Rationale: Reduces the number of colonizing microorganisms
- Gather soap, water, washcloth, towel, disposable pad, antiseptic solution, sterile gauze squares or cotton balls, antibiotic ointment, sterile cotton-tipped applicators, and clean and sterile gloves.
  Rationale: Facilitates organization and efficient time management
- Place a disposable pad beneath the hips of a female patient and beneath the penis of a male patient.
  Rationale: Prevents bed linen from becoming damp
- Don clean gloves and wash the genitalia and perineum with warm, soapy water, and dry afterward.
  Rationale: Removes gross secretions and transient microorganisms
- Remove gloves and wash hands.
  Rationale: Removes colonizing microorganisms
- Open sterile gauze squares or a package of cotton balls.
  Rationale: Reduces potential for transferring microorganisms

- Place antiseptic solution on the gauze squares or cotton balls.
  Rationale: Prepares supplies for additional cleansing
- Don sterile gloves.
  Rationale: Prevents contamination of sterile supplies
- Cleanse the meatus with antiseptic solution, following the techniques described for female and male catheterization.
  Rationale: Supports principles of asepsis
- Wipe the catheter with gauze or a cotton ball saturated with antiseptic from the meatus outward for several inches.
  Rationale: Removes colonizing microorganisms from the catheter
- Peel the cover from the cotton-tipped applicators, but protect the cotton tip from contamination.
  Rationale: Ensures sterility
- Squeeze a bit of antiseptic ointment onto the cotton applicators.
  Rationale: Provides a means for applying ointment using sterile technique
- Apply the ointment about the catheter at the meatus.
  Rationale: Reduces the local growth of microorganisms

(text continues on page 647)

SKILL 30-2
Applying a Condom Catheter

Suggested Action	Reason for Action
Assessment Assess the penis for swelling or skin breakdown.	Provides a database for future comparison or provides a basis for using some other method for urine collection
Determine how much the patient understands about the application and use of an external catheter.	Provides an opportunity for health teaching
Verify the willingness of the patient to use a condom catheter.	Respects the patient's right to participate in making decisions
Planning Gather supplies such as soap, water, towel, condom catheter, drainage tubing, collection device, and clean gloves. Some devices come packaged with an adhesive strip or Velcro device for securing the catheter.	Promotes organization and efficient time management
Provide privacy.	Demonstrates respect for dignity

(continued)

SKILL 30-2
Applying a Condom Catheter *(Continued)*

Suggested Action	Reason for Action
Place the patient in a supine position and cover him with a bath blanket.	Facilitates application of the catheter
Implementation Wash your hands and don clean gloves.	Reduces the transmission of microorganisms and follows the guidelines for Standard Precautions
Wash and dry the penis well.	Promotes skin integrity
Wind the adhesive strip in an upward spiral about the penis.	Reduces the potential for restricting blood flow

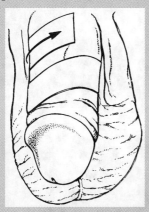

Applying adhesive strip in a spiral.

Suggested Action	Reason for Action
Roll the wider end of the sheath toward the narrow tip.	Facilitates application to the penis

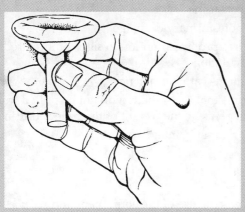

A rolled condom sheath.

(continued)

SKILL 30-2
Applying a Condom Catheter (Continued)

Suggested Action	Reason for Action
Hold approximately 1 to 2 inches (2.5–5 cm) of the lower sheath below the tip of the penis and unroll the sheath upward.	Leaves space below the urethra to prevent irritation of the meatus

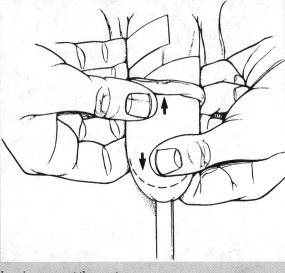

Leaving space at the meatus.

Suggested Action	Reason for Action
Secure the upper end of the unrolled sheath to the skin with a second strip of adhesive or a Velcro strap, but not so tight as to interfere with circulation.	Ensures that the catheter will remain in place
Connect the drainage tip to a drainage bag.	Collects urine
Keep the penis positioned in a downward position.	Promotes urinary drainage
Assess the penis at least every 2 hours.	Ensures prompt attention to signs of impaired circulation
Check that the catheter has not become twisted.	Maintains catheter patency
Empty the leg bag, if one is used, as it becomes partially filled with urine.	Ensures that the catheter will not be pulled from the penis by the weight of the collected urine
Remove and change the catheter daily or more often if it becomes loose or tight.	Maintains skin integrity
Substitute a waterproof garment during periods of nonuse.	Provides a mechanism for absorbing urine
Wash the catheter and collection bag with mild soap and water and rinse with a 1 : 7 solution of vinegar and water.	Extends the use of the equipment and reduces offensive odors

(continued)

SKILL 30-2
Applying a Condom Catheter (Continued)

Suggested Action	Reason for Action

Evaluation
- Catheter remains attached to the penis
- No evidence of skin breakdown, swelling, or impaired circulation
- Linen and clothing remain dry

Document
- Preapplication assessment data
- Hygiene measures performed
- Time of catheter application
- Content of teaching
- Postapplication assessment data

Sample Documentation

Date and Time	Penis washed with soap and water. Penile skin is intact. No discoloration or lesions noted. Condom catheter applied and connected to a leg bag. Instructed to report any swelling or local discomfort. _____ **Signature, Title**

Excess tubing is coiled on the bed, but the section from the bed to the collection bag is kept in a vertical orientation. Dependent loops in the tubing interfere with gravity flow. Care is also taken to avoid compressing the tubing, which can obstruct urinary drainage. Placing the tubing over the patient's thigh is an acceptable practice.

The drainage system is always positioned lower than the bladder to avoid backflow of urine. It may be difficult to follow this principle when transporting a patient in a wheelchair. Therefore, it is better to clamp the catheter and release it when the patient is returned to bed. It is important, however, to confirm that it is safe to clamp the catheter because there are situations in which this may be contraindicated.

To reduce the potential for the drainage system becoming a reservoir of pathogens, the entire drainage system is changed whenever the catheter is changed. It may be done more frequently, but care is taken that the end of the catheter is not contaminated in the process.

Providing Catheter Care

Catheter care is a term that applies to the hygiene measures used to keep the meatus and adjacent area of catheter clean. Because the catheter keeps the meatus slightly dilated, pathogens have a direct pathway to the bladder, where an infection could develop. Therefore, providing catheter care helps to deter the growth and spread of colonizing pathogens.

Catheter Irrigation

A **catheter irrigation** is a technique for maintaining a patent catheter. A catheter that drains well does not need irrigating. Providing a generous oral fluid intake is sometimes sufficient to produce dilute urine, thus keeping the catheter from becoming obstructed with small shreds of mucus or tissue debris. However, there are times when the catheter may need to be irrigated to maintain its patency, such as when there has been an operative procedure that results in bloody urine.

Depending on the type of indwelling catheter that is used, catheters may be irrigated periodically using an open system or closed system, or continuously through a three-way catheter.

USING AN OPEN SYSTEM

An open system is one in which the retention catheter is separated (ie, *opened*) from the drainage tubing to insert the tip of an irrigating syringe. Opening the system creates the potential for infection because it provides an opportunity for pathogens to enter the exposed connection. Consequently, it is the least desirable of the three methods, but remains the one most commonly used (Skill 30-5).

(text continues on page 662)

SKILL 30-3
Inserting a Foley Catheter in a Female Patient

Suggested Action	Reason for Action
Assessment	
Check the patient's record to verify that a medical order has been written.	Demonstrates the legal scope of nursing; catheterization is not an independent measure
Determine the type of catheter that has been prescribed.	Ensures selecting the appropriate catheter
Review the patient's record for documentation of genitourinary problems or an allergy to latex.	Provides data by which to modify the procedure or equipment
Assess the age, size, and mobility of the patient.	Influences the size of the catheter and the need for additional assistance
Assess the time of the last voiding.	Indicates how full the bladder may be
Determine how much the patient understands about catheterization.	Provides an opportunity for health teaching
Familiarize yourself with the anatomic landmarks.	Facilitates insertion in the appropriate location

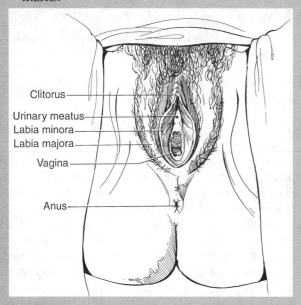

Female anatomic landmarks.

Planning	
Gather supplies, which include a catheterization kit, bath blanket, and additional light, if the room light is inadequate.	Promotes organization and efficient time management
Implementation	
Close the door and pull the privacy curtain.	Demonstrates concern for preserving the patient's dignity
Raise the bed to a high position.	Prevents back strain
Cover the patient with a bath blanket and pull the top linen to the bottom of the bed.	Avoids unnecessary exposure

(continued)

SKILL 30-3
Inserting a Foley Catheter in a Female Patient (Continued)

Suggested Action	Reason for Action
Position an additional light at the bottom of the bed or ask an assistant to hold a flashlight.	Ensures good visualization
Use the corners of the bath blanket to cover each leg.	Provides warmth and maintains modesty
Place the patient in a dorsal recumbent position with the feet about 2 feet apart.	Provides access to the female urinary system

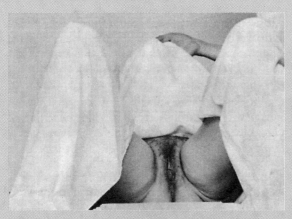

Draped and placed in dorsal recumbent position.

Suggested Action	Reason for Action
Use a lateral or Sims' position as alternatives for patients who have difficulty maintaining a dorsal recumbent position.	Provides access to the female urinary system, but neither is the preferred position
If the patient is soiled, don gloves, wash the patient, remove gloves, and rewash your hands.	Supports principles of asepsis
Remove the wrapper from the catheterization kit and position it nearby.	Provides a receptacle for collecting soiled supplies
Unwrap the sterile cover so as to maintain the sterility of the supplies inside (see Chapter 21).	Prevents contamination and the potential for infection
Remove and don the packaged sterile gloves (see Chapter 21).	Facilitates handling the remaining equipment without transferring any microorganisms

(continued)

Suggested Action	Reason for Action
Remove the sterile towel from the kit and place it beneath the patient's hips.	Provides a sterile field

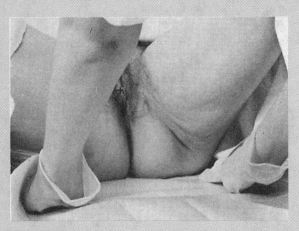

Placing a sterile towel.

Suggested Action	Reason for Action
Open and pour the packet of antiseptic solution (Betadine) over the cotton balls.	Prepares sterile supplies before contaminating one of two hands later in the procedure
Test the balloon on the catheter by instilling fluid from the prefilled syringe; then aspirate the fluid back within the syringe.	Determines if the balloon is intact or defective
Spread lubricant on the tip of the catheter.	Facilitates insertion

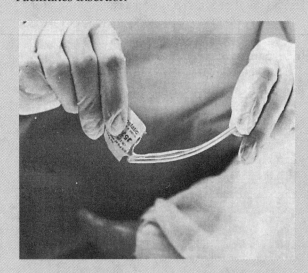

Lubricating the catheter.

Suggested Action	Reason for Action
Place the catheterization tray on top of the sterile towel between the patient's legs.	Promotes access to supplies and reduces the potential for contamination
Pick up a moistened cotton ball with the sterile forceps and wipe one side of the labia majora from an anterior to posterior direction.	Cleanses outer skin before cleansing deeper areas of tissue
Discard the soiled cotton ball in the outer wrapper of the catheterization kit; repeat cleansing the other side of the labia majora.	Completes bilateral cleansing

(continued)

SKILL 30-3
Inserting a Foley Catheter in a Female Patient *(Continued)*

Suggested Action	Reason for Action
Separate the labia majora and minora with the thumb and fingers of the nondominant hand, exposing the urinary meatus.	Facilitates visualization of anatomic landmarks and prevents the potential for contaminating the catheter during insertion

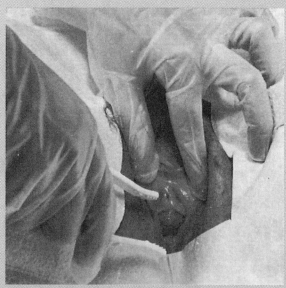

Separating the labia.

Suggested Action	Reason for Action
Consider the hand separating the labia to be contaminated.	Avoids transferring microorganisms to sterile equipment and supplies
Clean each side of the labia minora with a separate cotton ball while continuing to retract the tissue with the nondominant hand.	Removes colonizing microorganisms
Use the last cotton ball to wipe centrally, starting above the meatus down toward the vagina.	Completes the cleaning of external structures

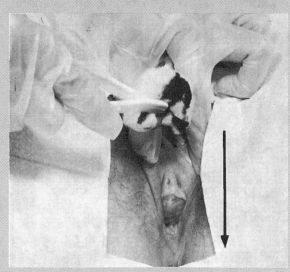

Wiping from above the meatus downward.

(continued)

SKILL 30-3
Inserting a Foley Catheter in a Female Patient (Continued)

Suggested Action	Reason for Action
Discard the forceps with the last cotton ball into the wrapper for contaminated supplies.	Follows principles of asepsis
Keep the clean tissue separated.	Prevents recontamination
Pick up the catheter, holding it approximately 3 to 4 inches (7.5–10 cm) from its tip.	Facilitates control during insertion

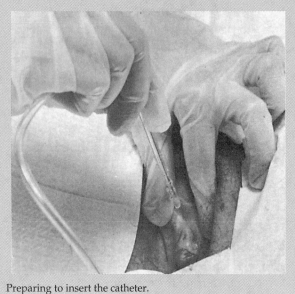

Preparing to insert the catheter.

Suggested Action	Reason for Action
Insert the tip of the catheter into the meatus approximately 2 to 3 inches (5–7.5 cm) or until urine begins to flow.	Locates the tip beyond the length of the female urethra, which is approximately 1.5 to 2.5 inches (4–6.5 cm)
Recheck anatomic landmarks if there is no evidence of urine; remove an incorrectly placed catheter and repeat, using another sterile catheter.	Indicates one of two possibilities: either the bladder is empty or the catheter has been placed within the vagina by mistake; ensures sterility of equipment
Advance the catheter another 1/2 to 1 inch (1.3–2.5 cm) after urine begins to flow.	Ensures that the catheter is well within the bladder, where the balloon can be safely inserted
Direct the end of the catheter so that it drains into the equipment tray or specimen container.	Avoids wetting the linen
Hold the catheter in place with the fingers and thumb that were separating the labia.	Stabilizes the catheter externally
Pick up the prefilled syringe with the sterile, dominant hand, insert it into the opening to the balloon, and instill the fluid.	Stabilizes the catheter internally
Withdraw the fluid from the balloon if the patient describes feeling pain or discomfort, advance the catheter a little more, and try again.	Prevents internal injury
Tug gently on the catheter after the balloon has been filled.	Tests whether the catheter is well anchored within the bladder

(continued)

Suggested Action	Reason for Action
Connect the catheter to a urine collection bag.	Provides a means of assessing the urine and its volume
Wipe the meatus and labia of any residual lubricant.	Demonstrates concern for the patient's comfort
Secure the catheter to the leg with tape or other commercial device.	Prevents pulling on the balloon within the catheter

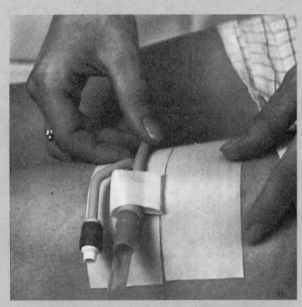

Securing the catheter to the thigh. (Courtesy of the MC Johnson Company, Inc., Leominster, MA.)

Suggested Action	Reason for Action
Hang the collection bag below the level of the bladder; coil excess tubing on the mattress.	Ensures gravity drainage
Discard the catheterization tray and wrapper with soiled supplies.	Follows principles of asepsis
Remove your gloves and wash your hands.	Removes colonizing microorganisms
Remove the drape, restore the top sheets, make the patient comfortable, and lower the bed.	Restores comfort and safety

Evaluation
- Catheter is inserted under aseptic conditions
- Urine is draining from the catheter
- No evidence of discomfort during or after insertion

Document
- Preassessment data
- Size and type of catheter
- Amount and appearance of urine
- Patient's response

Sample Documentation

Date and Time	Unable to void in past 8 hours. Bladder feels distended. Dr. Peter notified. 18 F Foley catheter inserted per order and connected to gravity drainage. 550 mL of urine drained from bladder at this time. Urine appears light amber. No discomfort reported. _____ **Signature, Title**

SKILL 30-4
Inserting a Foley Catheter in a Male Patient

Suggested Action	Reason for Action
Assessment	
Check the patient's record to verify that a medical order has been written.	Demonstrates the legal scope of nursing; catheterization is not an independent measure
Determine the type of catheter that has been prescribed.	Ensures selecting the appropriate catheter
Review the patient's record for documentation of genitourinary problems or an allergy to latex.	Provides data by which to modify the procedure or equipment
Assess the age, size, and mobility of the patient.	Influences the size of the catheter and the need for additional assistance
Assess the time of the last voiding.	Indicates how full the bladder may be
Determine how much the patient understands about catheterization.	Provides an opportunity for health teaching
Familiarize yourself with the anatomic landmarks.	Facilitates insertion

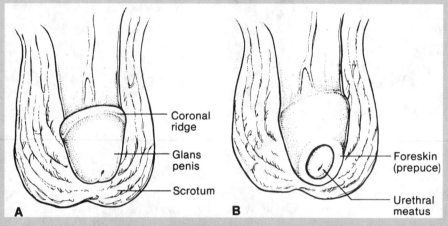

Male anatomic landmarks. (*A*) Circumcised. (*B*) Uncircumcised. (Fuller J, Schuller-Ayers J: Health Assessment: A Nursing Approach, 2nd ed, p 489. Philadelphia, JB Lippincott, 1994)

Planning	
Gather supplies, which include a catheterization kit, bath blanket, and additional light.	Promotes organization and efficient time management
Implementation	
Close the door and pull the privacy curtain.	Demonstrates concern for preserving the patient's dignity
Raise the bed to a high position.	Prevents back strain
Place the patient in a supine position.	Provides access to the male urinary system
Cover the patient's upper body with a bath blanket, and lower the top linen to expose just the penis.	Provides minimal exposure
Position an additional light at the bottom of the bed or ask an assistant to hold a flashlight.	Ensures good visualization

(continued)

SKILL 30-4
Inserting a Foley Catheter in a Male Patient *(Continued)*

Suggested Action	Reason for Action
If the patient is soiled, don gloves, wash the patient, remove gloves, and rewash your hands.	Supports principles of asepsis
Remove the wrapper from the catheterization kit and position it nearby.	Provides a receptacle for collecting soiled supplies
Unwrap the sterile inner cover so as to maintain the sterility of the supplies inside (see Chap. 21).	Prevents contamination and the potential for infection
Remove and don the packaged sterile gloves (see Chap. 21).	Facilitates handling the remaining equipment without transferring any microorganisms
Place the **fenestrated drape**, one with an open circle in its center, over the patient's penis without touching the upper surface of the drape.	Provides a sterile field

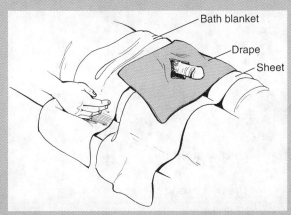

Placing a fenestrated drape.

Open and pour the packet of antiseptic solution (Betadine) over the cotton balls.	Prepares sterile supplies before contaminating one of two hands later in the procedure
Test the balloon on the catheter by instilling fluid from the prefilled syringe; then aspirate the fluid back within the syringe.	Determines if the balloon is intact or defective
Spread lubricant over 6 to 7 inches (15–18 cm) of the catheter.	Facilitates insertion
Place the catheterization tray on top of the sterile drape over the patient's thighs.	Promotes ease of access to supplies and reduces the potential for contamination
Lift the penis at its base with the nondominant hand; retract the foreskin, if the patient is uncircumcised.	Promotes visualization and support during catheter insertion
Consider the gloved hand holding the penis to be contaminated.	Avoids transferring microorganisms to sterile equipment and supplies

(continued)

Suggested Action	Reason for Action
Pick up a moistened cotton ball with the sterile forceps and wipe the penis in a circular manner from the meatus toward the base; repeat using a different cotton ball each time.	Moves microorganisms away from the meatus

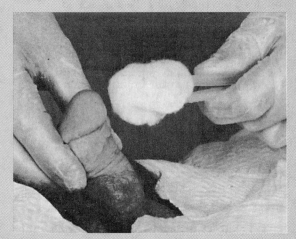

Cleaning the penis.

Suggested Action	Reason for Action
Discard the forceps with the last cotton ball into the wrapper for contaminated supplies.	Follows principles of asepsis
Apply gentle traction to the penis by pulling it straight up with the nondominant gloved hand.	Straightens the urethra
Insert the tip of the catheter into the meatus approximately 6 to 8 inches (15–20 cm) or until urine begins to flow.	Locates the tip beyond the length of the male urethra

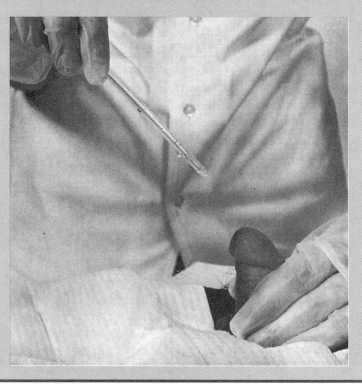

Preparing to insert the catheter.

(continued)

SKILL 30-4
Inserting a Foley Catheter in a Male Patient *(Continued)*

Suggested Action	Reason for Action
Never force the catheter; rather, rotate the catheter, apply more traction to the penis, encourage the patient to breathe deeply, or angle the penis toward the toes.	Adjusts for passing the catheter beyond the prostate gland

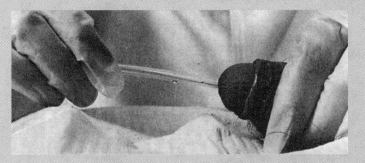

Angling the penis downward.

Suggested Action	Reason for Action
Advance the catheter another 1/2 to 1 inch (1.3–2.5 cm) or more until urine begins to flow.	Ensures that the catheter is well within the bladder, where the balloon can be safely inserted
Direct the end of the catheter so that it drains into the equipment tray or specimen container.	Avoids wetting the linen
Pick up the prefilled syringe with the sterile, dominant hand, insert it into the opening to the balloon, and instill the fluid.	Stabilizes the catheter internally
Withdraw the fluid from the balloon if the patient describes feeling pain or discomfort, advance the catheter a little more, and try again.	Prevents internal injury
Tug gently on the catheter after the balloon has been filled.	Tests whether the catheter is well anchored within the bladder
Connect the catheter to a urine collection bag.	Provides a means of assessing the urine and its volume
Wipe the meatus and penis of any residual lubricant.	Demonstrates concern for the patient's comfort
Secure the catheter to the leg with tape or other commercial device.	Prevents pulling on the balloon within the catheter

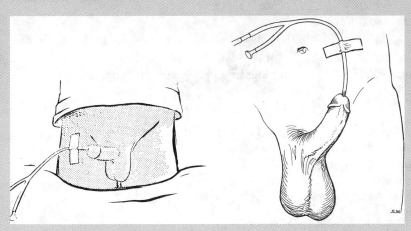

Methods for securing a catheter.

(continued)

Inserting a Foley Catheter in a Male Patient (Continued)

Suggested Action	Reason for Action
Hang the collection bag below the level of the bladder; coil excess tubing on the mattress.	Ensures gravity drainage
Discard the catheterization tray and wrapper with soiled supplies.	Follows principles of asepsis
Remove your gloves and wash your hands.	Removes colonizing microorganisms
Remove the drape, restore the top sheets, make the patient comfortable, and lower the bed.	Restores comfort and safety

Evaluation
- Catheter is inserted under aseptic conditions
- Urine is draining from the catheter
- No evidence of discomfort during or after insertion

Document
- Preassessment data
- Size and type of catheter
- Amount and appearance of urine
- Patient's response

Sample Documentation

Date and Time   #16 F Foley catheter inserted before surgery according to preoperative orders. 350 mL of urine obtained before connecting the catheter to gravity drainage. Urine appears light yellow and clear. _____ **Signature, Title**

SKILL 30-5

Irrigating a Foley Catheter

Suggested Action	Reason for Action
Assessment	
Check the patient's record to verify that a medical order has been written.	Demonstrates the legal scope of nursing; a catheter irrigation is not an independent measure
Verify the type of irrigating solution prescribed, or follow the standard for practice, which usually advises sterile normal saline solution.	Complies with medical directives or standards for care
Assess the urine characteristics.	Provides a baseline for assessing the outcome of the procedure
Determine how much the patient understands about a catheter irrigation.	Provides an opportunity for health teaching
Planning	
Gather the equipment and supplies that are needed. They include a flask of sterile irrigating solution, a 30- to 50-mL blunt-tipped syringe, sterile basin or container for holding the solution, alcohol swabs, a sterile cap for the tip of the drainage tubing, and a kidney basin.	Promotes organization and efficient time management

(continued)

SKILL 30-5
Irrigating a Foley Catheter (Continued)

Suggested Action	Reason for Action
Implementation	
Wash hands and don clean gloves.	Follows principles of asepsis and standards of practice
Raise the height of the bed.	Reduces back strain
Pull the privacy curtain.	Demonstrates concern for the patient's dignity
Unwrap the container for the irrigating solution and add 100 to 200 mL of solution.	Avoids contaminating and wasting all the solution in the flask

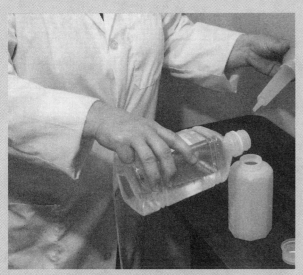

Preparing irrigation solution. (Courtesy of Ken Timby.)

Remove the cap on the tip of the irrigating syringe; fill the syringe with 30 to 60 mL of solution, and loosely replace the cap.	Maintains sterility but eases the cap's removal

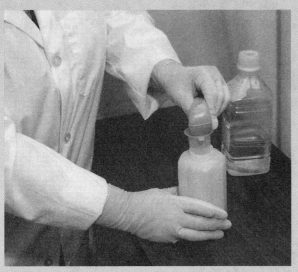

Filling the irrigation syringe. (Courtesy of Ken Timby.)

(continued)

SKILL 30-5
Irrigating a Foley Catheter (Continued)

Suggested Action	Reason for Action
Place the kidney basin nearby.	Facilitates collecting the drainage of irrigating solution and urine
Clean the area where the catheter and drainage tubing connect with an alcohol swab.	Removes gross debris and colonizing microorganisms
Separate the two tubes and place a cap on the exposed end of the drainage tube.	Prevents contamination
While holding the catheter with one hand, insert the syringe into the catheter with the other hand.	Maintains sterility

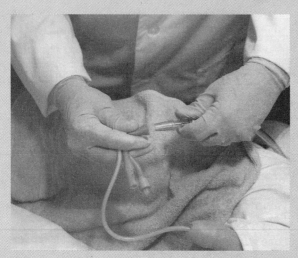

Capping the drainage tubing to ensure sterility. (Courtesy of Ken Timby.)

Gently instill the solution.	Clears the catheter of debris and dilutes particles within the bladder

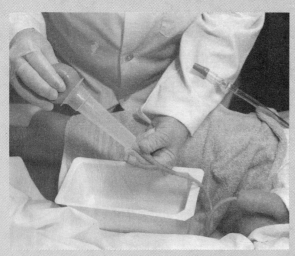

Instilling irrigation solution. (Courtesy of Ken Timby.)

(continued)

SKILL 30-5
Irrigating a Foley Catheter *(Continued)*

Suggested Action	Reason for Action
Pinch the catheter and remove the syringe.	Prevents leaking
Replace the tip of the syringe loosely within its cap or place it tip down in the basin of irrigating solution.	Maintains sterility
Direct the end of the catheter over the kidney basin and release the compression on the tubing.	Facilitates gravity drainage

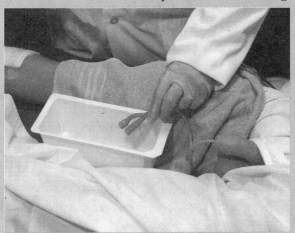

Draining the irrigation solution. (Courtesy of Ken Timby.)

Suggested Action	Reason for Action
Repeat the instillation and drainage if the urine appears to contain an appreciable amount of debris.	Promotes patency
Remove the cap on the drainage tubing and reconnect it to the catheter.	Reestablishes a closed system
Measure the amount of drained fluid. Record the volume of instilled solution as fluid intake and the drained volume as output.	Maintains accurate assessment data
Discard or protect the sterility of the irrigating equipment that may be reused for the next 24 hours as long as it is not contaminated.	Complies with principles of infection control

Evaluation
- The prescribed amount and type of solution are instilled
- Principles of asepsis have been maintained
- Urine continues to drain well through the catheter
- No discomfort noted

Document
- Preassessment data
- Volume, type of solution
- Volume and appearance of drainage

Sample Documentation

Date and Time Urine appears amber with some evidence of white particles. 60 mL of sterile normal saline solution instilled into catheter. 120 mL drainage returned. Urine appears to have less sediment. Catheter remains patent. _____ **Signature, Title**

USING A CLOSED SYSTEM

A closed system is one that can be irrigated without separating the catheter from the drainage tubing. To do so, the catheter or drainage tubing must have a self-sealing port. After cleansing the port with an alcohol swab, the port is pierced with an 18- or 19-gauge, 1.5-inch needle (see Chap. 34). The needle is attached to a 50-mL syringe containing sterile irrigation solution. The tubing is pinched or clamped beneath the port and the solution is instilled.

CONTINUOUS IRRIGATION

A **continuous irrigation** is one in which an irrigating solution is instilled by gravity over a period of days (Fig. 30-10). Continuous irrigations are usually used to keep a catheter patent after prostate or other urologic surgery in which blood clots and tissue debris collect within the bladder.

A three-way catheter is necessary to provide a continuous irrigation. The catheter gets its name from the fact that there are three lumens or channels within the catheter, each leading to a separate port.

To provide a continuous irrigation, the nurse would:

- Hang the sterile irrigating solution from an intravenous pole.
- Purge the air from the tubing.
- Connect the tubing to the catheter port for irrigation.
- Regulate the rate of infusion according to the medical order.

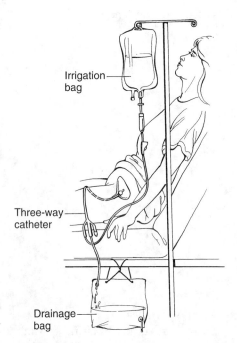

FIGURE 30-10
Bladder irrigation using a three-way catheter.

- Monitor the appearance of the urine and volume of urinary. drainage

Removing an Indwelling Catheter

A catheter may be removed when the current one needs to be replaced or when its use is being discontinued. Resnick (1993) suggests that the best time to remove a catheter is in the morning so that there is more opportunity to address any difficulties that may ensue.

NURSING GUIDELINES FOR REMOVING A FOLEY CATHETER

- Wash your hands and don clean gloves.
  Rationale: Follows Standard Precautions
- Empty the balloon by aspirating the fluid with a syringe.
  Rationale: Ensures that all the fluid has been withdrawn
- Gently pull the catheter near the point where it exits from the meatus.
  Rationale: Facilitates withdrawal
- Inspect the catheter and discard if it appears to be intact.
  Rationale: Ensures safety
- Clean the urinary meatus.
  Rationale: Promotes comfort and hygiene
- Monitor the patient's voiding, especially for the next 8 to 10 hours; measure the volume of each voiding.
  Rationale: Determines if normal elimination is occurring and the characteristics of the urine

URINARY DIVERSIONS

A **urinary diversion** is a procedure in which one or both ureters are surgically implanted elsewhere. The ureter(s) may be brought to and through the skin of the abdomen (Fig. 30-11), or implanted within the bowel. A urinary diversion that discharges urine from an opening on the abdomen is referred to as a **urostomy.** Managing a urostomy is the focus of this discussion.

Caring for a patient with a urostomy presents many challenges for the nurse, such as the collection of urine and care of the skin.

Caring for a Urostomy

Care for an ostomy, a surgically created opening, is discussed in more detail in Chapter 31 because those formed from the bowel are more common. The reader is referred to Chapter 31 for a more detailed description

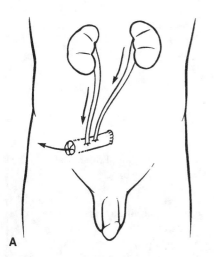
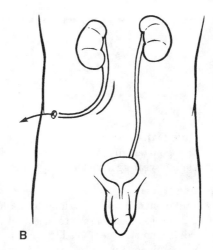

A   B

FIGURE 30-11
Examples of urinary diversions. (*A*) Ileal conduit. (*B*) Cutaneous ureterostomy. (Smeltzer SC, Bare BG: Brunner and Suddarth's Textbook of Medical-Surgical Nursing, 7th ed, p 1209. Philadelphia, JB Lippincott, 1992)

of an ostomy appliance, the device for collecting stool or urine, and the manner in which it is applied and removed from the skin.

For the purposes of this discussion, it is sufficient to say that caring for a urostomy and changing a urinary appliance is somewhat more challenging than in those covering intestinal stomas. Nursing management is complicated by the fact that urine drains continuously from a urostomy, which potentiates the risk for skin breakdown. In addition, because moisture and the weight of the collected urine tend to loosen the appli-

ance from the skin, a urinary appliance may need to be changed more frequently. When changing the appliance, it may help to place a tampon within the stoma to absorb urine temporarily while the skin is cleansed and prepared for another appliance application.

It often becomes very difficult to maintain the integrity of the peristomal skin (skin around the stoma) because of the frequent appliance changes and the ammonia that is present in urine. Consequently, skin barrier products are used, and sometimes antibiotic or steroid ointment is applied.

 FOCUS ON OLDER ADULTS

- Patterns of urinary elimination in older adults are often altered because of normal physiologic changes like a decrease in bladder capacity and a reduction in muscle elasticity and bladder tone.
- Age-related changes contribute to increased residual urine in the bladder, and incontinence.
- Enlargement of the prostate, a common problem among older men, can totally obstruct urinary outflow and make catheterization difficult or impossible. Sometimes a catheter must be inserted into the bladder through the abdominal wall when a urethral catheter cannot be passed beyond the narrowed pathway.
- Diuretic therapy, a common category of drugs prescribed for older adults, makes the problem of incontinence an even greater issue.
- Independent toileting is a developmental milestone in childhood; loss of bladder control therefore threatens an older adult's independence, body image, and social roles.

- Some older adults misguidedly attempt to control urge incontinence by restricting their oral fluid intake.
- Urinary tract infections are a common cause for urinary incontinence among older adults and one that is easily treated if it is diagnosed properly.
- When efforts to restore continence are unsuccessful, nurses can help older adults by encouraging verbalization of feelings and working jointly with them to develop acceptable methods for maintaining their lifestyle while disguising the loss of bladder control.
- Older adults with incontinence problems may choose to use products like disposable absorbent briefs or absorbent pads that are inserted within elastic underwear.
- In long-term care facilities, it is less expensive to toilet older adults regularly than to deal with the consequences of incontinence (Creason et al., 1993).

NURSING CARE PLAN:
Urge Incontinence

Assessment

Subjective Data
States, "I hope when this catheter comes out I don't wet myself again. I'd like to go home without wearing a leg bag or being connected to a drainage bag."

Objective Data
75-year-old woman admitted to long-term care facility for rehabilitation after repair of a fractured hip. Fracture occurred as a result of tripping on way to bathroom because of feeling an urgent need to void. Has had an indwelling catheter with continuous drainage for 4 weeks.

Diagnosis

Urge Incontinence related to reduced bladder capacity secondary to continuous urine drainage from an indwelling catheter.

Plan

Goal
The patient will be able to wait at least 3 hours between voidings without experiencing incontinence by 6/12.

Orders: 6/2
1. Before removing Foley catheter, perform bedside *cystometrogram* by instilling sterile water until the patient indicates feeling the need to void. Measure the volume instilled.
2. Remove the catheter and maintain a 3-day log of:
    * Time of each urination
    * Volume per voiding
    * Episodes of incontinence
    * Cause of incontinence
3. Maintain a total intake of approximately 2,500 mL/day, divided in the following amounts:
    * 1,200 mL on day shift
    * 1,200 mL on evening shift
    * 100 mL during the night
4. When there is an urge to void, help patient to:
    * Breathe deeply while waiting longer to void
    * Sing a song
    * Tell a story about her family as a distraction technique while proceeding to the toilet at a safe pace
5. Praise every urinary elimination that occurs without incontinence.
    _____F. WISNIECKI, RN

Implementation   6/2
(Documentation)

1000   Bedside cystometrogram performed. Felt an urge to void when 100 mL of sterile water was instilled through catheter. Reconnected to gravity drainage for 15 minutes and then catheter removed. Instructed to drink approximately one glass of fluid per hour. Explained the 3-day assessment log. Explored distraction techniques to avoid incontinence while increasing bladder capacity.
_____ N. ZAK, LPN

Evaluation
(Documentation)

2000   Feeling a need to void at approximately 2-hour intervals (see log for specifics). Has had two episodes of dribbling while getting onto toilet. Sings "Amazing Grace" as a distraction technique. States, "I was so hoping this wouldn't happen; I'm determined to avoid that catheter again." Praised for the two successful voidings without incontinence. Drinking fluids at scheduled intervals._____ S. BURKE, LPN

APPLICABLE NURSING DIAGNOSES

- Toileting Self-Care Deficit
- Altered Urinary Elimination
- Risk for Infection
- Stress Incontinence
- Urge Incontinence
- Reflex Incontinence
- Functional Incontinence
- Total Incontinence
- Urinary Retention
- Situational Low Self-Esteem
- Risk for Impaired Skin Integrity

NURSING IMPLICATIONS

Patients with urinary elimination problems may have one or more nursing diagnoses from the list of Applicable Nursing Diagnoses.

The accompanying Nursing Care Plan is developed for a patient with Urge Incontinence. In its 1994 taxonomy, the North American Nursing Diagnosis Association (NANDA) defines this diagnostic category as "The state in which an individual experiences involuntary passage of urine occurring soon after a strong sense of urgency to void."

KEY CONCEPTS

- The urinary system is composed of the kidneys, ureters, bladder, and urethra. Collectively, they serve to produce urine, collect it, and excrete it from the body.
- Various factors affect urination. Some examples include a person's neuromuscular development, the integrity of the spinal cord, the volume of fluid intake, fluid losses from other sources, and the amount and type of food consumed.
- The physical characteristics of urine include its volume, color, clarity, and odor.
- Nurses often collect voided urine specimens, clean-catch urine specimens, catheter specimens, and 24-hour urine specimens.
- Common abnormal patterns of urinary elimination include anuria, oliguria, polyuria, nocturia, dysuria, and incontinence.
- Other than a conventional toilet, urine may be eliminated in a commode, urinal, or bedpan.
- Continence training is the process for restoring the ability to empty the bladder at an appropriate time and place.

- There are three general types of catheters: external catheters, straight catheters, and retention catheters.
- When using a closed drainage system, it is important to avoid dependent loops in the tubing and to keep the collection bag below the level of the bladder.
- Catheter care is important because it helps to deter the growth and spread of colonizing pathogens.
- Catheters are irrigated to keep them patent, or free flowing. They may be irrigated using an open or closed system, or a three-way catheter may be used.
- A urinary diversion is a procedure in which one or both ureters are surgically implanted elsewhere.
- Skin impairment tends to be a major problem among patients with a urostomy because they require frequent appliance changes, and the contact of urine with the skin causes skin irritation.
- The self-esteem and socialization of older adults who are incontinent may be improved by using disposable absorbent briefs or absorbent pads inserted within elastic underwear.

CRITICAL THINKING EXERCISES

- An older adult patient confides that she would like to participate in activities outside her home, but she is worried her problem with incontinence will be noticed. What response might help this patient? What suggestions could you offer?
- A resident in a nursing home who has had a retention catheter for the last 6 months says, "I'd do anything if I didn't have to have this catheter." What suggestions would be appropriate at this time?

SUGGESTED READINGS

Brooks MJ. Urinary incontinence: assessment, treatment, and reimbursement. Home Healthcare Nurse July–August 1993;11:41–46.

Cooper C. What color is that urine specimen? American Journal of Nursing August 1993;93:37.

Creason NS, Burgener SC, Farrand L. Guidelines for assessment of incontinence in elderly institutionalized women. Geriatric Nursing March–April 1992;13:76–79.

Culbertson L. A comparison of Foley catheter types in home care use. Home Healthcare Nurse November–December 1992;10:45–47.

Hughes E, Anderson CL. The voiding record: a new approach to an old problem. Geriatric Nursing March–April 1992;13:90–93.

Incontinence . . . product focus. Journal of Gerontological Nursing May 1992;18:45–46.

Kee CC. Age-related changes in the renal system: causes, consequences, and nursing implications. Geriatric Nursing March–April 1992;13:80–83.

Lloyd C. Making sense of reagent strip urine testing. Nursing Times December 1–7, 1993;89:32, 35–36.

Madejski RM. LPN overview of urinary incontinence. Journal of Practical Nursing December 1992;42:24–33.

McConnell EA. Teaching a patient to perform Kegel exercises. Nursing August 1993;23:90.

McCormick KA, Newman DK, Colling J. Urinary incontinence in adults. American Journal of Nursing October 1992;92:75–76, 78–82, 84–86+.

Meehan JB. Guideline issued for urinary incontinence. American Nurse May 1992;24:2.

Moore KN. Indwelling catheters: problems and management. Canadian Nurse June 1992;88:33–35.

Powers I, Williams D. Urinary incontinence: helping a patient regain control. Nursing December 1992;22:46–47.

Resnick B. Retraining the bladder after catheterization. American Journal of Nursing November 1993;93:46–49.

Sherwood L. Fundamentals of Physiology: A Human Perspective. 2nd ed. Anaheim: West Publishing Company, 1995.

Warkentin R. Implementation of a urinary continence program. Journal of Gerontological Nursing January 1992;18:31–38.

Winslow EH. Myth of the clean catch. American Journal of Nursing August 1993;93:20.

CHAPTER 31

Bowel Elimination

Chapter Outline

Bowel Elimination
Assessing Bowel Elimination
Common Alterations in Bowel Elimination
Promoting Bowel Elimination
Ostomy Care
Nursing Implications
Key Concepts
Critical Thinking Exercises
Suggested Readings

 NURSING GUIDELINES

Testing Stool for Blood
Removing a Fecal Impaction
Administering a Hypertonic Enema Solution

 SKILLS

Inserting a Rectal Tube
Inserting a Rectal Suppository
Administering a Cleansing Enema
Changing an Ostomy Appliance
Irrigating a Colostomy

 NURSING CARE PLAN

Colonic Constipation

Key Terms

Anal Sphincters	Constipation
Appliance	Continent Ostomy
Colostomy	Defecation

Diarrhea	Gastrocolic Reflex
Enema	Ileostomy
Excoriation	Ostomates
Fecal Impaction	Peristalsis
Fecal Incontinence	Retention Enema
Feces	Stoma
Flatulence	Suppository
Flatus	Valsalva's Maneuver

Learning Objectives

An understanding of the content within this chapter will be evidenced by the student's ability to:

- Describe the process of defecation
- Name two components of a bowel elimination assessment
- List five common alterations in bowel elimination
- Name four types of constipation and identify the one whose treatment is within the scope of nursing practice
- Identify two interventions for promoting bowel elimination when it does not occur naturally
- Name two categories of enema administration
- List at least three common solutions for administering a cleansing enema
- Explain the purpose of an oil retention enema
- Name four nursing activities involved in ostomy care

This chapter reviews briefly the process of intestinal elimination and discusses measures to help promote it. Nursing skills that may assist patients with alterations in bowel elimination are also described.

Timby BK: *Fundamental Skills and Concepts in Patient Care, Sixth Edition* © 1996 Lippincott-Raven Publishers

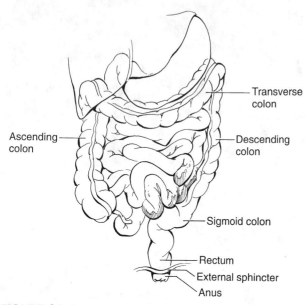

FIGURE 31-1
The large intestine.

BOWEL ELIMINATION

Bowel elimination, also known as **defecation**, is the act of expelling **feces**, or stool, from the body. To do so, all the structures of the gastrointestinal tract must function in a coordinated manner. This is especially true for the components of the large intestine, also referred to as the *bowel* or *colon* (Fig. 31-1); it is within these structures that a remarkable volume of water is removed from the remnants of digestion, causing the bowel's contents to become a consolidated mass of residue before being eliminated.

Defecation

Defecation is facilitated by **peristalsis**, rhythmic contractions of intestinal smooth muscle. Peristalsis moves fiber, water, and nutritional wastes along the ascend-ing, transverse, descending, and sigmoid colon toward the rectum. The process becomes even more active while eating, which explains the derivation of the term **gastrocolic reflex**.

The gastrocolic reflex usually precedes defecation. Its accelerated wave-like movements, sometimes perceived as slight abdominal cramping, propel stool forward, packing it within the rectum. As the rectum distends, there is an urge to defecate. Stool is eventually released when the ring-shaped band of muscles, called **anal sphincters**, relax. The process is further facilitated by performing **Valsalva's maneuver**, which involves closing the glottis and contracting the pelvic and abdominal muscles to increase abdominal pressure.

The bowel's mechanical functions just described are also influenced by dietary, physical, social, and emotional factors (Table 31-1).

ASSESSING BOWEL ELIMINATION

A comprehensive assessment includes collecting data about the patient's elimination patterns, or bowel habits, and the actual characteristics of the feces itself.

Elimination Patterns

Because there may be diverse, yet normal, variations in bowel elimination patterns, it is essential to determine what is unique to each patient. Therefore, it is appropriate to obtain a description of the frequency of elimination, effort required to expel the stool, and what elimination aids, if any, are used.

Stool Characteristics

More objective data result from inspecting the stool or having the patient describe its appearance. Information that is particularly diagnostic includes the stool's color, odor, consistency, shape, and unusual components (Table 31-2).

TABLE 31-1. *Common Factors Affecting Bowel Elimination*	
Factor	Effect
Types of food consumed	Affects color, odor, volume, and consistency of stool, and fecal velocity
Fluid intake	Influences moisture content of stool
Drugs	Slow or speed motility
Emotions	Alter bowel motility
Neuromuscular function	Affects the ability to control muscles about the rectum
Abdominal muscle tone	Affects the ability to increase intraabdominal pressure (Valsalva's maneuver)
Opportunity for defecation	Inhibits or facilitates elimination

TABLE 31-2. *Characteristics of Stool*

Characteristic	Normal	Abnormal
Color	Brown	Black
		Clay-colored (tan)
		Yellow
		Green
Odor	Aromatic	Foul
Consistency	Soft, formed	Soft, bulky
		Hard, dry
		Watery
		Paste-like
Shape	Round, full	Absent
		Flat
		Pencil-shaped
		Stone-like
Components	Undigested fiber	Worms
		Blood
		Pus
		Mucus

Whenever stool appears abnormal, a sample is saved in a covered container for the physician's inspection. In some instances, the nurse may independently perform screening tests on stool samples, like those that determine the presence of blood. The results, which can be falsely positive, are then reported to the physician, who may order more extensive laboratory or diagnostic tests.

NURSING GUIDELINES FOR TESTING STOOL FOR BLOOD

- Collect stool within a toilet liner or bedpan.
  Rationale: Prevents mixing stool with water or urine
- Don gloves and use an applicator stick.
  Rationale: Reduces the transmission of microorganisms
- Take a sample from the center area of the stool.
  Rationale: Provides more diagnostic findings because it is not superficially tainted with blood from local tissue
- Apply a thin smear of stool onto the test area supplied with the screening kit.
  Rationale: Facilitates thorough contact with the chemical reagent
- Take care to cover the entire test space.
  Rationale: Ensures more accurate findings
- Place two drops of chemical reagent onto the test space.
  Rationale: Promotes a chemical reaction

- Wait 60 seconds.
  Rationale: Allows time for chemical interaction with the stool
- Observe for a blue color.
  Rationale: Indicates blood is present

By analyzing the assessment findings, the nurse may help the physician diagnose a medical problem or use the conclusions to identify alterations that are within the scope of nursing management.

COMMON ALTERATIONS IN BOWEL ELIMINATION

Patients often experience temporary or chronic problems with bowel elimination and intestinal function such as constipation, fecal impaction, flatulence, diarrhea, and fecal incontinence. If these conditions are a component of a serious disorder, their relief is addressed by collaborative efforts between nurses and physicians. However, those alterations within the nurse's domain of practice may be treated independently.

Constipation

Constipation is an elimination problem that is characterized by dry, hard stool that is not easily passed. There may be other accompanying symptoms as well (Display 31-1). One must not automatically assume, however, that infrequent elimination of stool necessarily indicates that a person is constipated. Some may be constipated despite having a daily bowel movement, whereas others who defecate irregularly may have normal bowel function.

DISPLAY 31-1. *Chief Characteristics of Constipation*

- Abdominal distention or bloating
- Change in amount of gas passed rectally
- Less frequent bowel movements
- Oozing liquid stool
- Rectal fullness or pressure
- Rectal pain with bowel movement
- Small volume of stool
- Unable to pass stool

From McMillan SC, Williams FA: Validity and reliability of the Constipation Assessment Scale. Cancer Nurs 12(3):183–188, 1989

The incidence of constipation among Americans and people from other affluent countries tends to be quite extensive. Many authorities attribute this to dietary preferences that often exclude adequate sources of fiber like raw fruits and vegetables, whole grains, seeds, and nuts. Fiber, which becomes undigested cellulose, attracts water, resulting in the formation of bulkier stool that is more quickly and easily eliminated.

Researchers speculate that a shortened transit time—that is, the time from which food is consumed to the time that its undigested end products are eliminated—protects people from development of serious medical disorders (Burkitt, 1984). Supposedly, the longer stool is retained, the more contact with and absorption of toxic substances takes place.

TYPES OF CONSTIPATION

Constipation may be classified into one of four distinct types that are primarily based on their underlying etiology. They include primary, secondary, iatrogenic, and pseudo constipation.

Primary Constipation

Primary or simple constipation, which is well within the treatment domain of nurses, occurs as a result of lifestyle factors such as inactivity, inadequate dietary fiber, insufficient fluid intake, or ignoring the urge to defecate.

Secondary Constipation

Secondary constipation is a consequence of some pathologic disorder like a partial bowel obstruction. It usually resolves when the primary cause is treated.

Iatrogenic Constipation

Iatrogenic constipation is that which occurs as a consequence of other medical treatment. For example, prolonged use of narcotic analgesia tends to cause constipation. These and other drugs as well slow peristalsis, delaying transit time. The longer the stool remains within the colon, the drier it becomes, making it more difficult to pass.

Pseudo Constipation

"Pseudo constipation," which the North American Nursing Diagnosis Association (NANDA) refers to as *Perceived Constipation*, is a term that is used when patients believe themselves to be constipated, but this is not actually the case. Pseudo constipation is manifested by people who are fixated about having a daily bowel movement. In their zeal for regularity, they often overuse laxatives, suppositories, and enemas.

Unfortunately, these forms of unnecessary self-treatment may ultimately *cause* rather than treat constipa-tion. Chronic purging eventually weakens the tone of the bowel. Consequently, bowel elimination is less likely to occur unless it is artificially stimulated.

Fecal Impaction

A **fecal impaction** is a condition in which it is impossible to pass feces voluntarily because it has become a large, hardened mass. Fecal impactions may be the result of unrelieved constipation, retained barium from an intestinal x-ray, dehydration, and muscle weakness.

Affected patients usually report a frequent desire to defecate, but an inability to do so. Rectal pain may also be experienced as a result of the unsuccessful efforts to evacuate the lower bowel. Ironically, some impacted patients do pass liquid stool, which may be misinterpreted as a case of diarrhea. However, the liquid stool is caused by forceful waves of peristalsis in higher bowel areas where the stool is still quite fluid. The force of the muscular contractions sends the liquid around the margins of the impacted stool, but without relief of the initial condition.

To determine if the patient is impacted, it may be necessary to insert a lubricated, gloved finger into the rectum. If the rectum is filled with a mass of stool, the nurse implements measures that facilitate its removal. Sometimes enemas, first oil retention and then cleansing, may be administered. These therapeutic measures are discussed later in this chapter. Another intervention is to remove the stool digitally.

◄ NURSING GUIDELINES FOR REMOVING A FECAL IMPACTION

- Wash your hands.
  Rationale: Reduces the transmission of microorganisms
- Provide privacy.
  Rationale: Demonstrates respect for the patient's dignity
- Place the patient in a Sims' position (see Chap. 23).
  Rationale: Facilitates access to the rectum
- Cover the patient with a drape and place a disposable pad under the patient's hips.
  Rationale: Prevents soiling
- Place a bedpan conveniently on the bed.
  Rationale: Provides a container for removed stool
- Don clean gloves.
  Rationale: Reduces the transmission of microorganisms
- Lubricate the forefinger of your dominant hand.
  Rationale: Eases insertion within the rectum
- Insert your lubricated finger within the rectum to the level of the hardened mass.

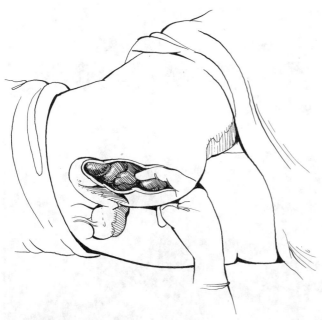

FIGURE 31-2
Removing impacted stool.

Rationale: Facilitates digital manipulation of the stool
• Move your finger about slowly and carefully so as to break up the mass of stool.
Rationale: Facilitates removal or voluntary passage

• Withdraw segments of the stool (Fig. 31-2) and deposit them in the bedpan.
Rationale: Reduces the internal mass of stool
• Provide periods of rest, but continue until the mass has been removed or sufficiently reduced.
Rationale: Restores patency to the lower bowel
• Clean the patient's rectal area; dispose of the stool and soiled gloves; wash your hands.
Rationale: Supports principles of medical asepsis

Flatulence

Flatulence is an excessive accumulation of intestinal gas, or **flatus**. Flatulence may be caused by swallowing air while eating or by sluggish peristalsis. However, it also may be caused by the gas that forms as a by-product of bacterial fermentation within the bowel. Some foods are notorious for producing gas, including various vegetables like cabbage, cucumbers, and onions. Beans are other gas-formers. They create intestinal gas because humans lack an enzyme to digest completely their particular form of complex carbohydrate.

Regardless of its cause, flatus may be expelled rectally, thus reducing intestinal accumulation and distention. However, sometimes this is not sufficient to eliminate the cramping pain or other symptoms. When patients are extremely uncomfortable, and ambulating does not help eliminate its passage, a rectal tube may be inserted to help the gas escape (Skill 31-1).

SKILL 31-1
Inserting a Rectal Tube

Suggested Action	Reason for Action
Assessment	
Check the medical orders.	Collaborates nursing activities with medical treatment
Inspect the abdomen, auscultate bowel sounds, and gently palpate its fullness.	Provides baseline data for future comparisons
Determine how much the patient understands about the procedure.	Provides an opportunity for health teaching
Planning	
Obtain a 22- to 32-F catheter and lubricant.	Eases insertion
Implementation	
Wash your hands and don gloves.	Reduces the transmission of microorganisms
Pull the privacy curtain.	Demonstrates respect for the patient's dignity
Place the patient in a Sims' position.	Facilitates access to the rectum

(continued)

Suggested Action	Reason for Action
Lubricate the tip of the tube generously.	Eases insertion

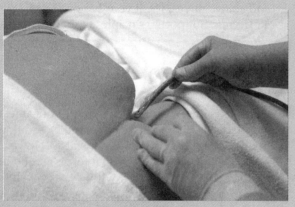

Preparing for insertion. (Courtesy of Ken Timby.)

Suggested Action	Reason for Action
Separate the buttocks well so that the anus is in plain view.	Helps visualize insertion location
Insert the tube 4 to 6 inches (10–15 cm) in an adult.	Places the distal tip above the sphincter muscles, stimulates peristalsis, and prevents displacement of the tube

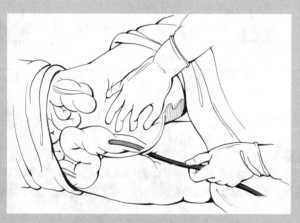

Inserting rectal tube.

Suggested Action	Reason for Action
Enclose the free end of the tube within a clean, soft washcloth or gauze square.	Provides a means for absorbing stool should it drain from the tube
Tape the tube to the buttocks or inner thigh.	Allows the patient to ambulate or change positions without tube displacement
Leave the rectal tube in place no longer than 20 minutes.	Reduces the risk of impairing the sphincters
Reinsert the tube every 3 to 4 hours if discomfort returns.	Reinstitutes therapeutic management

Evaluation
- Symptoms are relieved
- No ill effects are experienced

(continued)

SKILL 31-1
Inserting a Rectal Tube (Continued)

Suggested Action	Reason for Action
Document • Assessment data • Intervention • Length of time tube was in place • Patient response *Sample Documentation* **Date and Time** Abdomen round, firm, and tympanic. Bowel sounds present in all four quads, but difficult to hear because of distention. States, "I can't hardly stand the pain any more." Ambulated without relief. 26-F straight catheter inserted into rectum for 20 minutes. Flatus expelled during tube insertion. Abdomen softer. <div align="right">_____ **Signature, Title**</div>	

Diarrhea

Diarrhea is the urgent passage of watery stools accompanied by abdominal cramping. Simple diarrhea tends to have a sudden onset and last only a short period of time. Other associated signs and symptoms include nausea and vomiting and the presence of blood or mucus in the stools.

Usually diarrhea is a means for eliminating an irritating substance, like tainted food or intestinal pathogens. But diarrhea may also be an outcome of emotional stress, dietary indiscretions, laxative abuse, or bowel disorders.

Simple diarrhea may be relieved by temporarily resting the bowel. This means the person can drink clear liquids, but solid foods are avoided for 12 to 24 hours. When eating is resumed, it is best to start with bland foods and those that are low in residue like bananas, applesauce, and cottage cheese. If the diarrhea is not relieved within 24 hours, it may be best to consult a physician.

Fecal Incontinence

Fecal incontinence is the inability to control the elimination of stool. It does not necessarily imply that the stool is loose or watery, although that may be the case. In many cases of incontinence, bowel function is normal, but the incontinence results from neurologic changes that impair muscle activity, sensation, or thought processes. Even a fecal impaction may be an underlying cause of incontinence. In addition, there are always those isolated instances when a person cannot

postpone elimination until a toilet can be reached, as may be the case when a particularly harsh laxative is administered.

Most people are devastated socially and emotionally by chronic fecal incontinence. Therefore, incontinent patients and their families require much support and understanding when dealing with the problem.

PROMOTING BOWEL ELIMINATION

There are two interventions that promote elimination when it does not occur naturally or when the bowel must be cleansed for other purposes, like preparation for surgery and endoscopic or x-ray examinations. The interventions most commonly used include inserting a rectal suppository and administering an enema.

Inserting a Rectal Suppository

A **suppository** is a medicated oval or cone-shaped mass that is inserted into a body cavity like the rectum (Skill 31-2). The most frequent reason for inserting a suppository is to deliver a drug that will promote the expulsion of feces. Administering a suppository is a form of medication administration. For additional principles, refer to Chapters 32 and 33.

Suppositories are constructed so as to melt at body temperature. Medications released from the suppository can have either a local or systemic effect. Depending on the drug, local effects may include softening and lubricating dry stool, irritating the wall of the rec-

(text continues on page 676)

PATIENT TEACHING FOR MANAGING FECAL INCONTINENCE

Teach the patient and family to do the following:
- Eat regularly and nutritiously.
- Monitor the pattern of incontinence to determine if it occurs at a similar time on a daily basis.
- Sit on the toilet or bedside commode somewhat before the time when bowel elimination tends to occur.
- Consult the physician about inserting a suppository or administering an enema every 2 to 3 days to establish a pattern for bowel elimination.

- Use moisture-proof undergarments and absorbent pads to protect clothing and bed linen.

FOR CAREGIVERS:
- Control making any implication, verbal or nonverbal, that the person is to blame for the incontinence or that cleaning him or her is disgusting.
- Avoid anything that connotes diapering to preserve dignity and self-esteem.

SKILL 31-2
Inserting a Rectal Suppository

Suggested Action	Reason for Action
Assessment	
Check the medical orders.	Collaborates nursing activities with medical treatment
Compare the medication administration record (MAR) with the written medical order.	Ensures accuracy
Read and compare the label on the suppository with the MAR at least three times—before, during, and after preparing the drug.	Prevents errors
Determine how much the patient understands about the purpose and technique for administering a suppository.	Provides an opportunity for health teaching
Planning	
Prepare to administer the suppository according to the time prescribed by the physician.	Complies with medical orders
Obtain clean gloves and lubricant.	Facilitates insertion
Implementation	
Read the name on the patient's identification band.	Prevents errors
Pull the privacy curtain.	Demonstrates respect for the patient's modesty and dignity
Place the patient in a Sims' position.	Facilitates access to the rectum
Drape the patient so as to expose only the buttocks.	Ensures modesty and dignity
Wash hands and don gloves.	Reduces the transmission of microorganisms

(continued)

SKILL 31-2
Inserting a Rectal Suppository *(Continued)*

Suggested Action	Reason for Action
Lubricate the suppository and index finger of the dominant hand.	Reduces friction and tissue trauma
Separate the buttocks so that the anus is in plain view.	Enhances visualization

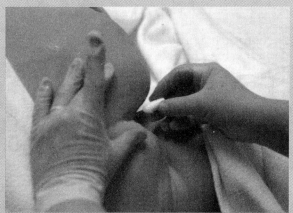

Lubricated suppository and insertion finger. (Courtesy of Ken Timby.)

Suggested Action	Reason for Action
Instruct the patient to take several slow, deep breaths.	Promotes muscle relaxation
Introduce the suppository, tapered end first, beyond the internal sphincter, about the distance of the finger.	Places the suppository in the best location for achieving a local effect

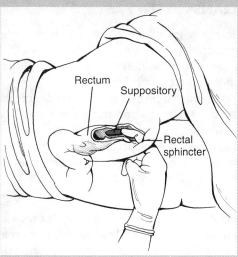

Inserting suppository.

Suggested Action	Reason for Action
Avoid placing the suppository within stool.	Reduces effectiveness

(continued)

SKILL 31-2
Inserting a Rectal Suppository *(Continued)*

Suggested Action	Reason for Action
Wipe the excess lubricant from about the anus with a paper tissue.	Promotes comfort
Tell the patient to try to retain the suppository at least 15 minutes.	Enhances effectiveness
Suggest contracting the gluteal muscles if there is a premature urge to expel the suppository.	Tightens the anal sphincters
Ask the patient to wait to flush the toilet until the stool has been inspected.	Provides an opportunity for evaluating the drug's effectiveness
Remove your gloves and wash your hands.	Reduces the transmission of microorganisms

Evaluation
- Suppository is retained
- Bowel elimination occurs

Document
- Drug, dose, route, and time (see Chap. 32)
- Outcome of drug administration

Sample Documentation

Date and Time   Dulcolax suppository inserted within rectum. Lg. brown formed stool expelled.
_____ **Signature, Title**

---

tum and anal canal to stimulate smooth muscle contraction, or liberating carbon dioxide, thus increasing rectal distention.

Occasionally drugs are administered in suppository form to achieve a systemic effect. This route may be chosen when patients are not likely to retain or absorb oral medications because of chronic vomiting, or their ability to swallow is somehow impaired.

Administering an Enema

An **enema** is the introduction of a solution within the rectum. Enemas may be given for several reasons, but the most common purpose is to cleanse the lower bowel (Skill 31-3). Here are some other common reasons:

- Cleanse the lower bowel
- Soften feces
- Expel flatus
- Soothe irritated mucous membranes
- Outline the colon during diagnostic x-rays
- Treat worm and parasite infestations

CLEANSING ENEMAS

Cleansing enemas are given to remove feces from the rectum with various types of solutions (Table 31-3). They usually cause defecation to occur within 5 to 15 minutes of their administration.

Large-volume cleansing enemas may create discomfort because they distend the lower bowel. They must be cautiously administered to patients with intestinal disorders like colitis (inflammation of the colon) because they may rupture the bowel or cause other secondary complications.

Tap Water and Normal Saline Enemas

Tap water and normal saline solutions may be preferred for their nonirritating effects, especially for patients with rectal diseases or those being prepared for rectal examinations. Tap water and normal saline appear to have about the same degree of effectiveness for cleansing the bowel.

Tap water, because it is hypotonic, can be absorbed through the bowel. Consequently, if several are ad-

(text continues on page 681)

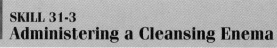

SKILL 31-3
Administering a Cleansing Enema

Suggested Action	Reason for Action
Assessment	
Check the medical orders for the type of enema and prescribed solution.	Collaborates nursing activities with medical treatment
Check the date of the patient's last bowel movement.	Helps determine the need to check for an impaction or the basis for realistic expected outcomes
Auscultate bowel sounds.	Establishes the status of peristalsis
Determine how much the patient understands about the procedure.	Provides an opportunity for health teaching
Planning	
Plan the location where the patient will expel the enema solution and stool.	Determines if a bedpan is necessary
Obtain appropriate equipment, which includes an enema set, solution, absorbent pad, lubricant, bath blanket, and gloves.	Facilitates organization and efficient time management
Plan to perform the procedure according to the time specified by the physician or when it is most appropriate during patient care.	Demonstrates collaboration and participation of the patient in decision-making
Prepare the solution and equipment in the utility room.	Provides access to supplies
Warm the solution to approximately 105°F to 110°F (40°C–43°C).	Promotes comfort and safety
Clamp the tubing on the enema set.	Prevents loss of fluid
Fill the container with the specified solution.	Provides the mechanism for cleansing the bowel
Implementation	
Pull the privacy curtain.	Demonstrates respect for the patient's dignity
Place the patient in a Sims' position.	Facilitates access to the rectum

(continued)

SKILL 31-3
Administering a Cleansing Enema (Continued)

Suggested Action	Reason for Action
Drape the patient, exposing the buttocks, and place a waterproof pad under the hips.	Preserves modesty and protects bed linen

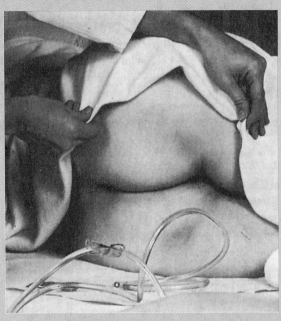

Draping for an enema.

Suggested Action	Reason for Action
Wash your hands and don gloves.	Reduces the transmission of microorganisms
Place (or hang) the solution container so that it is between 12 to 20 inches (30–50 cm) above the level of the patient's anus.	Facilitates gravity flow
Open the clamp and fill the tubing with solution. Reclamp.	Purges air from the tubing

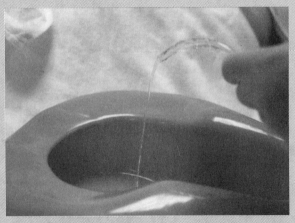

Purging air. (Courtesy of Ken Timby.)

(continued)

SKILL 31-3
Administering a Cleansing Enema *(Continued)*

Suggested Action	Reason for Action
Lubricate the tip of the tube generously.	Eases insertion

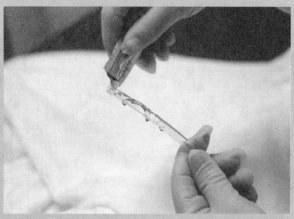

Lubricating tube. (Courtesy of Ken Timby.)

Suggested Action	Reason for Action
Separate the buttocks well so that the anus is in plain view.	Helps visualize insertion
Insert the tube 3 to 4 inches (7–10 cm) in an adult.	Places the distal tip above the sphincters
Direct the tubing at an angle pointing toward the umbilicus.	Follows the contour of the rectum

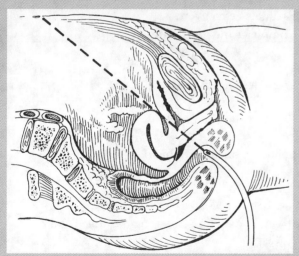

Direction for tube insertion.

(continued)

SKILL 31-3
Administering a Cleansing Enema (Continued)

Suggested Action	Reason for Action
Hold the tube in place with one hand.	Avoids displacement

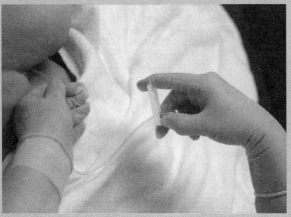

Holding the tube in place. (Courtesy of Ken Timby.)

Suggested Action	Reason for Action
Release the clamp.	Promotes instillation
Instill the solution gradually over 5 to 10 minutes.	Fills the rectum
Clamp the tube for a brief period while the patient takes deep breaths and contracts the anal sphincters if cramping occurs.	Avoids further stimulation
Resume instillation when cramping is relieved.	Facilitates effectiveness
Clamp and remove the tubing after sufficient solution has been instilled or the patient protests that he or she is unable to retain more.	Completes the procedure
Encourage the patient to retain the solution for 5 to 15 minutes.	Promotes effectiveness
Hold the enema tubing in one hand and pull a glove over the inserting end of the tubing.	Prevents direct contact
Remove and discard the remaining glove and dispose of the enema equipment.	Follows principles of medical asepsis
Assist the patient to sit while eliminating the solution and stool.	Aids defecation
Examine the expelled solution.	Provides data for evaluating the effectiveness of the procedure
Clean and dry the patient and help to a position of comfort.	Demonstrates concern for well-being

(continued)

SKILL 31-3
Administering a Cleansing Enema (Continued)

Suggested Action	Reason for Action
Evaluation • Sufficient amount of solution has been instilled • Comparable amount of solution has been expelled • Stool has been eliminated *Document* • Type of enema solution • Volume instilled • Outcome of procedure *Sample Documentation* **Date and Time**　　1,000 mL tap water enema administered. Lg. amt. of brown, formed stool expelled. _____ **Signature, Title**	

ministered in succession, it may cause fluid and electrolyte imbalances to occur (see Chap. 15). Therefore, to ensure patient safety, if stool continues to be expelled after the administration of three enemas, the physician is consulted before administering any more.

Soap Solution Enemas

A soap solution enema is a mixture of water and soap. Many disposable enema kits contain a prepackaged envelope of soap that is mixed with up to a quart (1,000 mL) of water. If these soap packets are not available, a comparable mixture would be 1 mL of mild liquid soap per 200 mL of solution, or a 1:200 ratio. Therefore, to prepare a volume of 1,000 mL, 5 mL of soap would be added.

Soap does cause chemical irritation of the mucous membrane, but that is part of the mechanism of its action. However, adding too much soap or strong soap can potentiate the irritating effect.

Hypertonic Saline Enemas

A hypertonic saline (sodium phosphate) enema draws fluid from body tissues into the bowel. This increases the fluid volume in the intestine beyond what was originally instilled. The concentrated solution also acts on the mucous membranes as a local irritant.

Hypertonic enema solutions are available in commercially prepared, disposable containers with a prelubricated tip (Fig. 31-3). The total amount of solution is about 4 ounces, or 120 mL. The container substitutes for enema equipment and tubing.

In many health agencies and in the home, disposable administration sets have become the method of choice for cleansing the bowel. Their smaller volume makes them less fatiguing and distressing than large-volume enemas, and they can be easily self-administered.

TABLE 31-3. *Types of Cleansing Enema Solutions*

Solution	Amount	Mechanism of Action
Tap water	500–1,000 mL	Distends rectum, moistens stool
Normal saline	500–1,000 mL	Distends rectum, moistens stool
Soap and water	500–1,000 mL	Distends rectum, moistens stool, irritates local tissue
Hypertonic saline	120 mL	Irritates local tissue
Mineral, olive, or cottonseed oil	120–180 mL	Lubricates and softens stool

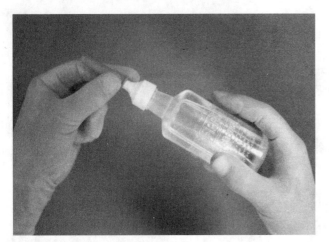

FIGURE 31-3
Hypertonic enema administration container. (Courtesy of Ken Timby.)

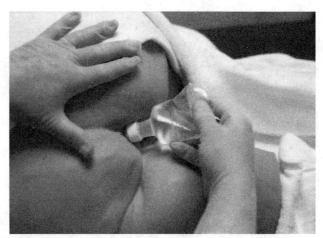

FIGURE 31-4
Compressing enema container. (Courtesy of Ken Timby.)

- Discard the container, remove gloves, and wash hands.
  Rationale: Follows principles of medical asepsis

NURSING GUIDELINES FOR ADMINISTERING A HYPERTONIC ENEMA SOLUTION

- Warm the container of solution by placing it in a basin or sink of warm water, if it is unusually cold.
  Rationale: Promotes comfort
- Assist the patient to a Sims' or use a knee–chest position (see Chap. 13).
  Rationale: The latter promotes gravity distribution of the solution
- Wash hands and don gloves.
  Rationale: Reduces the transmission of microorganisms
- Remove the cover from the prelubricated tip.
  Rationale: Facilitates administering the solution
- Cover the tip with additional lubricant.
  Rationale: Eases insertion
- Invert the container.
  Rationale: Causes air within the container to rise toward the upper end
- Insert the full length of the tip within the rectum.
  Rationale: Places the tip at a level that promotes effectiveness
- Apply gentle, steady pressure on the solution container for 1 to 2 minutes or until the solution has been completely administered.
  Rationale: Instills a steady stream of solution
- Compress the container as the solution instills (Fig. 31-4).
  Rationale: Provides positive pressure rather than gravity to instill fluid
- Clean the patient, and position for comfort.
  Rationale: Demonstrates concern for the patient's well-being

Occasionally it is necessary to administer a retention enema.

RETENTION ENEMAS

A **retention enema** is one that is held within the large intestine. Some are retained for a minimum of 30 minutes; others are not expelled at all. One type of enema is called an *oil retention enema* because the fluid instilled is either mineral, cottonseed, or olive oil. Oils are used to lubricate and soften the stool so it can be expelled more easily.

The oil may come in a prefilled container similar to those that contain hypertonic saline. If disposable equipment is not available, a 14- to 22-F tube is lubricated and inserted within the rectum. A small funnel or large syringe is attached to the tube, and approximately 100 to 200 mL of warmed oil is instilled.

The secret to achieving the best results is to instill the oil *slowly.* A slow administration avoids stimulating an urge to defecate. Premature defecation defeats the purpose of retaining the oil.

Additional skills are required when providing care for ostomy patients, also known as **ostomates** (also see Chap. 30).

OSTOMY CARE

Some ostomates have surgically created openings into intestinal structures through which stool is eliminated. An **ileostomy** is a surgically created opening to the

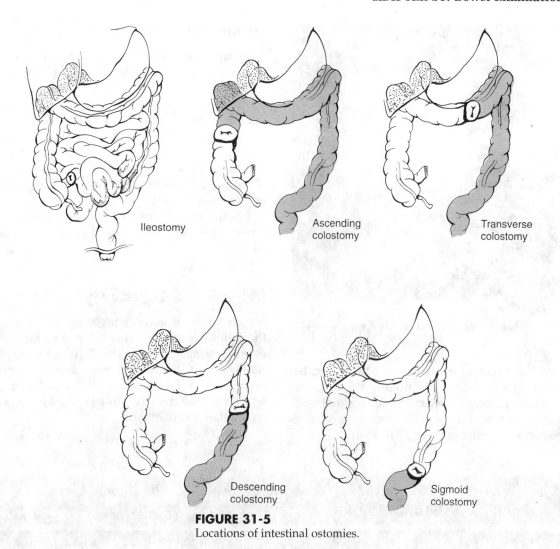

Ileostomy

Ascending colostomy

Transverse colostomy

Descending colostomy

Sigmoid colostomy

FIGURE 31-5
Locations of intestinal ostomies.

ileum; a **colostomy** is an opening to some portion of the colon (Fig. 31-5). The orifice or entrance to the opening is called a **stoma**.

Most ostomates wear an **appliance**, or bag, over their stoma to collect stool. Depending on the type and location of the ostomy, patient care may involve providing peristomal care, applying an appliance, draining a continent ileostomy, and in the case of colostomy patients, administering irrigations through the stoma.

Peristomal Care

Prevention of skin breakdown is one of the biggest challenges in ostomy care. Enzymes in stool can quickly cause **excoriation**, the chemical injury of skin. The integrity of the skin can be preserved by washing the stoma and surrounding skin with mild soap and water and patting it dry. There are also skin barrier substances like *karaya*, a plant substance that becomes gelatinous when moistened, that can be applied around the stoma.

Applying an Ostomy Appliance

Ostomy suppliers provide a variety of appliances to meet the individual needs of each ostomate. Basically, all appliances consist of a pouch for collecting stool and a faceplate, or disk, that attaches to the abdomen. An opening in the center of the appliance provides space through which the stoma protrudes (Fig. 31-6).

The pouch is designed to fasten into position when pressed over the circular support on the faceplate. Some ostomates prefer a type that is also fastened to an elastic belt worn about the waist. The belt helps support the weight of the fecal material and prevents the faceplate from being pulled away from the abdomen. Releasing the clamp at the bottom of the pouch facilitates emptying the appliance.

The faceplate is usually left in place for 3 to 5 days unless it becomes loose or causes skin discomfort. Pouches may be emptied and rinsed, or detached and replaced, periodically. It is wise to empty stool from the pouch whenever it becomes one-third to one-half full.

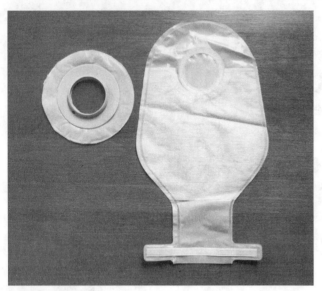

FIGURE 31-6
An ostomy appliance: faceplate and pouch. (Courtesy of Ken Timby.)

Following this regimen prevents the pouch from becoming excessively heavy and pulling the faceplate from the skin. Although there are variations in the design of the equipment, almost all types of appliances are changed in a similar manner (Skill 31-4).

Draining a Continent Ileostomy

A **continent ostomy** is a surgically created opening in which the drainage of liquid stool (or urine) is controlled by siphoning it from an internal reservoir. The continent ostomy is also referred to as a *Kock pouch*, after the surgeon who developed the technique.

The advantage of this procedure is that an appliance need not be worn. The disadvantage is that the patient must drain the accumulating liquid stool (or urine) about every 4 to 6 hours. A gravity drainage system can be used during the night.

Colostomy patients whose stool is more solid sometimes require an instillation of fluid to promote elimination.

Irrigating a Colostomy

A colostomy irrigation involves instilling solution through the stoma into the colon, a process similar to administering an enema (Skill 31-5). Its purpose is to remove formed stool and in some cases regulate the timing of bowel movements. With regulation, a patient with a sigmoid colostomy may choose to omit wearing an appliance altogether.

(text continues on page 694)

SKILL 31-4
Changing an Ostomy Appliance

Suggested Action	Reason for Action
Assessment	
Inspect the faceplate, pouch, and peristomal skin.	Determines the necessity for changing the appliance and provides data about the condition of the stoma and surrounding skin
Determine how much the patient understands about stomal care and changing an ostomy appliance.	Provides an opportunity for health teaching; prepares the patient for assuming self-care
Planning	
Obtain replacement equipment, supplies for removing the adhesive like the manufacturer's recommended solvent, and products for skin care.	Facilitates organization and efficient time management
Plan to replace the appliance immediately if the patient has localized symptoms.	Prevents complications
Schedule an appliance change for an asymptomatic patient before a meal and before a bath or shower.	Coincides with a time when the gastrocolic reflex is less active and prevents repeating hygiene
Empty the pouch just before the appliance will be changed.	Prevents soiling

(continued)

SKILL 31-4
Changing an Ostomy Appliance (Continued)

Suggested Action	Reason for Action
Implementation	
Pull the privacy curtain.	Demonstrates respect for the patient's dignity
Place the patient in a supine or dorsal recumbent position.	Facilitates access to the stoma
Wash your hands and don gloves.	Reduces the transmission of microorganisms
Unfasten the pouch and discard it in a lined receptacle or waterproof container.	Facilitates access to the faceplate
Gently peel the faceplate from the skin.	Prevents skin trauma

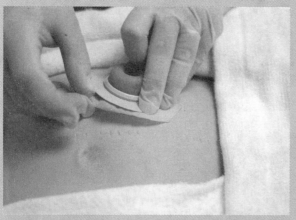

Removing faceplate. (Courtesy of Ken Timby.)

Wash the stoma and peristomal area with water or mild soapy water using a soft washcloth or gauze square.	Cleans mucus and stool from the skin and stoma
Suggest that the patient shower or bathe at this time.	Provides an opportunity for daily hygiene and will not affect the exposed stoma
After bathing or in lieu of bathing, pat the peristomal skin dry.	Promotes potential for adhesion when the faceplate is applied
Measure the stoma with a stomal guide.	Determines the size of the stomal opening in the faceplate

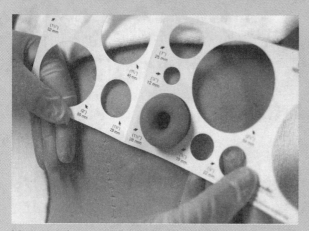

Measuring the stoma. (Courtesy of Ken Timby.)

(continued)

Suggested Action	Reason for Action
Trim the opening in the faceplate the measured diameter plus 1/8 to 1/4 inch larger (Paulford-Lecher, 1993).	Avoids pinching the stoma and causing circulatory impairment

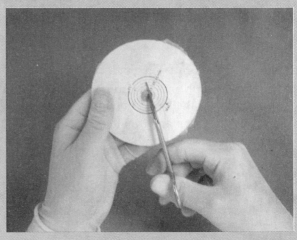

Trimming the stomal opening. (Courtesy of Ken Timby.)

Suggested Action	Reason for Action
Attach a new pouch to the ring of the faceplate.	Avoids pushing it into place after the faceplate has been applied

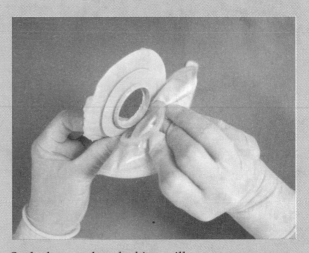

Attaching the pouch. (Courtesy of Ken Timby.)

Suggested Action	Reason for Action
Fold and clamp the bottom of the pouch.	Seals the pouch so leaking will not occur

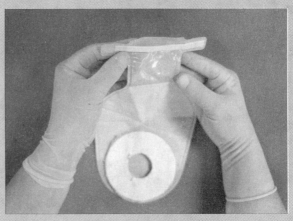

Sealing the pouch. (Courtesy of Ken Timby.)

(continued)

Changing an Ostomy Appliance (Continued)

Suggested Action	Reason for Action
Peel the backing from the adhesive on the face-plate.	Prepares the appliance for application

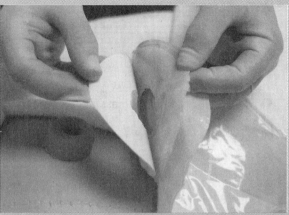

Removing adhesive backing. (Courtesy of Ken Timby.)

Suggested Action	Reason for Action
Have the patient stand or lie flat.	Keeps the skin taut and avoids wrinkles.
Position the opening over the stoma and press into place from the center outward.	Prevents air gaps and skin wrinkles

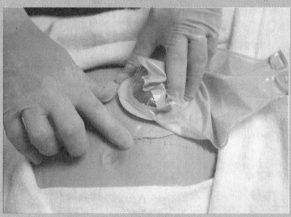

Attaching appliance. (Courtesy of Ken Timby.)

Evaluation

- Stoma appears healthy
- No impairment in skin
- New appliance adheres to the skin without wrinkles or gaps

Document

- Assessment data
- Peristomal care
- Application of new appliance

Sample Documentation

Date and Time   Ostomy appliance removed. Stoma and peristomal skin cleansed with soapy water and patted dry. Stoma is pink and moist. Peristomal skin is intact and painless. New appliance applied over stoma. _____ **Signature, Title**

Teach the patient or family to do the following:
- Assume a sitting position.
- Insert a lubricated 22- to 28-F catheter into the stoma.
- Expect resistance after the tube has been inserted approximately 2 inches; this is the location of the valve that controls the retention of liquid stool or urine.
- Gently advance the catheter through the valve at the end of exhalation, while coughing, or bearing down as if to pass stool.
- Lower the external end of the catheter at least 12 inches below the stoma.
- Direct the end of the catheter into a container or toilet as stool or urine begins to flow.
- Allow at least 5 to 10 minutes for complete emptying.
- Remove the catheter and clean it with warm, soapy water.

- Place the clean catheter in a sealable plastic bag until its next use.
- Cover the stoma with a gauze square or a large bandage.

IF THE CATHETER BECOMES PLUGGED WITH STOOL OR MUCUS:
- Bear down as if to have a bowel movement.
- Rotate the catheter tip inside the stoma.
- Milk the catheter.
- If these are not successful, remove the catheter, rinse it, and try again.
- Notify the physician if these efforts do not result in any drainage.
- Never wait longer than 6 hours without obtaining drainage.

SKILL 31-5
Irrigating a Colostomy

Suggested Action	Reason for Action
Assessment	
Check the medical orders to verify that a written order exists and the type of solution to use.	Collaborates nursing activities with medical treatment
Determine how much the patient understands about a colostomy irrigation.	Provides an opportunity for health teaching; prepares the patient for assuming self-care
Planning	
Obtain an irrigating bag and sleeve, lubricant, and belt. A bedpan will be needed if the patient is confined to bed.	Promotes organization and efficient time management

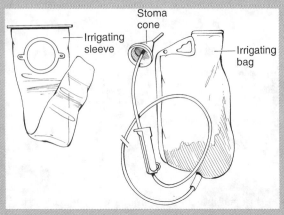

Irrigating sleeve and bag.

(continued)

SKILL 31-5
Irrigating a Colostomy *(Continued)*

Suggested Action	Reason for Action
Prepare the irrigating bag with solution in the same way as an enema set is prepared (see Skill 31-3).	Provides the mechanism for cleansing the bowel
Unclamp the tubing and fill it with solution.	Purges air from the tubing
Implementation	
Place the patient in a sitting position either in bed, in a chair in front or beside the toilet, or on the toilet itself.	Facilitates collecting drainage
Place absorbent pads or towels on the patient's lap.	Prevents having to change linen or clothing
Hang the container approximately 12 inches (30 cm) above the stoma.	Facilitates gravity flow
Wash your hands and don gloves.	Reduces the transmission of microorganisms
Empty and remove the pouch from the faceplate, if one is worn.	Provides access to the stoma
Secure the sleeve over the stoma and fasten it about the patient with an elastic belt.	Provides a pathway for drainage

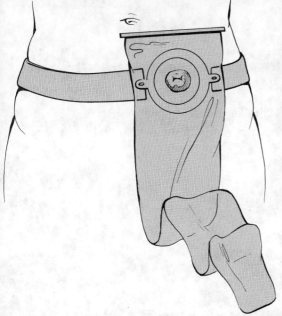

Positioning irrigation sleeve.

(continued)

SKILL 31-5
Irrigating a Colostomy (Continued)

Suggested Action	Reason for Action
Place the lower end of the sleeve into the toilet, commmode, or a bedpan.	Collects drainage

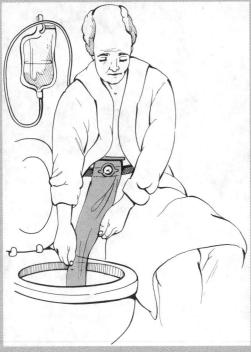

Placing distal end of sleeve.

Suggested Action	Reason for Action
Lubricate the cone at the end of the irrigating bag.	Facilitates insertion
Open the top of the irrigating sleeve.	Provides access to the stoma

(continued)

SKILL 31-5
Irrigating a Colostomy (Continued)

Suggested Action	Reason for Action
Insert the cone into the stoma.	Dilates the stoma and provides a means for instilling fluid

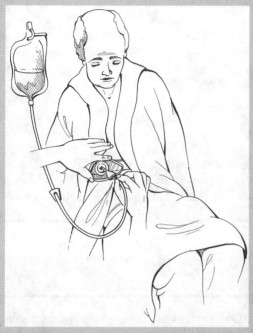

Inserting irrigation cone.

Suggested Action	Reason for Action
Hold the cone in place and release the clamp on the tubing.	Prevents expulsion of the cone and initiates the instillation
Clamp the tubing and wait if cramping occurs.	Interrupts the instillation while the bowel adjusts
Release the clamp and continue once the discomfort disappears.	Resumes instilling fluid
Clamp the tubing and remove the cone when the irrigating solution has been instilled.	Discontinues the administration of solution
Close the top of the irrigating sleeve.	Keeps drainage in a downward direction
Give the patient reading materials or hygiene supplies.	Provides diversion or uses time for other productive activities
Remove the belt and sleeve when draining has stopped.	Eliminates unnecessary equipment
Clean the stoma and pat it dry.	Maintains tissue integrity
If an appliance is worn, place a clean pouch over the stoma, or cover the stoma temporarily with a gauze square.	Collects fecal drainage

(continued)

SKILL 31-5
Irrigating a Colostomy (Continued)

Suggested Action	Reason for Action

Evaluation
- Sufficient amount of solution has been instilled
- Comparable amount of solution has been expelled
- Stool has been eliminated

Document
- Type of irrigation solution
- Volume instilled
- Outcome of procedure

Sample Documentation

Date and Time   Colostomy irrigated with 500 mL of tap water. Instilled without difficulty. Mod. amt. of semiformed stool expelled with solution. Stoma cleansed with soapy water and dried. Covered with a gauze square. _____ **Signature, Title**

FOCUS ON OLDER ADULTS

- Gastrointestinal motility, muscle tone, and digestive enzymes decrease with age, predisposing older adults to constipation.
- Older adults may implement various home remedies for promoting elimination, such as drinking hot water or prune juice in the morning. As long as the health beliefs are not harmful, and in some cases they are helpful, continue to implement them while caring for older adults.
- Older adults may be receptive to eating bran cereal or adding bran to casseroles or muffins as a healthier alternative to using laxatives to maintain bowel elimination.
- Older adults who live alone may rely on commercially prepared boxed or frozen meals that they can heat and eat. Consequently, older adults may not consume adequate amounts of dietary fiber to promote regular bowel elimination.
- Some older adults become very bowel-conscious and may overuse laxatives. When an elimination aid is necessary, those that form bulk like psyllium (Metamucil; Procter & Gamble, Cincinnati, OH) and polycarbophil (FiberCon; Lederle Laboratories, Pearl River, NY) may be less irritating to the intestinal system.

- Older adults who use mineral oil as a self-treatment for preventing or relieving constipation need to be informed that prolonged use interferes with the absorption of fat-soluble vitamins.
- The incidence of colorectal cancer rises with age. One of its early signs is a change in bowel patterns and stool characteristics. Therefore, older adults are advised to have regular endoscopic bowel examinations after the age of 50 years. Any change in bowel elimination that does not respond to simple dietary or lifestyle changes must be further investigated.
- Diarrhea can easily cause dehydration and electrolyte imbalances among older adults, who tend to have less body fluid reserve than younger people.
- Because many older adults have benign lesions like hemorrhoids or polyps in their lower bowel, removing an impaction must be done gently to prevent bleeding and tissue trauma.
- Arthritis of the hands may interfere with an older adult's ability to care for an ostomy appliance or perform colostomy irrigations. An enterostomal therapist, a nurse who is certified in caring for ostomies and related skin problems, may be able to offer suggestions for promoting self-care.

NURSING CARE PLAN:
Colonic Constipation

Assessment	**Subjective Data**
	States, "I've got a problem with constipation. I haven't had a bowel movement in 4 days even though I've felt like I need to pass stool. I sit and strain but I only pass a small amount of hard stool. I used to have a problem now and then when I was a kid; but since I'm living alone it's getting to be very frequent. Maybe its's because I don't eat regularly and when I do, it's a lot of convenience food."
	Objective Data
	21-year-old man recovering from a fractured ankle that occurred when he tripped on an area rug in his apartment yesterday. Plaster cast on L. leg that extends from toes to midcalf. Abdomen tympanic during percussion. Bowel sounds are hypoactive in all four quadrants.
Diagnosis	Colonic Constipation related to inadequate dietary habits.
Plan	**Goal**
	The patient will have a bowel movement within 24 hours and list three ways to improve the regularity of bowel elimination by 10/25.

Orders: 10/24

1. Give oil retention enema as ordered for prn administration.
2. Give prescribed laxative at HS if no bowel movement has occurred.
3. Encourage drinking at least 8 to 10 glasses of fluid per day; avoid carbonated beverages.
4. Instruct about high-fiber foods and inform that daily consumption should consist of at least four servings. _____ A. ZIMMERMAN, RN

Implementation (Documentation)

10/24 1300   Instructed to drink at least 5 more glasses of fluid today and 8 to 10 thereafter. Explained that soft drinks increase intestinal gas. Given paper and pencil to record his current eating pattern, food likes and dislikes._____ M. HASS, LPN

1330   200 mL oil retention enema administered. Instructed to remain in bed and re-tain solution for at least 30 minutes or longer if possible. _____ M. HASS, LPN

Evaluation (Documentation)

1400   Helped to bathroom using crutches and three-point non–weight-bearing gait. Passed a moderate amount of hard stool. Blood observed on stool and toilet paper. States, "It took a lot of straining but I feel much better now."
_____ M. HASS, LPN

1400   Reviewed dietary list. Noted the following: does not eat breakfast, usually eats lunch at fast-food establishment near campus, fixes frozen meals in evening, snacks on chips._____ M. HASS, LPN

1445   Recommended eating breakfast and waiting at home a little while for urge to eliminate. Include whole-grain bread/toast, cereal, fresh fruits, fruit juices, salads, and nuts or seeds as additions to diet for at least four servings each day. States, "I guess I could eat an apple or carrots between classes. I used to eat shredded wheat for breakfast. They sell salads where I eat lunch. I didn't realize soda pop could add to the bloating I've been feeling. Maybe I'll have to start shopping and eating a little differently from now on." _____ M. HASS, LPN

APPLICABLE NURSING DIAGNOSES

- Constipation
- Perceived Constipation
- Colonic Constipation
- Diarrhea
- Bowel Incontinence
- Toileting Self-Care Deficit
- Situational Low Self-Esteem

NURSING IMPLICATIONS

While assessing and caring for patients with altered bowel elimination, the nurse may identify one or more of the accompanying Applicable Nursing Diagnoses that are pertinent to the patient's problems.

The Nursing Care Plan for this chapter reflects the nursing process as it applies to a patient with Colonic Constipation. Colonic Constipation is defined as "The state in which an individual's pattern of elimination is characterized by hard, dry stool which results from a delay in passage of food residue" (NANDA, 1994).

KEY CONCEPTS

- Defecation, the elimination of stool, occurs when peristalsis moves fecal wastes toward the rectum, and the rectum distends, creating an urge to relax the anal sphincters, which releases stool.
- Two components of a bowel elimination assessment include assessing elimination patterns and stool characteristics.
- Constipation, fecal impaction, flatulence, diarrhea, and fecal incontinence are common alterations that occur in bowel elimination.
- There are four different types of constipation: primary constipation, which can be treated independently by nurses, secondary constipation, iatrogenic constipation, and pseudo constipation.
- When bowel elimination does not occur naturally, defecation can be promoted by inserting a rectal suppository or administering an enema.

- Cleansing enemas and oil retention enemas are two categories of enema administration.
- Cleansing enemas are administered by instilling tap water, normal saline, soap and water, and other solutions.
- Oil retention enemas are given for the purpose of lubricating and softening dry stool.
- When caring for patients with intestinal ostomies, nursing activities are likely to include providing peristomal care, applying an ostomy appliance, draining a continent ileostomy, and irrigating a colostomy.

CRITICAL THINKING EXERCISES

- Develop a list of suggestions designed to promote healthy bowel elimination.
- Formulate suggestions for promoting bowel continence among older adults with impaired cognition, like those affected by Alzheimer's disease.

SUGGESTED READINGS

Anastasi JK. AIDS update: caring for patients with diarrhea. Nursing August 1993;23:68–70.

Beverley L, Travis I. Constipation: proposed natural laxative mixtures. Journal of Gerontological Nursing October 1992;18:5–12.

Burkitt D. Fiber as protective against gastrointestinal diseases. American Journal of Gastroenterology April 1984;79:249–252.

Eliopoulos C. Gerontological Nursing. 3rd ed. Philadelphia: JB Lippincott, 1993.

Hogstel MO, Nelson M. Anticipation and early detection can reduce bowel elimination complications. Geriatric Nursing January–February 1992;13:28–33.

Kovach T. Managing geriatric constipation. Home Healthcare Nurse September–October 1992;10:57–58.

Krasner D. Six steps to successful stoma care. RN July 1993;56:32–38.

Murray S, Preuss M, Schultz F. How do you prep the bowel without enemas? American Journal of Nursing August 1992;92:66–67.

Paulford-Lecher N. Teaching your patient stoma care. Nursing September 1993;23:47–49.

Van Niel J. What's wrong with this peristomal skin? American Journal of Nursing December 1991;91:44–45.

Yen PK. An apple a day is not enough. Journal of Gerontological Nursing November–December 1992;13:336, 339.

Yen PK. The dark side of fiber. Geriatric Nursing January–February 1991;12:43.

UNIT X
Medication Administration

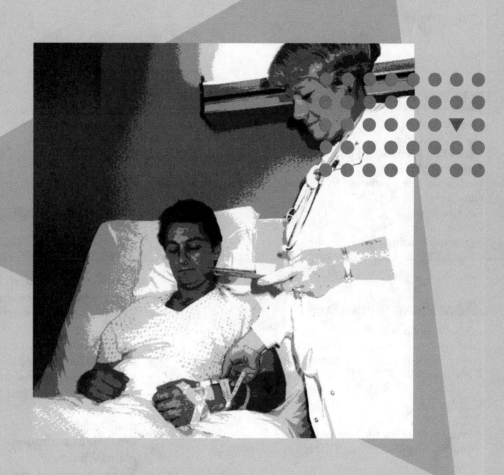

CHAPTER 32

Oral Medications

Learning Objectives

An understanding of the content within this chapter will be evidenced by the student's ability to:

- Describe a medication
- Name seven components of a drug order
- Explain the difference between a trade and generic drug name
- Name four common routes for administration
- Describe the oral route
- Explain the circumstances when oral medications are given by an enteral tube
- Name two general forms of medications that are administered by the oral route
- Describe a medication administration record and explain its purpose
- Name three ways that drugs are supplied
- Discuss two nursing responsibilities that apply to the administration of narcotics
- Name the five rights of medication administration
- Give the formula for calculating a drug dose
- Discuss at least one guideline that applies to the safe administration of medications
- Discuss one point to stress when teaching patients about taking medications
- Identify one common problem associated with administering medications through an enteral tube
- Describe three actions that are appropriate if a medication error occurs

Timby BK: *Fundamental Skills and Concepts in Patient Care, Sixth Edition* © 1996 Lippincott-Raven Publishers

• Discuss at least one unique consideration that applies to administering medications to older adults

Among one of the nurse's most important responsibilities is the administration of medications. This chapter emphasizes the safe preparation and administration of medications, particularly those given by the oral route. Information on specific drugs can be found in pharmacology texts or drug reference manuals.

MEDICATIONS

A **medication** is any chemical substance that changes body function. In this chapter, the terms "medication" and *drug* are used synonymously.

MEDICATION ORDERS

A **medication order** is the name and directions for giving a drug. A *drug prescription* is a type of medication order. Only medication orders given by a physician, dentist, or other person designated by statutes in each state, like a physician's assistant or certified nurse practitioner, are legal. Those written on the patient's medical record are used here for the purposes of discussion.

Components of a Medication Order

All medication orders must contain seven components:

1. The name of the patient
2. The date and time the order is written
3. The drug name
4. The dose to be administered
5. The route for administration
6. The frequency for administration
7. The signature of the person ordering the drug

If any one of these components is absent, the drug is withheld until the missing information is obtained. Medication errors are serious. *A questionable medication order is never implemented until after consulting with the physician.*

Drug Names

Each drug has both a trade, or proprietary, name and a generic, or nonproprietary, name. The **trade name** is the name used by the pharmaceutical company for the drug it sells. The drug's **generic name** is a chemical name that is not protected by a company's trademark. For example, Demerol (Winthrop Pharmaceuticals, New York, NY) is a trade name. It is a company's brand name for meperidine hydrochloride, the generic name.

Drug Dose

The **dose** of a drug is the amount that is prescribed. Drugs are prescribed using the metric and sometimes the apothecary systems of measurement. For home use, doses may be prescribed in household measurements, which are more easily interpreted by nonprofessionals.

Routes of Administration

The **route of administration** is the manner in which the drug is administered. Common routes of administration include oral, topical, inhalant, and parenteral routes (Table 32-1). Topical and inhalant routes of administration are discussed in Chapter 33; parenteral administration is described in Chapters 34 and 35.

THE ORAL ROUTE

The **oral route** refers to administering drugs that are swallowed or instilled through an enteral tube (see Chap. 29). Oral medications are intended for absorption in the gastrointestinal tract. The oral route is the most common and frequently used route for medication administration because it is safer, more economic, and comfortable than others.

Forms of Oral Medications

Oral medications come in both solid and liquid forms.

Solid Forms. Solid medications include tablets and capsules. Some tablets are scored. A **scored tablet** has a groove in its center that facilitates breaking it exactly in half. Scored tablets are convenient when only part of a tablet is needed. Others may be enteric coated. An **enteric-coated tablet** is one that is covered with a substance that does not dissolve until past the stomach. Enteric-coated tablets are never cut, crushed, or chewed because when the integrity of the coating is impaired, the drug is released too soon. Capsules may contain small beads or pellets of drugs that are designed for **sustained release**—that is, small portions of the drug dissolve at timed intervals.

Some tablets are placed in the mouth, but they are not swallowed (see section on Sublingual and Buccal Applications, Chap. 33).

TABLE 32-1. *Routes of Drug Administration*	
Route	Method of Administration
Oral	Swallowing
	Instillation through an enteral tube
Topical	Application to skin or mucous membrane
Inhalant	Aerosol
Parenteral	Injection

Liquid Forms. Liquid forms of oral drugs include syrups, elixirs, and suspensions. Liquid medications are measured and administered in calibrated cups, droppers, or syringes, or with a dosing spoon (Fig. 32-1).

Frequency of Administration

The frequency of drug administration refers to how often and how regularly the medication is to be administered. The frequency of administration is written using standard abbreviations that have their origin in Latin words (Display 32-1; also see Chap. 9 and Appendix A for other commonly used abbreviations). When the medication order is implemented, the drug administration is scheduled according to the prescribed frequency.

DRUG SCHEDULING

Drug administrations are scheduled according to a predetermined timetable set by the health agency. The hours of administration may vary from one place of employment to another. For example, if a physician orders a q.i.d. (four times a day) administration of a medication, it may be scheduled for administration at:

0800, 1200, 1600, and 2000, or
1000, 1400, 1800, and 2200, or
0600, 1200, 1800, and 2400

Verbal Orders

Verbal orders are instructions for patient care that are given during face-to-face conversation or by telephone. Verbal instructions are more likely to result in misinterpretation than those that are written. If the physician

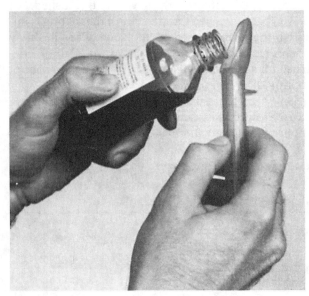

FIGURE 32-1
A dosing spoon.

DISPLAY 32-1. *Common Routines for Medication Administration*

Abbreviation	Meaning
Stat	Immediately
q.d.	Every day
q.o.d	Every other day
b.i.d.	Twice a day
t.i.d.	Three times a day
q.i.d.	Four times a day
q.h.	Hourly
q.4h	Every 4 hours

is physically present, it is appropriate to ask tactfully that the order be handwritten. In the physician's absence, it is sometimes necessary to obtain verbal orders by telephone.

NURSING GUIDELINES FOR TAKING TELEPHONE ORDERS

- Have a second nurse listen simultaneously on an extension.
  Rationale: Provides a witness to the communication
- Record the drug order directly on the patient's record.
  Rationale: Avoids errors in memory
- Repeat the written information back to the physician.
  Rationale: Clarifies understanding
- Make sure the order includes the essential components of a drug order.
  Rationale: Complies with standards for care
- Clarify any drug names that sound similar, such as Feldene (Pfizer Laboratories, New York, NY) and Seldane (Merrell Dow Laboratories, Cincinnati, OH), Nicobid (Rorer Pharmaceuticals, Fort Washington, PA) and Nitro-Bid (Marion Laboratories, Kansas City, MO).
  Rationale: Avoids medication errors
- Spell or repeat numbers that could be misinterpreted, such as fifteen (one, five) and fifty (five, zero).
  Rationale: Avoids medication errors
- Use the abbreviation "T.O." at the end of the order.
  Rationale: Indicates the order is a telephone order
- Write the physician's name and cosign with your name and title.
  Rationale: Complies with legal standards and demonstrates accountability for the communication

Once the medication order is obtained, the order is transcribed to the medication administration record.

MEDICATION ADMINISTRATION RECORD

The **medication administration record** (MAR) is a form used to document drug administration. Each agency adopts the type of record it thinks will ensure the timely and safe administration of medications. Some use a form on which the drug order is transcribed by hand; others use a computer-generated form (Fig. 32-2). Regardless of the type used, all MARs provide a space for documenting when a drug is administered, along with a place for the signature and initials of each nurse who administers a medication. The current MAR is usually kept separate from the patient's medical record, but it eventually becomes a permanent part of it.

After the medication order is transcribed to the MAR, the drug is requested from the pharmacy.

SUPPLYING MEDICATIONS

Drugs are supplied, or dispensed, in three different ways: in an individual supply, in unit doses, and stock supply. An **individual supply** is a single container with several days' or weeks' supply of the prescribed drug (Fig. 32-3). More often, however, drugs are dispensed in unit doses. A **unit dose** is a self-contained packet that holds one tablet or capsule (Fig. 32-4). When the unit dose system is used, the pharmacist supplies sufficient unit dose packets for 1 day's worth of drug administration. The supply is replenished each day. A **stock supply** consists of drugs that are commonly prescribed or needed in an emergency. They are replaced as they are used.

Storing Medications

In each health agency, there is one area where drugs are stored. Some agencies keep medications in a mobile cart, whereas others may store them in a separate room. Each patient has a separate drawer or cubicle in which their prescribed medications are kept. Regardless of their location, medications are kept locked until they are administered.

Accounting for Narcotics

Narcotics are controlled substances. This means that there are federal laws regulating their possession and administration. In health agencies, narcotics are kept in a *double-locked* drawer, box, or room on the nursing unit. Because narcotics are usually delivered by stock supply, nurses are responsible for an accurate account of their use. A record is kept of each narcotic that is used from the stock supply.

Narcotics are counted at each change of shift. One nurse counts the number in the supply, while another checks the record of their administration. Both counts must agree. Inconsistencies are accounted for as soon as possible.

MEDICATION ADMINISTRATION

Safety is the main concern underlying medication administration. By taking various precautions before, during, and after the administration of medications (Skill 32-1), the potential for making medication errors is reduced. Some of the precautions include ensuring the five rights of medication administration, calculating drug dosages accurately, preparing medications carefully, and recording their administration.

The Five Rights

To ensure that medication errors do not occur, nurses follow the **five rights** of medication administration (Fig. 32-5). Some nurses have added a sixth right, the right to refuse. Every rational adult patient has the right to refuse medication. If this happens, the nurse identifies the reason for the omission of the drug's administration, circles the scheduled time on the MAR, and reports the situation to the physician.

Calculating Dosages

One of the major nursing responsibilities, and one of the five rights, is preparing the dose accurately. Preparing an accurate dose sometimes requires that nurses convert doses into the metric, apothecary, and household equivalents. Once the prescribed and supplied amounts are in the same measurements and system of measurement, the quantity for administration can be easily calculated using a standard formula (Display 32-2).

DISPLAY 32-2. *Drug Calculation Formula*

$$\frac{D}{H} \times Q = \frac{Desired\ \text{dose}}{Dose\ on\ hand\ \text{(supplied dose)}} \times Quantity = \text{Amount to administer}$$

Example
   Drug order: Tetracycline 500 mg (*desired dose*) by mouth q.i.d.
   Dose supplied: 250 mg (*dose on hand*) per 5 mL (*quantity*)
Calculation: $\frac{500\ mg}{250\ mg} \times 5\ mL = 10\ mL$

MEDICATION ADMINISTRATION RECORD

PAGE 1

SHIFT	FULL NAME/TITLE	INITIAL
0701 - 1500		
0701 - 1500		
0701 - 1500		
1501 - 2300		
1501 - 2300		
1501 - 2300		
2301 - 0700		
2301 - 0700		

10/02/90 00010 PHARMACY/CHART
TESTDP DON'T DISC AGE: 041
00000000107 DEMPSEY. JAMES
ACCT #: 000000108 ADMIT DATE 04/21/88
DIAG.: ASTHMA-EXACERBATED BY PNEUMONIA
ALL: CODEINE TETRACYCLINE

	1501 10/02/90 THRU 1500 DATE 10/03/90	1501-2300 (0701-1500)	2301-0700 (1501-2300)	0701-1500 (2301-0700)	COMMENTS
1	(01016) 10/01/90 1800 SOLU-CORTEF 100 MG/2ML-HYDROCORT DOSE: 100 MG. IP Q6H IP RATE = 500 MG. OVER 1 MIN. ABBOTT	1800	0000 0600	1200	
2	(03090) 09/27/90 0900 ACETAMINOPHEN EXTRA ST.CAP DOSE: 1 PO Q DAY TYLENOL			0900	
3	(04841) 10/01/90 0900 TENORMIN TAB. 50 MG. DOSE: 50 MG. PO Q DAY			0900	
4	(03096) 10/01/90 0900 LANOXIN (DIGOXIN) TAB. 0.25 MG. DOSE: 0.25 MG. PO Q DAY			0900	
5	(00543) 10/01/90 1800 BRETHINE AMP. 1 MG./ML. 1 ML. DOSE: 0.25MG SC Q6H (TERBUTALINE)	1800	0000 0600	1200	
6					
7					
8					
9					
10					
11					
12					
13					

TESTDP DON'T DIS 00000000107 DEMPSEY. JAMES THRU 1500 10/03/90

FIGURE 32-2
A computer-generated medication administration record (MAR).

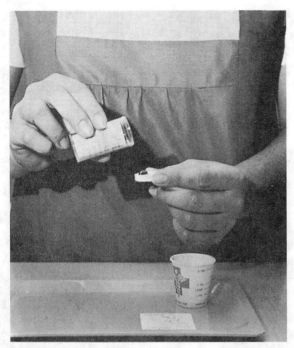

FIGURE 32-3
Medication from an individual supply.

Careful Preparation

There are additional precautions to take when preparing medications that may avoid errors.

◄ NURSING GUIDELINES FOR THE SAFE PREPARATION OF MEDICATIONS

- Prepare medications under well lighted conditions.
  Rationale: Improves the ability to read labels accurately

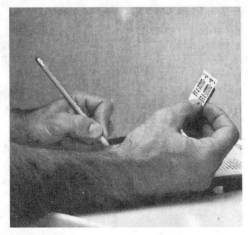

FIGURE 32-4
Unit dose medications.

BE SURE YOU HAVE THE

1. RIGHT DRUG
2. RIGHT DOSE
3. RIGHT ROUTE
4. RIGHT TIME
5. RIGHT PATIENT

FIGURE 32-5
The five rights of medication administration.

- Work alone, without interruptions and distractions.
  Rationale: Promotes concentration
- Check the label of the drug container three times: (1) when reaching for the medication, (2) just before placing the medication into an administration cup, and (3) when returning the medication to the patient's drawer.
  Rationale: Ensures attention to important information
- Avoid using medications from containers with a missing or obliterated label.
  Rationale: Eliminates speculating on the drug name or dose
- Return medications with dubious or obscured labels to the pharmacy.
  Rationale: Facilitates replacement or new labeling
- Never transfer medications from one container to another.
  Rationale: Avoids mismatching contents
- Check the expiration dates on liquid medications.
  Rationale: Ensures administration at desired potency
- Inspect the medication and reject those that appear to be decomposing in any manner.
  Rationale: Promotes appropriate absorption

Administering Oral Medications

Oral medications are prepared and brought to the patient's bedside in a paper souffle cup or plastic medication cup. Only those medications that one has personally prepared are administered to patients; *never*

(text continues on page 706)

SKILL 32-1
Administering Oral Medications

Suggested Action	Reason for Action
Assessment	
Compare the medication administration record (MAR) with the written medical order.	Prevents medication errors

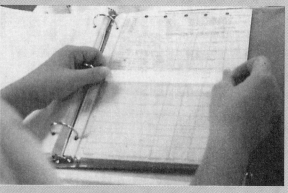

Checking the MAR. (Courtesy of Ken Timby.)

Suggested Action	Reason for Action
Review the patient's drug, allergy, and medical history.	Avoids potential complications
Consult a current drug reference concerning the drug's action, side effects, contraindications, and administration information.	Ensures appropriate administration
Planning	
Plan to administer medications within a half-hour to an hour of the time they are scheduled.	Demonstrates timely administration and compliance with the medical order
Allow sufficient time to prepare the medications in a location where there are minimal distractions.	Promotes safe preparation of drugs
Make sure that there is a sufficient supply of paper and plastic medication cups.	Facilitates organization and efficient time management
Chill oily medications.	Reduces their unpleasant odor and improves palatability
Implementation	
Wash your hands.	Removes colonizing microorganisms

(continued

SKILL 32-1
Administering Oral Medications

Suggested Action	Reason for Action
Read and compare the label on the drug with the MAR at least three times—before, during, and after preparing the drug.	Ensures that the *right drug* is given at the *right time* by the *right route*

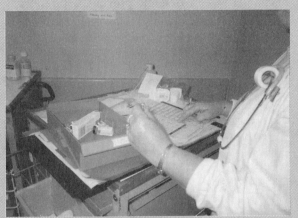

Comparing the drug label and MAR. (Courtesy of Ken Timby.)

Suggested Action	Reason for Action
Calculate doses.	Complies with the medical order and ensures that the *right dose* is given
Place medications or unit dose packets within a paper or plastic cup without touching the medication itself.	Supports principles of asepsis
Keep drugs that require special assessments or administration techniques in a separate cup.	Helps identify drugs that require special nursing actions
Pour liquids from the opposite side of the drug label.	Prevents liquid from running onto the label
Hold the cup for liquid medications at eye level when pouring.	Facilitates accurate measurement

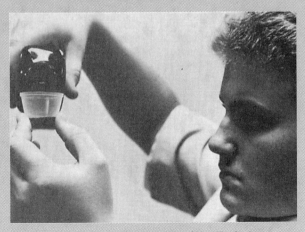

Pouring liquid medication. (Courtesy of Ken Timby.)

(continued)

SKILL 32-1
Administering Oral Medications

Suggested Action	Reason for Action
Prepare a supply of soft-textured food like apple-sauce or pudding, according to the patient's individual needs.	Facilitates administration for patients with impaired swallowing
Help the patient to a sitting position.	Facilitates swallowing and prevents aspiration
Identify the patient by checking the wristband or asking the patient's name.	Ensures that medications are given to the *right patient*

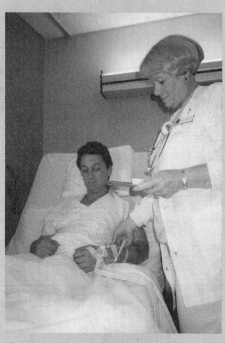

Checking the identification band. (Courtesy of Ken Timby.)

Suggested Action	Reason for Action
Prepare fresh water in a glass with or without a straw.	Facilitates swallowing the medication
Offer water before giving solid forms of oral medications.	Moistens mucous membranes and prevents medication from sticking
Advise patients to take medications one at a time or in amounts they can easily swallow.	Prevents choking

(continued)

SKILL 32-1
Administering Oral Medications *(Continued)*

Suggested Action	Reason for Action
Encourage patients to keep their head in a neutral position or one of slight flexion, rather than hyperextending the neck.	Protects the airway

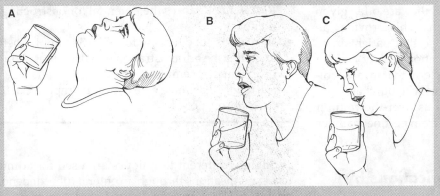

(*A*) Inappropriate neck position; (*B*) and (*C*) appropriate neck positions.

Suggested Action	Reason for Action
Remain with patients until their medications are swallowed.	Ensures appropriate administration
Restore the patient to a position of comfort and safety.	Shows concern for the patient's well-being
Record the volume of fluid consumed on the intake and output record.	Demonstrates responsibility for accurate fluid assessment
Record the administration of the medication.	Prevents medication errors
Assess the patient in 30 minutes for desired and undesired drug effects.	Aids in evaluating the patient's response and effect of drug therapy

Evaluation
- The five rights are upheld
- No choking or aspiration occurs
- There is a therapeutic response to the medication
- Side effects are absent or minimized

Document
- Preassessment data, if indicated
- Date, time, drug, dose, route, signature, initials (usually on the MAR)
- Evidence of patient's response, if it can be determined

Sample Documentation
Date and Time   Temp. 103.8°F. Tylenol tabs ii given by mouth for relief of fever. Fever reduced to 103°F 30 minutes later. _____ **Signature, Title**

administer medications prepared by another nurse. Once at the bedside, it also is important to remain with the patient while medications are taken. If the patient is unavailable, the medications are returned to the medication cart or room. Leaving medications unattended may result in their loss or accidental ingestion by some other patient.

PATIENT TEACHING

Before patients are discharged, they are often given prescriptions for oral medications. This provides an opportunity for health teaching so that patients may self-administer their own medications safely and remain compliant. **Compliance** is a term that means "following instructions." Even patients who purchase nonprescription drugs, also known as **over-the-counter** (OTC) **medications**, may benefit from pertinent advice about drug-taking.

Administering Oral Medications by Enteral Tube

Oral medications can be instilled by enteral tube when they cannot be swallowed orally (Skill 32-2). Because the lumen of a tube is smaller than the esophagus, special techniques may be required to avoid obstructing the tube.

◄········ **NURSING GUIDELINES FOR PREPARING MEDICATIONS FOR ENTERAL TUBE ADMINISTRATION**

- Use liquid form of the drug whenever possible.
  Rationale: Promotes tube patency
- Add 15 to 60 mL of water to liquid medications that are thick.
  Rationale: Dilutes the medication and facilitates instillation
- Pulverize tablets, except those that are enteric coated.
  Rationale: Creates small granules that may instill more readily
- Open the shell of a capsule to release the powdered drug.
  Rationale: Facilitates mixing into a liquid form
- Avoid crushing sustained-release pellets.
  Rationale: Ensures their sequential rate of absorption
- Mix each drug separately with at least 15 to 30 mL of water.
  Rationale: Provides a medium and dilute volume for administration
- Use warm water when mixing powdered drugs.

Rationale: Promotes dissolving the solid form
- Pierce the end of a sealed gelatin capsule and squeeze the liquid medication inside or aspirate it with a needle and syringe.
  Rationale: Facilitates access to the medication
- Soak a soft gelatin capsule in 15 to 30 mL of warm water, as an alternative, for approximately 1 hour.
  Rationale: Dissolves the gelatin seal
- Avoid administering bulk-forming laxatives through an enteral tube.
  Rationale: Reduces the potential for obstructing the tube
- Interrupt a tube feeding for 15 to 30 minutes before and after the administration of a drug that should be given on an empty stomach.
  Rationale: Facilitates the drug's therapeutic action or its absorption

---

Slightly different techniques are used for administering medications through an enteral tube, depending on whether the tube is being used for decompression or nourishment.

TUBES USED FOR DECOMPRESSION

Medications may be given through gastric tubes used for decompression (ie, suctioning; see Chap. 29), but afterward the tube is clamped for at least one half-hour. This prevents removing the drug before it leaves the stomach.

TUBES USED FOR ENTERAL FEEDING

Medications can be given while a patient is receiving tube feedings, but the medications are instilled separately—that is, they are not added to the formula. This is done for two reasons. First, some drugs may physically interact with the components in the formula, causing it to curdle or otherwise change its consistency. Also, a slow infusion would alter the drug's dose and rate of absorption.

Documentation

Medication administration is documented either on the MAR, the patient's chart, or both as soon as possible. Timely documentation prevents medication errors in which someone may assume that a patient has not received medication and gives a second dose. Documentation also demonstrates that the medication order has been implemented.

If a medication is withheld, its omission is documented according to agency policy. This is commonly done by circling the time of administration and initialing the entry. The reason for the omission may be doc-

(text continues on page 710)

PATIENT TEACHING ABOUT TAKING MEDICATIONS

Teach the patient and family to do the following:

- Inform your physician of all the other drugs that are currently prescribed or being taken.
- Have prescriptions filled at the same pharmacy all the time so that the pharmacist can advise on any potential drug interactions.
- Ask for a partial-fill of a newly prescribed drug. This provides an opportunity to evaluate the drug's effect and potential for side effects before purchasing the full amount.
- Read and follow label directions carefully.
- Take prescription medication for the full time that it has been prescribed.
- Check with your physician before combining nonprescription drugs with those that have been prescribed.
- Dispose of old prescription drugs and outdated over-the-counter medications because they tend to disintegrate or change in potency.
- Consult with your physician if a prescribed drug does not relieve your symptoms or causes additional discomfort.
- Ask your physician or pharmacist if it is appropriate to take specific medications with food or on an empty stomach.
- Drink a liberal amount of water or other fluids each day so that drugs can be absorbed and eliminated appropriately.

- Refrain from taking prescription drugs that have been prescribed for someone else, even if your symptoms are similar.
- Wear a Medic-Alert tag if prescription drugs are taken on a regular and long-term basis.
- Use a pill organizer if it is difficult to remember when, or if, medications are taken.

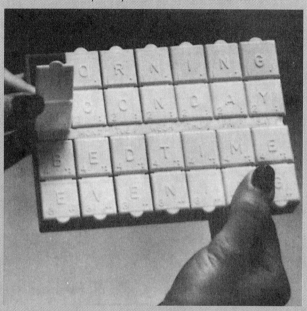

A pill organizer. (Courtesy of Apex Medical Corporation, Bloomington, MN.)

SKILL 32-2
Administering Medications Through an Enteral Tube

Suggested Action	Reason for Action
Assessment	
Check the medication administration record (MAR) and compare the information with the written medical order.	Prevents medication errors
Review the patient's drug, allergy, and medical history.	Avoids potential complications
Consult a current drug reference concerning the drug's action, side effects, contraindications, and administration information.	Ensures appropriate administration
Verify the location of the tube by auscultating instilled air or aspirating secretions.	Ensures airway protection
Compare the length of the external tube with its measurement at the time of insertion.	Determines if the tube has migrated
Inspect the patient's mouth and throat.	Determines if the tube has been displaced and coiled at the back of the throat

(continued)

SKILL 32-2
Administering Medications Through an Enteral Tube

Suggested Action	Reason for Action
Planning	
Plan to administer medications within a half-hour to an hour of the time they are scheduled.	Demonstrates timely administration and compliance with the medical order
Separate and clamp a gastric tube for 15 to 30 minutes if the drug will interact with food.	Ensures that the stomach will be relatively empty.
Allow sufficient time to prepare the medications in a location where there are minimal distractions.	Promotes safe preparation of drugs
Make sure that there is a sufficient supply of plastic medication cups.	Facilitates organization and efficient time management
Implementation	
Wash your hands.	Removes colonizing microorganisms
Read and compare the label on the drug with the MAR at least three times—before, during, and after preparing the drug	Ensures that the *right drug* is given at the *right time* by the *right route*
Prepare each drug separately.	Prevents potential physical changes when some drugs are combined
Take the cups containing diluted medications to the bedside with water for flushing, a 30- to 50-mL syringe, a towel or disposable pad, and clean gloves.	Facilitates instillation
Identify the patient by checking the wristband or asking the patient's name.	Ensures that medications are given to the *right patient*
Help the patient into a Fowler's position.	Prevents gastric reflux
Don clean gloves.	Prevents contact with body fluids
Insert the syringe into the tube and instill 15 to 30 mL of water by gravity.	Flushes the tube and reduces the surface tension of the tube
Add the diluted medication to the syringe as it becomes nearly empty.	Prevents instilling air
Apply gentle pressure with the plunger or bulb of a syringe if the medication fails to instill easily.	Provides positive pressure

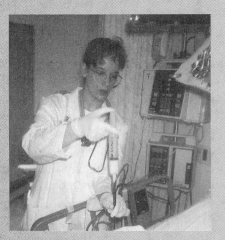

Instilling medication. (Courtesy of Ken Timby.)

(continued)

SKILL 32-2
Administering Medications Through an Enteral Tube (Continued)

Suggested Action	Reason for Action
Flush with at least 5 mL of water between each instillation of medication and as much as 30 mL after all the medications have been instilled.	Prevents drug interactions and obstruction of the tube; fully instills all of the prescribed drug
Pinch the tube as the syringe empties.	Prevents distending the abdomen with air; maintains patency of the tube
Clamp or plug the tube for 30 minutes before reconnecting a tube to suction.	Prevents removing the medication after it has been instilled

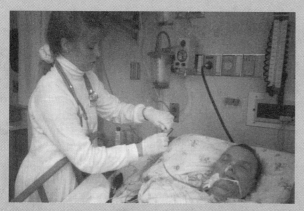

Plugging a gastric tube. (Courtesy of Ken Timby.)

Connect a tube used for nourishment immediately if the medication and formula will not interact.	Facilitates the primary purpose of the enteral tube
Keep the head of the bed elevated for at least 30 minutes.	Reduces the potential for aspiration

Evaluation
- Tube placement is verified
- The five rights are upheld
- Medications instill freely and are flushed afterward
- No abdominal distention, nausea, vomiting, or other undesirable effects occur
- Tube remains patent

Document
- Preadministration assessment data
- Medication administration on the MAR
- Volume of fluid instilled with the medication as well as for flushing the tube on the bedside intake and output record
- Response of the patient

Sample Documentation

Date and Time   Placement of NG tube verified by auscultation. No evidence of tube migration. Medications administered (see MAR) per NG tube. Flushed with 30 mL after instilling medications. Tube clamped at this time. No evidence of nausea or distention.

_____ **Signature, Title**

FOCUS ON OLDER ADULTS

- Older adults often are victims of polypharmacy. **Polypharmacy** is the administration of multiple drugs, which often interact and may cause more harm than good.
- Because older adults have age-related changes in their organs of digestion, metabolism, and elimination, they are observed closely for adverse and toxic reactions to medications.
- Stroke patients generally have an impaired ability to swallow. Administering oral medications can be facilitated by mixing the drug with a small amount of soft food rather than giving it as a liquid.
- A second responsible person is included in the discharge instructions regarding medications if an older adult cannot be relied on to comprehend the information or assume unsupervised responsibility for their administration.
- To ensure the best conditions for teaching, older patients are provided with their glasses or hearing aids before beginning instructions. Written instructions should be printed in large letters.
- After providing instructions on medications, it is best to have patients repeat the information to evaluate their comprehension.
- It may be more economic for some older adults with group prescription plans to have their prescriptions filled with a 3-month supply.
- Suggest that older adults discuss whether they can obtain generic forms of their prescribed drugs as a cost-saving measure.
- Older adults who are weak or suffer from arthritis of the hands are told that they may request caps on prescription medications that are easily removed, rather than those that are childproof.
- Older adults who are visually impaired may benefit from suggestions on how to identify bottles other than by their labels. Some suggestions include using rubber bands on the outside of the container or putting each medication container in a different place.
- Hearing-impaired adults are given written instructions for the self-administration of their medications.

APPLICABLE NURSING DIAGNOSES

- Knowledge Deficit
- Risk for Aspiration
- Ineffective Management of Therapeutic Regimen
- Altered Health Maintenance
- Noncompliance

umented in a comment section on the MAR or elsewhere in the patient's medical record.

MEDICATION ERRORS

Medication errors do happen. When they do, nurses have an ethical responsibility to report them so that the patient's safety is maintained.

As soon as an error is recognized, the patient's condition is checked and the mistake is reported to the physician and the supervising nurse immediately. Health care agencies have a special form for reporting medication errors, called an incident sheet or accident sheet (see Chap. 3). The incident sheet is not a part of the patient's permanent record, nor is any reference made in the chart to the fact that an incident sheet has been compiled.

NURSING IMPLICATIONS

Whenever nursing care involves the administration of medications, it is likely that one or more of the accompanying Applicable Nursing Diagnoses may be made.

The accompanying Nursing Care Plan reflects how the steps in the nursing process have been followed to manage the care of a patient with the diagnosis of Noncompliance. Noncompliance is defined in the NANDA taxonomy (1994) as "A person's informed decision not to adhere to a therapeutic recommendation."

KEY CONCEPTS

- A medication is any chemical substance that changes body function.
- A complete drug order contains the date and time of the order, the name of the patient, the name of the drug, its dose, route, and frequency of administration, and the signature or name of the writer.
- A drug's trade name is the name used by the pharmaceutical company for the drug it sells. The drug's generic name is a chemical name that is not protected by a company's trademark.

NURSING CARE PLAN:
Noncompliance

Assessment	**Subjective Data**
	States, "I didn't get my prescription refilled. I wasn't having any chest pain and I didn't think I needed to take my pills anymore. I figured the surgery fixed my heart."
	Objective Data
	63-year-old man admitted for chest pain and dyspnea. Lives with widowed sister who remains employed. Was discharged 6 weeks ago after coronary bypass surgery. Was to continue taking a beta-blocker (Tenormin 50 mg PO daily) and a diuretic (Lasix 20 mg PO q.o.d.). Abruptly stopped taking both medications 1 week ago. Pulse rate is presently 94 at rest and BP is 178/94 in R. arm while sitting.
Diagnosis	Noncompliance related to inaccurate health belief.
Plan	**Goal**
	The patient will explain the consequences that can occur if medications are not taken by 3/7.

Orders: 3/5
1. Explain the following at separate times during the next two days:
   - The purpose for reducing myocardial oxygen consumption
   - The benefit for lowering blood pressure
   - The advantage of reducing blood volume
   - The therapeutic actions of Tenormin and Lasix
2. Have patient repeat explanations and note his level of understanding; clarify any misunderstanding immediately.
3. Go over schedule of medication administration on 3/7 with patient and again with patient and his sister before discharge.
4. Advise the patient to discuss any deviations in medication schedule or dosage with his physician. _____ M. MOHNEY, RN

Implementation 3/5   0930   Chest pain relieved by sublingual nitroglycerin administered 30 minutes
(Documentation) earlier. Has voided 700 mL of urine in past hour after IV Lasix. Resting comfortably. Pulse =90 bpm, BP 156/90 R. arm in semi-Fowler's position. _____ B. VIANNY, LPN

1000   Explained that the nitroglycerin dilates blood vessels and eases the work of the heart. Used the analogy of blowing air through a very narrow straw vs. a very wide one. Informed that one of the actions of Tenormin is to reduce blood pressure and therefore reduce the work of the heart and its need for oxygen. _____ B. VIANNY, LPN

Evaluation 1015   Could paraphrase explanation correctly. States, "I know people take nitro-
(Documentation) glycerin for chest pain, but I didn't know how it helped relieve it. I'd rather take a pill once a day and prevent chest pain than have to take a pill to get rid of it." _____ B. VIANNY, LPN

- Common routes for medication administration include the oral, topical, inhalant, and parenteral routes.
- The oral route is used to administer drugs that are intended for absorption in the gastrointestinal tract. Oral medications can be instilled by enteral tube when they cannot be swallowed.
- A medication administration record (MAR) is a form used to document drug administration so as to ensure timely and safe administration.
- Drugs are dispensed to nursing units in the forms of an individual supply, a supply of unit dose packets, and a stock supply.

- With regard to narcotic medications, nurses are responsible for keeping the supply locked and maintaining an accurate record of their use.
- The five rights refer to making sure that the right patient receives the right drug, in the right dose, at the right time, and by the right route.
- Once drug doses are converted to the same system of measurement and the same measurement within that system, the amount that is to be administered can be calculated by dividing the desired dose by the dose on hand and then multiplying it by the quantity of the supply.
- One important guideline for the safe preparation of medications is to check the drug label three times before administering the medication.
- One point to stress when teaching patients about taking medications is to inform each physician of other prescribed and nonprescribed drugs that are currently being taken.
- A common problem when administering drugs through an enteral tube is maintaining the tube's patency.
- If a medication error occurs, nurses have an obligation to report the error to the physician and supervisor, check the patient, and document the situation on an incident or accident sheet.
- Because older adults have age-related changes in their organs of digestion, metabolism, and elimination, they are observed closely for adverse and toxic reactions to medications.

CRITICAL THINKING EXERCISES

- While you are administering medications to a patient, the patient says, "I've never taken that little yellow pill before." What action(s) would be appropriate to take next?

- A patient who lives alone says, "You have to be a genius to keep all these pills straight." How could you help this patient organize this aspect of taking medications?

SUGGESTED READINGS

Calculating drug dosages: self-test. Nursing February 1993;23:87, 89–90.

Carson W. Gains and challenges in prescriptive authority. American Nurse June 1993;25:19–20.

Cohen MR. 12 ways to prevent medication errors. Nursing February 1994;24:3–9, 41–42.

Cohen MR. Help new nurses avoid making errors. Nursing April 1992;22:21.

Cohen MR. Medication errors: don't let doctors intimidate you. January 1992;22:18.

Cornish JL. Color coding patient medications. Caring November 1992;11:46–48, 51.

Drake AC, Romano E. How to protect your older patient from the hazards of polypharmacy. Nursing June 1995;25:34–39.

Hicks W. Taking the right approach to a drug error . . . what to do when an error occurs—how to avoid making another one. Nursing March 1995;25:72.

Kluckowski JC. Solving medication noncompliance in home care. Caring November 1992;11:34–41.

Lehmann S, Barber JR. Giving medications by feeding tube: how to avoid problems. Nursing November 1991;21:58–61.

Long T. Pointing out medication errors. American Journal of Nursing February 1992;92:76, 78.

Masson V. Prescriptive ambivalence. American Journal of Nursing February 1993;93:14.

McKenney JM, Dorn MR, DeSalvo AF. Helping the noncompliant, forgetful patient: a case history. Home Healthcare Nurse January–February 1992;10:43–45.

Merkatz R, Couig MP. Helping America take its medicine . . . educating patients about medicines. American Journal of Nursing June 1992;92:56, 59–60, 62.

Teplitsky B. Avoiding the hazards of look-alike drug names. Nursing January 1992;22:60–61.

CHAPTER 33

Topical and Inhalant Medications

Chapter Outline

Topical Route
Inhalant Route
Nursing Implications
Key Concepts
Critical Thinking Exercises
Suggested Readings

 NURSING GUIDELINES

Applying an Inunction
Applying Nitroglycerin Paste

 SKILLS

Instilling Eye Medications
Administering Nasal Medications

 NURSING CARE PLAN

Risk for Impaired Gas Exchange

Key Terms

Aerosol	Ophthalmic Application
Buccal Application	Otic Application
Cutaneous Application	Paste
Inhalant Route	Rebound Effect
Inhalers	Skin Patches
Inunction	Spacer
Metered Dose Inhaler	Sublingual

Topical Route	Transdermal Application
Turbo-inhaler	Vehicle

Learning Objectives

An understanding of the content within this chapter will be evidenced by the student's ability to:

- Explain how topical medications are administered
- Give at least five examples of where topical medications are commonly applied
- Describe an inunction and give three examples
- Name two forms of drugs that are used when applying medications by the transdermal route
- Discuss at least two principles that are followed when applying a skin patch
- Describe where eye medications are applied
- Explain how the administration of ear medications differs for adults compared to young children
- Explain the rebound effect as it applies to the administration of nasal decongestants
- Describe the difference between a sublingual and buccal administration
- Explain why inhalation provides a good route for medication administration
- Describe the mechanism for creating an aerosol
- Name two types of inhalers and describe the manner in which each is used to administer medication
- Name a device that can potentiate the effect of an inhaled medication

Drugs may be administered by other than the oral route. This chapter describes the unique techniques that apply to the administration of drugs by the topical and inhalant routes.

TABLE 33-1. Common Routes of Topical Administration		
Routes	Location	Vehicles
Cutaneous	To the skin	Ointment Cream Lotion Patch Paste
Sublingual	Under the tongue	Tablet Sprays
Buccal	Between the cheek and gum	Lozenge
Vaginal	Within the vagina	Douche Suppository
Rectal	Within the rectum	Irrigation Suppository
Otic	Within the ear	Drops Irrigation
Ophthalmic	Within the eye	Drops Ointment
Nasal	Within the nose	Spray Ointment

TOPICAL ROUTE

The **topical route** refers to a method of drug administration in which medications are applied to the skin or mucous membranes. Drugs administered topically may be applied externally or internally (Table 33-1). Topically applied drugs may have a local or systemic effect; however, many are administered to achieve a direct effect on the tissue to which they are applied.

Cutaneous Applications

Cutaneous applications are those in which drugs are rubbed into or placed in contact with the skin. Inunctions, pastes, and patches are examples of cutaneously applied drugs.

APPLYING AN INUNCTION

An **inunction** is a medication that is incorporated into a **vehicle**, or transporting agent, like ointment, oil, lotion, or cream. Inunctions are administered by rubbing the vehicle into the skin.

It may be acceptable for alert patients to self-administer an inunction after they have been instructed. The nurse's role, then, becomes one of teaching proper application techniques and checking that the medication has been applied appropriately as often as it has been prescribed. For patients who are unable to assume responsibility for their own skin applications, the nurse may be required to do so.

NURSING GUIDELINES FOR APPLYING AN INUNCTION

- Wash your hands.
  Rationale: Removes colonizing microorganisms
- Check the identity of the patient.
  Rationale: Prevents administering medication to the wrong patient
- Don clean gloves if your skin or that of the patient is not intact.
  Rationale: Provides a barrier to pathogens
- Cleanse the area of application with soap and water.
  Rationale: Promotes absorption
- Warm the inunction, if it will be applied to a sensitive area of skin, by holding it temporarily within your hands or placing its sealed container in warm water.
  Rationale: Promotes comfort
- Shake the contents of liquid inunctions.
  Rationale: Mixes the contents uniformly
- Apply the inunction to the skin with the fingertips, a cotton ball, or gauze square.
  Rationale: Provides a means of distributing the application over a wide area
- Rub the inunction into the skin.
  Rationale: Promotes absorption
- Apply local heat to the area if desired (see Chap. 28).
  Rationale: Dilates peripheral blood vessels and speeds absorption

TRANSDERMAL APPLICATIONS

A **transdermal application** is a method of applying a drug on the skin and allowing it to become passively absorbed. Drugs incorporated into patches or paste are administered in this manner. After the application, the drug migrates through the skin and is eventually absorbed into the bloodstream.

Skin Patches

Skin patches contain drugs that are bonded to an adhesive bandage (Fig. 33-1). Several drugs are now prepared for transdermal applications, including nitroglycerin, a medication used to dilate the coronary arteries; scopolamine, a drug that is used to relieve motion sickness; and estrogen, a hormone used to treat menopausal symptoms.

Skin patches can be applied to any skin area where there is adequate circulation. Most patches are applied to the upper body in places like the chest, shoulders,

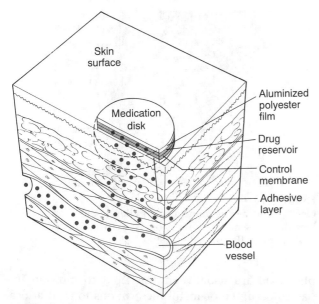

FIGURE 33-1
Pathway for absorption from a transdermal skin patch.

and upper arms (Fig. 33-2). Small patches can be applied behind the ear. Each time a new patch is applied, it is placed in a slightly different location. It may help adhesion to clip extremely hairy skin areas.

After the patch is applied, it may take approximately 30 minutes for the drug to reach a therapeutic level. Thereafter, however, the patch provides a continuous supply of medication. In fact, the drug may still be active for up to 30 minutes after the patch is removed. It is always best to date and initial a patch so that others can determine when it was applied.

Drug Paste

A **paste** is a vehicle that contains a drug within a viscous (thick) base. A paste is applied to the skin, but it is not rubbed into it. Nitroglycerin is a drug that can be applied as a paste. Although sometimes the product is referred to as an ointment, the term is actually a misnomer because the skin is not massaged once the drug

is applied. Although nitroglycerin paste is prepared by several pharmaceutical companies, the technique for its application is similar.

◄ NURSING GUIDELINES FOR APPLYING NITROGLYCERIN PASTE

- Wash your hands.
  Rationale: Removes colonizing microorganisms
- Check the identity of the patient.
  Rationale: Prevents administering medication to the wrong patient
- Squeeze a ribbon of paste (ointment) from the tube onto an application paper (Fig. 33-3).
  Rationale: Complies with the medication order, which usually specifies the dose in inches
- Fold the paper or use a wooden applicator to spread the paste over approximately a $2\frac{1}{4} \times 3\frac{1}{2}$-inch (5.6 × 8.8-cm) area of the paper.
  Rationale: Facilitates distributing the drug over a wider area for quicker absorption
- Take care not to touch the paste with your bare fingers.
  Rationale: Prevents potential self-administration of the drug
- Place the application paper on a clean, nonhairy area of skin.
  Rationale: Facilitates drug absorption
- Cover the paper with a square of plastic kitchen wrap or tape all the edges of the paper to the skin.
  Rationale: Seals the drug between the paper and the skin
- Remove one application before applying another and remove any residue remaining on the skin.
  Rationale: Prevents excessive drug levels
- Rotate the sites where the medication is placed.
  Rationale: Reduces the potential for skin irritation.

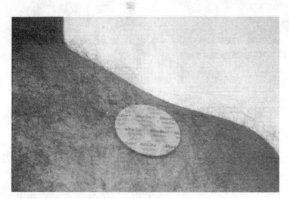

FIGURE 33-2
Transdermal skin patch. (Courtesy of Ken Timby.)

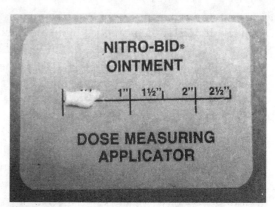

FIGURE 33-3
Paste and applicator paper. (Courtesy of Ken Timby.)

Ophthalmic Applications

An **ophthalmic application** is a method of applying drugs onto the mucous membrane of one or both eyes (Skill 33-1). The mucous membrane of the eyes is called the *conjunctiva*. It lines the inner eyelids and anterior surface of the *sclera* (Fig. 33-4).

Ophthalmic medications are usually supplied in liquid form and instilled as drops, or as ointments that are applied along the lower lid margin. Blinking, rather than rubbing, distributes the drug over the surface of the eye.

The eye is a delicate structure, and it is susceptible to infection and injury just like any other tissue. Therefore, care is taken to keep the applicator tip of the medication container sterile. As long as the tissue of the eye is intact, medications can be instilled without the use of gloves. There have been no reported cases of human immunodeficiency virus being transmitted through conjunctival secretions, even when patients are known to have AIDS.

Otic Applications

An **otic application** is one in which a drug is instilled within the outer, external portion of the ear. Otic ap-

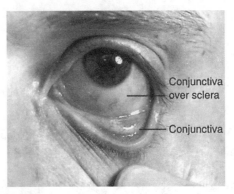

FIGURE 33-4
Ophthalmic application sites. (Fuller J, Schuller-Ayers J: Health Assessment: A Nursing Approach, 2nd ed, p 320. Philadelphia, JB Lippincott, 1994)

plications are usually administered to moisten impacted cerumen or instill medications to treat a local bacterial or fungal infection.

When ear medication is instilled, the ear is first manipulated to straighten the auditory canal. The technique varies depending on whether the patient is a young child or adult (see Chap. 12).

With the head tilted away from the nurse, the prescribed number of drops of medication are instilled

SKILL 33-1
Instilling Eye Medications

Suggested Action	Reason for Action
Assessment	
Compare the medication administration record (MAR) with the written medical order.	Prevents medication errors
Review the patient's drug, allergy, and medical history.	Avoids potential complications
Consult a current drug reference concerning the drug's action, side effects, contraindications, and administration information.	Ensures appropriate administration
Planning	
Plan to administer medications within a half-hour to an hour of the time they are scheduled.	Demonstrates timely administration and compliance with the medical order
Allow sufficient time to prepare the medications in a location where there are minimal distractions.	Promotes safe preparation of drugs
Warm eye drops and ointments by holding them between the hands if they have not been stored at room temperature.	Promotes comfort
Read and compare the label on the drug with the MAR at least three times—before, during, and after preparing the drug.	Ensures that the *right drug* is given at the *right time* by the *right route*

(continued)

SKILL 33-1
Instilling Eye Medications *(Continued)*

Suggested Action	Reason for Action
Implementation	
Wash your hands.	Removes colonizing microorganisms
Identify the patient by checking the wristband or asking the patient's name.	Ensures that medications are given to the *right patient*
Position the patient supine or sitting with the head tilted back and slightly to the side into which the medication will be instilled.	Prevents passage of the drug into the naso-lacrimal duct or from being blinked onto the cheek
Clean the lids and lashes if they contain debris. Use a cotton ball or tissue that has been moistened with water.	Promotes comfort and maximizes the potential for absorption
Wipe the eye from the corner by the nose, called the *inner canthus*, toward the *outer canthus*, the corner of the eye near the temple.	Moves debris away from the nasolacrimal duct
Instruct the patient to look toward the ceiling.	Prevents looking directly at the applicator, which usually causes a blinking reflex as it comes close to the eye
Make a pouch in the lower lid by pulling the skin over the bony orbit downward.	Provides a natural reservoir for depositing liquid medication

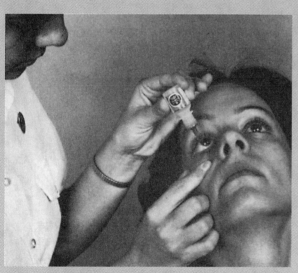

Instilling eyedrops.

Suggested Action	Reason for Action
Move the container of medication from below the patient's line of vision or from the side of the eye.	Prevents a blink reflex
Steady the container above the location for instillation without touching the surface of the eye.	Prevents injury
Instill the prescribed number of drops into the appropriate eye within the conjunctival pouch.	Complies with the medical order by administering the *right dose*

(continued)

SKILL 33-1
Instilling Eye Medications (Continued)

Suggested Action	Reason for Action
If ointment is used, squeeze a ribbon onto the lower lid margin.	Applies the ointment to the conjunctiva

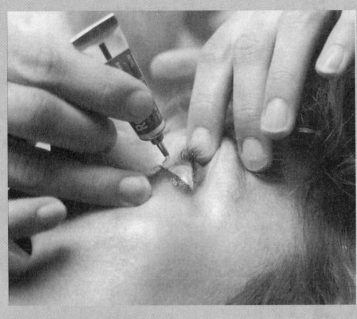

Instilling eye ointment. (Scherer JC, Timby BK: Introductory Medical-Surgical Nursing, 6th ed, p 621. Philadelphia, JB Lippincott, 1995)

Instruct the patient to close the eyelids gently and then blink several times.	Distributes the drug
Wipe the eyes with a clean tissue.	Removes excess drug and promotes comfort

Evaluation
- The five rights are upheld
- The tip of the container remains uncontaminated
- Sufficient drug is distributed within the eye

Document
- Assessment data
- Medication administration on the MAR

Sample Documentation

Date and Time	Prescribed eye medication instilled into L. eye before cataract surgery (see MAR). Conjunctiva appears pink and intact. Lens is opaque. Eyelashes have been clipped.
	_____ **Signature, Title**

within the ear. The patient remains in this position briefly as the solution travels toward the eardrum. A small cotton ball can be placed *loosely* in the ear to absorb excess medication. It is appropriate to wait at least 15 minutes if medication must be instilled in the opposite ear.

Nasal Applications

Topical medications may be dropped or sprayed within the nose (Skill 33-2). Proper instillation is important to avoid displacing the medication into nearby structures like the back of the throat. Adults often self-administer their own nasal medications, but sometimes nurses must assist older adults and very young children.

Patients who purchase over-the-counter decongestant nasal sprays are warned that if used too frequently, or if more than the recommended amount is administered, the nasal mucosa may swell within a short time of administration, a phenomenon referred to as a **rebound effect**. Rebound effect can be avoided by following labeled directions or by using nasal sprays containing just normal saline solution.

Sublingual and Buccal Applications

The term **sublingual** literally translates as "under the tongue," which is exactly where a sublingual application is placed. The tablet is left to dissolve slowly and become absorbed by the rich blood supply within the area. Some drugs in spray or liquid form may also be administered sublingually.

A **buccal application** is one in which a drug is placed against the mucous membranes of the inner cheek. When buccal or sublingual administrations are given, patients are instructed not to chew or swallow the medication. Eating and smoking are also con-

traindicated during the brief time that it takes for the medication to dissolve.

Vaginal Applications

Topical vaginal applications are most often used to treat local infections. Vaginal infections are fairly common. They are usually the result of colonization of the vaginal tissue by microorganisms, like yeasts, that are abundant in the stool. The microorganisms usually become transferred at the time of bowel elimination if the rectal area is not wiped away from the vagina.

The Food and Drug Administration has lifted the prescription requirement on several drugs that are useful in the treatment of vaginal yeast infections. When women recognize the symptoms of a yeast infection, such as intense vaginal itching and white, cheese-like vaginal discharge, they can purchase appropriate over-the-counter drugs in suppository, tablet, or cream form. Early and appropriate self-treatment restores the normal integrity to the tissue.

It may be helpful to provide patients with instructions on how to administer vaginal medications for their most effective action.

SKILL 33-2
Administering Nasal Medications

Suggested Action	Reason for Action
Assessment	
Compare the medication administration record (MAR) with the written medical order.	Prevents medication errors
Review the patient's drug, allergy, and medical history.	Avoids potential complications
Consult a current drug reference concerning the drug's action, side effects, contraindications, and administration information.	Ensures appropriate administration
Planning	
Plan to administer medications within a half-hour to an hour of the time they are scheduled.	Demonstrates timely administration and compliance with the medical order
Allow sufficient time to prepare the medications in a location where there are minimal distractions.	Promotes safe preparation of drugs
Read and compare the label on the drug with the MAR at least three times—before, during, and after preparing the drug.	Ensures that the *right drug* is given at the *right time* by the *right route*

(continued)

SKILL 33-2
Administering Nasal Medications (Continued)

Suggested Action	Reason for Action
Implementation	
Wash your hands.	Removes colonizing microorganisms
Identify the patient by checking the wristband or asking the patient's name.	Ensures that medications are given to the *right patient*
Help the patient to a sitting position with his or her head tilted backward, or to the side if the drug needs to reach one or the other sinuses.	Facilitates depositing the drug where its effect is desired
If the patient cannot sit, place a rolled towel or pillow beneath the neck.	Provides support and aids in positioning
Remove the cap from liquid medication, to which a dropper is usually attached.	Provides a means for administering the drug
Aim the tip of the dropper toward the nasal passage and squeeze the rubber portion of the cap to administer the number of drops prescribed.	Deposits the drug within the nose rather than into the throat and ensures administering the *right dose*

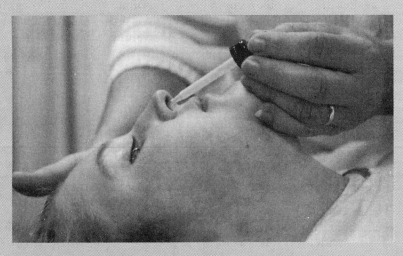

Instilling nasal medication. (Courtesy of Ken Timby.)

Suggested Action	Reason for Action
Instruct the patient to breathe through the mouth as the drops are instilled.	Prevents inhaling large droplets
If the drug is in a spray form, place the tip of the container just inside the nostril.	Confines the spray within the nasal passage
Occlude the opposite nostril.	Administers medication to one and then the other nasal passage
Instruct the patient to inhale as the container is squeezed.	Distributes the aerosol
Repeat in the opposite nostril.	Deposits the drug bilaterally for maximum effect
Advise the patient to remain in position for approximately 5 minutes.	Promotes local absorption
Recap the container and replace where medications are stored.	Supports principles of asepsis and demonstrates responsibility for the patient's property

(continued)

SKILL 33-2
Administering Nasal Medications (Continued)

Suggested Action	Reason for Action
Evaluation • The five rights are upheld • Sufficient drug is distributed within the nose *Document* • Assessment data • Medication administration on the MAR *Sample Documentation* **Date and Time** Indicates nasal passages are congested. Observed to be breathing through the mouth. Nasal medication administered (see MAR). States symptoms are relieved. —————————————————————————— **Signature, Title**	

If the patient is not able to instill vaginal medication, the nurse always wears gloves to avoid contact with secretions. After the gloves are removed, conscientious handwashing is performed. The same advice holds true of rectal applications.

Rectal Applications

Drugs that are administered rectally are usually in the form of suppositories (see Chap. 31). However, creams and ointments may also be prescribed. Internal applications require the use of an applicator. The technique for using a rectal applicator is similar to that for using a vaginal applicator.

INHALANT ROUTE

The **inhalant route** is used for medication administration because the lungs provide an extensive area of tissue from which drugs may be absorbed quickly into the circulatory system. To distribute the medication to the distal areas of the airways, liquid medication is converted to an aerosol.

An **aerosol** is the mist that results after forcing a liquid drug through a narrow channel using pressurized air or an inert gas. The same principle is incorporated into cosmetic and household products like canisters of hairspray and furniture polish. A simple method of administering aerosolized medications is to use an inhaler.

Inhalers

Inhalers are hand-held devices for delivering medication into the respiratory passages. An inhaler consists of a canister, which holds medication, and a mouthpiece or nosepiece through which the aerosol is inhaled (Fig. 33-5).

There are two types of inhalers, those that deliver a metered dose and those referred to as turbo-inhalers. A **turbo-inhaler** contains an internal propeller that spins and suspends a finely powdered medication. The propellers are activated during a patient's inhalation. Because turbo-inhalers are much less common, a metered dose inhaler is used for the purposes of discussion.

METERED DOSE INHALERS

A **metered dose inhaler** (Fig. 33-6) contains medication under pressure. Each time the container is com-

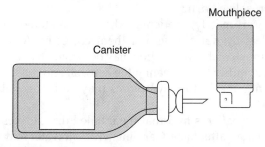

FIGURE 33-5
Parts of an inhaler.

PATIENT TEACHING FOR ADMINISTERING MEDICATIONS VAGINALLY

Tell the patient to do the following:
- Obtain a form of medication that is to your personal preference; all come with a vaginal applicator.

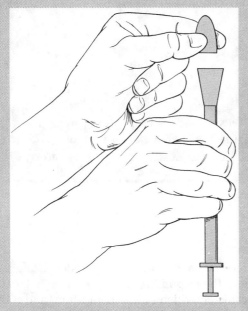

Example of a vaginal applicator.

- Plan to instill the medication before retiring for sleep to facilitate retention of the medication for a prolonged period of time.
- Empty your bladder just before inserting the medication.
- Place the drug within the applicator.
- Lubricate the applicator tip with a water-soluble lubricant like K-Y Jelly.
- Lie down, bend your knees, and spread your legs.

- Separate the labia and insert the applicator within the vagina to the length recommended in the package directions, which is usually 2 to 4 inches (5–10 cm).

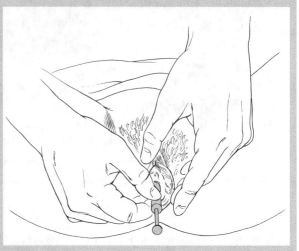

Vaginal insertion.

- Depress the plunger to insert the medication.
- Remove the applicator and place it on a clean tissue; discard the applicator if it is disposable.
- Apply a sanitary pad if you prefer.
- Remain recumbent for at least 10 to 30 minutes.
- Wash a reusable applicator when handwashing and hygiene are performed.
- Consult a physician if, after following the package directions, symptoms continue to persist.

---

pressed, it releases a measured volume (metered dose) of aerosolized drug.

Unfortunately, patients who use metered dose inhalers do not always use them correctly. As a result, much of the medication may be wasted from swallowing rather than inhaling the aerosol, and the patient's respiratory symptoms may be inadequately relieved.

Some patients find that the inhaled drug leaves an unpleasant after taste. Gargling with salt water may diminish this undesirable effect. The mouthpiece of an inhaler may also accumulate drug residue. Conse-

quently, it is best to rinse the mouthpiece in warm water after it is used.

Even with instruction, some patients continue to have problems coordinating their breathing so as to receive the full dose of aerosol. In situations like this, a spacer may be used.

Spacers

A **spacer** is a holding chamber that is attached to an inhaler. (Fig. 33-7) It provides a reservoir for the aerosol medication. Consequently, as patients take additional

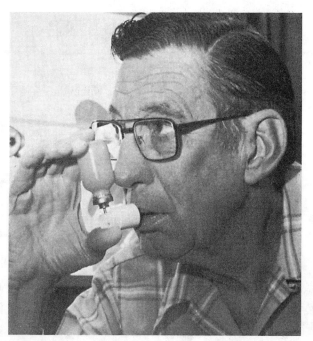

FIGURE 33-6
Metered dose inhaler.

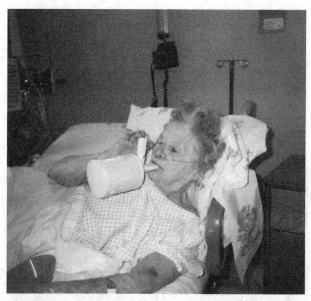

FIGURE 33-7
A spacer and inhaler. (Courtesy of Ken Timby.)

breaths, they continue to inhale medication held within the reservoir. This tends to maximize drug absorption because it prevents drug loss . Some patients also find that by prolonging the time over which the drug is inhaled, undesirable side effects, like a burst of tachycardia or tremulousness, are reduced.

 PATIENT TEACHING FOR USING A METERED DOSE INHALER

Teach the patient to do the following:
- Attach the stem of the canister into the hole of the mouthpiece so that the inhaler looks like an "L."
- Shake the canister to distribute the drug within its pressurized chamber.
- Exhale slowly through pursed lips (see Chap. 20).
- Seal your lips around the mouthpiece.
- Compress the canister between your thumb and fingers and slowly inhale at the same time.
- Release the pressure on the canister, but continue inhaling as much as possible.
- Withdraw the mouthpiece.
- Hold your breath for a few seconds.
- Exhale slowly, again through pursed lips.

NURSING IMPLICATIONS

When administering topical or inhalant drugs, nursing management often involves assessing and maintaining the integrity of the skin and mucous membranes. It may also require attention to health teaching to prevent the consequences of improper self-administration. Therefore, nursing diagnoses may include those listed in the accompanying Applicable Nursing Diagnoses.

The Nursing Care Plan for this chapter demonstrates the use of the steps of the nursing process in managing the care of a patient with the diagnosis of Risk for Impaired Gas Exchange. Impaired Gas Exchange, according to the NANDA taxonomy (1994), is "The state in which an individual's inhalation and/or exhalation pattern does not enable adequate pulmonary inflation or emptying."

 APPLICABLE NURSING DIAGNOSES

- Knowledge Deficit
- Ineffective Management of Therapeutic Regimen
- Impaired Gas Exchange
- Impaired Skin Integrity
- Impaired Tissue Integrity

✳ **FOCUS ON OLDER ADULTS**

- Some older adults have difficulty instilling eye medications independently. There are other devices that may be used if another person is unavailable. For example, one type of medication used to treat glaucoma is inserted inside the lower eyelid. It releases medication for 7 days before it needs to be replaced.
- Some older adults may take two or more types of eye medications each day. Unfortunately, most eye medications come packaged in containers that look quite similar. Older adults may benefit from suggestions on how to distinguish one container from another because vision problems may interfere with reading the small print on each container's label.
- The onset of drug action may be atypical when topical medications are administered to older adults because they tend to have less subcutaneous fat. The lack of subcutaneous fat may cause the topical medication to be absorbed more rapidly than in a younger person.
- Older adults may have difficulty reaching areas of the body to which some topical drugs are applied. For example, arthritis may interfere with applying medications within the vagina or rectum, or to skin lesions on the lower extremities.
- The mechanics of inhaling and compressing the inhaler at the same time may be awkward for some older adults. Spacer devices may compensate for less-than-optimum administration techniques.
- Sometimes two inhalers containing different drugs may be prescribed. During health teaching, it is important to stress how and when each is used.
- Patients who self-administer topical and inhalant drugs are instructed on the name of the drug, dosage, how the drug is to be administered, and its desired and undesired effects.
- It is important to monitor the heart rate and blood pressure of older adults who use inhalers containing bronchodilating drugs. These types of medications often cause tachycardia and hypertension. Either or both may increase risks for complications among those who may also have cardiovascular diseases.

KEY CONCEPTS

- Topical medications are applied to the skin or mucous membranes.
- Common locations where topical medications are applied include the skin, eye, ear, nose, vagina, rectum, and mouth.
- An inunction is a medication that is incorporated into a vehicle, or transporting agent, like ointment, oil, lotion, or cream.
- Skin patches and applications of paste are two methods for administering medications by the transdermal route.
- Skin patches can be applied to any skin area where there is adequate circulation, and each time a new patch is applied, it is placed in a slightly different location.
- Eye medications are applied onto the mucous membrane, or conjunctiva, of the eye, which lines the inner eyelids and anterior surface of the sclera.
- The manner in which the ear is manipulated to straighten the auditory canal is the major difference in the technique for administering ear medications to adults and younger children.
- The rebound effect is a phenomenon characterized by rapid swelling of the nasal mucosa. It is more apt to occur when more than the recommended amount of nasal decongestant is chronically administered, or if it is administered too frequently.
- When administering medication sublingually, the drug is placed under the tongue. For buccal administration, the medication is placed in contact with the mucous membrane of the cheek.
- The inhalant route is used for medication administration because the lungs provide an extensive area of tissue from which drugs may be absorbed.
- To create an aerosol, liquid medication is forced through a narrow channel under high pressure.
- Drug are commonly inhaled with turbo-inhalers or metered dose inhalers. A turbo-inhaler delivers a burst of fine powder at the time of inhalation. A metered dose inhaler releases a measured volume of aerosolized drug when its canister is compressed.
- A spacer provides a reservoir for aerosol medication, which can then be inhaled beyond the time of the first initial breath.

NURSING CARE PLAN:
Risk for Impaired Gas Exchange

Assessment

Subjective Data
States, "I have trouble breathing even though I use my inhaler when my chest starts getting tight."

Objective Data
Patient is a 56-year-old man who smoked two packs of cigarettes a day for the last 30 years. Chronic emphysema recently aggravated by pneumonia. Given a prescription two days ago for albuterol (Ventolin) to be administered by a metered dose inhaler. Appears to exhale quickly rather than retaining the inhaled aeosol for a brief time.

Diagnosis

Risk for Impaired Gas Exchange related to improper technique using metered dose inhaler.

Plan

Goal
The patient's ventilations will maintain an SaO_2 of no less than 90% with appropriate use of an inhaler.

Orders: 8/02
1. Redemonstrate the correct use of a metered dose inhaler.
2. Observe patient's technique at least four times after demonstration.
3. Monitor SaO_2 with pulse oximeter before and after use of metered dose inhaler.
   _____ D. FORTIS, RN

Implementation (Documentation)

8/02   1000   Short of breath. Sitting up to breathe. Lung sounds are diminished bilaterally. SaO_2 @ 88% per pulse oximeter. Shown how to use metered dose inhaler. Emphasized enclosing the mouthpiece within the lips. Coached to hold the inhaled breath for several seconds. _____ J. BENTHIN, LPN

Evaluation (Documentation)

1030   Observed to perform technique appropriately with each of two puffs from the inhaler. SaO_2 @ 90% within 15 minutes of using the inhaler.   J. BENTHIN, LPN

CRITICAL THINKING EXERCISES

- Before Mr. Rumsey, who has had a heart attack, is discharged, he says, "You nurses always put my nitroglycerin patches on my back. How can I do that when I have to do it myself?" How would you respond?
- How might you help Mrs. Fuller, who is legally blind and lives alone, identify two different containers of eye medication?

SUGGESTED READINGS

Cornish JL. Color coding patient medications. Caring November 1992;11:46–48, 51.

Kluckowski JC. Solving medication noncompliance in home care. Caring November 1992;11:34–41.

Lewis M. Aerosol medication administration. Emergency September 1992;24:18–22.

Marley R, Mullineaux T. Postoperative administration of aerosolized medications. Part II: the techniques. Journal of Post Anesthesia Nursing December 1994;9:360–370.

McKenney JM, Dorn MR, DeSalvo AF. Helping the noncompliant, forgetful patient: a case history. Home Healthcare Nurse January–February 1992;10:43–45.

Merkatz R, Couig MP. Helping America take its medicine . . . educating patients about medicines. American Journal of Nursing June 1992;92:56, 59–60, 62.

Using a metered-dose nebulizer correctly. Nursing February 1992; 22:18.

CHAPTER 34
Parenteral Medications

NURSING GUIDELINES

Withdrawing Medication From an Ampule
Withdrawing Medication From a Vial
Combining Insulins
Giving an Injection by Z-Track Technique

SKILLS

Administering Intradermal Injections
Administering Subcutaneous Injections
Administering Intramuscular Injections

NURSING CARE PLAN

Ineffective Management of Therapeutic Regimen

Key Terms

Ampule
Barrel
Deltoid Site
Diluent

Dorsogluteal Site
Gauge
Induration
Insulin Syringe

Learning Objectives

An understanding of the content within this chapter will be evidenced by the student's ability to:

- Name three parts of a syringe
- List five factors to consider when selecting a syringe and needle
- Explain why conventional syringes and needles are being redesigned
- Name three ways parenteral drugs are prepared by pharmaceutical companies
- Discuss an appropriate action to take before combining two drugs in a single syringe
- List four injection routes
- Identify one common injection site for an intradermal, subcutaneous, and intramuscular injection
- Name a type of syringe that is commonly used to administer an intradermal, subcutaneous, and intramuscular injection
- Describe the angle of entry for an intradermal, subcutaneous, and intramuscular injection
- Discuss why most insulin combinations must be administered within 15 minutes of being mixed
- Describe two techniques for preventing bruising when administering heparin subcutaneously

Timby BK: *Fundamental Skills and Concepts in Patient Care, Sixth Edition* © 1996 Lippincott-Raven Publishers

- Name five intramuscular injection sites and their general anatomic locations
- Explain two reasons for giving an intramuscular injection using the Z-track technique

This chapter discusses the techniques for administering injections. Injections are prepared and administered following principles of asepsis and infection control (see Chaps. 21 and 22).

PARENTERAL ROUTE

The term **parenteral** refers to all routes of drug administration other than oral. It is used most commonly, however, to indicate medications that are given by injection.

PARENTERAL ADMINISTRATION EQUIPMENT

Parenteral injections are administered with various types of syringes and needles.

Syringes

All syringes contain a **barrel**, which holds the medication, a **plunger**, which is used to withdraw and instill the medication, and a **tip** to which the needle is attached (Fig. 34-1). Syringes may be calibrated in milliliters (mL) or cubic centimeters (cc), units (U), and, in some cases, minims (m). When drugs are administered parenterally, syringes that hold 1 mL, or its equivalent in units, and up to 3- to 5-mL volumes are most commonly used.

Needles

Needles are supplied in various lengths and gauges. The length, or **shaft** of the needle, depends on the depth to which the medication will be instilled. Needle lengths vary from 0.5 to 2.5 inches. The tip of the shaft is beveled, or slanted, so as to pierce the skin more easily (see Chap. 15, Skill 15-3, Starting an Intravenous Infusion).

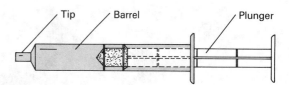

FIGURE 34-1
Parts of a syringe. (Earnest VV: Clinical Skills in Nursing, 2nd ed, p 862. Philadelphia, JB Lippincott, 1992)

The needle **gauge** refers to the diameter, or width, of the needle. For most injections, 18- to 27-gauge needles are used; the smaller the number, the larger the diameter. For example, an 18-gauge needle is wider than a 27-gauge needle. A wider diameter provides a larger lumen, or opening, through which drugs are administered into the tissue.

Several factors are considered when selecting an appropriate syringe and needle. They include:

- Type of medication
- Depth of tissue
- Volume of prescribed drug
- Viscosity of the drug
- Size of the patient

Table 34-1 identifies common sizes of syringes and needles used for various types of injections.

Modified Injection Equipment

Conventional syringes and needles are being redesigned to avoid needlestick injuries. The thrust for modifying traditionally used equipment is to reduce the potential risk for acquiring a blood-borne viral disease like hepatitis or AIDS.

Some health agencies are already using one or several types of modified equipment. Basically, these are blunt substitutes for needles that can pierce laser-cut rubber ports, and syringes with shields that allow for recessing the needle (Gurevich, 1994).

PREVENTING NEEDLESTICK INJURIES

If newer types of equipment are not available, there are two techniques that may be used for preventing needlestick injuries with standard equipment. Before administering an injection, the protective cap covering

TABLE 34-1. *Common Sizes of Syringes and Needles*

Type of Injection	Size of Syringe	Size of Needle
Subcutaneous	2, 2.5, or 3 mL calibrated in 0.1 mL	23-, 25-, or 26-gauge, ½- or ⅝-inch
Intramuscular	3 or 5 mL calibrated in 0.2 mL	20-, 21-, 22-, or 23-gauge, 1½- or 2-inch
Intradermal (tuberculin)	1 mL calibrated in 0.1 mL or 0.01 mL or in minims	25-, 26-, or 27-gauge, ½- to ⅝-inch
Insulin, given subcutaneously	1 mL calibrated in units	25-, 26-, or 27-gauge, ½- or ⅝-inch

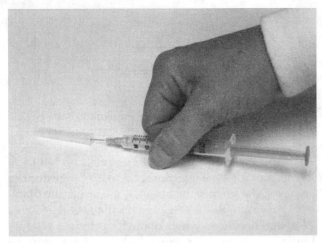

FIGURE 34-2
Scoop method for covering needle. (Courtesy of Ken Timby.)

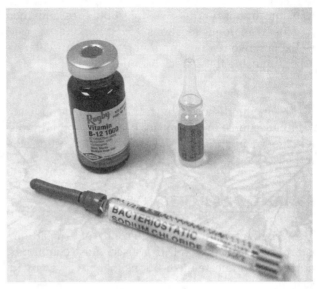

FIGURE 34-3
Vial, ampule, and prefilled cartridge. (Courtesy of Ken Timby.)

a needle can be replaced by using the **scoop method**. The scoop method is performed by threading the needle within the cap without touching the cap itself (Fig. 34-2). After giving an injection, the needle is left uncapped and deposited within the nearest biohazard container, which is usually at the patient's bedside.

Should an accidental injury occur, health care workers are advised to follow certain postexposure recommendations to determine their infectious status (Display 34-1).

Ampules

An **ampule** is a sealed glass container. To withdraw the medication, the ampule must be broken.

DRUG PREPARATION

Drug preparation involves withdrawing medication from an ampule or vial, or assembling a prefilled cartridge (Fig. 34-3).

DISPLAY 34-1. *Post-Needlestick Recommendations*

- Report the injury to one's supervisor
- Document the injury in writing
- Identify the patient, if possible
- Obtain human immunodeficiency virus and hepatitis B virus patient status results, if it is legal to do so
- Obtain counseling on the potential for infection
- Receive the most appropriate postexposure prophylaxis
- Be tested for the presence of antibodies at appropriate intervals
- Receive instructions on monitoring potential symptoms and medical follow-up

---

NURSING GUIDELINES FOR WITHDRAWING MEDICATION FROM AN AMPULE

- Select an appropriate syringe and needle.
  Rationale: Ensures appropriate drug administration
- Tap the top of the ampule.
  Rationale: Distributes all the medication to the lower portion of the ampule
- Protect your thumb and fingers with a gauze square or alcohol swab.
  Rationale: Reduces the potential for injury
- Snap the neck of the ampule away from your body.
  Rationale: Avoids accidental injury
- Insert the needle into the ampule, being careful to avoid touching the outside of the ampule.
  Rationale: Ensures sterility of the needle
- Invert the ampule (Fig. 34-4).
  Rationale: Facilitates withdrawing medication
- Pull back on the plunger.
  Rationale: Fills the syringe

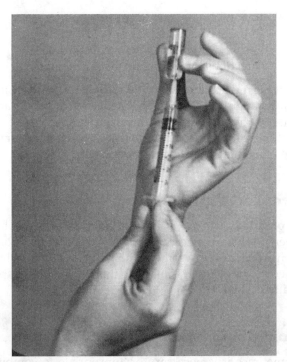

FIGURE 34-4
Withdrawing drug.

- Remove the needle from the ampule when a sufficient volume has been withdrawn.
  Rationale: Prepares for drug administration
- Tap the barrel of the syringe near the hub.
  Rationale: Moves air toward the needle
- Push carefully on the plunger.
  Rationale: Expels air or excess medication
- Scoop the needle within its protective cap, or extend a guard that recesses the needle.
  Rationale: Reduces the risk of a needlestick injury
- Empty the unused portion of medication from the syringe.
  Rationale: Prevents illegal drug use
- Discard the glass ampule in a puncture-resistant container.
  Rationale: Prevents accidental injury

A slightly different technique is used for medication supplied in vials.

Vials

A **vial** is a glass or plastic container of medication with a self-sealing rubber stopper. Medication is removed from a vial by piercing the rubber stopper with a needle or needleless adapter. The amount of drug within a vial may be enough for one or several doses. Any unused drug for future use is dated before it is stored.

NURSING GUIDELINES FOR WITHDRAWING MEDICATION FROM A VIAL

- Select an appropriate syringe and needle.
  Rationale: Ensures appropriate drug administration
- Remove the metal cover from the rubber stopper.
  Rationale: Facilitates inserting the needle or adapter
- Clean a preopened vial by swabbing it with an alcohol square.
  Rationale: Removes colonizing microorganisms
- Fill the syringe with a volume of air equal to the volume that will be withdrawn from the vial.
  Rationale: Provides a means for increasing pressure within the vial
- Pierce the rubber stopper with the needle and instill the air.
  Rationale: Facilitates drug withdrawal
- Invert the vial, hold, and brace it while pulling on the plunger (Fig. 34-5).
  Rationale: Locates medication near the tip of the needle to facilitate its withdrawal
- Remove the needle when the desired volume has entered the barrel of the syringe.
  Rationale: Leaves remaining drug for additional administrations

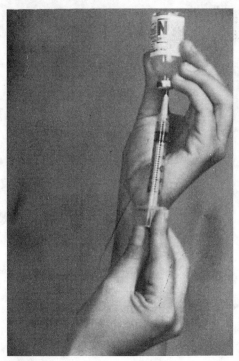

FIGURE 34-5
Withdrawing drug.

- Or, if the medication is a controlled substance like a narcotic, aspirate the entire contents from the vial.
  Rationale: Prevents illegal drug use
- Discard any excess volume of medication; if the drug is a narcotic, have someone witness wasting the medication.
  Rationale: Complies with federal laws to prevent illegal drug use
- Cover the needle and care for used supplies as described in the guidelines for withdrawing from an ampule.
  Rationale: Follows similar principles
- Date and initial the vial if the remaining drug will be used in the near future.
  Rationale: Supports principles of asepsis

Most of the time, the drugs within vials are in liquid form. Occasionally they are supplied as powders that must be dissolved.

RECONSTITUTING MEDICATIONS

Reconstitution is the process of adding liquid, known as **diluent**, to a powdered substance. Common diluents for injectable drugs are sterile water or sterile normal saline.

Reconstituting a drug just before it is needed ensures that the drug's potency is at its maximum. When reconstitution is necessary, the drug label provides directions for the:

- Type of diluent to add
- Amount of diluent to use
- Dosage per volume after reconstitution
- Directions for storing the drug

If the medication will be used for more than one administration, the label on the vial is dated, timed, and initialed by the preparer. In some cases, when the directions provide several options in diluent volumes, the amount added is also written on the vial.

Prefilled Cartridges

A **prefilled cartridge** is a sealed glass cylinder that has been filled with medication by a pharmaceutical company. The cartridge comes supplied with a preattached needle. The cylinder is made so that it fits within a specially designed syringe (Fig. 34-6).

Combining Medications

Sometimes it is necessary or appropriate to combine more than one drug within a single syringe. Before mixing any drugs, however, a drug reference or compatibility chart is consulted because some drugs may interact chemically when combined. The chemical reaction often causes a precipitate to form.

Care is taken to withdraw and fill the syringe with the exact amounts from each drug container to avoid excess volumes of either drug. Once the drugs are within the barrel of the syringe, there is no way to expel one of the drugs without also expelling some of the other (see the discussion on Combining Insulins later in this chapter).

INJECTION ROUTES

There are four **routes** or locations where injections are administered. They include **intradermal injections**, given between the layers of the skin; **subcutaneous injections**, given beneath the skin, but above the muscle; **intramuscular injections**, placed within muscle tissue; and **intravenous injections**, those instilled into veins (Fig. 34-7). Each site requires a slightly different injection technique. Intravenous medication administration is discussed separately in Chapter 35.

Intradermal Injections

Intradermal injections are commonly used for diagnostic purposes. Examples include tuberculin tests and allergy testing. Small volumes, usually 0.01 mL (cc) to no more than 0.05 mL (cc) are injected because of the small tissue space.

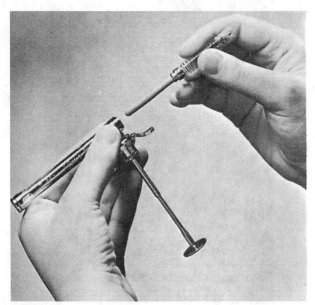

FIGURE 34-6
Inserting a prefilled cartridge.

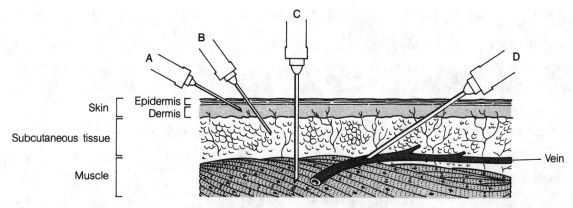

FIGURE 34-7
Injection routes. (*A*) Intradermal, (*B*) subcutaneous, (*C*) intramuscular, (*D*) intravenous. (Scherer JC: Introductory Clinical Pharmacology, 5th ed, p 18. Philadelphia, JB Lippincott, 1992)

INJECTION SITES

A common site for an intradermal injection is the inner aspect of the forearm. Other areas that may be used are the back and upper chest.

INJECTION EQUIPMENT

A tuberculin syringe is used to administer intradermal injections. A **tuberculin syringe** is narrow and holds 1 mL of fluid. The syringe is calibrated in 0.01-mL increments (Fig. 34-8). A 25- to 27-gauge needle measuring 1/2 inch in length is commonly used when administering an intradermal injection.

INJECTION TECHNIQUE

When giving an intradermal injection, the technique requires that the medication be instilled quite shallowly (Skill 34-1).

Subcutaneous Injections

A subcutaneous injection is administered somewhat more deeply than an intradermal injection. Medication instilled between the skin and muscle is absorbed fairly rapidly and begins acting within one half-hour of being administered. The volume of a subcutaneous injection is usually up to 1 mL (cc).

The subcutaneous route is commonly used to administer insulin and heparin.

INJECTION SITES

The sites for giving a subcutaneous injection include the upper arm, thigh, abdomen, and back (Fig. 34-9).

INJECTION EQUIPMENT

Equipment used for subcutaneous injection may depend on the type of medication that has been prescribed. Insulin is prepared in an insulin syringe (see section on Administering Insulin). Heparin may be

(*text continues on page 737*)

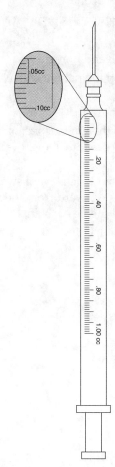

FIGURE 34-8
A tuberculin syringe.

SKILL 34-1
Administering Intradermal Injections

Suggested Action	Reason for Action
Assessment	
Check the medical orders.	Collaborates nursing activities with medical treatment
Compare the medication administration record (MAR) with the written medical order.	Ensures accuracy
Read and compare the label on the drug with the MAR at least three times—before, during, and after preparing the drug.	Prevents errors
Check for any documented allergies to food or drugs.	Ensures safety
Determine how much the patient understands about the purpose and technique for administering the injection.	Provides an opportunity for health teaching
Planning	
Prepare to administer the injection according to the schedule prescribed by the physician.	Complies with medical orders
Obtain clean gloves, tuberculin syringe, appropriate needle, and alcohol swabs.	Facilitates drug preparation and administration
Prepare the syringe with the medication.	Fills the syringe with the appropriate volume
Implementation	
Wash your hands and don gloves.	Reduces the transmission of microorganisms
Read the name on the patient's identification band.	Prevents errors
Pull the privacy curtain.	Demonstrates respect for the patient's dignity
Select an area on the inner aspect of the forearm, about a hand's breadth above the patient's wrist.	Provides a convenient and easy location for accessing intradermal tissue
Cleanse the area with an alcohol swab using a circular motion outward from the site where the needle will pierce the skin.	Removes microorganisms, following principles of asepsis
Allow the skin to dry.	Reduces tissue irritation
Hold the patient's arm and stretch the skin taut.	Helps control the placement of the needle

(continued)

SKILL 34-1
Administering Intradermal Injections *(Continued)*

Suggested Action	Reason for Action
Hold the syringe almost parallel to the skin at a 10° to 15° angle with the bevel pointing upward.	Facilitates delivering the drug between the layers of the skin

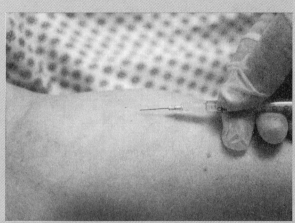

Entering the skin. (Courtesy of Ken Timby.)

Suggested Action	Reason for Action
Insert the needle about ⅛ inch.	Advances the needle to the depth desired
Push the plunger of the syringe and watch for a small **wheal**, or elevated circle, to appear.	Verifies that the drug has been injected correctly

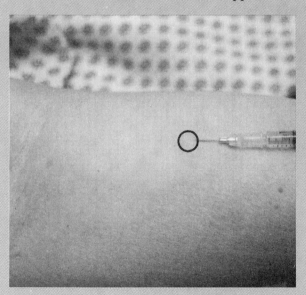

Forming a wheal. (Courtesy of Ken Timby.)

Suggested Action	Reason for Action
Withdraw the needle at the same angle at which it was inserted.	Minimizes tissue trauma and discomfort
Do not massage the area after removing the needle.	Prevents interfering with test results
Deposit the uncapped needle and syringe in a puncture-resistant container.	Prevents injury

(continued)

SKILL 34-1
Administering Intradermal Injections (Continued)

Suggested Action	Reason for Action
Remove your gloves and wash your hands.	Reduces the transmission of microorganisms
Observe the patient's condition for at least the first half-hour after performing an allergy test.	Ensures that emergency treatment can be quickly administered
Observe the area for signs of a local reaction at standard intervals, such as at 24 and 48 hours after the injection.	Determines if and the extent to which the patient responds to the injected substance

Evaluation
- Injection is administered with no untoward effects

Document
- The date, time, drug, dose, route, and specific site
- Response of the patient

Sample Documentation

Date and Time Tuberculin skin test administered intradermally in L. forearm with no immediate untoward effects. Instructed to return in 48 hours for inspection of site.

_____ **Signature, Title**

SKILL 34-2
Administering Subcutaneous Injections

Suggested Action	Reason for Action
Assessment	
Check the medical orders.	Collaborates nursing activities with medical treatment
Compare the medication administration record (MAR) with the written medical order.	Ensures accuracy
Read and compare the label on the drug with the MAR at least three times—before, during, and after preparing the drug.	Prevents errors
Check for any documented allergies to food or drugs.	Ensures safety
Determine where the last injection was given if the site must be rotated.	Prevents tissue injury
Determine how much the patient understands about the purpose and technique for administering the injection.	Provides an opportunity for health teaching
Inspect the potential injection site for signs of bruising, swelling, redness, warmth, or tenerness.	Indicates tissue injury
Planning	
Prepare to administer the injection according to the schedule prescribed by the physician.	Complies with medical orders

(continued)

Administering Subcutaneous Injections

Suggested Action	Reason for Action
Obtain clean gloves, appropriate syringe and needle, and alcohol swabs.	Facilitates drug preparation and administration
Prepare the syringe with the medication.	Fills the syringe with the appropriate volume
Add 0.1 to 0.2 mL of air to the syringe.	Flushes all of the medication from the syringe at the time of the injection
Implementation	
Wash your hands and don gloves.	Reduces the transmission of microorganisms
Read the name on the patient's identification band.	Prevents errors
Pull the privacy curtain.	Demonstrates respect for the patient's dignity
Select and prepare an appropriate site by cleansing it with an alcohol swab.	Removes colonizing microorganisms
Allow the skin to dry.	Reduces tissue irritation
Bunch the skin at the site or spread it taut.	Facilitates placement within the subcutaneous level of tissue according to the patient's body composition
Pierce the skin at either a 45° or 90° angle of entry.	Facilitates placement within the subcutaneous level of tissue according to the length of the needle being used

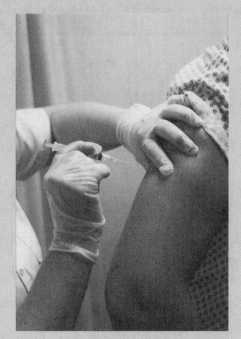

Entering the tissue at a 45° angle. (Courtesy of Ken Timby.)   Entering the tissue at a 90° angle. (Courtesy of Ken Timby.)

Release the tissue once the needle is inserted and use the hand to support the syringe at its hub.	Steadies the syringe
Pull back gently on the plunger* with a free hand and observe for blood in the barrel.	Determines if the needle lies within a blood vessel
Inject the medication by pushing on the plunger if there is no blood after aspiration.	Ensures subcutaneous administration
Withdraw the needle quickly while applying pressure against the medication site.	Controls bleeding

(continued)

Suggested Action	Reason for Action
Massage the site, unless contraindicated.	Promotes absorption and relieves discomfort
Deposit the uncapped needle and syringe in a puncture-resistant container.	Prevents injury
Remove your gloves and wash your hands.	Reduces the transmission of microorganisms
Assess the patient's condition at least 30 minutes after giving the injection.	Aids in evaluating the drug's effectiveness

Evaluation

• Injection is administered with no untoward effects

Document

• The date, time, drug, dose, route, and specific site
• Site assessment data
• Response of the patient

Sample Documentation[†]

Date and Time 25 U of regular insulin administered into L. upper arm. Site appears free of redness, swelling, warmth, tenderness, and bruising. Alert and oriented one half-hour after injection. _____ **Signature, Title**

* Skip this step if administering heparin.

† The administration of drugs is usually documented on the MAR.

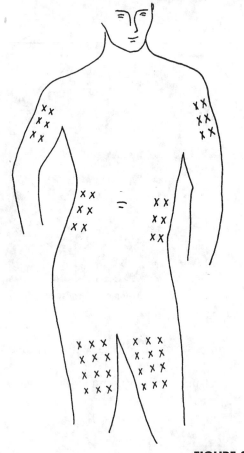

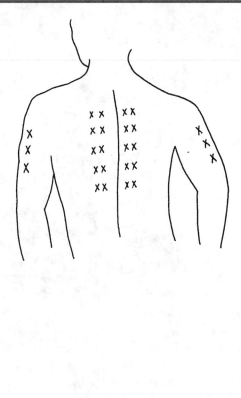

FIGURE 34-9
Subcutaneous injection sites.

prepared in a tuberculin syringe or it may be supplied in a prefilled cartridge in some agencies. A 25-gauge needle is most often used because the medications administered by the subcutaneous route usually are not viscous. Needle lengths may vary from 1/2 to 5/8 inch.

INJECTION TECHNIQUE

To reach subcutaneous tissue in a person of average weight, a 1/2-inch needle is inserted at a 90° angle; for larger or obese patients, a 5/8-inch needle is inserted at a 45° angle (Fig. 34-10). For a description of the technique for administering a subcutaneous injection, see Skill 34-2.

There are also situations in which it may be preferable to bunch the tissue between the thumb and fingers or stretch the tissue taut before administering the injection. The technique usually depends on the size of the patient. For thin, dehydrated patients and most children and infants, bunching is preferred.

Other modifications are involved when the drug administered is either insulin or heparin.

Administering Insulin

Insulin is a hormone that can be administered only by injection. Usually insulin is administered subcutaneously, but it can also be administered intravenously. Because insulin is supplied and prescribed in a dosage strength called units, a special syringe called an insulin syringe is used to measure the prescribed dose. An **insulin syringe** holds a volume of 0.5 to 1 mL, but it is calibrated in units (Fig. 34-11). Because the standard dosage strength of supplied insulin is 100 U/mL, one or the other syringes can be used to administer up to 50 or 100 U of prescribed insulin.

Patients who require insulin often receive one or more daily injections. Over time, the injection sites tend to undergo changes that interfere with the absorption of the insulin. To avoid **lipoatrophy**, a condition in which the subcutaneous fat breaks down at the site of repeated insulin injections, and **lipohypertrophy**, a build-up of subcutaneous fat at insulin injection sites, the sites are rotated each time an injection is administered.

Insulin must also be prepared for administration in unique ways.

Preparing Insulin. Various types of insulin vary in their onset, peak effect, and duration of action. The nurse must take care to read the labeled vials carefully because they look similar to one another.

Some preparations of insulin also contain an additive that delays its absorption. The two tend to separate on standing. Therefore, when preparing other than regular insulin, the vial is rotated between the palms to redistribute the two before the insulin is withdrawn.

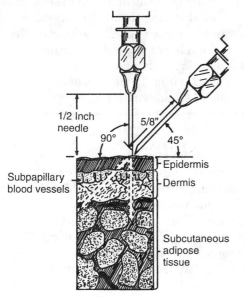

FIGURE 34-10
Angles and needle lengths for subcutaneous injections.

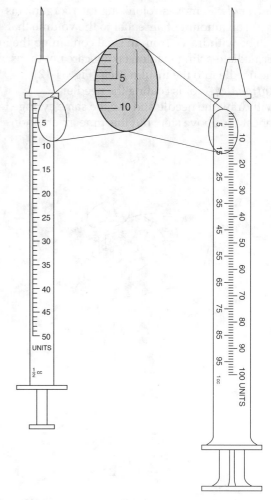

FIGURE 34-11
Low-dose and standard insulin syringe.

Combining Insulins. Insulins, when they are mixed together, tend to bind and become equilibrated. This means that each one's unique characteristics are offset by the other. For this reason, most types of insulin are combined just before they are administered. When injected within 15 minutes of being combined, they act as if they had been injected separately.

Regular insulin, which is additive-free, often is combined with an intermediate-acting insulin like Humulin N. When they are combined, they are mixed in a particular sequence to avoid contaminating one with the other.

NURSING GUIDELINES FOR COMBINING INSULINS

- Roll the vial of insulin containing an additive between the palms of the hands.
  Rationale: Mixes the insulin without damaging the protein molecules
- Cleanse the rubber stoppers of both vials of insulin.
  Rationale: Removes colonizing microorganisms
- Instill an amount of air equal to the volume that will be withdrawn from the vial containing the intermediate-acting insulin, taking care not to insert the needle into the insulin itself (Fig. 34-12).
  Rationale: Avoids coating the needle
- Withdraw the needle and use the same syringe to repeat the above step, but this time invert and

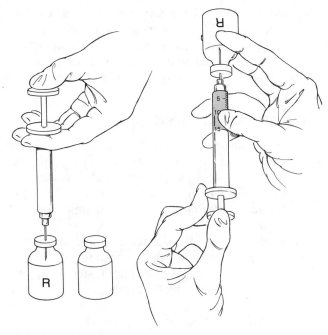

FIGURE 34-13
Instilling air then withdrawing from additive-free vial.

withdraw the prescribed number of additive-free units (Fig. 34-13).
Rationale: Prepares the partial dose
- Ask another nurse to check the label on the insulin and the number of units in the syringe.
  Rationale: Prevents a medication error
- Swab the rubber stopper of the other vial and pierce it with the needle of the partially filled syringe.
  Rationale: Facilitates withdrawing the other type of insulin
- Withdraw the specified number of units from the vial containing the insulin with the additive.
  Rationale: Prepares the full prescribed dose
- Ask another nurse to check the label on the insulin and the number of units in the syringe.
  Rationale: Prevents a medication error
- Administer within 15 minutes of mixing.
  Rationale: Avoids equilibration

Administering Heparin

Heparin is an anticoagulant drug—that is, it prolongs the time it takes for blood to clot. Heparin is frequently administered subcutaneously as well as intravenously. The unique characteristics of the drug require special techniques when using the subcutaneous route for its administration.

Heparin may be supplied in multiple-dose vials or prefilled cartridges. The dosages are measured in tenths and hundredths of a milliliter. These very small

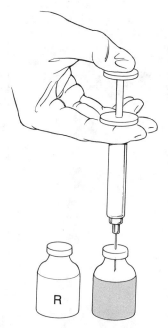

FIGURE 34-12
Instilling air into vial with additive insulin.

volumes require a tuberculin syringe to ensure accuracy. The needle is changed after withdrawal of the drug from a multidose vial and replaced with another before administration.

Various techniques may be used to prevent bruising in the area of the injection. The sites are rotated with each injection to avoid a previous area where there has been local bleeding. Sometimes a rubber glove filled with ice is applied to the site to promote vasoconstriction. The plunger is not aspirated once the needle is in place, and massaging the site is contraindicated because this can increase the tendency for local bleeding.

Intramuscular Injections

An intramuscular injection is the administration of up to 3 mL of medication into one muscle or a muscle group. Because very few nerve endings are in deep muscles, irritating medications are commonly given intramuscularly. Except for medications injected directly into the bloodstream, absorption from an intramuscular injection occurs more rapidly than from other routes.

INJECTION SITES

There are five common injection sites; most are named for the muscles into which the medications are injected. They include the dorsogluteal, ventrogluteal, vastus lateralis, rectus femoris, and deltoid muscle sites.

Dorsogluteal Site

The **dorsogluteal site** is located in the upper outer quadrant of the buttocks. The primary muscle in this site is the *gluteus maximus*, which is large and therefore capable of holding a fair amount of injected medication with minimal postinjection discomfort. This site is avoided in patients younger than 3 years of age because their muscle is not sufficiently developed at this age.

If the site is not identified correctly, damage to the sciatic nerve with subsequent paralysis of the leg can result. To palpate the landmarks appropriately (Fig. 34-14), the nurse:

* Divides the buttock into four imaginary quadrants
* Palpates the posterior iliac spine and the greater trochanter
* Draws an imaginary diagonal line between the two landmarks, and inserts the needle superiorly and laterally to the midpoint of the diagonal line

Ventrogluteal Site

The **ventrogluteal site** is located in the hip area. It uses the *gluteus medius* and *gluteus minimus* muscles for injection. This site has several advantages over the dorsogluteal site. There are no large nerves or blood vessels in the injection area, and it is usually less fatty and cleaner because fecal contamination is rare at this site. The ventrogluteal site is also safe for use in children.

To locate the ventrogluteal site:

* Place the palm of the hand on the greater trochanter and the index finger on the anterior superior iliac spine (Fig. 34-15).
* Move the middle finger away from the index finger as far as possible along the iliac crest.
* Inject into the center of the triangle formed by the index finger, middle finger, and iliac crest.

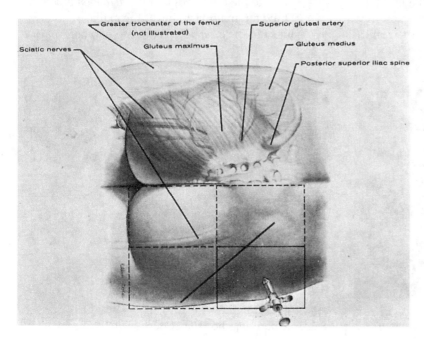

FIGURE 34-14

Dorsogluteal site. (Courtesy of Wyeth Laboratories, Philadelphia, PA.)

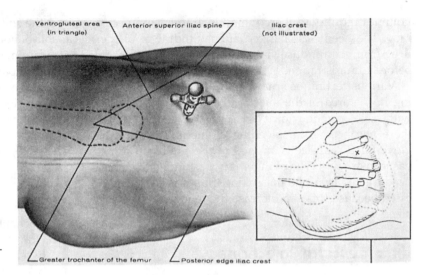

FIGURE 34-15
Ventrogluteal site. (Courtesy of Wyeth Laboratories, Philadelphia, PA.)

Vastus Lateralis Site

The **vastus lateralis site** is located within the outer thigh in a muscle for which the site is named. The *vastus lateralis* muscle is one of the muscles in the quadriceps group. Large nerves and blood vessels usually are absent in this area, which ensures relative safety for the patient. It is a particularly desirable site for administering injections to infants and small children and other thin or debilitated people whose gluteal muscles are poorly developed.

The vastus lateralis site is located by placing one hand just below the *greater trochanter* at the top of the thigh. The needle is then inserted into the lateral area of the thigh (Fig. 34-16).

Rectus Femoris Site

The **rectus femoris site** is located in the anterior aspect of the thigh. The muscle is quite visible in infants and is the preferred injection site for this age group. An injection in this site is placed in the middle third of the thigh with the patient in a sitting or supine position (Fig. 34-17).

Deltoid Site

The **deltoid site** is in the lateral aspect of the upper arm (Fig. 34-18). It is the least-used intramuscular injection site because it is a small muscle compared with the others. The site is used only for adults because the muscle is not sufficiently developed in infants and children. Because of its small capacity, intramuscular injections into this site are limited to no more than 1 mL of solution.

There is a potential risk for damaging the radial-nerve and artery if the deltoid site is not well identified. To use this site safely:

- Have the patient lie down, sit, or stand with the shoulder well exposed.
- Palpate the lower edge of the *acromion process*.
- Draw an imaginary line at the axilla.
- Inject in the area between these two landmarks.

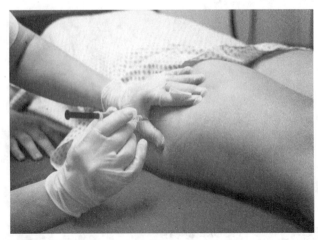

FIGURE 34-16
Vastus lateralis injection site. (Courtesy of Ken Timby.)

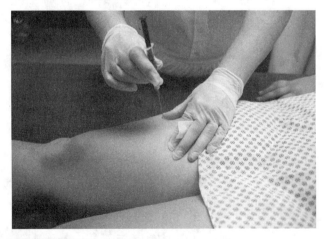

FIGURE 34-17
Rectus femoris injection site. (Courtesy of Ken Timby.)

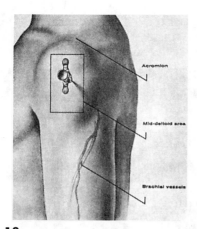

FIGURE 34-18
Deltoid site. (Courtesy of Wyeth Laboratories, Philadelphia, PA.)

INJECTION EQUIPMENT

Generally 3- to 5-mL syringes are used to administer medications by the intramuscular route. A 22-gauge needle that is 1½ to 2 inches long usually is adequate for depositing medication within most sites.

INJECTION TECHNIQUE

When administering intramuscular injections, a 90° angle is used for piercing the skin (Skill 34-3). Drugs that may be irritating to the upper levels of tissue may be administered by Z-track or zig-zag technique.

Z-Track Technique

The **Z-track technique**, sometimes called the *zig-zag technique*, is a technique for manipulating the tissue in such a way as to seal medication, especially that which is irritating, within the muscle. It acquired its name because the maneuver resembles forming the letter "Z."

◄ NURSING GUIDELINES FOR GIVING AN INJECTION BY Z-TRACK TECHNIQUE

- Fill the syringe with the prepared drug, but change the needle.
  Rationale: Prevents tissue contact with the irritating drug
- Attach a needle that is at least 1½ to 2 inches in length.
  Rationale: Helps deposit the drug deep within the muscle
- Add a 0.2-mL bubble of air within the syringe.
  Rationale: Flushes all of the medication from the syringe during the injection
- Select a large muscular injection site, like the ventrogluteal site.

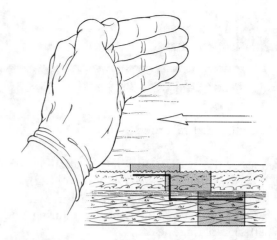

FIGURE 34-19
Stretching tissue laterally.

Rationale: Provides a location with a large capacity where the drug can be deposited and absorbed
- Wash your hands and don gloves.
  Rationale: Reduces the transmission of micro-organisms
- Use the side of the hand to pull the tissue laterally about 1 inch (2.5 cm) until it is taut (Fig. 34-19).
  Rationale: Creates the mechanism for sealing the drug within the muscle
- Insert the needle at a 90° angle while continuing to hold the tissue laterally.
  Rationale: Directs the tip of the needle well within the muscle
- Steady the barrel of the syringe with the fingers and use the thumb to manipulate the plunger (Fig. 34-20).
  Rationale: Avoids releasing the tissue held taut by the nondominant hand

(text continues on page 744)

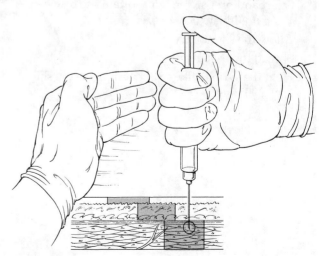

FIGURE 34-20
Manipulating the plunger.

SKILL 34-3
Administering Intramuscular Injections

Suggested Action	Reason for Action
Assessment	
Check the medical orders.	Collaborates nursing activities with medical treatment
Compare the medication administration record (MAR) with the written medical order.	Ensures accuracy
Read and compare the label on the drug with the MAR at least three times—before, during, and after preparing the drug.	Prevents errors
Check for any documented drug allergies.	Ensures safety
Determine where the last injection was given.	Prevents tissue injury
Determine how much the patient understands about the purpose and technique for administering the injection.	Provides an opportunity for health teaching
Inspect the potential injection site for signs of bruising, swelling, redness, warmth, tenderness, or **induration** (hardness).	Indicates tissue injury
Planning	
Prepare to administer the injection according to the schedule prescribed by the physician.	Complies with medical orders
Obtain clean gloves, appropriate syringe and needle, and alcohol swabs.	Facilitates drug preparation and administration
Prepare the syringe with the medication.	Fills the syringe with the appropriate volume
Add 0.2 mL of air to the syringe.	Flushes all of the medication from the syringe at the time of the injection
Implementation	
Wash your hands and don gloves.	Reduces the transmission of microorganisms
Read the name on the patient's identification band.	Prevents errors
Pull the privacy curtain.	Demonstrates respect for the patient's dignity
Select and prepare an appropriate site by cleansing it with an alcohol swab.	Removes colonizing microorganisms
Allow the skin to dry.	Reduces tissue irritation
Spread the tissue taut.	Facilitates placement within the muscle
Hold the syringe like a dart and pierce the skin at a 90° angle.	Reduces discomfort

(continued)

SKILL 34-3
Administering Intramuscular Injections *(Continued)*

Suggested Action	Reason for Action

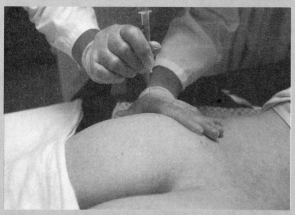

Holding syringe like a dart. (Courtesy of Ken Timby.)

Steady the syringe and aspirate to observe for blood.

Determines if the needle is within a blood vessel

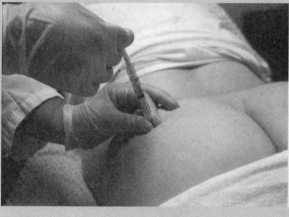

Aspirating for blood. (Courtesy of Ken Timby.)

Instill the drug if no blood is apparent.

Deposits the drug into the muscle

Withdraw the needle quickly at the same angle it was inserted while applying pressure against the site.

Reduces discomfort and controls bleeding

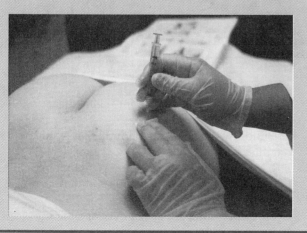

Withdrawing the needle. (Courtesy of Ken Timby.)

(continued)

SKILL 34-3
Administering Intramuscular Injections (Continued)

Suggested Action	Reason for Action
Massage the injection site with the alcohol swab, unless contraindicated.	Distributes the medication and reduces discomfort

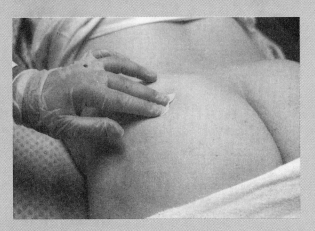

Massaging the site. (Courtesy of Ken Timby.)

Suggested Action	Reason for Action
Deposit the uncapped needle and syringe in a puncture-resistant container.	Prevents injury
Remove your gloves and wash your hands.	Reduces the transmission of microorganisms
Assess the patient's condition at least 30 minutes after giving the injection.	Aids in evaluating the drug's effectiveness

Evaluation
- Injection is administered with no untoward effects

Document
- The date, time, drug, dose, route, and specific site
- Site assessment data
- Response of the patient

Sample Documentation*

Date and Time   Demerol 50 mg given IM into R. ventrogluteal site for pain rated as #8 on a scale of 0–10. No signs of irritation at the site. Rates pain at #5, 30 min. after injection.
_____ **Signature, Title**

* The administration of drugs is usually documented on the MAR; prn drugs may be documented both in the nurse's notes and the MAR.

- Aspirate for a blood return.
  Rationale: Determines if the needle is within a blood vessel
- Instill the medication by depressing the plunger with the thumb.
  Rationale: Deposits the medication into the muscle
- Wait 10 seconds with the needle still in place and the skin still held taut.

Rationale: Provides time for the medication to be distributed in a larger area
- Withdraw the needle and immediately release the taut skin.
  Rationale: Creates a diagonal path that prevents leaking into the subcutaneous and dermal layers of tissue (Fig. 34-21)
- Apply pressure, but *do not* massage the site.

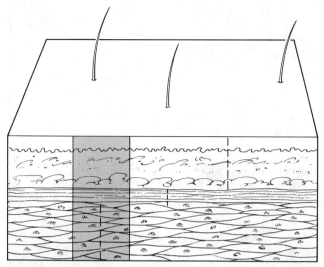

FIGURE 34-21
Interrupted pathway to sealed medication.

Rationale: Ensures that the medication remains sealed
- Discard the syringe without recapping the needle.
Rationale: Reduces the potential for needlestick injury
- Remove your gloves and wash your hands.
Rationale: Reduces the transmission of micro-organisms
- Document the medication administration.
Rationale: Maintains a current record of patient care

Any intramuscular injection can be given by Z-track. Patients report slightly less pain during and the next day after a Z-track injection compared with the usual intramuscular injection technique.

REDUCING INJECTION DISCOMFORT

All injections cause discomfort, some more than others. There is one product currently available that produces anesthesia when applied to the skin or mucous membranes. The product is called EMLA (**E**utectic **M**ixture of **L**ocal **A**nesthetic). It reduces or eliminates the local discomfort of invasive procedures in which the skin is pierced. Its disadvantage is that the effect may not be effectively achieved until 60 to 120 minutes after its application (Givens et al., 1993).

Because time constraints make EMLA somewhat impractical, there are several alternative techniques that may reduce the discomfort associated with injections:

 PATIENT TEACHING FOR REDUCING INJECTION DISCOMFORT

Teach the patient to do the following:
- Lie prone and point the toes inward when receiving an injection into the dorsogluteal site.
- Perform deep breathing and other relaxation techniques before receiving an injection.
- Avoid watching when the injection is given.
- Ambulate or move the extremity where the injection was given as much as possible.

- Use the smallest gauge that is appropriate.
- Change the needle before administering a drug that is irritating to tissue.
- Select a site that is free of irritation.
- Rotate injection sites.
- Numb the skin with an ice pack.
- Insert and withdraw the needle without hesitation.
- Instill the medication slowly and steadily.
- Use the Z-track method for all intramuscular injections.
- Apply pressure to the site during needle withdrawal.
- Massage the site afterward.

NURSING IMPLICATIONS

Nurses who administer parenteral medications may identify nursing diagnoses like the ones included in the accompanying Applicable Nursing Diagnoses.

The Nursing Care Plan for this chapter demonstrates the nursing process as it applies to a patient with Ineffective Management of Therapeutic Regimen. In the NANDA taxonomy (1994), this diagnostic category is defined as "A pattern of regulating and integrating into daily living a program for treatment of illness and the sequelae of illness that is unsatisfactory for meeting specific health goals."

 APPLICABLE NURSING DIAGNOSES

- Pain
- Anxiety
- Fear
- Risk for Trauma
- Knowledge Deficit
- Ineffective Management of Therapeutic Regimen

NURSING CARE PLAN:
Ineffective Management of Therapeutic Regimen

Assessment

Subjective Data
States, "I don't know what happened. I gave myself my insulin and then I started cleaning the house. All of a sudden I fainted."

Objective Data
70-year-old newly diagnosed diabetic woman discharged 2 days earlier. Brought by ambulance to the Emergency Department after having been found unconscious at home by spouse. Blood sugar was 55 mg/dL on admission; current blood sugar is 85 mg per glucometer.

Diagnosis

Ineffective Management of Therapeutic Regimen related to misunderstanding of how to balance insulin and dietary needs.

Plan

Goal
The patient will describe the need to eat food within ½ to 1 hour of insulin administration and ways to raise blood sugar if symptoms reappear.

Orders: 5/28
1. Request consult with dietition.
2. Review onset, peak, and duration of Humulin N.
3. Review the signs and symptoms of low blood sugar.
4. Suggest ways of raising blood sugar quickly.
5. Have patient demonstrate use of glucometer and self-administration of insulin
   before discharge. _____ J. FULCHER, RN

Implementation 5/28
(Documentation)
1345 Consult request sent to dietary department. Reviewed Humulin onset as 1 to 1½ hours after eating; peak in 4 to 12 hours; and duration of 18 to 28 hours. Explained the meaning of terms. _____ K. DAMON, LPN

Evaluation 5/28
(Documentation)
1800 Could explain purpose for eating within the onset time, but could not identify the time of peak and duration of action. Information repeated. K. DAMON, LPN

 FOCUS ON OLDER ADULTS

- Because older adults tend to have less subcutaneous fat, it may be best to bunch the tissue when administering an intramuscular injection to avoid striking the bone.
- Older adults with diabetes often have visual problems that interfere with their ability to self-administer their own insulin injections. It may be appropriate to collaborate with the physician about teaching blind or nearly blind patients how to use a loading gauge that prevents filling a syringe with more than the prescribed dose.
- Older adults tend to experience more adverse effects from drugs because of their compromised ability to absorb and metabolize them

at the same rate as younger adults.
- Older adults may require lower dosages of parenteral medications to avoid untoward effects.
- Injections are avoided in limbs that are paralyzed or inactive. The deltoid site may be best for older adults with impaired mobility.
- Contractures and arthritis complicate techniques for positioning older adults to identify injection site landmarks appropriately.
- It may be wise to investigate the possibility of drug interactions or toxicity when older adults have a dramatic change in behavior that coincides with the administration of a new drug.

KEY CONCEPTS

- Three parts of a syringe include the barrel, plunger, and tip.
- When selecting a syringe and needle, the following factors are considered: type of medication, depth of tissue, volume of prescribed drug, viscosity of the drug, and size of the patient.
- Conventional syringes and needles are being redesigned to reduce the potential for needlestick injuries and the transmission of blood-borne pathogens.
- Pharmaceutical companies supply drugs for parenteral administration in ampules, vials, and prefilled cartridges.
- Before combining any two drugs within a single syringe, it is important to consult a drug reference or a compatibility chart to determine if a chemical interaction may occur.
- There are four parenteral injection routes: intradermal, subcutaneous, intramuscular, and intravenous.
- A common site for an intradermal injection is the inner forearm; subcutaneous injections are commonly given in the thigh, arm, or abdomen; intramuscular injections may be given in the buttocks, hip, thigh, and arm.
- An intradermal injection is commonly given with a tuberculin syringe; insulin is administered subcutaneously with an insulin syringe; and intramuscular injections are usually given with a syringe that holds a volume of 3 mL (cc).
- When administering an intradermal injection, the needle is inserted at a 10° to 15° angle; a 45° to 90° angle is used when giving a subcutaneous injection; and a 90° angle is used when administering an intramuscular injection.
- When two insulins are combined, they must be administered within 15 minutes to avoid equilibration, that is, the loss of each type of insulin's unique time of onset, peak, and duration of action.
- To prevent bruising when heparin is administered, the nurse avoids aspirating with the plunger and massaging the site afterward.
- Five sites used for administering intramuscular injections include the dorsogluteal site, ventrogluteal site, vastus lateralis site, rectus femoris site, and deltoid site.
- Intramuscular injections are given by Z-track technique to seal irritating substances within the muscle and to reduce discomfort after an injection.

CRITICAL THINKING EXERCISES

- Discuss the differences between administering injections by the intradermal, subcutaneous, and intramuscular routes.
- Discuss how an intramuscular injection would be different if given to a 3-year-old compared to a 33-year-old.
- You are to administer an intramuscular injection to a 76-year-old patient. Discuss the factors you will consider before choosing your equipment and injection site.

SUGGESTED READINGS

Calculating drug dosages: self-test. Nursing February 1993;23:87, 89–90.

Drass J. What you need to know about insulin injections. Nursing November 1992;22:40–45.

Farrell J. Nursing Care of the Older Person. Philadelphia: JB Lippincott, 1990.

Fowler-Kerry S. Relieving needle puncture pain. Canadian Nurse December 1992;88:35.

Givens B, Oberle S, Lander J. Taking the jab out of needles. Canadian Nurse November 1993;89:37–40.

Gurevich I. Preventing needlesticks: A market survey. RN November 1994;11:44–49, 52.

Matteson MA, McConnell ES. Gerontological Nursing: Concepts and Practice. Philadelphia: WB Saunders, 1988.

McConnell EA. How to administer a Z-track injection. Nursing April 1993;23:18.

Moorhouse A, Bolen R, Evans J. Needlestick injuries: the shock and the reality. Canadian Nurse November 1993;89:29–33.

Murphy JI. Reducing the pain of intramuscular injections. Advancing Clinical Care July–August 1991;6:35.

Newton M, Newton DW, Fudin J. Reviewing the "big three" injection routes. Nursing February 1992;22:34–32.

CHAPTER 35

Intravenous Medications

Key Terms

Bolus Administration	Intravenous Push
Central Venous Catheter	Piggyback Infusion
Chemotherapy	Port
Continuous Infusion	Secondary Infusion
Intermittent Infusion	Volume-control Set
Intravenous Route	

Learning Objectives

An understanding of the content within this chapter will be evidenced by the student's ability to:

- Name two types of veins into which intravenous medications are administered
- Describe at least three situations for which it is appropriate to administer intravenous medications
- Name two ways intravenous medications are administered
- Describe two methods for giving bolus administrations of intravenous medications
- Describe two methods for administering medicated solutions intermittently
- Explain the technique for administering a piggyback infusion
- Discuss two purposes for using a volume-control set
- Describe a central venous catheter
- Name three types of central venous catheters
- Discuss three techniques for protecting oneself when administering antineoplastic drugs

Administering intravenous solutions, which is discussed in Chapter 15, can be considered a form of intravenous medication administration. The focus of this chapter, however, is on the methods for administering intravenous drugs, not fluid replacement solutions, and the techniques for using various venous access devices.

INTRAVENOUS ROUTE

The **intravenous** (IV) **route** includes peripheral and central veins. Medications administered intravenously have an immediate effect, and consequently it is the most dangerous route for drug administration. Drugs administered in this manner cannot be recalled once they have been given. For this reason, only selectively qualified nurses are permitted to administer IV medications. Even those who are responsible for IV medication administration must exercise extreme caution in preparation and instillation.

Despite its inherent risks, there are legitimate reasons for using the IV route.

INTRAVENOUS MEDICATION ADMINISTRATION

Intravenous administration is the route chosen when:

- A quick response is needed during an emergency
- Patients have disorders that affect absorption or metabolism of drugs, like a seriously burned patient
- Blood levels of drugs need to be maintained at a consistent therapeutic level, such as when treat-

ing infections caused by drug-resistant pathogens or when providing postoperative pain relief
- It is in the patient's best interests to avoid the discomfort of repeated intramuscular injections
- A mechanism is needed to administer drug therapy over a prolonged period of time, as in the case of patients with cancer

When drugs are administered intravenously, they may be given either continuously or intermittently.

Continuous Administration

A **continuous infusion** is one that is instilled over several hours. Sometimes this method of administration is called a *continuous drip.*

Continuous infusions involve adding medication to a large volume (500–1,000 mL) of IV solution (Skill 35-1). Drugs may be added to a new container of IV solution or to an existing infusion if there is a sufficient volume to dilute the drug.

(text continues on page 754)

SKILL 35-1
Administering Intravenous Medication by Continuous Infusion

Suggested Action	Reason for Action
Assessment Check the medical orders.	Collaborates nursing activities with medical treatment
Compare the medication administration record (MAR) with the written medical order.	Ensures accuracy

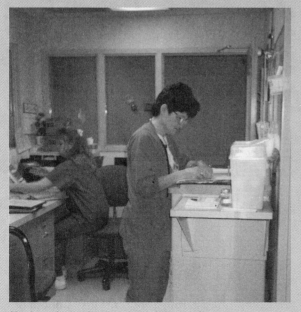

Checking the MAR. (Courtesy of Ken Timby.)

(continued)

SKILL 35-1
Administering Intravenous Medication by Continuous Infusion (Continued)

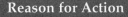

Suggested Action	Reason for Action
Read and compare the label on the drug with the MAR	Prevents errors
Make sure the drug label indicates that it is for IV use.	Prevents patient injury
Check for any documented drug allergies.	Ensures safety
Inspect the current infusion site for swelling, redness, and tenderness.	Determines if a site change is needed

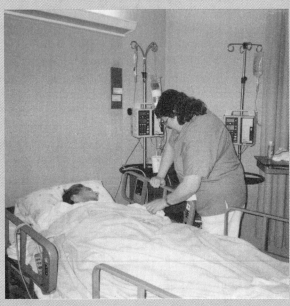

Assessing the infusion site. (Courtesy of Ken Timby.)

Suggested Action	Reason for Action
Review the drug action and side effects.	Promotes safe patient care
Consult a compatibility chart or drug reference.	Determines if the solution and drug are known to interact when mixed
Determine how much the patient understands about the purpose and technique for administering the medication.	Provides an opportunity for health teaching
Perform assessments that will provide a basis for evaluating the drug's effectiveness.	Provides a baseline for future comparisons

Planning

Prepare the medication, taking care to read the medication label at least three times.	Avoids medication errors
Have a second nurse double-check your drug calculations.	Ensures accuracy

Implementation

Wash your hands.	Reduces the transmission of microorganisms
Check the patient's identification band.	Prevents a medication error
Clamp or stop the current infusion of fluid.	Prevents administering a concentrated amount of medication as it is being added

(continued)

SKILL 35-1
Administering Intravenous Medication by Continuous Infusion (Continued)

Suggested Action	Reason for Action
Swab the appropriate port on the container of IV fluid.	Removes colonizing microorganisms

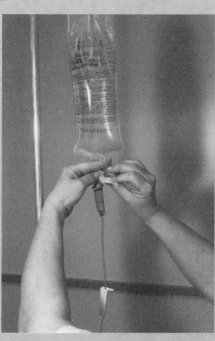

Swabbing the port on the container. (Courtesy of Ken Timby.)

Suggested Action	Reason for Action
Instill the medication through the port into the full container of infusing fluid.	Promotes dilution of concentrated additive

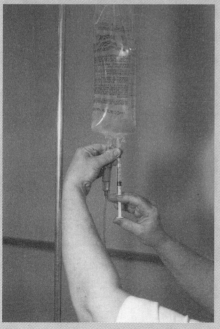

Instilling medication. (Courtesy of Ken Timby.)

(continued)

Suggested Action	Reason for Action
Lower the bag and gently rotate it back and forth.	Distributes the medication equally throughout the fluid

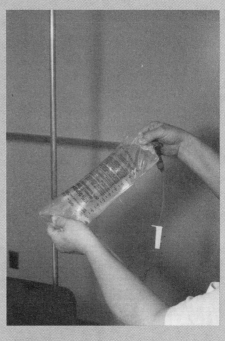

Rotating the container. (Courtesy of Ken Timby.)

Suggested Action	Reason for Action
Suspend the solution and release the clamp.	Facilitates infusion
Regulate the rate of flow by using the roller clamp or programming the rate on the electronic infusion device.	Promotes continuous infusion at prescribed rate

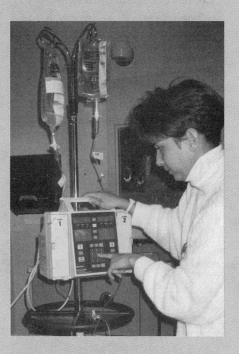

Programming the rate. (Courtesy of Ken Timby.)

(continued)

SKILL 35-1
Administering Intravenous Medication by Continuous Infusion (Continued)

Suggested Action	Reason for Action
Attach a label to the container of fluid identifying the drug, its dose, time it was added, and your initials.	Provides information for others and demonstrates accountability for nursing actions

Attaching the label. (Courtesy of Ken Timby.)

Suggested Action	Reason for Action
Record the medication administration in the MAR.	Documents nursing care; avoids medication errors
Check the patient and the progress of the infusion at least hourly.	Promotes early intervention for complications

Evaluation
- Medication instills at prescribed rate without any adverse effects

Document
- Patient and site assessment data
- The date, time, drug, dose, and initials
- Solution to which drug has been added
- Response of the patient

*Sample Documentation**

Date and Time   IV infusing in L. forearm. No tenderness, swelling, or redness observed. KCl 20 mEq added to 1,000 mL of D5/W. IV infusing at 125 mL/hr. Heart rate is regular and ranges between 65 and 75 bpm. _____ **Signature, Title**

* The administration of drugs is usually documented on the MAR.

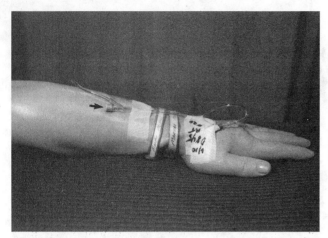

FIGURE 35-1
An intravenous port. (Courtesy of Ken Timby.)

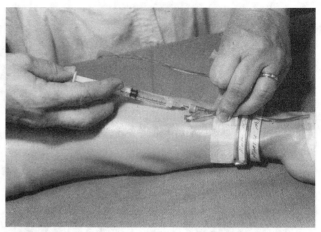

FIGURE 35-2
Instilling medication. (Courtesy of Ken Timby.)

After the medication has been added, the solution is administered by gravity infusion or with an electronic infusion device like a controller or pump (see Chap. 15).

Intermittent Administration

An **intermittent infusion** is one in which IV medication is given within a relatively short period of time. Medications given in this manner may instill in a matter of minutes or up to 1 hour.

There are three ways in which intermittent infusions are administered: bolus administrations, secondary administrations, and those in which a volume-control set is used.

BOLUS ADMINISTRATION

The term *bolus* refers to a substance that is given all at one time. A **bolus administration** is one in which undiluted medication is given fairly quickly into a vein.

Sometimes the term **IV push** (IVP) is used to describe a bolus administration. Although the term "push" is used, the standard is to administer the medication at the rate specified in an authoritative drug reference or at a rate of 1 mL (cc) per minute if there is no information available.

Bolus administrations are given in one of two ways: through a port in an existing IV line or through a medication lock (see Chap. 15).

Using an IV Port

A **port** is a sealed protrusion that extends from IV tubing (Fig. 35-1). The seal is made of latex or another substance that can be pierced with a needle or needleless adapter.

NURSING GUIDELINES FOR ADMINISTERING MEDICATIONS THROUGH AN INTRAVENOUS PORT

- Prepare the medication within a syringe.
  Rationale: Provides a means for accessing the port
- Locate the port nearest the IV insertion site.
  Rationale: Facilitates the most rapid placement of medication within the circulatory system
- Swab the port with an alcohol square.
  Rationale: Removes colonizing microorganisms
- Pierce the port with the needle or needleless adapter.
  Rationale: Gains access to inside the tubing
- Pinch the tubing above the access port.
  Rationale: Temporarily stops the flow of IV fluid
- Pull back on the plunger of the syringe.
  Rationale: Creates negative pressure
- Observe for blood in the tubing near the IV catheter or insertion device.
  Rationale: Validates that the IV catheter is within the vein
- Gently instill a few tenths of a milliliter of medication (Fig. 35-2).
  Rationale: Initiates the bolus administration
- Release the tubing.
  Rationale: Allows some IV fluid to flow
- Continue the pattern of pinching the tubing,* instilling a small amount of drug, and releasing the tubing until the medication has been administered over the specified period of time.
  Rationale: Delivers the drug gradually; keeps the catheter or venous insertion device patent when medication is not being instilled

---

*Pinching the tubing while instilling drug ensures that the drug is administered to the patient rather than backfilling the tubing.

Because the entire dose is administered so fast, bolus administration has the greatest potential for causing life-threatening changes should a drug reaction occur. If the patient's condition changes for any reason, the administration is immediately ceased and emergency measures are taken to protect the patient's safety.

Using a Medication Lock

A medication lock is also called a saline or heparin lock. The insertion and technique for maintaining the patency of a medication lock are described in Chapter 15.

Briefly, a medication lock is a plug that, when inserted into the end of an IV catheter, allows instant access to the venous system. One of its best features is that it eliminates the need for a continuous, and sometimes unnecessary, administration of IV fluid.

Instilling IV medication through a lock is similar to the routine for keeping it patent (see Skill 15-6, Chap. 15). The technique varies somewhat depending on whether it is the agency's policy to maintain patency with saline or heparin. The trend is to use saline.

Basically, most nurses use the mnemonic "SAS" or "SASH" as a guide to the steps involved in administering IV medication into a lock. SAS stands for **S**aline—**A**dminister drug—**S**aline; whereas SASH refers to **S**aline—**A**dminister drug—**S**aline—**H**eparin. These steps are implemented in the following way.

NURSING GUIDELINES FOR ADMINISTERING MEDICATIONS THROUGH A LOCK

- Prepare three syringes, two with at least 1 mL of sterile normal saline, one with the prescribed medication.
  Rationale: Facilitates flushing the lock before and after the administration of the medication
- Prepare a fourth syringe with heparin (10 Units/mL), if it is the policy of the agency to use it.
  Rationale: Maintains patency by interfering with clot formation
- Label all the syringes in some way, such as attaching a piece of tape with the letters "S" and "H" according to the substance each syringe contains.
  Rationale: Identifies contents of syringes
- Check the identity of the patient.
  Rationale: Prevents medication errors
- Wipe the medication port with an alcohol swab.
  Rationale: Removes colonizing microorganisms
- Insert the needle from a syringe containing saline through the "bull's eye" of the rubber seal on the medication lock (Fig. 35-3).
  Rationale: Provides the least resistance when introducing the needle

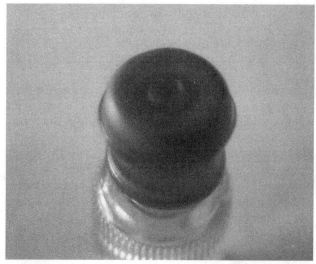

FIGURE 35-3
Bull's eye on a medication lock. (Courtesy of Ken Timby.)

- Hold the lock and pull back on the plunger of the syringe.
  Rationale: Stabilizes the lock while aspirating for blood
- Observe for blood within the barrel of the syringe.
  Rationale: Verifies that the lock is still patent and within the vein (depending on the gauge of the needle, a blood return may not always be observed)
- Instill the saline (represents the first "S" in the mnemonic).
  Rationale: Clears the lock and venous access device
- Remove the syringe when empty, wipe the tip of the lock, and insert the syringe containing the drug.
  Rationale: Facilitates administering the medication
- Gently and gradually administer the medication over the specified time period (represents the letter "A" in the mnemonic).
  Rationale: Ensures safety when recommendations from an authoritative source are followed
- Remove the syringe when it is emptied, wipe the lock again, insert the second syringe with saline, and instill the fluid (represents the second "S" in the mnemonic).
  Rationale: Facilitates moving the medication that remains within the lock into the venous system and filling the lock with saline
- Begin to withdraw the syringe while instilling the last of the fluid within the syringe.
  Rationale: Prevents drawing blood, which may clot, within the lumen of the IV catheter, and ensures future patency
- Wipe, insert, and instill the heparin, if that is agency policy, following the same technique for withdrawal (represents the "H" in the mnemonic).
  Rationale: Maintains patency using an anticoagulant

• Deposit all uncapped syringes in the nearest puncture-resistant biohazard container.
Rationale: Prevents needlestick injuries

To maintain the continued patency of medication locks, they are usually flushed every 8 hours with saline or heparin. The flushing technique is the same, except only one syringe of flush solution is required. Medication locks are changed when the IV site is changed, or at least every 72 hours. If patency cannot be verified by obtaining a blood return, and if there is resistance when administering the flush solution, the IV catheter is removed, the site is changed, and the lock is replaced.

SECONDARY INFUSIONS

A **secondary infusion** involves administering a drug that has been diluted in a small volume of IV solution, usually 50 to 100 mL (cc), over a period of 30 to 60 minutes. Secondary infusions are also called **piggyback infusions** when they are administered in tandem with an infusing primary solution (Fig. 35-4).

Actually, both names are misnomers when the small volume of medicated solution is administered through a medication lock or the port of a central venous catheter

(discussed later in this chapter). When administered in this way, the medications are independent of a primary infusion. There are also instances when small volumes of medicated solution are given alongside of and simultaneously with a primary infusion. This method involves using certain types of electronic infusion devices.

Skill 35-2, however, describes how secondary infusions are administered by gravity in tandem with a currently infusing primary solution.

USING A VOLUME-CONTROL SET

A **volume-control set** is a chamber within IV tubing that holds a portion of the solution from a larger container (Fig. 35-5). Other commercial names for a volume-control set include *Volutrol*, *Soluset* (Abbott, North Chicago, IL), and *Buretrol*.

A volume-control set may be used for two purposes: (1) to administer IV medication in a small volume of solution at intermittent intervals, and (2) to avoid overloading the circulatory system. The volume-control set essentially substitutes for the separate secondary container of solution, and therefore eliminates the need for additional fluid.

When caring for patients who are at risk for or manifest signs of fluid excess, it may be appropriate to collaborate with the physician and pharmacy department

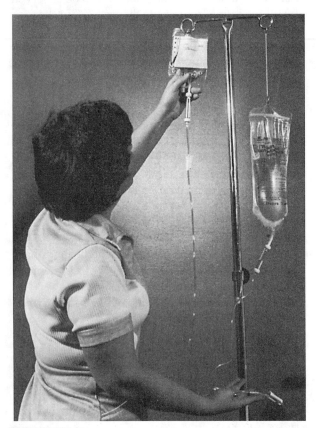

FIGURE 35-4
Piggyback arrangement.

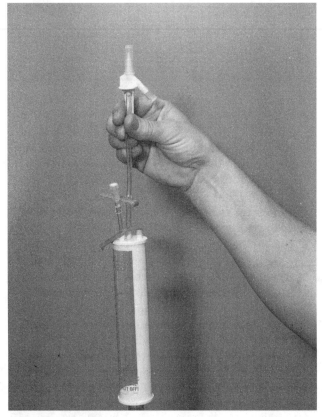

FIGURE 35-5
Volume-control set. (Courtesy of Ken Timby.)

on the feasibility of giving intermittent IV medications with a volume-control set (Skill 35-3).

CENTRAL VENOUS CATHETERS

A **central venous catheter** (CVC) is a venous access device that extends to the vena cava or right atrium. A CVC is used when patients require long-term IV fluid or medication administration, when IV medications are irritating to peripheral veins, or when it is difficult to insert or maintain a peripherally inserted catheter.

Central venous catheters may have single or multiple lumens (Fig. 35-6). The advantage of multiple lumens is that incompatible substances or more than one solution or drug can be given simultaneously. Each infuses through a separate channel and exits the catheter at a different location near the heart. Thus, the drugs or solutions never interact with one another. When a lumen is used only intermittently, it can be capped with a medication lock. The unused lumen is kept patent by scheduled flushes with normal saline or heparin.

There are basically three types of central catheters: percutaneous, tunneled, and implanted.

(text continues on page 761)

35-2
Administering an Intermittent Secondary Infusion

Suggested Action	Reason for Action
Assessment	
Check the medical orders.	Collaborates nursing activities with medical treatment
Compare the medication administration record (MAR) with the written medical order.	Ensures accuracy
Read and compare the label on the medicated solution with the MAR.	Prevents errors
Check for any documented drug allergies.	Ensures safety
Inspect the current infusion site for swelling, redness, and tenderness.	Determines if a site change is needed
Review the drug action and side effects.	Promotes safe patient care
Consult a compatibility chart or drug reference.	Determines if the drug in the secondary solution may interact when mixed with the solution in the primary tubing
Determine how much the patient understands about the purpose and technique for administering the medication.	Provides an opportunity for health teaching
Perform assessments that will provide a basis for evaluating the drug's effectiveness.	Provides a baseline for future comparisons
Planning	
Plan to administer the secondary infusion within 30 to 60 minutes of the scheduled time for drug administration established by the agency.	Complies with agency policy
Remove a refrigerated secondary solution at least 30 minutes before administration.	Warms the solution slightly to promote comfort during its instillation
Check the drop factor on the package of secondary (short) IV tubing and calculate the rate for infusion (see Chap. 15).	Ensures that the secondary infusion will be instilled within the specified time
Have a second nurse double-check your calculations for the rate of infusion.	Ensures accuracy

(continued)

SKILL 35-2
Administering an Intermittent Secondary Infusion (Continued)

Suggested Action	Reason for Action
Attach the tubing to the solution (see Skill 15-2), fill the drip chamber, and purge air from the tubing.	Prepares the medicated solution for administration

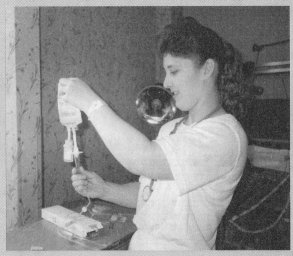

Preparing secondary infusion equipment. (Courtesy of Ken Timby.)

Suggested Action	Reason for Action
Attach a needle, recessed needle, or needleless adaptor.	Facilitates piercing the port

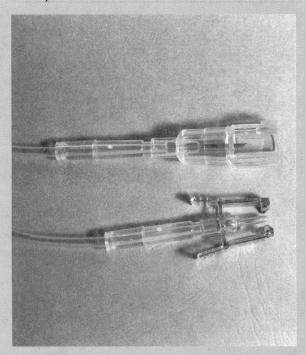

Recessed needle and needleless adaptors. (Courtesy of Ken Timby.)

(continued)

SKILL 35-2
Administering an Intermittent Secondary Infusion (Continued)

Suggested Action	Reason for Action
Implementation	
Wash your hands.	Reduces the transmission of microorganisms
Check the identity of the patient.	Prevents medication errors
Hang the secondary solution on the IV pole or standard.	Prepares the solution for administration
Lower the container of primary solution approximately 10 inches (25 cm) below the height of the secondary solution using a plastic or metal hanger.	Positions the secondary solution so as to instill under greater hydrostatic pressure
Wipe the *uppermost port* on the primary tubing with an alcohol swab.	Removes colonized microorganisms

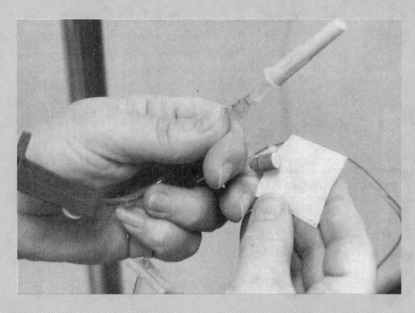

Swabbing the port. (Courtesy of Ken Timby.)

(continued)

SKILL 35-2
Administering an Intermittent Secondary Infusion (Continued)

Suggested Action	Reason for Action
Insert the needle or modified adaptor within the port.	Provides access to the venous system

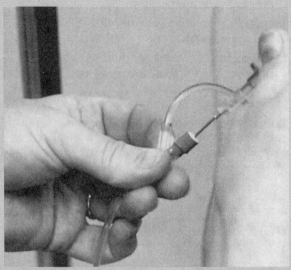

Inserting the needle. (Courtesy of Ken Timby.)

Suggested Action	Reason for Action
Tape the needle, if one is used, within the port; adaptors are usually self-securing.	Prevents separation from the port

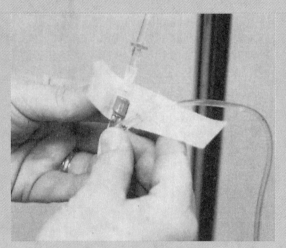

Taping the connection. (Courtesy of Ken Timby.)

Suggested Action	Reason for Action
Release the roller clamp on the secondary solution.	Initiates the infusion
Regulate the rate of flow by counting the drip rate and adjusting the roller clamp.	Establishes the maintenance rate of flow to instill the solution in the time specified
Clamp the tubing when the solution has instilled.	Prevents backfilling with solution from the primary solution

(continued)

SKILL 35-2
Administering an Intermittent Secondary Infusion *(Continued)*

Suggested Action	Reason for Action
Rehang the primary container of solution and readjust the rate of flow.	Continues fluid replacement therapy at its appropriate rate
Leave the secondary tubing in place within the port if another secondary infusion of the same medication is scheduled again within the next 24 to 72 hours.	Controls health care costs without jeopardizing patient safety; different tubing, however, is used if other drugs are administered as secondary infusions

Evaluation

• Secondary infusion instills at prescribed rate without any adverse effects

Document

• Patient and site assessment data
• The date, time, drug, dose, and initials
• Response of the patient

*Sample Documentation**

Date and Time   IV infusing in L. forearm. No tenderness, swelling, or redness observed. Vancomycin 1 g administered in 100 mL of NSS as a secondary infusion over 60 minutes without signs of a reaction. _____ **Signature, Title**

* The administration of drugs is usually documented on the MAR.

Percutaneous Catheters

A percutaneous catheter is one that is inserted through the skin in a peripheral vein like the jugular or subclavian vein (see Chap. 15). This type is used when patients require short-term fluid or medication therapy, lasting a few days or weeks. Most are inserted by a physician and then sutured to the skin.

Tunneled Catheters

Tunneled catheters are inserted into a central vein with a portion of the catheter secured within subcutaneous tissue. The end of the catheter exits from the skin lateral to the xiphoid process (Fig. 35-7). Tunneled catheters are used when patients require extended therapy. Tunneling helps stabilize the catheter and also reduces

(text continues on page 766)

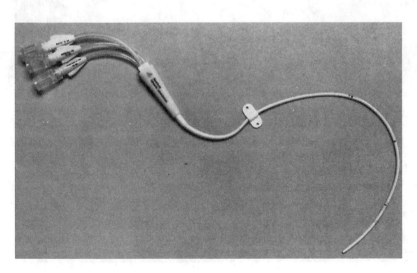

FIGURE 35-6
A triple-lumen central venous catheter. (Courtesy of Ken Timby.)

Suggested Action	Reason for Action
Assessment	
Check the medical orders.	Collaborates nursing activities with medical treatment
Compare the medication administration record (MAR) with the written medical order.	Ensures accuracy
Review the drug action and side effects.	Promotes safe patient care
Consult a compatibility chart or drug reference.	Determines if the medication may interact when diluted with the IV solution
Read and compare the label on the medication with the MAR at least three times.	Prevents errors
Check for any documented drug allergies.	Ensures safety
Assess the patient's fluid status (see Chap. 15) and perform other assessments that will provide a basis for evaluating the drug's effectiveness.	Provides a baseline for making future comparisons
Inspect the current infusion site for swelling, redness, and tenderness.	Determines if a site change is needed
Determine how much the patient understands about the purpose and technique for administering the medication.	Provides an opportunity for health teaching
Planning	
Plan to administer the medication within 30 to 60 minutes of the scheduled time for drug administration established by the agency.	Complies with agency policy
Obtain a volume-control set	Provides the means for instilling an intermittent infusion
Determine the drop factor on the volume-control set and calculate the rate of infusion.	Differs, in some instances, from the drop size on IV tubing
Have a second nurse double-check your calculations for the rate of infusion.	Ensures accuracy
Implementation	
Wash your hands and don gloves.	Reduces the transmission of microorganisms
Close all the clamps on the volume-control set and insert the spike into the IV solution.	Prepares the equipment for medication administration

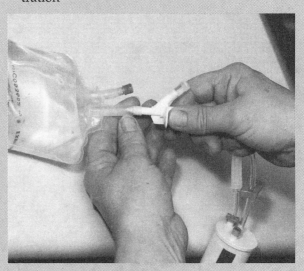

Inserting the spike. (Courtesy of Ken Timby.)

(continued)

SKILL 35-3
Using a Volume-Control Set *(Continued)*

Suggested Action	Reason for Action
Seal the air vent located to the side of the spike on the volume-control set if the solution is in a plastic bag; if the container is glass, leave the air vent open.	Facilitates the administration of fluid from collapsible or noncollapsible containers

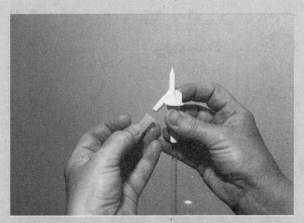

Capping the air vent. (Courtesy of Ken Timby.)

Suggested Action	Reason for Action
Release the clamp above the fluid chamber.	Permits fluid to enter the calibrated container
Fill the calibrated chamber with approximately 30 mL of IV solution and retighten the clamp.	Provides a small volume with which to fill the drip chamber and purge air from the distal tubing
Squeeze and release the drip chamber until it is half full.	Fills the drip chamber with fluid

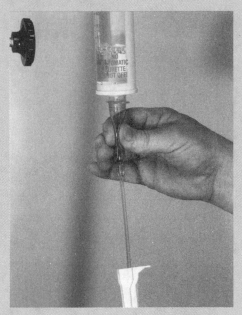

Squeezing the drip chamber. (Courtesy of Ken Timby.)

(continued)

SKILL 35-3
Using a Volume-Control Set (Continued)

Suggested Action	Reason for Action
Note: *For volume-control sets with a membrane filter, the clamp below the drip chamber must be open when the drip chamber is filled or the set will be damaged.*	
Open the lower clamp until the tubing is filled with fluid; then reclamp.	Purges air from the tubing
Open the clamp above the calibrated container, fill the chamber with the desired volume of fluid, and reclamp.	Provides diluent for the medication
Swab the injection port on the calibrated container.	Removes colonizing microorganisms
Instill the prepared medication.	Prepares the drug for administration

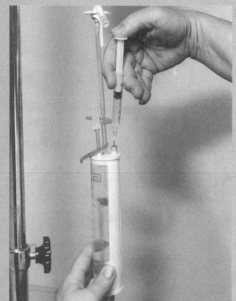

Instilling medication. (Courtesy of Ken Timby.)

Suggested Action	Reason for Action
Rotate the fluid chamber back and forth.	Mixes the drug throughout the fluid
Connect the tubing to the patient's IV catheter.	Completes the circuit for administering IV medication
Release the lower clamp and regulate the drip rate.	Continues the administration of fluid replacement

(continued)

SKILL 35-3
Using a Volume-Control Set *(Continued)*

Suggested Action	Reason for Action
Add a label to the fluid chamber identifying the name of the drug, dose, time it was added, and your initials.	Provides information for other health professionals

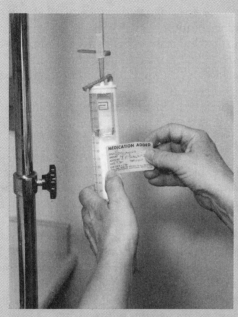

Attaching a drug label. (Courtesy of Ken Timby.)

Suggested Action	Reason for Action
Return before the time the medication is due to finish instilling.	Facilitates further fluid therapy
Release the upper clamp when the fluid chamber is empty and refill it with the next hour's worth of fluid.	Continues the administration of fluid replacement
Readjust the rate, if that is required.	Accommodates for differences between the rates for medication and fluid administration
Remove the drug label from the fluid chamber.	No longer applies after the medication is instilled

Evaluation
• Medicated solution instills within the specified period of time with no adverse effects

Document
• Patient and site assessment data
• The date, time, drug, dose, and initials
• Solution to which drug has been added
• Response of the patient

*Sample Documentation**

Date and Time   Azactam 1 g added to 100 mL of D5/W within volume-control chamber and instilled IV over 60 min. Site is not irritated, tender, or swollen. Lungs sound clear. 100 mL urine output in the past hour. _____ **Signature, Title**

* The administration of drugs is usually documented on the MAR.

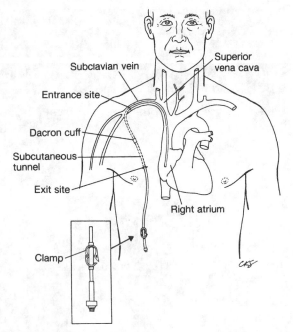

FIGURE 35-7
A tunneled catheter. (Ellis JR, Nowlis EA, Bentz PM: Modules For Basic Nursing Skills, 5th ed, p 477. Philadelphia, JB Lippincott, 1992)

the potential for infection because an internal cuff acts as a barrier against migrating microorganisms. Some examples of tunneled catheters include the Hickman, Broviac, and Groshong catheters.

Implanted Catheters

An implanted catheter, like the Porta-Cath, is one that is totally sealed beneath the skin (Fig. 35-8). Consequently, it provides the greatest protection against infection.

Implanted catheters have a self-sealing port that is pierced through the skin with a special needle when administering IV medications or solutions. To reduce skin discomfort, a local anesthetic is first applied topically. Implanted ports can sustain approximately 2,000 punctures, making it possible for the catheter to remain in place for several years, barring any complications. A dressing is applied only when the catheter is being used. Implanted catheters remain patent with monthly flushing with heparin.

Medication Administration

Intravenous medications may be instilled through any of the types of central venous catheters. They are usually administered by continuous or intermittent infusions; percutaneous and tunneled catheters are more commonly used.

NURSING GUIDELINES FOR USING A CENTRAL VENOUS CATHETER

- Prepare the IV solution, tubing, and drug following those steps described for administering a continuous or secondary infusion.
  Rationale: Principles for preparation remain the same
- Prepare a syringe with 3 to 5 mL of sterile normal saline solution.
  Rationale: Facilitates clearing the catheter of heparin if that is used to maintain patency
- Release the clamp, if there is one, on the exposed section of catheter.
  Rationale: Facilitates flushing the catheter
- Swab the sealed port at the end of the catheter with alcohol.
  Rationale: Removes colonizing microorganisms
- Pierce the port with the syringe containing the saline and instill the flush solution (Fig. 35-9).
  Rationale: Clears the catheter of previous flush solution
- Swab again, and insert the needle, recessed needle, or needleless adapter through the port.
  Rationale: Provides access to the circulatory system
- Tape the needle in place for a continuous infusion; adapters are usually self-securing.
  Rationale: Prevents displacement
- Release the clamp on the tubing and regulate the rate of infusion.
  Rationale: Administers the medication according to the prescribed rate
- Remove the needle or adapter from the port when the medicated solution has instilled.
  Rationale: Terminates the current use of the catheter
- Flush the catheter with saline or heparin according to the agency's protocol.
  Rationale: Maintains patency of the catheter
- Reclamp the catheter.
  Rationale: Prevents complications such as air embolism (see Chap. 15)

Central venous catheters are often used to administer antineoplastic drugs to cancer patients. Administration of these drugs requires special safety precautions.

ADMINISTERING ANTINEOPLASTIC DRUGS

Antineoplastic drugs are those medications that are used to destroy or slow the growth of malignant cells. Patients and nurses sometimes refer to the use of anti-

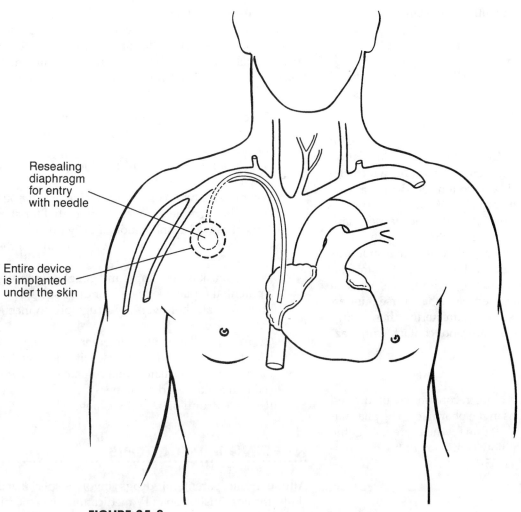

Resealing
diaphragm
for entry
with needle

Entire device
is implanted
under the skin

FIGURE 35-8
Placement of an implanted catheter. (Ellis JR, Nowlis EA, Bentz PM: Modules For Basic Nursing Skills, 5th ed, p 476. Philadelphia, JB Lippincott, 1992)

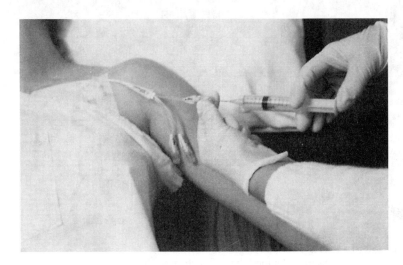

FIGURE 35-9
Flushing the lumen. (Courtesy of Ken Timby.)

neoplastic drugs as **chemotherapy**; some shorten the term to "chemo."

Administration Hazards

Antineoplastic drugs are toxic to both normal and abnormal cells. It has been found that these drugs can even cause adverse effects in the pharmacists who mix them and the nurses who administer them.

Antineoplastic drugs can be absorbed by health care professionals through skin contact, inhalation of tiny fluid droplets or dust particles on which the droplets fall, or oral absorption of drug residue during hand-to-mouth contact. When transferred to the caregiver, these drugs can cause headaches, nausea, dizziness, and burning or itching of the skin. Long-term, unprotected exposure to small amounts of antineoplastic drugs can lead to changes in fast-growing body cells, including sperm, ova, or fetal tissue. It is important, therefore, that nurses understand safety measures for administering these drugs and how to avoid exposure and contact with hazardous materials.

Drug Preparation

In most cases, drugs are reconstituted or diluted with sterile IV solutions in the pharmacy. The pharmacist wears protective clothing when preparing the drugs under a vertical flow containment hood or biologic safety cabinet (Fig. 35-10).

Drug Administration

To warn nurses to take special precautions during drug administration, the pharmacist usually attaches a special label (Fig. 35-11). Some common recommendations for avoiding self-contamination with antineoplastic drugs include the following:

- Cover the drug preparation area with a disposable paper pad that will absorb a small drug spill, if it should occur.
- Don a long-sleeved, cuffed, low-permeability gown with a closed front.
- Wear one or two pairs of surgical latex, *nonpowdered* gloves, which reduce the potential for skin contact as well as inhalation of drug powder.
- Cover the cuffs of the gown with the cuffs of the gloves.
- Wear a mask or respirator and goggles if there is a potential for aerosolization or drug splash.
- Pour 70% alcohol over any drug spill to inactivate the drug.
- Clean the spill area with detergent and water at least three times and then rinse with clean water.
- Dispose of all substances that contain drug material into a biohazard container.
- Perform scrupulous handwashing.

NURSING IMPLICATIONS

Although all parenteral drugs involve specialized skills, the administration of IV medications, in general, and antineoplastic drugs, in particular, requires extreme caution. During the period of patient care, some of the accompanying Applicable Nursing Diagnoses may be identified.

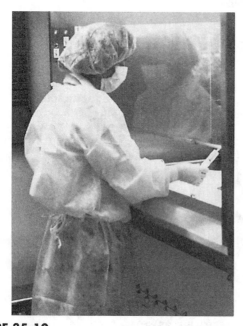

FIGURE 35-10
Pharmacy preparation of antineoplastic drugs. (Courtesy of Ken Timby.)

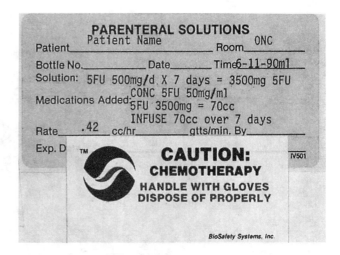

FIGURE 35-11
Drug warning label. (Courtesy of Ken Timby.)

NURSING CARE PLAN:
Risk for Altered Protection

Assessment	**Subjective Data** States, "I haven't been eating much. It's difficult to swallow; as a result I'm losing weight and feeling very weak." **Objective Data** 26-year-old man admitted with enlarged cervical and axillary lymph nodes. Medical diagnosis is Hodgkin's lymphoma. Has had a Hickman central venous catheter inserted and will begin chemotherapy. Potential side effect is thrombocytopenia.
Diagnosis	Risk for Altered Protection related to debilitated state and tendency to bleed secondary to side effect of chemotherapy.
Plan	**Goal** Blood loss will be minimal as evidenced by normal red blood cell count and negative hemoccult tests on urine and stool throughout hospitalization. **Orders:** 2/10 1. Obtain all blood samples from central line. 2. Monitor platelet count and hold chemotherapy if count is < 100,000 until physician is consulted. 3. Assess skin for bruising, catheter site for bleeding, and test urine and stool for occult blood q day. 4. Avoid aspirin or products containing salicylates. 5. Use a soft-bristle toothbrush or swabs for mouth care. 6. Substitute oral forms of medications rather than IM whenever possible. 7. If injections must be given, apply pressure for at least 3 minutes or longer to control bleeding. _____ N. HURDER, RN
Implementation (Documentation)	2/10 1300 Blood for CBC and chemistry profile obtained from central venous catheter. Catheter flushed following blood draw. Results of blood tests unavailable at this time. _____ A. VALERIONI, LPN
Evaluation (Documentation)	1300 Skin is intact except at catheter insertion site. No evidence of bleeding from site. No bruises noted on skin. Urine and stool test negative for occult blood. Has not taken any over-the-counter aspirin products in the last 2 weeks. Soft-bristle toothbrush used for mouth care. No evidence of active bleeding from gums after mouth care. Not currently scheduled for injectable medications except those that will infuse through the central line. _____ A. VALERIONI, LPN

APPLICABLE NURSING DIAGNOSES

- Anxiety
- Fear
- Risk for Injury
- Risk for Infection
- Fluid Volume Excess
- Altered Protection

The Nursing Care Plan for this chapter demonstrates the nursing process as it applies to a patient with the nursing diagnosis of Risk for Altered Protection. This diagnosis may be associated with the undesirable consequences of antineoplastic medication therapy. It is defined in the 1994 NANDA taxonomy as "The state in which an individual experiences a decrease in the ability to guard the self from internal or external threats such as illness or injury." An example might be deficient immunity or an altered ability to control bleeding.

FOCUS ON OLDER ADULTS

- Early discharges may require teaching older adults how to flush venous access equipment like medication locks on peripheral and central venous catheters because some may be discharged and resume treatment on an outpatient basis.
- Older adults are the largest age group of patients cared for in acute and long-term health care agencies. Therefore, it is quite common for them to be recipients of IV medications.
- Older adults require frequent and comprehensive assessment both before and after IV medication administration because they are more likely to manifest adverse reactions due to age-related changes.
- The veins of older adults tend to be quite fragile. A percutaneous central venous catheter is often better than risking the trauma of repeated attempts at restarting or changing IV sites.
- To avoid the hazards of infiltrating tissue with medications that should be delivered intravenously, it may be appropriate to collaborate with the physician on administering the same drug by another route.
- It is important to explain the purpose for each drug that is administered because some older adults have a tendency not to ask questions of health care professionals.
- A portion of many drugs is bound to protein in the blood. Drugs that are protein bound are basically inactive. That which is not bound is called *free drug*; it is the free portion of drugs that is physiologically active. Older adults tend to have more free drug in proportion to bound drug. Therefore, they are more likely to experience adverse drug effects.
- Another cause for adverse drug effects among older adults is the fact that they tend to metabolize and excrete drugs at a slower rate. This factor may predispose older adults to toxic effects from the accumulation of normal doses of medication.
- With the revocation of the Medicare Catastrophic Coverage Act of 1988, the costs for administering IV drugs during home care are not currently reimbursed (Rice, 1992).

KEY CONCEPTS

- Intravenous medications can be given into peripheral or central veins.
- The IV route is appropriate when a quick response is needed during an emergency; when patients have disorders that affect absorption or metabolism of drugs; and when blood levels of drugs need to be maintained at a consistent therapeutic level.
- Intravenous medications can be administered continuously or intermittently.
- Two methods for administering a bolus of IV medication are using a port on an IV tubing or using a medication lock.
- Medicated solutions may be administered intermittently using secondary, piggyback infusions or a volume-control set.
- A piggyback solution is a small volume of diluted medication that is connected to, and positioned higher than, the primary solution.
- A volume-control set is used to administer IV medication in a small volume of solution at intermittent intervals, and to avoid overloading the circulatory system.
- A central venous catheter is a venous access device that extends to the vena cava or right atrium.
- There are three general types of central venous catheters: percutaneous, tunneled, and implanted.
- When administering antineoplastic drugs, it is best to wear a cover gown, one or two pairs of gloves, and a disposable or respirator mask as a means of protecting oneself from contact with or inhalation of the medication.

CRITICAL THINKING EXERCISES

- Discuss the advantages and disadvantages of giving IV medications to older adults.
- When preparing to administer an IV medication through an IV port or lock, you find there is no blood return on aspiration. Discuss the significance of this finding and what actions are appropriate.

SUGGESTED READINGS

Gurevich I. Preventing needlesticks. RN November 1994;57:44–49.

Hendrickson ML. How to access an implanted port. Nursing January 1993;23:50–53.

Howard MP, Eisenberg PG, Gianino MS. Dressing a central venous catheter: a better way. Nursing March 1992;22:60–61.

Larson EL, Cheng G, Choo JTE. In vitro survival of skin flora in heparin locks and needleless valve infusion devices. Heart and Lung September–October 1993;22:459–462.

McMullen A, Fioravanti ID, Pollack V. Heparinized saline or normal saline as a flush solution in intermittent intravenous lines in infants and children. MCN: The American Journal of Maternal–Child Nursing March–April 1993;18:78–85.

Munz N. Evaluating needleless IV tubing. American Journal of Nursing February 1993;93:74–75.

Murray EW. Probing the safety of central venous catheters. American Journal of Nursing May 1993;93:72, 74–76.

Parker GG. Chemotherapy administration in the home. Home Healthcare Nurse January–February 1992;10:30–36.

Rice R. Home Health Nursing Practice: Concepts and Application. St. Louis: Mosby Year Book, 1992.

Tillman KR. Venous access devices: guidelines for home healthcare nurses. Home Healthcare Nurse September–October 1991;9:13–17.

UNIT XI

Intervening in Emergency Situations

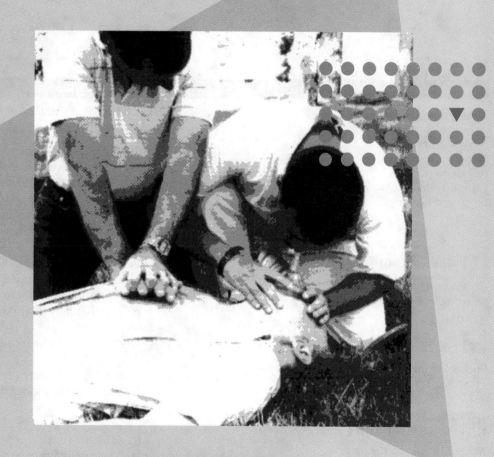

CHAPTER 36
Airway Management
CHAPTER 37
Resuscitation

773

CHAPTER 36
Airway Management

Key Terms

Airway	Oropharyngeal Suctioning
Airway Management	Percussion
Chest Physiotherapy	Postural Drainage
Inhalation Therapy	Sputum
Mucus	Suctioning
Nasopharyngeal Suctioning	Tracheostomy
Nasotracheal Suctioning	Tracheostomy Care
Oral Airway	Tracheostomy Tube
Oral Suctioning	Vibration

Learning Objectives

An understanding of the content within this chapter will be evidenced by the student's ability to:

- Describe the airway and its function
- List structures that make up the airway
- Discuss three natural mechanisms that protect the airway
- Describe what airway management includes
- Name two techniques for liquefying respiratory secretions
- Explain chest physiotherapy and name three techniques that are included
- Describe at least three types of suctioning techniques that may be used to clear secretions from the airway
- Discuss two indications for inserting an artificial airway
- Name two examples of artificial airways
- Name three components of tracheostomy care

The primary function of the respiratory system is to facilitate ventilation so that there is appropriate exchange of oxygen and carbon dioxide at the cellular level (see Chap. 20). Adequate ventilation, however, depends on clear air passages from the nose to the alveoli. This chapter focuses on the nursing skills that help to ensure that the structures of the airway remain open and clear.

THE AIRWAY

The **airway** is the collective system of tubes in the upper and lower respiratory tract through which gases travel during their passage to and from the alveoli (Fig. 36-1).

Timby BK: *Fundamental Skills and Concepts in Patient Care, Sixth Edition* © 1996 Lippincott-Raven Publishers

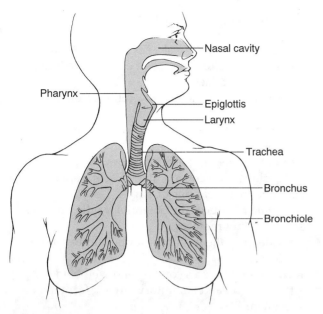

FIGURE 36-1
The airway and related structures.

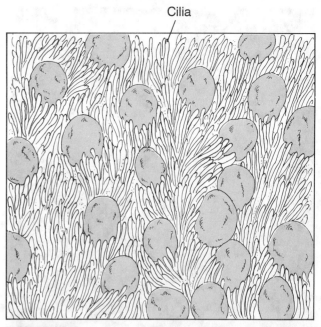

FIGURE 36-2
Cilia and mucous producing cells.

The upper airway consists of the nose and pharynx, which is subdivided into the nasopharynx, oropharynx, and laryngopharynx. The lower airway is made up of the trachea, bronchi, and bronchioles. Additional structures and mechanisms keep the airway open and protect it from a wide variety of inhaled substances.

Airway Protection

The main structures that protect the airway are the epiglottis, tracheal cartilage, mucous membrane, and cilia. The epiglottis is a protrusion of flexible cartilage located above the larynx. It acts as a lid that closes during swallowing so that fluid and food is directed toward the esophagus rather than the respiratory tract. The rings of tracheal cartilage ensure that the trachea, the portion of the airway beneath the larynx, remains open.

The respiratory passages are lined with mucous membrane, a type of tissue from which mucus is secreted. The sticky mucus acts to trap particulate matter. In the nose, the debris can be cleared by sneezing or blowing. That which collects in the lower airway is beaten upward on hair-like projections called cilia (Fig. 36-2). Once it is raised to the level of the upper airway, the mucus, now referred to as **sputum**, is cleared from the upper airway by coughing, expectoration, or swallowing.

Certain factors may jeopardize the patency of the airway. Some examples may include:

- Increased volume of mucus
- Thick mucus
- Fatigue or weakness

- Decreased level of consciousness
- Ineffective cough
- Impaired airway

Consequently, it may become necessary to assist patients with measures that support or replace their own natural efforts.

AIRWAY MANAGEMENT

Airway management refers to those skills that maintain natural or artificial airways for compromised patients.

Maintaining the Natural Airway

The natural airway is most often maintained by keeping respiratory secretions liquefied, promoting their expectoration with chest physiotherapy, or mechanically clearing mucus from the airway by means of suctioning.

LIQUEFYING SECRETIONS

Mucus is a mixture of mucin, white blood cells, electrolytes, cells that have been shed through the natural process of tissue replacement, and water. The volume of water affects the *viscosity*, or thickness, of the mucus.

To keep the mucus at a consistency that will facilitate expectoration, nurses keep patients adequately hydrated (see Chap. 15). Hydration, the process of providing an adequate fluid intake, tends to keep the mucous membranes moist and the mucus thin.

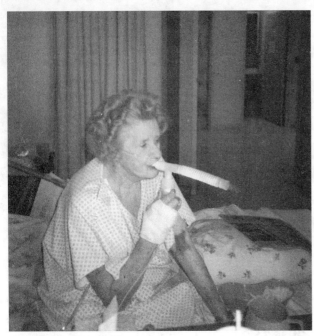

FIGURE 36-3
Aerosol therapy. (Courtesy of Ken Timby.)

Rationale: Avoids inconclusive or invalid test results
- Instruct the patient to take several deep breaths, attempt a forceful cough, and expectorate into the specimen container.
Rationale: Helps mobilize secretions from the lower airway
- Collect at least a 1- to 3-mL (nearly ½ teaspoon) specimen.
Rationale: Ensures sufficient quantity
- Wear gloves and cover and enclose the specimen container in a clear plastic bag.
Rationale: Reduces the potential for the transmission of microorganisms
- Provide the patient with the opportunity for oral hygiene.
Rationale: Promotes comfort and well-being
- Attach a label and laboratory request form to the specimen.
Rationale: Ensures correct specimen identification and test procedure
- Take the specimen to the laboratory immediately.
Rationale: Facilitates prompt and accurate analysis of the specimen

In addition, nurses may assist with inhalation therapy. **Inhalation therapy**, also known as *aerosol therapy*, refers to respiratory treatments that provide a mixture of oxygen, humidification, and aerosolized medications directly to the lungs. The aerosol is delivered through a mask or hand-held mouthpiece (Fig. 36-3). Aerosol therapy improves breathing, facilitates spontaneous coughing, and helps patients raise sputum so that it can be analyzed for diagnostic purposes.

◄ NURSING GUIDELINES FOR COLLECTING A SPUTUM SPECIMEN

- Plan to collect a sputum specimen just after the patient awakens or after an aerosol treatment.
Rationale: Correlates with a time when there is a greater volume of mucus available or it is in a thinner state
- Obtain a sterile sputum specimen cup.
Rationale: Prevents extraneous contamination of the specimen
- Encourage the patient to rinse his or her mouth with tap water.
Rationale: Removes some microorganisms and food residue from the mouth
- Explain that the desired specimen should be from deep within the respiratory passages, not saliva from within the mouth.

CHEST PHYSIOTHERAPY

Chest physiotherapy refers to techniques for mobilizing secretions from within distal airways using postural drainage, percussion, and vibration. Chest physiotherapy is usually indicated for patients with chronic respiratory diseases who have difficulty coughing or raising thick mucus.

Postural Drainage
Postural drainage is a physical technique in which patients are positioned so as to facilitate gravity drainage from various lobes or segments of their lung(s) (Fig. 36-4). In most hospitals, respiratory therapists are responsible for postural drainage. In long-term care facilities and home health care, however, nurses may teach or supervise this intervention.

The effectiveness of postural drainage can be further enhanced by performing percussion and vibration.

Percussion
Percussion refers to a rhythmic striking of the chest wall. The object is to dislodge respiratory secretions that adhere to the bronchial walls. When done appropriately, the hands are cupped by flexing and keeping the fingers and thumb together as if to carry water. The cupped hands are then applied to the chest as though trapping air between the hands and the patient's tho-

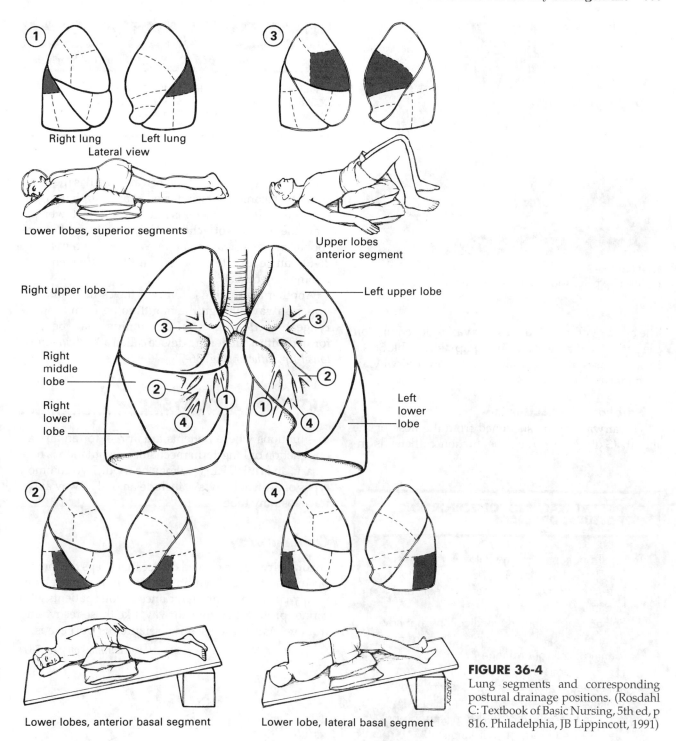

Right lung   Left lung
Lateral view

Lower lobes, superior segments

Upper lobes
anterior segment

Right upper lobe — ——— Left upper lobe

Right
middle
lobe —

Right
lower
lobe —

Left
lower
lobe

Lower lobes, anterior basal segment   Lower lobe, lateral basal segment

FIGURE 36-4

Lung segments and corresponding postural drainage positions. (Rosdahl C: Textbook of Basic Nursing, 5th ed, p 816. Philadelphia, JB Lippincott, 1991)

racic wall (Fig. 36-5). Percussion may be performed for 3 to 5 minutes in each position of postural drainage. When percussion is performed, care is taken to avoid striking the breasts of female patients and any areas where there is a concurrent chest injury or bone disease.

Vibration

Vibration is a technique in which the flat surfaces of the hands are used to shake the underlying tissue to loosen retained secretions. The hands are positioned during inhalation and vibrated as the patient exhales so as to increase the intensity of expiration. Vibration may be used with or as an alternative to percussion, especially for patients who are frail.

SUCTIONING

Suctioning is a technique for removing liquid secretions with a catheter using negative (vacuum) pressure.

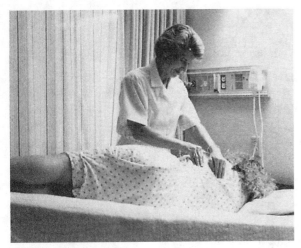

FIGURE 36-5
Performing percussion. (Courtesy of Ken Timby.)

The amount of negative pressure varies depending on the patient and type of suction equipment (Table 36-1). In some cases, the upper airway, the lower airway, or both may be suctioned.

Nasal and Oral Suctioning

The airway can be suctioned from the nose or the mouth (Skill 36-1). When the suction catheter is in-

---

TABLE 36-1. *Variations in Suction Pressure*		
Age	Wall Suction	Portable Suction Machine
Adults	100–140 mm Hg	10–15 mm Hg
Children	95–100 mm Hg	5–10 mm Hg
Infants	50–95 mm Hg	2–5 mm Hg

serted nasally into the upper airway, which is the more common technique, it is referred to as **nasopharyngeal suctioning**. If the catheter is advanced to the lower airway, the term **nasotracheal suctioning** is used. A nasopharyngeal airway, sometimes called a *trumpet* (Fig. 36-6), can be used to protect the nostril if frequent suctioning is necessary.

Another alternative is to insert the catheter into the upper airway through the mouth to perform **oropharyngeal suctioning**. **Oral suctioning** may be performed with a suctioning device called a *Yankeur-tip*, or *tonsil-tip*, *catheter* (Fig. 36-7).

ARTIFICIAL AIRWAYS

In situations where patients are at risk for an airway obstruction or long-term mechanical ventilation is necessary, an artificial airway may be used. Two common types of artificial airways include an oral airway and a tracheostomy tube.

Oral Airway

An **oral airway** is a curved device that keeps the tongue positioned forward within the mouth. It is most commonly used when caring for unconscious patients who cannot protect their own airway, like those recovering from general anesthesia or a seizure. Its purpose is to

(text continues on page 784)

┌─────────────────────────────────────┐
│ ◈ **PATIENT TEACHING FOR PERFORMING** │
│   **POSTURAL DRAINAGE**   │
└─────────────────────────────────────┘

Teach the patient to do the following:
* Plan to perform postural drainage two to four times each day, such as before meals and bedtime.
* Self-administer inhaled medications that have been prescribed (see Chap. 33) before performing postural drainage.
* Have paper tissues and a waterproof container nearby for collecting expectorated sputum.
* Position yourself so as to drain the appropriate diseased areas of your lung(s).
* Cough and expectorate the secretions that drain into the upper airway.
* Remain in each of the prescribed positions for at least 15 to 30 minutes, but no longer than 45 minutes.
* Resume a position of comfort after the usual volume of sputum has been expectorated, or if you experience fatigue, lightheadedness, rapid pulse rate, difficulty breathing, or chest pain.

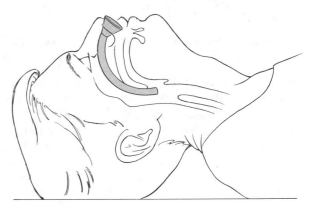

FIGURE 36-6
Placement of a nasopharyngeal trumpet.

Suggested Action	Reason for Action
Assessment	
Assess the patient's lung sounds, respiratory effort, and oxygen saturation level.	Determines the need for suctioning
Determine how much the patient understands about suctioning the airway.	Provides an opportunity for health teaching
Inspect the nose to determine if one or the other nostril is more patent.	Eases insertion of the catheter
Planning	
Obtain a suction kit. Equipment may vary, but all contain a basin and one or two sterile gloves. Some kits may also contain a sterile suction catheter.	Promotes organization and efficient time management
Select a catheter size, if one is not included, that will not occlude the diameter of the nostril; usually a 12- to 18-F catheter is appropriate for an adult.	Promotes comfort and reduces the potential for injury
Secure a flask of sterile normal saline and a suction machine, if a wall outlet is unavailable.	Provides items that are not prepackaged
Attach the suction canister to the wall outlet or plug a portable suction machine into an electrical outlet.	Provides a source for negative pressure
Connect the suction tubing to the canister.	Provides a means for connecting the canister to the suction catheter
Turn on the suction machine, occlude the suction tubing, and adjust the pressure gauge to the desired amount.	Ensures safe pressure during suctioning
Open the container of saline.	Reduces the risk for contamination later

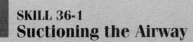

Adjusting the suction pressure. (Courtesy of Ken Timby.)

(continued)

SKILL 36-1
Suctioning the Airway *(Continued)*

Suggested Action	Reason for Action
Implementation	
Pull the privacy curtains.	Demonstrates respect for the patient's dignity
Elevate the head of the bed unless contraindicated.	Aids ventilation
Preoxygenate the patient for 1 to 2 minutes until the SaO_2 is maintained at 95% to 100%.	Reduces the risk of causing hypoxemia
Wash your hands.	Reduces the transmission of microorganisms
Open the suction kit without contaminating the contents.	Follows principles of asepsis
Don sterile glove(s). If only one is provided, don a clean glove on the nondominant hand and then don the sterile glove.	Prevents the transmission of microorganisms
Pour sterile normal saline into the basin with your nondominant hand.	Prepares solution for wetting and rinsing the suction catheter

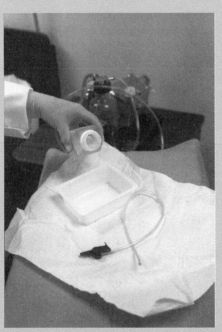

Pouring sterile saline. (Courtesy of Ken Timby.)

(continued)

SKILL 36-1
Suctioning the Airway *(Continued)*

Suggested Action	Reason for Action
Consider the nondominant hand contaminated.	Follows principles of asepsis
Pick up the suction catheter with your sterile (dominant) hand and connect it to the suction tubing.	Completes the circuit for applying suction

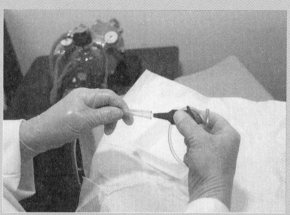

Connecting the catheter. (Courtesy of Ken Timby.)

Place the catheter tip within the saline and occlude the vent.	Wets the outer and inner surfaces of the catheter; reduces friction and facilitates insertion

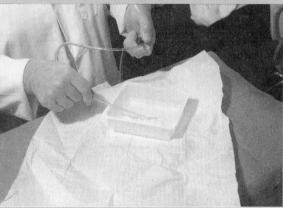

Wetting the catheter. (Courtesy of Ken Timby.)

Insert the catheter without applying suction along the floor of the nose or the side of the mouth.	Reduces the potential for sneezing or gagging
Advance the catheter to a depth of 5 to 6 inches (12.5–15 cm) in the nose or 3 to 4 inches (7.5–10 cm) in the mouth.	Places the distal tip in the pharynx

(continued)

SKILL 36-1
Suctioning the Airway (Continued)

Suggested Action	Reason for Action

Catheter placement. (*A*) Nasopharyngeal, (*B*) Oropharyngeal, and (*C*) Nasotracheal.

Suggested Action	Reason for Action
For tracheal suctioning, wait until the patient takes a breath and advance the tubing 8 to 10 inches (20–25 cm).	Eases insertion below the larynx
Encourage the patient to cough if it does not occur spontaneously.	Breaks up mucus and raises secretions
Occlude the air vent and rotate the catheter as it is withdrawn.	Maximizes effectiveness of suctioning
Complete the process in no more than 15 seconds from the time of insertion of the catheter to its removal; the vent is occluded no longer than 10 seconds.	Prevents hypoxemia
Rinse the secretions from the catheter by inserting the tip within the basin of saline and applying suction.	Flushes the mucus from the inner lumen
Provide a 2- to 3-minute period of rest while the patient continues to breathe oxygen.	Reoxygenates the blood
Suction again if it appears necessary.	Bases decision on individual assessment data
Pull the gloves off so as to enclose the suction catheter within an inverted glove.	Encloses the soiled catheter so as to reduce transmission of microorganisms

(continued)

SKILL 36-1
Suctioning the Airway (Continued)

Suggested Action	Reason for Action

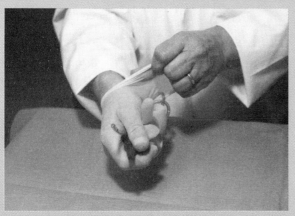

Enclosing the catheter. (Courtesy of Ken Timby.)

Discard suction kit, catheter, and gloves in a lined waste receptacle.   Follows principles of asepsis

Evaluation
- The airway is cleared of secretions
- The SaO_2 level remains at 95% or more
- Breathing requires less effort

Document
- Preassessment data
- Type of suctioning performed
- Appearance of secretions
- Patient's response

Sample Documentation

Date and Time   Respirations sound moist and noisy. SaO_2 shows a drop from 95% to 93% during last 15 minutes. Coughing effort is weak and ineffective. Raised to a high Fowler's position and oxygenated at 4 L per nasal cannula. Tracheal suctioning performed and reoxygenated. Lungs sound clear at this time. Pulse oximeter indicates SaO_2 at 95% at this time. _____ **Signature, Title**

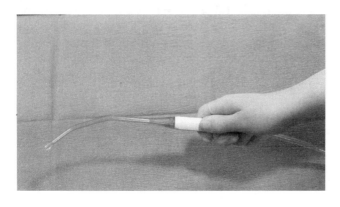

FIGURE 36-7
Yankeur-tip suction device for oral suctioning. (Courtesy of Ken Timby.)

prevent an upper airway obstruction caused by a relaxed tongue.

Oral airways are inserted by nurses. They are usually used for a very brief amount of time.

◄ NURSING GUIDELINES FOR INSERTING AN ORAL AIRWAY

- Gather the following supplies: various sizes of oral airways (most adults can accommodate an 80-mm airway), gloves, tongue blade, and suction equipment.
  Rationale: Promotes organization and efficient time management
- Place the airway on the outside of the cheek so that the front is parallel with the front teeth and note if the back of the airway reaches the angle of the jaw.
  Rationale: Determines the appropriate size to use (if the airway is too short, it will be ineffective; if it is too long, it will depress the epiglottis, potentiating the risk for an airway obstruction)
- Wash your hands and don clean gloves.
  Rationale: Reduces the transmission of microorganisms
- Explain what is about to be done.
  Rationale: Provides information that some unconscious patients may comprehend even though they may not respond verbally
- Perform oral suctioning if necessary.
  Rationale: Clears saliva from the mouth and prevents aspiration
- Place the patient in a supine position with the neck hyperextended, unless contraindicated.
  Rationale: Opens the airway and facilitates insertion

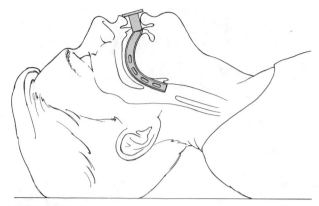

FIGURE 36-9
Final position of an oral airway after rotation.

- Open the patient's mouth using a gloved finger and thumb, or use a tongue blade.
  Rationale: Prevents injury to the teeth during insertion
- Hold the airway so that the curved tip points upward toward the roof of the mouth (Fig. 36-8) or toward the side of the cheek, and insert it about halfway.
  Rationale: Prevents pushing the tongue into the pharynx during insertion
- Rotate the airway over the top of the tongue and continue inserting it until the front flange is flush with lips (Fig. 36-9).
  Rationale: Ensures that the artificial airway follows the natural curve of the upper airway
- Assess breathing.
  Rationale: Indicates that the natural airway is patent
- Remove the airway every 4 hours; provide oral hygiene; clean and reinsert the airway.
  Rationale: Removes transient bacteria; promotes integrity of the oral mucosa

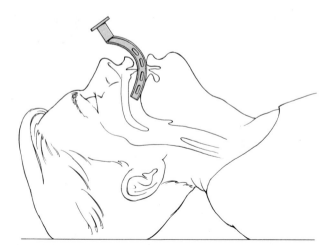

FIGURE 36-8
Initial insertion position for an oral airway.

As the level of consciousness becomes elevated, many patients extubate, or remove, an oral airway independently. Patients who are less stable, have an upper airway obstruction, or require prolonged ventilation and oxygenation are more likely candidates for a tracheostomy.

Tracheostomy

A **tracheostomy** is an opening into the trachea that is surgically created. A tube is inserted through the opening to maintain the airway and provide a new route for ventilation.

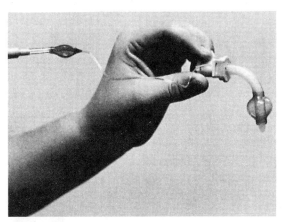

FIGURE 36-10
A cuffed tracheostomy tube. (Courtesy of Ken Timby.)

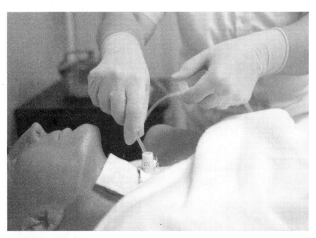

FIGURE 36-11
Suctioning through a tracheostomy tube. (Courtesy of Ken Timby.)

TRACHEOSTOMY TUBE

A **tracheostomy tube** consists of a curved, plastic, hollow tube called a *cannula*. Some are constructed with an inner and an outer cannula. The tracheostomy tube may also have a balloon cuff (Fig. 36-10) that, when inflated, seals the upper airway to prevent aspiration of oral fluids and provides more efficient ventilation. During the initial insertion of a tracheostomy tube, another component, called an *obturator*, is used. The obturator is a curved guide that facilitates placement of the tube within the trachea. Once the tube is in place, the obturator is removed because it is no longer needed.

Because a tracheostomy tube is below the level of the larynx, patients are usually unable to speak in their natural voice. Communication is facilitated by writing or reading the patient's lips. Being unable to call verbally for help, if it may be needed, is very frightening for most patients with a tracheostomy. Therefore, it is important to check these patients frequently and respond immediately when they signal.

TRACHEOSTOMY SUCTIONING

Most tracheostomy patients require frequent suctioning. Although they can cough, the force of the cough may be ineffective in completely clearing their airway, or the cough may be inadequate considering the volume of their respiratory secretions. Therefore, suctioning is necessary whenever there are copious secretions.

Tracheostomy suctioning is performed similarly to nasotracheal suctioning, except that the catheter is inserted within the tracheostomy tube rather than the nose (Fig. 36-11). The catheter is also inserted a shorter distance because the tube lies within the trachea. A rule of thumb that some nurses use is to insert the catheter approximately 4 to 5 inches (10–12.5 cm) or until there

is resistance. The resistance is caused by contact between the catheter tip and the *carina*, the ridge at the lower end of the tracheal cartilage where the main bronchi are located. The catheter is then raised about ½ inch (1.25 cm) and suction is applied.

Tracheal suctioning may be done separate from or at the same time as tracheostomy care is provided.

TRACHEOSTOMY CARE

Tracheostomy care involves cleaning the skin around the stoma, changing the dressing, and cleaning the inner cannula (Skill 36-2). Tracheostomy care is performed at least every 8 hours or as often as needed to keep the secretions from becoming dried, thus narrowing the airway.

NURSING IMPLICATIONS

Maintaining an open and patent airway is a priority for nursing care. Lack of oxygen for more than 4 to 6 minutes can result in death or permanent brain damage. Therefore, it is essential to identify nursing diagnoses that apply to respiratory problems and plan care accordingly for patients who are at risk. Some diagnoses that are possible include those listed in the accompanying Applicable Nursing Diagnoses.

The Nursing Care Plan for this chapter has been developed to illustrate how the nursing process applies to a patient with Ineffective Airway Clearance. This diagnostic problem is defined in the 1994 NANDA taxonomy as "A state in which an individual is unable to clear secretions or obstructions from the respiratory tract to maintain airway patency."

(text continues on page 791)

Suggested Action	Reason for Action
Assessment	
Check the nursing care plan to determine the schedule for providing tracheostomy care.	Provides continuity of care
Review the patient's record for documentation concerning previous tracheostomy care.	Provides a data base for comparison
Assess the condition of the dressing and the skin around the tracheostomy tube.	Determines need for skin care and dressing change
Determine the patient's understanding of tracheostomy care.	Provides an opportunity for health teaching
Planning	
Consult with the patient on an appropriate time for performing tracheostomy care if only routine care is needed.	Demonstrates respect for the patient's right to participate in decisions
Obtain a tracheostomy care kit, which usually includes sterile gloves, two basins, a drape, gauze squares, pipe cleaners, cotton-tipped applicators, forceps, stomal dressing, and twill ties.	Promotes organization and efficient time management
Secure a container of hydrogen peroxide and a flask of normal saline. Remove the cap from each container.	Provides items that are not prepackaged and prevents contamination of one gloved hand later in the procedure
Implementation	
Wash your hands.	Removes colonizing microorganisms
Raise the bed to an appropriate height.	Prevents back strain
Place the patient in a supine or low Fowler's position.	Facilitates access to the tracheostomy tube
Don a clean glove and remove the soiled stomal dressing and discard it, glove and all, within a lined waste receptacle.	Follows principles of asepsis
Wash your hands again.	Reduces the transmission of microorganisms
Open the tracheostomy kit, taking care not to contaminate its contents.	Provides access to supplies and maintains their sterility
Don sterile gloves, one of which—usually the one on the dominant hand—must remain sterile.	Prevents transferring microorganisms to the lower airway
Lip the containers of solution and add sterile normal saline to one basin and sterile hydrogen peroxide to the other.	Follows principles of asepsis; the hand used to pour the liquids is now considered contaminated

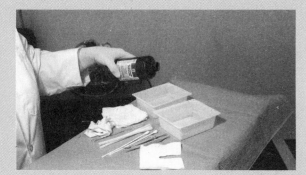

Adding cleaning solutions. (Courtesy of Ken Timby.)

(continued)

SKILL 36-2
Providing Tracheostomy Care *(Continued)*

Suggested Action	Reason for Action
Unlock the inner cannula by turning it counter-clockwise and deposit it within the basin of hydrogen peroxide.	Loosens protein secretions and reduces the numbers of colonizing microorganisms

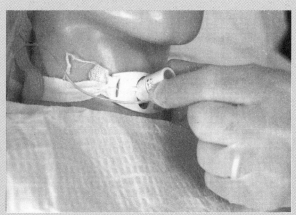

Removing the inner cannula. (Courtesy of Ken Timby.)

Suggested Action	Reason for Action
Clean the inside and outside of the cannula with pipe cleaners.	Removes gross debris

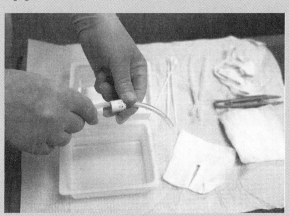

Cleaning the inner cannula. (Courtesy of Ken Timby.)

Suggested Action	Reason for Action
Deposit contaminated supplies in a lined or waterproof waste receptacle.	Reduces the potential for contaminating sterile supplies
Rinse the cleaned cannula in the basin of normal saline.	Removes remnants of hydrogen peroxide
Tap the rinsed cannula against the edge of the basin and wipe the excess solution with a gauze square.	Removes large droplets of fluid

(continued)

SKILL 36-2
Providing Tracheostomy Care (Continued)

Suggested Action	Reason for Action
Replace the inner cannula and turn it clockwise within the outer cannula.	Secures the inner cannula

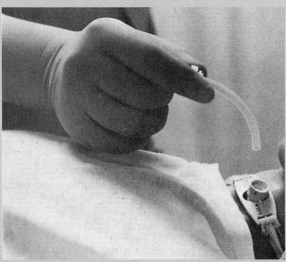

Replacing the inner cannula.

Suggested Action	Reason for Action
Clean around the stoma with an applicator moistened with peroxide. Never go back over an area once it has been cleaned.	Removes secretions and colonizing microorganisms from the tracheal opening

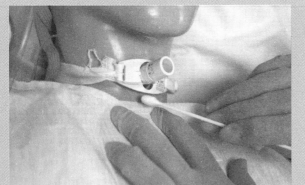

Cleaning the stoma. (Courtesy of Ken Timby.)

Suggested Action	Reason for Action
Wipe the same area in the same manner with another applicator moistened with saline.	Removes the hydrogen peroxide from the skin

(continued)

SKILL 36-2
Providing Tracheostomy Care *(Continued)*

Suggested Action	Reason for Action
Place the sterile stomal dressing around the tracheostomy tube.	Absorbs secretions and keeps the stomal area clean

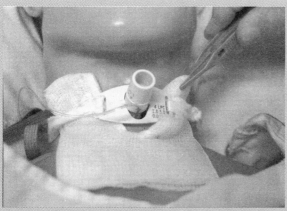

Applying the stomal dressing. (Courtesy of Ken Timby.)

Suggested Action	Reason for Action
Change the tracheostomy ties by threading them through the slits on the flange of the tracheostomy tube and tying them in place.	Holds the tracheostomy tube in place

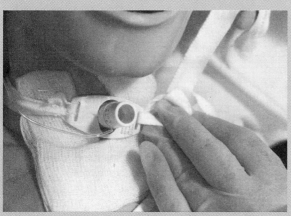

Securing the tracheostomy ties. (Courtesy of Ken Timby.)

Suggested Action	Reason for Action
Wait to remove the previous ties until after the new ones are secure, if working alone. Otherwise have an assistant stabilize the tracheostomy tube while the soiled ones are cut and the new ones are applied.	Prevents accidental extubation
Tie the two ends snugly, but not tightly, at the side of the neck.	Prevents skin impairment
Discard all soiled supplies, remove your gloves, and wash your hands.	Follows principles of asepsis
Return the patient to a position of comfort and safety.	Demonstrates concern for the patient's well-being

(continued)

SKILL 36-2
Providing Tracheostomy Care *(Continued)*

Suggested Action	Reason for Action

Evaluation

- The tracheostomy tube remains patent
- The stomal opening is cleansed and there is no evidence of infection
- The dressing is clean and dry
- The skin about the neck is intact

Document

- Preassessment data
- Procedure as it was performed
- Appearance of skin and secretions
- Response of the patient

Sample Documentation

Date and Time   Respirations are quiet and effortless. Routine tracheostomy care provided. Moderate amount of mucus removed from inner cannula during cleaning. Stomal skin is pink but there is no redness, tenderness, swelling, or purulent drainage. Skin about the neck is intact; skin color is comparable to surrounding areas. __ **Signature, Title**

 FOCUS ON OLDER ADULTS

- Conditions that affect the respiratory system are among the most common life-threatening disorders experienced by older adults.
- The severity of chronic pulmonary diseases increases with age. Many older adults with pathologic pulmonary changes have a history of having smoked cigarettes since their youth, working in occupations where air pollution was not controlled, or living a greater share of their lives in industrial areas known for their toxic emissions.
- When assessing older adults, it is important to inquire about their current history of coughing, determine how long the cough has been present, and obtain a description of sputum that is raised.
- Persistent, dry coughing consumes energy and may cause fatigue among older adults if it is not relieved.
- Some older adults may be unable to cough

- effectively because they experience decreased strength of accessory muscles for respiration and increased rigidity of the chest wall.
- The production of respiratory secretions is often influenced by weather, such as high humidity or damp conditions.
- The muscular structures of the pharynx and larynx also tend to atrophy with age, which can affect the ability to clear the airway.
- There usually is less ventilation at the bases of the lungs in older adults, which contributes to the retention of secretions and compromised ventilation.
- The respiratory cilia become less efficient with age, predisposing older adults to a higher incidence of pneumonia.
- Older adults are at higher risk for developing cardiac dysrhythmias when being suctioned because many have preexisting hypoxemia due to age-related changes in ventilation.

APPLICABLE NURSING DIAGNOSES

- Ineffective Airway Clearance
- Impaired Gas Exchange
- Risk for Infection
- Anxiety
- Knowledge Deficit

KEY CONCEPTS

- The airway is the collective system of tubes in the upper and lower respiratory tract through which gases travel during their passage to and from the alveoli.
- The airway is composed of the nose, pharynx, trachea, bronchi, and bronchioles.
- The airway is protected by the epiglottis, which seals

NURSING CARE PLAN:
Ineffective Airway Clearance

Assessment

Subjective Data
States, "I've had such a hard time breathing this past week. I stayed home from work. Most of the time I slept in my recliner chair. I couldn't even eat or drink much."

Objective Data
48-year-old man with a history of smoking 2 packs of cigarettes per day admitted with possible bacterial pneumonia. T—101° (oral) P—100. Breathing is rapid (30/min) and shallow. Uses accessory muscles and demonstrates nasal flaring. Bronchial breath sounds and inspiratory gurgles heard in distal R. upper lobe both anteriorly and posteriorly; all other areas of lungs sound clear. Has a persistent cough but does not raise sputum. Skin is hot and dry. Urine is a dark, concentrated amber color.

Diagnosis

Ineffective Airway Clearance related to weak cough and retained secretions.

Plan

Goal
The patient's lungs will sound clear throughout by 12/4.

Orders: 12/1
1. Auscultate lungs q shift, and before and after coughing or other respiratory therapy.
2. Elevate head of bed at all times.
3. Maintain 2,000–3,000 mL fluid intake of patient's choice (avoid milk) for 24 hours.
4. Instruct to take 3 deep breaths in through nose and out mouth, lean forward, and cough forcefully. Repeat q 1–2 hr while awake.
5. Perform oral/pharyngeal suctioning if secretions are loosened but not expectorated. _____ L. HOWARD, RN

Implementation 12/1
(Documentation)

0730   Continues to demonstrate effort at breathing. Sitting upright, nostrils flare, and physical activity is limited. Lungs clear except for inspiratory gurgles in RUL. Receiving 36% O_2 per nasal cannula at 4 L/min. IV of 1,000 mL of 5% D/W c̄ 800 mg of aminophyllin infusing at 30 mL per hour through infusion pump. Respiratory department contacted concerning new order for aerosol therapy. Instructed on deep breathing and coughing technique. _____ A. SANTINI, LPN

Evaluation
(Documentation)

0800   Breathing and coughing performed 3 times with no change in lung assessments. Able to drink a pot (240 mL) of hot tea with sugar and lemon. _____ A. SANTINI, LPN

1000   Able to raise a small amount of tenacious, purulent sputum after breathing and coughing. Specimen sent to laboratory for culture and sensitivity. Lung sounds remain unchanged. _____ A. SANTINI, LPN

the airway when swallowing food and fluids, by the rings of tracheal cartilage that keep the trachea from collapsing, by the mucous membrane that traps particulate matter, and by the cilia that beat debris upward in the airway so it can be coughed, expectorated, or swallowed.

- Airway management refers to those skills that maintain natural or artificial airways for compromised patients. It includes measures for liquefying secretions, promoting their expectoration with chest physiotherapy, or mechanically clearing mucus from the airway by means of suctioning.
- When suctioning the airway, any one of several approaches may be used. Examples include nasopharyngeal suctioning, nasotracheal suctioning, oropharyngeal suctioning, oral suctioning, and tracheal suctioning.
- Artificial airways are indicated for managing the care of patients who are at risk for an airway obstruction or those for whom long-term mechanical ventilation is necessary.
- Two examples of artificial airways include an oral airway and a tracheostomy tube.
- Tracheostomy care includes cleaning the skin around the stoma, changing the dressing, and cleaning the inner cannula.

CRITICAL THINKING EXERCISES

- Some tracheostomy patients learn to suction themselves. Develop a plan for teaching this procedure that would promote independence yet avoid overwhelming patients.

- Discuss ways to relieve the anxiety of a tracheostomy patient who needs frequent suctioning yet is fearful that he or she will be unable to obtain assistance when needed.

SUGGESTED READINGS

Ebersole P, Hess P. Toward Healthy Aging: Human Needs and Nursing Response. St. Louis: CV Mosby, 1990.

Eliopoulos C. Gerontological Nursing. 3rd ed. Philadelphia: JB Lippincott, 1993.

Ellstrom J. What's causing your patient's respiratory distress? Nursing November 1990;20:57–61

Finesilver C. Perfecting the art of respiratory assessment. RN February 1992;55:22–29.

Foyt MM. Impaired gas exchange in the elderly. Geriatric Nursing September–October 1993;13:262–268.

Gift AG, Pugh LC. Dyspnea and fatigue. Nursing Clinics of North America June 1993;28:373–384.

Hough A. Making sense of sputum retention. Nursing Times September 2–8, 1992;88:33–35.

Karper WB, Boschen MB. Effects of exercise on acute respiratory tract infections and related symptoms. Geriatric Nursing May–June 1993;14:15–18.

Kuhn JK, McGovern M. Respiratory assessment of the elderly. Journal of Gerontological Nursing May 1992;18:40–43.

Managing pulmonary patients . . . self-test. Nursing May 1992;22:108–112.

Mathews PJ, Mathews LM, Mitchell RR. Artificial airways: resuscitation guidelines you can follow. Nursing January 1992;22:53–59.

McConnell EA. Preventing postop complications: minimizing respiratory problems. Nursing November 1991;21:33–39.

Musser V. How do you use shallow-suction technique in children? American Journal of Nursing May 1992;92:79–80, 82.

Odom JL. Airway emergencies in the post anesthesia care unit. Nursing Clinics of North America September 1993;28:483–491.

CHAPTER 37

Resuscitation

 ### SKILLS

Relieving an Airway Obstruction
Performing Basic Cardiopulmonary Resuscitation

 ### NURSING CARE PLAN

Risk for Inability to Sustain Spontaneous Ventilation

Key Terms

Automated External Defibrillator	Finger Sweep
	Head Tilt–chin Lift
Back Blows	Technique
Cardiopulmonary	Heimlich Maneuver
Resuscitation	Jaw-thrust Technique
Chest Compression	Recovery Position
Chest Thrusts	Subdiaphragmatic Thrust

Learning Objectives

An understanding of the content within this chapter will be evidenced by the student's ability to:

- Explain why an airway obstruction is life threatening
- Give at least three signs of an airway obstruction
- Describe two actions that are appropriate when a patient experiences a partial airway obstruction
- Explain the term "Heimlich maneuver," and the procedure's purpose
- Describe the circumstances under which subdiaphragmatic thrusts are used and when chest thrusts are used
- Discuss the technique used to dislodge an object from an infant's airway
- Explain the meaning of cardiopulmonary resuscitation
- Explain to what the ABCs of resuscitation refer
- Name two techniques for opening the airway
- List three ways to administer rescue breathing
- Describe the purpose of chest compression
- Identify the maximum time allowed for interrupting cardiopulmonary resuscitation
- Name at least three criteria that are used for deciding to discontinue resuscitation efforts

Nurses are often the first responders when patients experience pulmonary or cardiac emergencies. This chapter reviews the most recent guidelines from the Emergency Cardiac Care Committee and Subcommittees of the American Heart Association for performing basic life support techniques.

AIRWAY OBSTRUCTION

The upper airway, an area that includes the pharynx and trachea, may become occluded for various reasons. Sometimes the airway swells because of injury and may require an artificial airway to promote and sustain breathing (see Chap. 36). However, there are other instances in which the airway becomes mechanically obstructed with a bolus of food or some other foreign object.

When the airway becomes obstructed, air exchange and subsequent oxygenation of cells and tissue become compromised. Therefore, recognizing signs of an airway obstruction and responding appropriately are essential to sustaining the life of the victim.

Signs of Airway Obstruction

Although the signs of an airway obstruction may be somewhat similar to those seen in someone having a heart attack, there are some discernible differences. First and foremost, if distress occurs while a person is eating, airway obstruction is a probability. The victim may also be observed to:

- Grasp his or her throat with the hands (Fig. 37-1)
- Make aggressive efforts to cough and breathe
- Produce a high-pitched sound while inhaling
- Turn pale and then blue
- Be unable to speak, breathe, or cough

If an airway obstruction exists, and is unrelieved, the victim will collapse, become unconscious, and eventually die.

Relieving an Obstruction

As long as the victim can speak or cough, there is some air being exchanged, indicating only a partial obstruction. No additional resuscitation efforts, other than encouraging and supporting the victim, are indicated for the time being.

If the victim's independent efforts to relieve the partial obstruction are unsuccessful or the situation begins to worsen, however, it is appropriate to activate the emergency medical system. In the hospital, this may be done by calling a **code**, the term given for summoning a team of personnel who are trained to administer advanced life support techniques. In the community, assistance is acquired by dialing 911 or calling another designated emergency number.

In the meantime, if the obstruction does become complete, actions are taken immediately to dislodge the obstructing substance (Skill 37-1). The method used to relieve a mechanical obstruction using **subdiaphragmatic thrusts**, also called abdominal thrusts, or **chest thrusts**, is referred to as the **Heimlich maneuver**, after the physician who proposed these techniques. Depending on the age of the victim, there are some differences in the manner in which it is performed.

AGE-RELATED DIFFERENCES

Adults and children older than the age of 1 year are given *five* abdominal subdiaphragmatic thrusts, to provide an increase in intrathoracic pressure equivalent to a cough. For obese adults or those victims with an advanced pregnancy, *five* chest thrusts can be administered as an alternative (see Skill 37-1).

When the victim of a partial or complete airway obstruction is younger than the age of 1 year, the emergency measures are performed somewhat differently. Because infants are unable to talk or provide a universal choking sign, the ability to cry is the best evidence that the obstruction is currently incomplete.

To assist an infant, it is best to support him or her over a forearm. In a prone position with the head held downward, the rescuer administers *five* **back blows** between the shoulder blades with the heel of one hand (Fig. 37-2). Or, if the infant is positioned supine, *five*

(text continues on page 799)

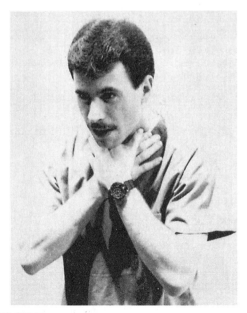

FIGURE 37-1
Universal sign for choking.

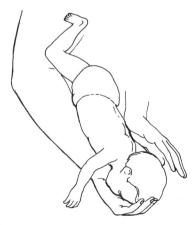

FIGURE 37-2
Giving back blows.

SKILL 37-1
Relieving an Airway Obstruction

Suggested Action	Reason for Action
Assessment	
Ask the victim who is still conscious if he or she is choking.	Identifies the nature of the problem
Look for the universal sign for choking.	Provides information nonverbally
Determine if the victim can speak.	Indicates whether the obstruction is partial or complete
Planning	
Call for stat respiratory assistance, or if the crisis happens in the community, dial 911 or another emergency number.	Communicates that there is an emergency situation
Prepare to respond if the obstruction becomes complete or the situation becomes worse.	Demonstrates anticipation of performing life-saving measures
Implementation	
Stand behind the victim and lean the head lower than the chest.	Increases intrathoracic pressure and uses gravity to best advantage
If the victim is in a chair, grasp the person about the abdomen from behind.	Facilitates resuscitation
Place the fist of one hand with the thumb facing inward in the middle of the victim's abdomen, above the navel, and grasp it with the other hand.	Reduces the potential for injury to internal organs

Giving subdiaphragmatic thrusts.

(continued)

SKILL 37-1
Relieving an Airway Obstruction *(Continued)*

Suggested Action	Reason for Action
Lay an unconscious victim supine on the floor and perform a **finger sweep** by inserting the index finger into the throat; use a hooking motion to remove the substance.	Facilitates resuscitation

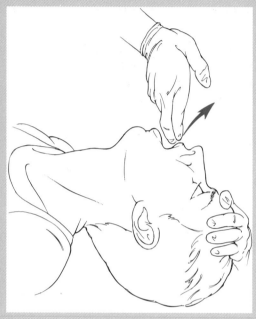

Performing a finger sweep.

(continued)

SKILL 37-1
Relieving an Airway Obstruction (Continued)

Suggested Action	Reason for Action
For an unconscious victim, place the hands in midline above the navel with the heel of one hand above the other and the fingers interlocked.	Provides an alternative for hand positioning when the victim cannot be grasped

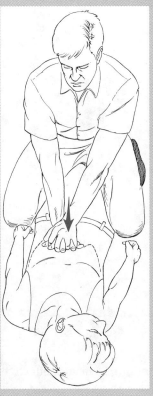

Assisting an unconscious victim.

Suggested Action	Reason for Action
Deliver up to five forceful thrusts to the abdomen, one after the other.	Simulates the force of coughing

(continued)

SKILL 37-1
Relieving an Airway Obstruction (Continued)

Suggested Action	Reason for Action
For a pregnant or obese victim, administer chest thrusts after positioning the fists in the middle of the victim's breastbone.	Provides an alternative when it is impossible to encircle the victim's abdomen

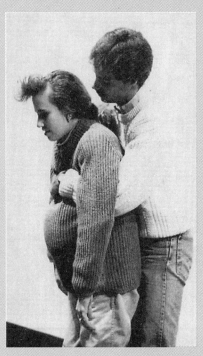

Chest thrusts.

Suggested Action	Reason for Action
Reassess a conscious victim after each of the five thrusts, and repeat until the obstruction is relieved or the victim loses consciousness.	Provides continued safe and effective resuscitation efforts
Proceed to perform a finger sweep when the victim loses consciousness.	Aids in clearing the airway
Continue performing a series of five abdominal thrusts followed by finger sweeps until exhausted or until emergency assistance arrives.	Provides continuous resuscitation efforts

Evaluation
• Victim clears the airway independently
• Thrusts or finger sweep dislodge obstructing substance
• Resuscitation efforts are sustained until personnel with advanced life support skills can assist

(continued)

SKILL 37-1
Relieving an Airway Obstruction (Continued)

Suggested Action	Reason for Action

Document
- Time of discovery
- Assessment data
- Resuscitation efforts that were performed
- Time when request for assistance was made
- Outcome of resuscitation

Sample Documentation

Date and Time   Found unconscious in chair @ 0745. No evidence of breathing. Food on breakfast tray partially eaten. Placed supine on floor. Finger sweep performed and a stewed prune was removed from the throat. Spontaneous breathing resumed. Lifted to bed and oxygen administered at 8 L with a simple mask. Conscious and oriented at this time. Dr. Wells notified. _____ **Signature, Title**

---

chest thrusts may be given with two fingers to the middle of the breastbone at about the level of the nipples (Fig. 37-3).

Other efforts, like cardiopulmonary resuscitation (CPR), are required if the cause of distress is other than an airway obstruction.

CARDIOPULMONARY RESUSCITATION

Cardiopulmonary resuscitation refers to the techniques used to restore breathing and circulation for lifeless victims (Skill 37-2). To determine the status of the victim, a quick assessment is performed.

Initial Assessment

The initial assessment involves determining responsiveness. This is easily performed by shaking the victim and shouting the victim's name, if it is known. If the victim is unresponsive and older than 8 years of age, the next step is to activate the emergency medical system before attempting resuscitation. The exception to this rule involves pediatric emergencies. In that case, resuscitation is attempted for a full minute before soliciting emergency assistance.

Obtaining Assistance

The sooner advanced life support measures are administered, the more likely the victim will survive. If there is another person present, this task may be delegated. The type of information that will provide the best assistance includes:

- The address (or room number) where assistance is needed, as accurately as possible
- The telephone number (or nursing unit) where the call is being made
- A description of the situation
- The current condition of the victim
- What actions have been taken up to the current time

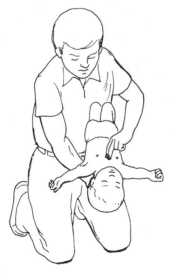

FIGURE 37-3
Delivering chest thrusts.

(text continues on page 803)

SKILL 37-2
Performing Basic Cardiopulmonary Resuscitation

Suggested Action	Reason for Action
Assessment	
Shake patient and shout name.	Determines responsiveness
Planning	
Plan to administer CPR after calling for assistance.	Potentiates successful outcome
Implementation	
Open the airway.	Facilitates spontaneous breathing
Look, listen, and feel for air.	Indicates the need to provide rescue breathing
Seal the nose and give two quick breaths lasting 1½ to 2 seconds through the patient's mouth, if there is no spontaneous breathing.	Initiates ventilations

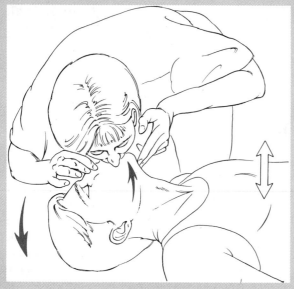

Mouth-to-mouth rescue breathing.

(continued)

SKILL 37-2
Performing Basic Cardiopulmonary Resuscitation (Continued)

Suggested Action	**Reason for Action**
Use a face shield, if there is one available, or a one-way valve mask.	Reduces the potential for acquiring an infectious disease

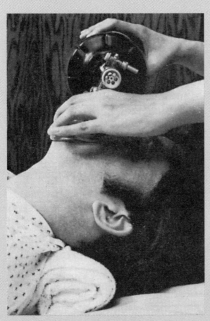

Using a one-way valve mask.

Reposition the head and reattempt ventilation if breathing is met with resistance or the chest does not rise.	Indicates narrowed or obstructed airway
Perform a finger sweep if the ventilation continues to be unsuccessful. Attempt the Heimlich maneuver.	Promotes relief of mechanical airway obstruction
Place in the recovery position if breathing resumes.	Prevents respiratory complications

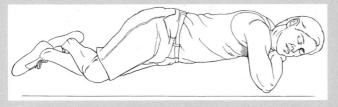

Recovery position

Check for a pulse.	Determines the need for chest compressions
Place a backboard beneath the pulseless patient.	Promotes the efficiency of chest compressions

(continued)

SKILL 37-2
Performing Cardiopulmonary Resuscitation (Continued)

Suggested Action	Reason for Action
Position hands and body over the patient's chest.	Facilitates administering chest compressions

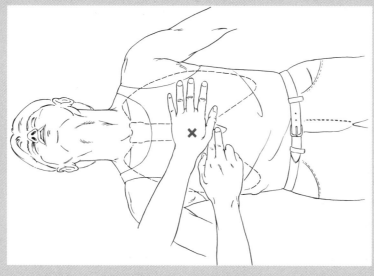

Location for chest compression.

Suggested Action	Reason for Action
Administer 15 compressions.	Circulates blood through the heart to the systemic circulation
Give two rescue breaths after each set of 15 chest compressions.	Meets the needs for ventilation and circulation
Reassess the patient after four cycles of chest compressions and ventilations.	Evaluates the patient's response
Continue CPR in the absence of breathing and pulse.	Promotes resuscitation
Reassess every few minutes.	Evaluates the patient's response
Assist code team with defibrillation, intubation, and administration of emergency drugs.	Enhances the successful outcome of resuscitation

Evaluation
- Spontaneous breathing occurs; circulation is maintained or resumes
- Ventilation is assisted and defibrillation restores heart beat
- No response or improvement occurs during resuscitation

(continued)

SKILL 37-2
Performing Basic Cardiopulmonary Resuscitation *(Continued)*

Suggested Action	Reason for Action

Document

- Time patient is discovered to be unresponsive
- Time the code is called
- Length of time CPR is administered, and if performed by one or two rescuers
- Time the code team arrives
- Methods used to restore ventilation and heart rate, including names of drugs, dose, route, and time given
- Names and results of laboratory tests to determine physiologic progress
- Response of the patient
- Time resuscitation is terminated

*Sample Documentation**

Date and Time   Unresponsive to shaking and shouting. Code called @ 1830. No breathing with opening of airway. Two rescue breaths given. No carotid pulse palpated. Backboard placed beneath patient. Cardiac compressions administered. No response after four cycles of compressions and ventilations. Code team arrived @ 1840. See resuscitation documentation form. _____ **Signature, Title**

* Special documentation forms are used to record the resuscitation activities of the code team.

Performing ABCs

The letters "ABC" stand for **A**irway, **B**reathing, and **C**irculation. They represent the sequence of steps in providing CPR.

OPENING THE AIRWAY

To verify that a victim is not breathing, it is essential to open the airway. This may be all that is necessary to restore ventilation.

The victim is first positioned supine on a firm surface, taking care not to twist the spine in case there is unidentified trauma. In the absence of a head or neck injury, the method of choice for opening the airway is the **head tilt–chin lift technique** (Fig. 37-4). As an alternative, the **jaw-thrust technique** may be used. It is performed by grasping the lower jaw and lifting it while tilting the head backward (Fig. 37-5). If there is evidence of material within the mouth, it is removed at this time.

Once the airway is opened, the victim is assessed for spontaneous breathing. Appropriate assessment techniques include observing for rising and falling movements of the chest, and listening and feeling for air escaping from the nose or mouth.

A breathing victim is then placed in the recovery position. The **recovery position** is a side-lying position that helps to maintain an open airway and prevent as-

piration of liquids. If breathing is not restored, it is appropriate to keep the victim supine and attempt rescue breathing.

RESCUE BREATHING

Rescue breathing refers to the process of ventilating a nonbreathing victim's lungs. This may be done

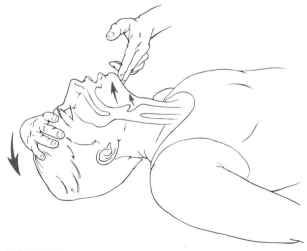

FIGURE 37-4
Head tilt–chin lift technique.

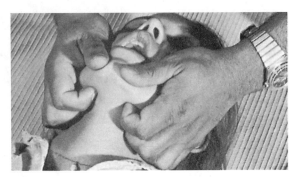

FIGURE 37-5
Jaw-thrust technique.

through the mouth, nose, or stoma of a victim. It is best to use a one-way valve mask or other protective face shield, if that is possible. These devices theoretically reduce the potential for acquiring infectious diseases like hepatitis and AIDS. However, lack of a barrier type of ventilation device should not interfere with attempting rescue breathing.

Mouth-to-Mouth Breathing

Mouth-to-mouth breathing involves:

- Maintaining an open airway
- Sealing the victim's nose
- Covering the victim's mouth with the rescuer's mouth
- Blowing air into the victim

Initially, two quick breaths are given before checking the victim's pulse. Rescue breathing resumes at a rate of 10 to 12 breaths per minute for adult victims.

Mouth-to-Nose Breathing

Mouth-to-nose breathing is an alternative method of providing rescue breathing in which the mouth is sealed and the breaths are delivered through the nose. Mouth-to-nose breathing is provided when the victim is an infant or small child or when mouth-to-mouth rescue breathing is impossible or unsuccessful.

Regardless of which method of rescue breathing is used, each breath is delivered (for an adult) over 1½ to 2 seconds. This rate reduces the potential for distending the esophagus and stomach, which may promote regurgitation and aspiration.

Mouth-to-Stoma Breathing

Patients with a laryngectomy or tracheostomy may require resuscitation. Laryngectomy patients can be given rescue breathing by sealing the mouth over the stoma. Because the upper airway is essentially a blind pathway, the nose does not require sealing.

For patients with a mechanical tracheostomy tube, rescue breathing may be given through the tube with the mouth or a one-way valve mask. If the tra-

cheostomy tube does not have an inflated cuff (see Chap. 36), however, the nose will need to be sealed.

PROMOTING CIRCULATION

To determine if circulation requires support, the rescuer must determine if the victim is pulseless. This assessment is performed by compressing the carotid artery to the side of the trachea with two fingers on adult victims (Fig. 37-6). The carotid artery is the most accessible site, but the femoral artery in the groin is also an appropriate site for assessment. The brachial artery in the upper arm is assessed when the victim is an infant. If the victim is pulseless, chest compressions are indicated.

Chest Compression

Circulation is promoted by compressing the chest. **Chest compressions** circulate blood in one of two ways. It has been proposed that squeezing the heart between the sternum and vertebrae increases the pressure in the heart's ventricles. Supposedly this pushes blood into the pulmonary arteries and aorta. However, there are others who propose that it increases the pressure in blood vessels within the thorax, which promotes systemic blood flow (Coleman, 1992).

To be effective, however, cardiac compressions must be delivered at a rate of 80 to 100 times a minute for adult victims. For a one-person rescue, 15 chest compressions are given followed by 2 breaths, or a ratio of 15:2. For a team of two, the ratio is five compressions to one breath, or 5:1. After the completion of successive compressions, there is an obvious pause in compressions as the rescue breath is delivered.

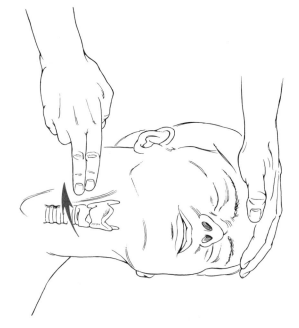

FIGURE 37-6
Assessing the carotid artery.

Besides an appropriate rate, adequate circulation also depends on proper placement of the hands and body position.

Hand and Body Placement. The heel of one hand is placed over the lower half of the sternum, but above the xiphoid process. The other hand is placed on top with the fingers interlocked or extended.

The rescuer's body is positioned over the hands so as to deliver a straight-downward motion with each compression (Fig. 37-7). The compression is given with sufficient force to cause a pulsation in the carotid artery. This may not occur unless the chest is depressed at least 1½ to 2 inches or more. However, assessment of carotid pulsation requires the assistance of a second rescuer.

Whenever chest compressions are delivered, the hands remain in contact with the chest, and the elbows are kept locked to avoid rocking back and forth over the victim. Once CPR is initiated, it is not interrupted for more than 7 seconds except when:

- There is a pulse and the victim resumes breathing
- Exhaustion of the rescuer occurs.
- Deterioration progresses despite resuscitation efforts.
- There is written evidence that resuscitation is contrary to the victim's wishes.
- Advanced cardiac life support measures are administered, such as an automated external defibrillator.

An **automated external defibrillator** is a device that delivers an electrical charge when the heart is not beating effectively. However, this equipment is not currently included among the techniques for basic life support.

AGE-RELATED DIFFERENCES

There are variations that must be made in rescue breathing and chest compressions to accommodate for the anatomic differences and physiologic needs that exist in various age groups (Table 37-1).

Assessing Effectiveness

Periodically, the victim is assessed to determine if CPR is effective. Assessment is recommended after four cycles of compressions and ventilations, and every few minutes thereafter. Signs of spontaneous breathing can be assessed only by interrupting chest compressions; such interruptions should last no more than 3 to 5 seconds.

Discontinuing Resuscitation

Unfortunately, not every resuscitation attempt is successful. Success is more appropriately measured by the victim's quality of life rather than its quantity after resuscitation. Severe neurologic deficits often result even when a victim's life is saved. Therefore, there often comes a time when a decision must be made to discontinue both basic and advanced life support efforts.

Eventually, there may be clear-cut guidelines for suspending resuscitation. At present, however, none exist. Consequently, resuscitation efforts may extend for long periods of time on the possibility that the victim will be saved. The decision to cease is a medical judgment made by the physician leading the code.

The decision to stop resuscitation efforts often is based on the time that elapsed before resuscitation began, the length of time that resuscitation has continued without any change in the victim's condition, the age and diagnosis of the victim, and the results of objective data like arterial blood gas results and electrolyte studies. Regardless of the basis for the decision, it is not made lightly. And those involved in an unsuccessful code need the support of their colleagues as much as the survivors of the victim do. Yet, the code team is less likely than the survivors to receive it.

NURSING IMPLICATIONS

When it comes to resuscitation, nurses have several responsibilities. First, they must learn to perform basic cardiac life support measures and maintain their certification to do so. If the skills are not used or refreshed on at least a 2-year basis, the nurse-rescuer's skills may be less than adequate.

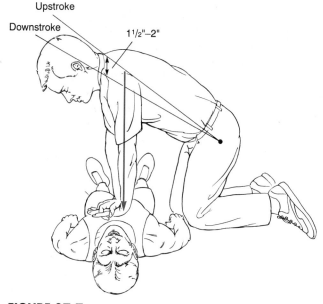

FIGURE 37-7
Correct hand and body position.

TABLE 37-1. *Differences in Cardiopulmonary Resuscitation Among Infants, Children, and Adults*

Technique	Infant (≤1 year of age)	Child (1–8 years of age)	Adult (≥8 years of age)
Rescue breaths			
Initial	2 breaths	2 breaths	2 breaths
Subsequent breaths	1 every 3 seconds	1 every 3 seconds	1 every 5 seconds
Rate	20/minute	20/minute	10–12/minute
Duration	1–1½ seconds	1–1½ seconds	1–1½ seconds
Compressions			
Location	In the midline, one finger-width below the nipples	Two fingerwidths above the tip of the sternum	Two fingerwidths above the tip of the sternum
Hand use	Two or three fingers	Heel of one hand	Two hands
Rate	At least 100/minute	100/min	80–100/min
Depth	½–1 in	1–1½ in	1½–2 in or more

Second, nurses must support and participate in efforts to teach lay people, both adults and children, how to perform CPR. Statistics show that most victims who are saved are those for whom CPR was initiated early in their demise.

Third, it is best to discuss the necessity for preparing advance directives (see Chap. 3). Honoring the patient's right to participate in the decision-making process is a noble goal.

Considering resuscitation from all of these perspectives, nurses may identify one or more of the accompanying Applicable Nursing Diagnoses.

The Nursing Care Plan for this chapter has been developed to demonstrate how the steps in the nursing process are used in the management of a patient with a nursing diagnosis of Risk for Inability to Sustain Spontaneous Ventilation. This diagnostic category is defined in the NANDA taxonomy (1994) as "A state in which the response pattern of decreased energy reserves results in an individual's inability to maintain breathing adequate to support life."

 APPLICABLE NURSING DIAGNOSES

- Ineffective Airway Clearance
- Inability to Sustain Spontaneous Ventilation
- Impaired Gas Exchange
- Decreased Cardiac Output
- Impaired Cardiopulmonary Tissue Perfusion
- Impaired Cerebral Tissue Perfusion
- Impaired Renal Tissue Perfusion
- Health Seeking Behaviors
- Decisional Conflict

 FOCUS ON OLDER ADULTS

- The resuscitation status of each patient is documented somewhere within the medical record. If no information is documented, CPR is administered in any life-threatening situation.
- Some older adults fear that if they specify that they do not wish to be resuscitated, they will receive less-than-appropriate care and treatment of their illness.
- It is possible to identify in an advance directive exactly the type of resuscitation that is allowed. For example, some may approve of emergency drugs, but refuse to allow mechanical ventilation.
- Older adults are informed that they may change their mind about their advance directives at any time. All changes are communicated with the physician.
- There is always the risk for fracturing ribs when performing CPR, but when the victim is elderly the risk is even greater because of the likelihood that many have osteoporosis.
- An emergency pacemaker, a device that initiates an electrical impulse that causes the heart to contract, may be inserted in patients who are resuscitated, yet remain in unstable condition.
- Some patients with a history of chronic life-threatening dysrhythmias that are unresponsive to drug therapy may have an automatic cardiac defibrillator (ACD) inserted surgically within their chest. The device senses the dys-

(continued)

within their chest. The device senses the dysrhythmia and almost instantaneously delivers an electrical current to restore normal heart rhythm.

- Older patients who take daily doses of aspirin or other anticoagulant drugs are more apt to bleed internally when chest compressions are administered.

- An airway obstruction may be suspected when a person grasps his or her throat with the hands, makes an aggressive effort to cough and breathe, and produces a high-pitched sound while inhaling.
- When a partial airway obstruction occurs, it is best to encourage and support the victim's efforts to clear the obstruction independently, and prepare to call for emergency assistance if the victim's condition worsens.
- The Heimlich maneuver is the name of the technique used to relieve a complete airway obstruction by performing a series of subdiaphragmatic thrusts or chest thrusts.
- Subdiaphragmatic thrusts are appropriate for almost all adults and children beyond the age of infancy. Chest thrusts are used for obese adults and those in advanced pregnancy.

KEY CONCEPTS

- An airway obstruction is potentially life threatening because it interferes with ventilation and subsequently deprives cells and tissues of oxygen.

NURSING CARE PLAN:
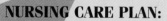
Risk for Inability to Sustain Spontaneous Ventilation

Assessment	**Subjective Data** States, "It has been more and more difficult for me to breathe. My doctor told me that's the usual outcome from this disease." **Objective Data** 34-year-old man with a history of amyotrophic lateral sclerosis (Lou Gehrig's disease) diagnosed 18 months ago. Admitted after being resuscitated by paramedics who responded to the family's 911 call for assistance. Currently has shallow respirations of 32 per min. SaO$_2$ is 80% with oxygen at 6 L per Venturi mask. Demonstrates difficulty talking and swallowing.
Diagnosis	Risk for Inability to Sustain Spontaneous Ventilation related to respiratory muscle weakness.
Plan	**Goal** The patient will receive assisted ventilation when SaO$_2$ falls below 60% or the PaO$_2$ is less than 50 mm Hg. **Orders:** 9/18 1. Monitor SaO$_2$ with pulse oximeter at all times. 2. Place in Fowler's position. 3. Administer oxygen at 45% using Venturi mask. 4. Replace Venturi mask with a nonrebreather mask if SaO$_2$ falls below 60%. 5. Obtain arterial blood gas when SaO$_2$ is sustained at 60% for more than 10 minutes. 6. Perform CPR if respiratory and/or cardiac arrest occurs. 7. Withhold advanced cardiac life support per advance directive. J. MANGOLD, RN.
Implementation 9/18 *(Documentation)*	1345 In Fowler's position. Monitored with pulse oximeter. Oxygen administered at 45% via Venturi mask. _____ S. OWENS, LPN
Evaluation 9/18 *(Documentation)*	1500 SaO$_2$ ranges from 80% to 84%. Heart rate is 120 bpm. Alert and oriented. _____ S. OWENS, LPN

- To dislodge an object from an infant's airway, a series of back blows is delivered, followed by a series of chest thrusts.
- Cardiopulmonary resuscitation refers to the techniques used to restore breathing and circulation for lifeless victims.
- The ABCs of resuscitation refer to the sequence of actions that involve opening the airway and assessing and initiating breathing and circulation.
- The airway can be safely opened under most circumstances by using the head tilt–chin lift technique or jaw-thrust technique.
- Rescue breathing is administered mouth-to-mouth, mouth-to-nose, or mouth-to-stoma.
- Chest compressions are used to circulate blood systemically.
- Once CPR is begun, it is never interrupted for more than 7 seconds, except in certain circumstances such as when advanced electronic equipment is used.
- The decision to stop resuscitation efforts often is based on the time that elapsed before resuscitation began, the length of time that resuscitation has continued without any change in the victim's condition, and the age and diagnosis of the victim.

CRITICAL THINKING EXERCISES

- Rearrange the resuscitation steps in the list that follows in the sequence in which they are performed: administer 15 compressions; open the airway; activate the emergency medical system; check the carotid pulse; shake and shout; give two rescue breaths; tilt the head and lift the chin; look, listen, and feel for air.
- Discuss the possible consequences, positive and negative, of resuscitating a patient who has a written advance directive to the contrary.

SUGGESTED READINGS

Bailey MM, Arbour R. Getting through your first code. Nursing June 1993;23:60–61.

Braun AE. Emergency cardiac care, fine-tuning for the '90s. RN September 1993;56:50–55.

Coleman A. Cardiac issues in C.P.R. Nursing April 1992;22:54–57.

Emergency Cardiac Care Committee and Subcommittees, American Heart Association. Guidelines for cardiopulmonary resuscitation and emergency cardiac care: Part II. Adult basic life support. Journal of the American Medical Association October 28 1992; 268:2184–2198.

Emergency Cardiac Care Committee and Subcommittees, American Heart Association. Guidelines for cardiopulmonary resuscitation and emergency cardiac care: Part V. Pediatric basic life support. Journal of the American Medical Association October 28 1992; 268:2251–2261.

Mathews PJ, Mathews LM, Mitchell RR. Artificial airways: resuscitation guidelines you can follow. Nursing January 1992;22:53–59.

Neimann JT. Cardiopulmonary resuscitation. New England Journal of Medicine October 8 1992;327:1075–1079.

Pengra H, Morgan D, Warren L. Nursing implementation of do not resuscitate policy into home healthcare. Home Healthcare Nurse March–April 1992;10:32–39

Sommers MS. The shattering consequences of C.P.R.: how to assess and prevent complications. Nursing July 1992;22:34–42.

Willens JS. B.C.L.S. forecast: big changes in the wind. Nursing November 1991;21:52–56.

Willens JS. Strengthen your life-support skills. Nursing April 1993; 23:54–58.

UNIT XII

Caring for the Terminally Ill

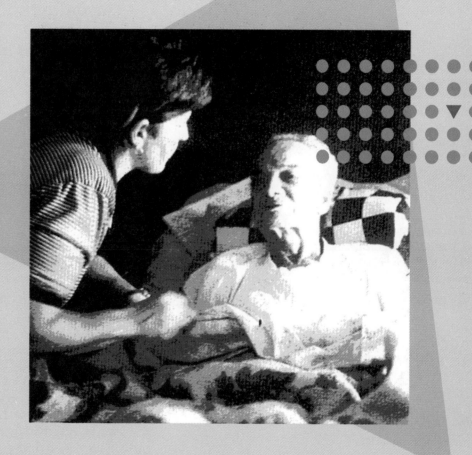

CHAPTER 38
Death and Dying

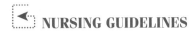

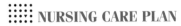
Learning Objectives

An understanding of the content within this chapter will be evidenced by the student's ability to:

- Explain the meaning of a terminal illness
- Name five stages of dying
- Describe two methods for promoting acceptance
- Explain the meaning of respite care
- Discuss the philosophy of hospice care
- List at least five aspects of care that are addressed when providing terminal care
- Name at least five signs of multiple organ failure
- Explain why a discussion of organ donation must take place as expeditiously as possible
- Name three components of postmortem care
- Discuss the benefit of grieving
- Describe one sign that a person's grief is becoming resolved

Life expectancy continues to lengthen year by year (Fig. 38-1), yet death is a certainty. The only unknowns are when, where, and how it will occur. Nurses and other health personnel are probably involved more than any other group with people who experience impending

Timby BK: *Fundamental Skills and Concepts in Patient Care, Sixth Edition* © 1996 Lippincott-Raven Publishers

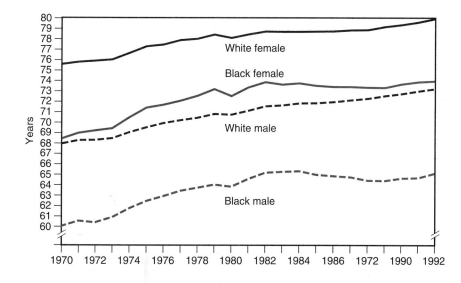

FIGURE 38-1
Life expectancy in the United States, 1970 to 1992. (Source: Centers for Disease Control and Prevention. Monthly Vital Statistics Report. National Center for Health Statistics December 4, 1994; 43:5.)

death. This chapter deals with aspects of caring for terminally ill patients and the grieving experience.

TERMINAL ILLNESS

A **terminal illness** is one from which recovery is beyond reasonable expectation. On learning that death is soon to be inevitable, patients tend to go through several stages as they process the information.

STAGES OF DYING

Dr. Elisabeth Kübler-Ross (1969), a recognized authority on the subject of dying, has described stages through which many terminally ill patients progress. They include sequential periods of *denial, anger, bargaining, depression*, and *acceptance* (Table 38-1).

Denial

Denial is a psychological defense mechanism in which a person refuses to believe that certain information is true. Terminally ill patients may first reject that their diagnosis is accurate. They may speculate that the test results are in error or that the reports have been confused with those of another.

Anger

Anger is an emotional response to feeling victimized. Because there is no way to retaliate against fate, patients often displace their anger onto others like nurses, the physician, family, and even God. Anger may be expressed in less-than-obvious ways, like complaining about the care or overreacting to even the slightest aggravation.

Bargaining

Bargaining is a psychological mechanism for delaying the inevitable. It involves a process of negotiation, usually with God or some higher power. Usually, the dying patient is willing to accept death, but wants to extend his or her life temporarily until some event takes place in the future. The future event usually has personal significance to the dying patient, like a son's or daughter's wedding.

Depression

Depression is a sad mood. It indicates the dying patient's realization that his or her death will come sooner, rather than later, than anticipated. The sad mood is a result of dealing with potential losses.

Acceptance

Acceptance is an attitude of complacency. Most patients arrive at the stage of acceptance after having dealt with their losses and completed their unfinished business.

Kübler-Ross describes **unfinished business** in two ways. Literally, it refers to completing legal and financial matters so as to provide the best security for sur-

TABLE 38-1. *Stages of Dying*		
Stage	Typical Emotional Response	Typical Comment
First stage	Denial	"No, not me."
Second stage	Anger	"Why me?"
Third stage	Bargaining	"Yes, me, but . . ."
Fourth stage	Depression	"Yes, me."
Fifth stage	Acceptance	"I am ready."

vivors. However, it also can refer to social and spiritual matters, such as making "peace with God" and saying "good-byes" to loved ones. It is as important for dying patients as it is for their families to say, "Thank you for . . . ," and "I'm sorry for . . ."

When all of the loose ends are tied, dying patients feel prepared to die. Some even happily anticipate death, viewing it as a bridge to another, better dimension.

PROMOTING ACCEPTANCE

Nurses can facilitate the passage from one stage to another by being available for emotional support and by supporting the patient's personal choices concerning terminal care.

Emotional Support

Patients who are dying require emotional support perhaps more than at any other time during their lives. Sometimes all dying patients want is an opportunity to vent their feelings and verbally work through their emotions. Nurses may be the nonjudgmental sounding board they need.

NURSING GUIDELINES FOR HELPING DYING PATIENTS COPE

- Accept patients' behavior no matter what it is.
  Rationale: Demonstrates respect for individuality
- Provide opportunities during which patients can express their feelings freely.
  Rationale: Demonstrates devotion to meeting individual needs
- Work toward understanding patients' feelings.
  Rationale: Reinforces that each person is unique
- Use statements with broad openings such as, "It must be difficult for you," and "Do you want to talk about it?"
  Rationale: Facilitates communication and allows patients to choose the topic or manner of their response

---

Besides being available for verbal interactions, nurses provide emotional support to dying patients by acknowledging them as unique and worthwhile individuals. When dying patients are cared for with an attitude of respect, no matter what their emotional, physical, or cognitive state, it is referred to as **dying with dignity**—a concept incorporated within the Dying Person's Bill of Rights (Display 38-1).

DISPLAY 38-1. *The Dying Person's Bill of Rights*

I have the right to be treated as a living human being until I die.

I have the right to maintain a sense of hopefulness, however changing its focus may be.

I have the right to be cared for by those who can maintain a sense of hopefulness, however changing this might be.

I have the right to express my feelings and emotions about my approaching death in my own way.

I have the right to participate in decisions concerning my care.

I have the right to expect continuing medical and nursing attention even though "cure" goals must be changed to "comfort" goals.

I have the right not to die alone.

I have the right to be free from pain.

I have the right to have my questions answered honestly.

I have the right not to be deceived.

I have the right to have help from and for my family in accepting my death.

I have the right to die in peace and dignity.

I have the right to retain my individuality and not be judged for my decisions which may be contrary to beliefs of others.

I have the right to discuss and enlarge my religious and/or spiritual experiences, whatever these may mean to others.

I have the right to expect that the sanctity of the human body will be respected after death.

I have the right to be cared for by caring, sensitive, knowledgeable people who will attempt to understand my needs and will be able to gain some satisfaction in helping me face my death.

From Barbus AJ. The dying person's bill of rights, © 1975, American Journal of Nursing Company. Reprinted with permission from the American Journal of Nursing January 1975;75:99.

Respect for dying patients' rights includes helping them choose how and where they most want to be cared for before their death.

Arranging for Care

Patients may find it extremely comforting to learn about preparing an advance directive if they have not already done so (see Chap. 3). Many also are appreciative of being informed about the various options available as to where they may receive care.

In general, patients have four choices for care: home care, hospice care (which may be the same as home care), residential care, and acute care.

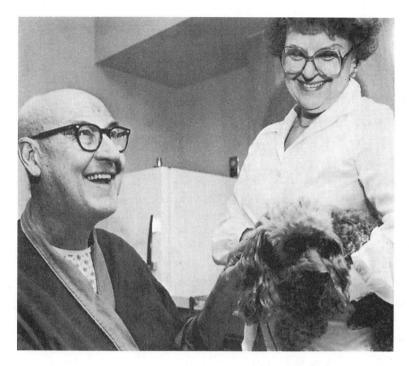

FIGURE 38-2
Home care.

HOME CARE

In the early stages of a terminal illness, most patients remain at home (Fig. 38-2). They may travel to and from a hospital or clinic for brief periods of treatment, tests, and medical evaluations. Nurses may help coordinate community services, secure home equipment, and arrange for home nursing visits.

Because the major burden of home care often falls on the shoulders of a spouse or significant other, nurses who care for home-bound patients need periodically to assess the toll this burden takes. The focus of support may shift back and forth from the patient to the caregiver. Respite care, in some instances, may be appropriate.

Respite Care

Respite care is care, or relief, for the caregiver. With the help of a surrogate, the spouse or relative most responsible within the network of care is given an opportunity to enjoy brief periods away from home.

HOSPICE CARE

A **hospice**, in the literal sense, is a place of refuge for travelers, but the term has come to mean a facility for the care of terminally ill patients.

The hospice movement in the United States is modeled after those established by Dr. Cicely Saunders in England during the late 1960s. Philosophically, whether the hospice is a free-standing building or a service that is provided in homes, hospice care involves helping patients live out their final days in comfort and with dignity and meaningfulness in a caring environment (Fig. 38-3).

In general, only those terminal patients who have 6 months or less to live are accepted for hospice care in the United States. Most are cared for in their own homes. The family's care, however, is supported by a multidisciplinary team of hospice professionals and volunteers.

Hospice organizations also provide support programs for family members and significant others. Individual and group counseling is offered both during and after the death of hospice patients to help survivors cope with their grief.

RESIDENTIAL CARE

Residential care is a form of intermediate care. It is provided in nursing homes or long-term care facilities where the level of care is usually subacute. These facilities provide around-the-clock nursing care for patients who cannot maintain independent living (Fig. 38-4).

Family members have the peace of mind that their loved one is being cared for and enjoy the opportunity to visit them as much as possible. Residential care tends to be quite costly. It may range between $1,500 to $2,000 per month, depending on the extent of nursing care that is required (Taeuber, 1992). Once a person has exhausted his or her savings, they may be financially assisted by state welfare programs like Medicaid.

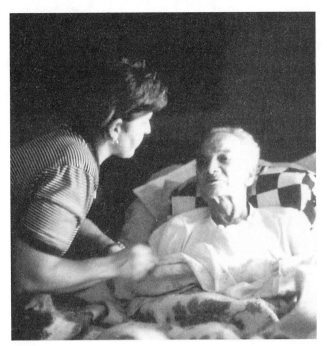

FIGURE 38-3
A hospice patient and nurse. (Courtesy of Visiting Nurse Association of Southwest Michigan.) (Scherer JC, Timby BK: Introductory Medical-Surgical Nursing, 6th ed, p 66. Philadelphia, JB Lippincott, 1995)

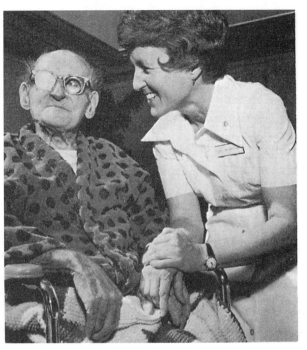

FIGURE 38-4
Residential care.

ACUTE CARE

Acute care, which is mainly provided in a hospital, is that which demands the most sophisticated technology or most labor-intensive care as the result of a patient's unstable condition. For these reasons, it is also the most expensive form of care. There are major costs involved in acute care over the hours, days, or weeks before a patient's death.

PROVIDING TERMINAL CARE

Immediately preceding death, the nurse continues to meet the patient's basic physical needs for hydration, nourishment, elimination, hygiene, positioning, and comfort. It is at this time that many of the skills described throughout this text may be implemented to meet the multiple problems experienced by dying patients.

Hydration

Hydration involves the maintenance of an adequate fluid volume. If the swallowing reflex is present, water and other beverages are offered at frequent intervals. As swallowing becomes impaired, there is the risk for aspiration, followed by pneumonia. Sucking, however, is one of the last reflexes to disappear as death approaches. Therefore, a possible alternative may be to provide a moist cloth or wrapped ice cubes that can be sucked. Eventually, intravenous fluids may be administered.

Nourishment

Terminally ill patients may have little interest in eating. The effort may simply be too exhausting, or nausea and vomiting may result in inadequate consumption of food. Poor nutrition leads to weakness, infection, and other complications, such as the development of pressure sores. Consequently, tube feedings or total parenteral nutrition may be used to maintain nutritional and fluid intake.

Elimination

Some terminally ill patients may be incontinent of urine and stool; others may experience urinary retention and constipation—all of which are uncomfortable. Cleansing enemas or suppositories may be ordered. Catheterization may also become necessary. Care of the skin becomes particularly important if patients are incontinent. Urine and stool, if left in contact with the skin, contribute to skin breakdown as well as produce foul odors.

Hygiene

The dignity of patients is largely the result of their personal appearance. Therefore, there is more than one reason for keeping dying patients clean, well groomed, and free of unpleasant odors.

Mouth care may be necessary at more frequent intervals. Mucus that cannot be swallowed or expectorated needs to be removed. The mouth can be wiped with gauze or suctioned. Using a lateral position helps keep the mouth and throat free of accumulating secretions. The lips may need periodic lubrication because they may be dried from mouth breathing or the administration of oxygen.

Positioning

Even though the lateral position is beneficial for preventing choking and aspiration, it cannot be the sole position that is used. For the sake of comfort and promoting circulation, the dying patient's position is changed at least every 2 hours, the same as with any other patient's care.

Comfort

Relieving pain may be the single most challenging problem involved in caring for dying patients. The goal is to keep patients free from pain, yet not dull their consciousness or ability to communicate.

Most patients initially are given nonnarcotics. The drug order may be changed to a narcotic later. The route may also change from oral to parenteral, with the administration taking place according to a routine schedule. Giving pain medication regularly, like every 4 hours, rather than on a *prn* basis, helps to maintain a consistent level of pain relief.

It is expected that the dosage will need to be increased to accommodate for drug tolerance (see Chap.

17). The possibility of addiction, however, does not stand in the way of pain control.

Unfortunately, although tolerance develops to the pain-relieving property of the drug, tolerance to the drug's other actions does not appear as quickly. Therefore, respirations may become depressed and constipation may be more common with regular use of narcotic drugs.

Involving the Family

Family members may appreciate helping with the patient's care. They often feel helpless and welcome an opportunity to assist, but it is unfair to burden them with major responsibilities. Occasional involvement, however, tends to maintain a family bond (Fig. 38-5) and helps survivors cope with their grief in the future.

APPROACHING DEATH

The signs of approaching death are the result of multiple organ failure.

Multiple Organ Failure

Multiple organ failure is a condition in which two or more organ systems gradually cease to function. Multiple organ failure is directly related to the quality of cellular oxygenation. When the supply of oxygen falls below what cells need, cells, followed by tissues and organs, begin to die. According to Reilly and Yucha (1994), the cardiovascular, pulmonary, hepatic, and renal systems are most vulnerable to failure.

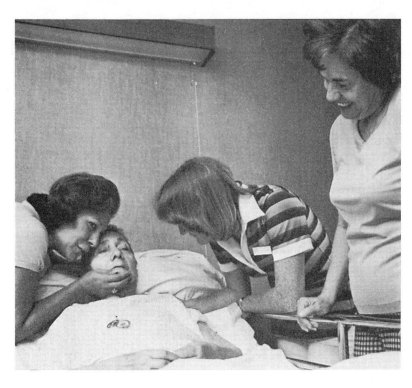

FIGURE 38-5
Family involvement.

As the cells die, their intracellular chemicals are released. The preexisting hypoxia is then complicated by a localized and then generalized inflammatory response (see Chap. 28) that causes the signs of multiple organ failure heralding approaching death (Table 38-2). The process itself may take place gradually over a period of hours or days.

Summoning the Family

As the signs of approaching death appear, it is important to make the family aware that the end is near. The physician is informed first, however.

If the death has already occurred, the physician is responsible for contacting the family and releasing that information. Sometimes the news is delayed until the family can be approached in person so as to avoid precipitating desperate acts like suicide, or contributing to a traffic accident.

NURSING GUIDELINES FOR SUMMONING THE FAMILY OF A DYING PATIENT

- Plan to notify the family in a timely manner.
  Rationale: Facilitates being with the dying patient at the time of death
- Check the patient's medical record for the name of the patient's next of kin or a responsible party.
  Rationale: Ensures notifying a person significantly involved in the patient's well-being
- Identify yourself by name, title, and location.
  Rationale: Provides more personal communication
- Ask for the family member by name.
  Rationale: Ensures clear communication of the information to the appropriate person
- Speak in a calm and controlled voice.
  Rationale: Communicates a serious, yet competent demeanor
- Use short sentences to provide small bits of information.
  Rationale: Facilitates processing and comprehending the news
- Explain that the patient's condition is deteriorating.
  Rationale: Clarifies the purpose for the call
- Pause after giving the most essential information.
  Rationale: Allows the family member to respond
- Give brief answers to questions, but emphasize the kind and level of care that is being given.
  Rationale: Reinforces that the patient is receiving appropriate care
- Urge the family members to come as soon as possible.

Rationale: Ensures that the most important people to the patient are there at the time of death
- Document the time, the individual to whom the information was communicated, and a description of the message.
  Rationale: Provides a permanent record of the communication that transpired

Meeting Relatives

Relatives of the dying patient are met by the nurse who informed them, if at all possible. When everyone has the benefit of first-hand communication, it promotes a smooth transition. If that is not possible, some other support person is designated to be available.

On arrival, the family may appreciate being shown to a room or area that provides privacy, or they may want to go directly to the patient's bedside. Either choice is facilitated.

Privacy allows people the freedom to express their feelings without any social inhibitions. It is not unusual for family members to weep and sob uncontrollably. However, if that does not happen, it is wrong to assume that their grief is less than genuine.

Discussing Organ Donation

Some patients have had the foresight to communicate whether they are interested in organ donation; others have not. In either case, if the dying or dead patient meets donation criteria (Table 38-3), the possibility of

TABLE 38-2. *Signs of Multiple Organ Failure*	
Organ	Signs
Heart	• Hypotension • Irregular, weak, rapid pulse • Cold, clammy, mottled skin
Liver	• Internal bleeding • Edema • Jaundice • Impaired digestion, distention, anorexia, nausea, vomiting
Lungs	• Dyspnea • Accumulation of fluid (eg, death rattle)
Kidneys	• Oliguria • Anuria • Pruritus (itching skin)
Brain	• Fever • Confusion and disorientation • Hypoesthesia (reduced sensation) • Hyporeflexia (reduced reflexes) • Stupor • Coma

TABLE 38-3. *Age Criteria for Organ Donation*	
Organ	Age Range
Kidney	6 months–55 years
Liver	<50 years
Heart	<40 years
Pancreas	2–50 years
Corneas	Acceptable at any age
Skin	15–74 years

Guidelines established by the Organ Procurement Agency of Michigan, Ann Arbor, MI.

harvesting organs after death is discussed with the next of kin. This must be delicately done because family members are under extreme duress when dealing with the death of a loved one.

Unfortunately, the matter cannot be delayed indefinitely because some organs must be harvested within a certain amount of time to ensure a successful transplant (Table 38-4). To protect the health care facility from any legal consequences, permission is always obtained in writing (Fig. 38-6).

CONFIRMING DEATH

Basically, death is determined on the basis that breathing and circulation have ceased. In most cases, when these criteria are met, there is no question that the patient is dead. Legally, a physician is responsible for pronouncing the patient dead, but there are a few states in which nurses are authorized to do so (Harris, 1992).

Brain Death

Sometimes there are situations involving irreversible brain damage in which breathing can be sustained with a mechanical ventilator and circulation continues reflexively. In essence, the person is "brain dead," and continued life support may only sustain a **persistent vegetative state**, a condition in which there is no cognitive function or capacity to experience emotions.

Consequently, brain function is now considered the most incontestable criterion for establishing whether a person is dead or alive. To ensure that brain activity is consistently and accurately assessed, the Harvard Ad Hoc Committee (1968) established some standards that are used as guidelines (Display 38-2).

Once death has been confirmed, the physician issues a death certificate and obtains written permission for an autopsy, if one is desirable.

Issuing a Death Certificate

A **death certificate** is a legal document attesting to the fact that the person named on the form has been examined and found to be dead. The certificate also indicates the presumptive cause of the person's death.

Death certificates are sent to local health departments, which use the information to compile mortality statistics. The statistics are important in identifying trends, needs, and problems in the fields of health and medicine.

The **mortician**, a person who prepares the body for burial or cremation, is responsible for filing the death certificate with the proper authorities. The death certificate also caries the mortician's signature and, in some states, his or her license number.

Obtaining Permission for an Autopsy

An **autopsy**, sometimes called a *postmortem examination*, is an examination of the organs and tissues of a human body after death. An autopsy is not necessary after all deaths, but it is useful for determining more conclusively the exact cause of death. The findings may

TABLE 38-4. *Times From Organ Removal to Transplantation*	
Type of Transplant	Transplant Time
Organs	
Heart and lung	Within 2 hours
Heart	Within 3–4 hours
Liver	Within 8–12 hours
Pancreas	Within 24 hours
Kidneys	Within 72 hours
Tissues	
Bones, dura mater, arteries, veins, heart valves, cartilage, ligaments, skin, and corneas	Within 6–36 hours after circulation has ceased; if freeze dried or fresh frozen, can be transplanted up to 5 years after removal.

From Howard S. How do I ask? Requesting tissue and organ donations from bereaved families. Nursing January 1989;19:70–73.

Organ Procurement Agency of Michigan

Subsidiary Of
TRANSPLANTATION SOCIETY OF MICHIGAN
2203 Platt Road, Ann Arbor, Michigan 48104
(313) 973-1577

1-800-482-4881

Detroit—464-7988

ANATOMICAL GIFT DONATION STATEMENT

I understand that in the present state of medical practice, several organs and tissues are being removed from persons who have died unexpectedly, and are being used for transplantation to living persons or for medical or scientific research. I understand that organs are removed after my relative has died, and before the organs suffer any damage, (usually within eight [8] hours) and that this gift authorizes all examinations of the body which are necessary to assure the medical acceptability of the gift.

I appreciate the benefits that come from organ donation and also understand the criteria used in determining death in the case of decedent. I am the surviving:

(1) _____ Spouse
(2) _____ Adult son or daughter
(3) _____ Mother or Father
(4) _____ Adult brother or sister
(5) _____ Guardian of the patient at the time of death
(6) _____ Other person authorized or obligated to
            dispose of the body

_____
Relationship

Relatives or persons in a class before my class are not available to sign this form (or have already signed such a form). I have no knowledge that during his or her lifetime the decedent, _____, was opposed to or said things against making an anatomical gift or organ donation such as the one described below. I do not know of any relative or person in a class before mine who is opposed to this gift, nor do I know of any person in the same class as myself who is opposed to this gift.

I hereby make the following anatomical gift from the body of _____:

( ) Any needed organs or parts, or
( ) Only the following organs or parts:

_____
(Please specify the organ(s) or part(s))

The specified organ(s) and/or part(s) may be used for any of the purposes allowed by law, i.e. transplantation, therapy, medical research and education.

WITNESSES:

_____   _____
                                         Name

_____   _____
                                        Relation

                                _____
                                         Date

FIGURE 38-6
Organ procurement form.

affect the medical care of blood relatives who may be at risk for a similar disorder, or contribute to medical science. It is usually the physician's responsibility to obtain permission for an autopsy.

A **coroner**, someone legally designated to investigate deaths that may not be the result of natural causes, has the right to order that an autopsy be performed. The coroner, who may or may not be a physician, does not need permission from the next of kin to do so. In general, a coroner orders an autopsy if the death involved a crime, was of a suspicious nature, or occurred without any prior medical consultation.

In the absence of hypothermia or central nervous system depressants, there is:

- Unreceptiveness and unresponsiveness to even intense painful stimuli
- No movement or spontaneous respiration for 3 minutes off of a mechanical ventilator
- Complete absence of central and deep tendon reflexes
- Flat electroencephalogram for at least 10 minutes
- No change in response with repeated assessment 24 hours later

PERFORMING POSTMORTEM CARE

Postmortem care refers to the care of the body after death. It involves cleaning and preparing the body in a manner that will enhance its appearance during viewing at the funeral home, ensuring proper identification, and releasing the body to mortuary personnel (Skill 38-1).

GRIEVING

Grieving is the process of feeling acute sorrow over a loss. Although it is a painful experience, it facilitates resolving the loss. For some, grieving begins before the loss occurs, in which case it is referred to as **anticipatory grieving**. It has been observed that the longer peo-

SKILL 38-1
Performing Postmortem Care

Suggested Action	Reason for Action
Assessment	
Determine that the patient is dead by assessing breathing and circulation.	Confirms that the patient is lifeless in all but those cases in which life support equipment is used
Determine if the physician and family have been notified.	Establishes the chain of communication
Notify the nursing supervisor and switchboard of the patient's death.	Makes others aware of a change in the status of the patient
Check the medical record for the name of the mortuary where the body will be taken.	Facilitates collaboration
Planning	
Contact the mortuary and inform them that the family has chosen them to manage the burial.	Communicates a need for services
Ask when mortuary personnel may be expected to arrive.	Facilitates efficient time management
Contact any individuals involved in organ procurement.	Promotes timely harvesting of organs
Obtain a postmortem kit or supplies for cleaning, wrapping, and identifying the body.	Promotes organization
Implementation	
Pull the curtains about the bed.	Ensures privacy
Don gloves.	Provides a barrier from contact with blood and body substances
Place the body supine with the arms extended at the side or folded over the abdomen.	Prevents skin discoloration in areas that will be visible in a casket

(continued)

SKILL 38-1
Performing Postmortem Care (Continued)

Suggested Action	Reason for Action
Remove all medical equipment* such as an intravenous catheter, urinary catheter, dressings, and so on.	Eliminates unnecessary equipment
Remove hairpins or clips.	Prevents accidental trauma about the face
Close the eyelids.	Ensures that they will close at the time the body is prepared
Replace or keep dentures within the mouth.	Maintains the natural contour of the face
Place a small rolled towel beneath the chin to close the mouth.	Promotes a natural appearance
Cleanse secretions and drainage from the skin.	Ensures delivery of a hygienic body
Apply one or more disposable pads between the legs and under the buttocks.	Absorbs stool or urine should they escape
Attach an identification tag to the ankle or wrist; pad the wrist first if it is used.	Facilitates accurate identification of the body; prevents damage to tissue that will be visible, if and when the body is publicly viewed
Wrap the body in a paper **shroud**, a covering for the body, and cover the body with a sheet.	Demonstrates respect for the dignity of the deceased person
Tidy the bedside area and dispose of soiled equipment.	Follows principles of medical asepsis
Remove your gloves and wash your hands.	Removes colonizing microorganisms
Leave the room and close the door, or transport the body to the **morgue**, an area where dead bodies are temporarily held or examined.	Provides a temporary location for the body until mortuary personnel arrive

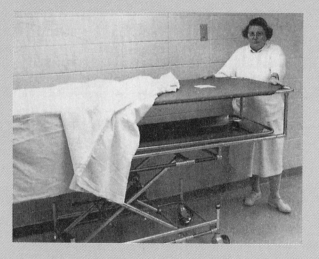

A morgue cart.

Make an inventory of valuables and send them to an administrative office where they are placed within a safe.	Ensures safekeeping and accountability for valuables until they can be claimed by a family member
Notify housekeeping after the body is removed from the room.	Facilitates cleaning and preparation for another admission

(continued)

SKILL 38-1
Performing Postmortem Care (Continued)

Suggested Action	Reason for Action

Evaluation
- The body is cleaned and prepared appropriately
- The body is transferred to mortuary personnel

Document
- Assessments that indicate the patient is dead
- Time of death
- People notified of death
- Care of the body
- Time body is transported to the morgue or transferred to mortuary personnel

Sample Documentation

Date and Time — No breathing noted and no pulse @ 1400. Dr. Williams notified @ 1415. Dr. Williams to call patient's wife. Foster's Funeral Home notified. Mortuary personnel unavailable until 1800. Postmortem care provided. Body transported to morgue after wife and children arrived. _____ **Signature, Title**

* Except in coroner's cases.

---

ple have to anticipate a loss, the faster they eventually come to resolve it.

Grief work, on the other hand, refers to the activities that are involved in grieving. It often includes participating in the burial rituals common within the culture. Although the rituals may be different, the grief response is universal.

Grief Response

A **grief response** involves both psychological and physical phenomena that are experienced by those who are grieving.

PSYCHOLOGICAL REACTIONS

Psychological reactions are those behaviors that commonly accompany grieving (Table 38-5). There are also sufficient anecdotal reports of what some may call **paranormal experiences** (ie, experiences outside scientific explanation). For example, some claim to see, hear, or feel the continued presence of the deceased. Currently there is no way to document the nature of these experiences. Some propose that they are nothing more than wishful thinking.

Physical symptoms also occur, but they are felt more acutely immediately after the death of a loved one.

PHYSICAL REACTIONS

Grieving people report experiencing physical symptoms like anorexia, tightness in the chest and throat, difficulty breathing, lack of strength, and sleep disturbances. Strangely, there is no identifiable pathologic state other than grief that can explain their etiology.

PATHOLOGIC GRIEF

Pathologic grief, also called *dysfunctional grief*, is a term that describes a condition in which a person is not able to accept someone's death. Sometimes pathologic grief is manifested by bizarre or morbid behavior. For

TABLE 38-5. *Stages of Grief*

Stage	Description
Shock and disbelief	Refusal to accept the fact that a loved one is about to die or has died
Developing awareness	Physical and emotional responses, like feeling sick, sad, empty, or angry
Restitution	Period during which the loss is recognized
Idealization	Exaggeration of the good qualities of the deceased

example, some may retain all of the deceased's possessions exactly as they were at the time of death. Others may attempt to make contact with the deceased through various forms of spiritualism, like attending seances. In rare instances, some may keep a dead body within their home for an extended period after death.

Resolution of Grief

Mourning is not finished immediately after a funeral. It may take longer for some than for others. However, one sign that grief is becoming resolved is when a person is able to talk about the dead person without becoming emotionally overwhelmed. Another sign is that the grieving person describes the good and bad qualities of the deceased.

NURSING IMPLICATIONS

Nurses who care for dying patients, their family, and friends may identify many different nursing diagnoses, some of which are listed in the accompanying Applicable Nursing Diagnoses.

The Nursing Care Plan for this chapter applies the nursing process to the care of a patient with a diagnosis of Hopelessness. In its 1994 taxonomy, NANDA defines this diagnostic category as "A subjective state in which an individual sees limited or no alternatives or personal choices available and is unable to mobilize energy on (his) own behalf." Lynda Carpenito (1995) further explains that "Hopelessness differs from powerlessness in that a hopeless person sees no solution to his problem and/or way to achieve what is desired, even if he has control of his life. A powerless person, on the

other hand, may see an alternative or answer to the problem, yet be unable to do anything about it because of lack of control and resources."

FOCUS ON OLDER ADULTS

- It has been shown that within 6 months of having experienced the death of a spouse, some survivors also develop life-threatening illnesses and die.
- It is unrealistic to expect that older adults will have a peaceful and accepting attitude toward death. Just as no two lives are the same, death also is an individualized experience.
- Older adults, including those who are dying, are included in as many aspects of their care as possible, which maintains their self-esteem and personal dignity.
- Older patients, and others as well, may feel their dignity is diminished with the use of machines and equipment designed to maintain life support.
- Many older adults are preparing advance directives concerning their health care and identifying a durable power of attorney at the same time that they prepare a will.
- Heart disease, cancer, and stroke are the leading causes of death in the United States. Together they account for 7 of every 10 deaths among older adults (United States Senate Special Subcommittee on Aging et al., 1991).
- Suicide is a more frequent cause of death among older adults than among any other age group (United States Senate Special Subcommittee on Aging et al., 1991).

APPLICABLE NURSING DIAGNOSES

- Pain
- Fear
- Spiritual Distress
- Social Isolation
- Altered Role Performance
- Altered Family Processes
- Ineffective Individual Coping
- Ineffective Family Coping
- Decisional Conflict
- Hopelessness
- Powerlessness
- Dysfunctional Grieving
- Anticipatory Grieving
- Caregiver Role Strain

KEY CONCEPTS

- A terminal illness is one from which recovery is beyond reasonable expectation.
- The five stages of dying as described by Dr. Elisabeth Kübler-Ross include denial, anger, bargaining, depression, and acceptance.
- Acceptance can be promoted by providing emotional support to dying patients and helping them to arrange their care.
- Respite care is care, or relief, for the caregiver.
- Hospice care involves helping patients live out their final days in comfort and with dignity and meaningfulness in a caring environment.

NURSING CARE PLAN:
Hopelessness

Assessment

Subjective Data
States, "It doesn't matter what's done or not done anymore. One of these days you won't be able to stop the infections."

Objective Data
26-year-old man about to be discharged from acute care hospital after successful treatment of *Pneumocystis* pneumonia secondary to HIV infection. During interview patient made little eye contact; stared out window. Will be followed up with home health care. Significant other expressed, "I'm afraid he'll just stop eating and taking his medications."

Diagnosis

Hopelessness related to eventual terminal outcome of illness.

Plan

Goal
The patient will identify one future-related goal and participate in one goal-directed activity by time of discharge.

Orders: 1/14
1. Reinforce at appropriate times that although his illness is terminal his current health status is stable.
2. After periodic physical examinations, verbalize normal as well as abnormal findings.
3. Present reality, during interactions, that each day provides an opportunity that can be used or ignored.
4. Explore with patient the goals he hoped to accomplish before his illness.
5. Ask patient to identify those goals that he could achieve in the next year.
6. Encourage patient to develop a daily schedule and set aside time for working toward at least one goal. _____ E. HILLYARD, RN

Implementation (Documentation) 1/15 0800 Head-to-toe assessment performed. Stated that lungs sound clear and heart rate is normal at 78 beats/min. Skin is intact. Discussed that there has been a ½ lb. weigh loss since yesterday. Indicated that date of discharge remains unchanged. Offered one can of Ensure as dietary supplement. Encouraged to perform oral hygiene and use Mycostatin mouthwash to prevent yeast infection._____ T. ROMIG, LPN

Evaluation (Documentation) 0830 Stated, "I think mouth care and anything else is futile. What a time for me to get sick. I'm a writer. . .or should I say, I was a writer. A publisher was interested in an idea I had; but it's past the deadline I was given." Encouraged to contact the publisher by phone before being discharged tomorrow.
_____ T. ROMIG, LPN

- Some of the aspects of care that are addressed when providing terminal care include hydration, nourishment, elimination, hygiene, positioning, and comfort.
- Many terminal illnesses result in death from multiple organ failure. Signs of multiple organ failure include, but are not limited to hypotension, rapid heart rate, difficulty breathing, cold and mottled skin, and a low urinary output.
- When a dying or recently deceased patient meets criteria for organ donation, permission for their removal must be obtained in a timely manner to ensure a successful transplant.
- Criteria that are used to confirm that a patient has died include cessation of breathing and heartbeat and absence of brain function.
- Postmortem care involves cleaning and preparing

the body, ensuring proper identification, and releasing the body to mortuary personnel.

- Although grieving is a painful experience, it facilitates resolution of the loss.
- One sign that a person's grief is becoming resolved is that the person can talk about the deceased person without becoming emotionally overwhelmed.

CRITICAL THINKING EXERCISES

- Discuss if being maintained with life support equipment supports or contradicts the right to die in peace and dignity (see the Dying Person's Bill of Rights).
- Select any right from the Dying Person's Bill of Rights and explain, hypothetically, how it might be violated. Propose how the same right can be protected.

SUGGESTED READINGS

A lethal injection: who's responsible? Nursing November 1992;22:79.

Benner KL. Terminal weaning: a loved one's vigil. American Journal of Nursing May 1993;93:22–25.

Carpenito LJ. Nursing Diagnosis: Application to Clinical Practice. 6th ed. Philadelphia: JB Lippincott, 1995.

Evans JV. Crisis, grief and loss. Canadian Nurse September 1993;89: 40–43.

Fry ST. Are new proposals to increase organ donations ethical? Nursing Outlook July–August 1991;39:192.

Grant A. Questions of life and death. Canadian Nurse May 1993; 89:31–34.

Harris MD. Death pronouncement by registered nurses. Home Healthcare Nurse March–April 1992;10:57–59.

Haddad AM, Kapp MB. Legal implications of withholding and withdrawing medical treatment. Caring September 1991;10:14–19.

Harvard Ad Hoc Committee. A definition of irreversible coma. Journal of the American Medical Association August 5 1968;205:337–340.

Kovach CR. Euthanasia: let nursing's voice be heard. Journal of Gerontological Nursing April 1992;18:5.

Kübler-Ross E. On Death and Dying. New York: Macmillan, 1969.

McCracken AL, Gerdsen L. Sharing the legacy: hospice care principles for terminally ill elders. Journal of Gerontological Nursing December 1991;17:4–8, 36–37.

Meyer C. "End of life" care: patients' choices, nurses' challenges. American Journal of Nursing February 1993;93:40–47.

Reilly E, Yucha CB. Multiple organ failure syndrome. Critical Care Nurse April 1994;14:25–31.

Simpson R. Nursing ethics and euthanasia . . . the "right to die." Canadian Nurse December 1992;88:36–38.

Speck P. Care after death . . . cleansing and shrouding the body. Nursing Times February 5–11 1992;88:20.

Stephany TM. Place of death: home or hospital. Home Healthcare Nurse May–June 1992;10:62.

Taeuber CM. Sixty-five plus in America. Washington, DC: U.S. Department of Commerce, 1992.

United States Senate Special Subcommittee on Aging, American Association of Retired Persons, Federal Council on the Aging, U.S. Administration on Aging. Aging America, Trends and Projections. DHHS Publication #91-28001. Washington, DC: U.S. Department of Health and Human Services, 1991.

Glossary

abduction   moving away from midline
active exercise   exercise performed independently
acute   sudden onset; severe, but short-term symptoms
adduction   moving toward midline
advance directive   written statement identifying a competent person's wishes concerning terminal care
aerobic   requiring oxygen
aerosol   small liquid droplets
afebrile   absence of fever
anabolism   process of building tissue
anaerobic   surviving in the absence of oxygen
analgesic   drug that relieves pain
anorexia   loss of appetite
antiseptic   an agent that inhibits, but does not kill, microorganisms
anxiety   vague, uneasy feeling
apnea   absence of breathing
arrhythmia   irregular heart contraction; also dysrhythmia
artery   blood vessel that carries oxygenated blood
asepsis   without infection; practices that reduce the potential for infection
aspiration   inhaling fluid into the respiratory tract
assessment   collection of data
auscultation   to examine by listening
bactericidal   ability to kill bacteria
bilateral   on both sides
bradycardia   heart rate below 60 bpm in adults
bradypnea   respiratory rate below 12 per minute in adults
cachexia   wasting away of body tissue
cannula   channel or tube
capillary   blood vessel that connects arteries to veins
catabolism   process of breaking down tissue
catheterization   inserting a tube
cerumen   ear wax
chart   medical record
chronic   slow onset; symptoms last a relatively long time
circadian   cycling at 24-hour, or daily, intervals
circumduction   turning in a circular fashion
colloid   undissolved substance that does not diffuse through a semipermeable membrane

colonization   presence of microorganisms
communication   the exchange of information
congenital   present at birth
constipation   stasis of stool
contracture   shortening of muscle, restricting joint motion
contrast medium   substance used to improve visualization of body structures
culture   technique for growing and identifying microorganisms
cutaneous   pertaining to the skin
cyanosis   blue discoloration of the skin or mucous membranes
decompression   relieving pressure
deciliter   one hundred milliliters; one hundredth of a liter
defecation   bowel elimination
dehiscence   wound separation
dehydration   result of inadequate fluid volume
dermis   skin
diaphoresis   excessive perspiration
diastole   period when the heart is filling with blood
diastolic pressure   arterial pressure at the time of diastole
disinfectant   an agent that kills microorganisms, but not spores
distal   furthest away
diurnal   on a daily basis
dorsal recumbent position   reclining with knees bent, hips rotated outward, and the feet flat on the bed or examination table
dorsiflexion   position in which the toes point toward the head
drape   cover
dressing   wound cover
dysphagia   difficulty swallowing
dyspnea   labored breathing
dysrhythmia   irregular heart contraction
edema   excess or trapped fluid
electrolyte   dissolved substances that conduct an electrical charge; synonym: ion
emaciation   extreme thinness

embolus   circulating blood clot

emesis   contents from the stomach lost during vomiting; synonym: vomitus

endoscopy   to examine internal structures with the use of a lensed instrument

enteral   through the digestive tract

epidermis   outer layer of skin

eructation   belching

erythema   redness

exacerbation   reactivation of signs and symptoms

extension   straight position with 180° between two adjoining bones

external rotation   turning outward

extracellular   outside the cells

febrile   presence of a fever

feces   stool

fever   elevated body temperature

flatus   intestinal gas that is passed from the rectum

flexion   bending so as to decrease the angle between two adjoining bones

Fowler's position   a body position in which the upper body is elevated, as in a sitting position

gait   manner of walking

gastric reflux   upward movement of gastric secretions into the esophagus

gavage   feeding by means of a tube

granulation   tissue formed during wound healing

glucometer   instrument used to measure capillary blood sugar

health   state of complete physical, mental, and social well-being

hereditary   transmitted through genetic codes

Homans' sign   pain in the calf on dorsiflexion of the foot

hygiene   practices that involve cleaning

hyperextension   an angle of more than 180° between two adjoining bones

hypertension   high blood pressure

hyperthermia   elevated body temperature

hypervolemia   excessive fluid volume

hypnotic   producing sleep

hypopnea   slower than normal breathing rate

hypotension   low blood pressure

hypothermia   low body temperature

hypovolemia   low fluid volume

hypoxemia   insufficient oxygen in arterial blood

hypoxia   inadequate oxygen at the cellular level

idiopathic   unknown cause

illness   state of discomfort that results when a person's health becomes impaired

implementation   carrying out a plan

incident report   written account of an unusual event

incontinence   inability to control bowel or bladder elimination

inflammation   response to cellular injury

inspection   to examine by looking

integument   skin and mucous membranes

internal rotation   turning inward toward the midline

interstitial   between cells

intracellular   within cells

intravascular   within blood

intubation   insertion of a tube into a body structure

isometric exercise   stationary exercise performed against a resistive force

isotonic exercise   exercise that involves movement and work

knee–chest position   one in which the patient lays on his or her abdomen and rests on flexed knees

lavage   wash out by means of a tube

lithotomy position   similar to the dorsal recumbent position, except that the feet are elevated and supported

lumen   channel or pathway

malaise   lack of energy

meatus   opening

medical asepsis   clean technique

microorganisms   living plants or animals that can be seen only with a microscope

milligram   one thousandth of a gram

morbidity   incidence of a disease, disorder, or injury

mortality   deaths associated with a condition

mucus   secretion from mucous membranes

nausea   a sensation that often precedes vomiting

nonpathogens   usually harmless microorganisms

nonverbal communication   the exchange of information without using words

nosocomial   acquired after admission to a health care agency

nursing diagnosis   a health problem that can be prevented, reduced, or resolved through independent nursing measures

nursing process   method for identifying and resolving health problems

obesity   state in which there are excessive fat cells

objective data   information that is observable and measurable

orthopnea   breathing that is facilitated by sitting or standing

palpation   to examine by feeling

palpitation   awareness of heartbeat

parenteral   other than the oral route

passive exercise   exercise performed with assistance

patent   unobstructed

pathogens   microorganisms that cause disease

percussion   to examine by tapping

phagocytosis   to engulf or eat

plantar flexion   position in which the toes point downward

postural hypotension   fall in blood pressure when rising quickly

primary   occurring first

prosthesis   artificial body part

proximal   nearest to a point of reference

pruritus   itching

pulse deficit   difference between the apical and radial pulse rate

pulse pressure   difference between systolic and diastolic blood pressure

pulse rhythm   pattern of arterial pulsations and pauses

pulse volume   quality of arterial pulsations

purulent   containing pus

radiograph   x-ray

range-of-motion exercise   exercise in which the joints are moved through all potential positions

regurgitation bringing stomach contents to the mouth

reflux backward movement

remission disappearance of signs and symptoms

resident microorganisms microorganisms that inhabit the skin and are more difficult to remove

secondary occurs as a consequence of something else

sedative drug that produces a calming effect

sepsis infection

signs objective data

Sims' position left lateral side-lying position with the chest leaning slightly forward

sphygmomanometer instrument for measuring blood pressure

Standard Precautions measures used to prevent the transmission of microorganisms regardless of the infectious status of patients

stasis stagnation

sterile free of microorganisms, including spores

stethoscope instrument for assessing sounds

stoma opening

subcutaneous beneath the skin

subjective data that which the patient feels and describes

sump tube one that is vented

surgical asepsis sterile technique

symptoms subjective data

systole period of heart contraction

systolic pressure arterial pressure during heart contraction

tachycardia rapid heart rate, between 100 to 150 bpm in adults

tachypnea rapid respirations; over 20 per minute in adults

tamponade compression

terminal no potential for cure

therapeutic communication using words and gestures to accomplish a particular objective

thermometer instrument for measuring temperature

thrombus stationary blood clot

tinnitus ringing in the ears

tolerance reduced drug effect from a previously effective dose

traction pull

transient microorganisms microorganisms that are easily removed from the skin

transcutaneous through the skin

Transmission-Based Precautions measures used to prevent transmission of pathogens from patients whose infectious status is known or suspected

trauma injury

turgor resiliency of the skin

unilateral one side

urination the act of passing urine; also known as voiding and micturition

vasoconstriction narrowing of blood vessels

vasodilation widening of blood vessels

vein blood vessel that carries deoxygenated blood

venipuncture pierce a vein

ventilation breathing

verbal communication communication that uses words

viscous thick

vital signs measurements of temperature, pulse, respiratory rate, and blood pressure

void urinate

vomiting forceful loss of stomach contents through the mouth

wound damaged skin or soft tissue

xerostomia dry mouth

APPENDIX A

Common Abbreviations

Symbols

⊂	less than
⊆	equal to or less than
⊃	more than
⊇	equal to or more than
±	plus or minus
°	degree

Words

ADL	activities of daily living
AHCPR	Agency for Health Care Policy and Research
AIDS	acquired immune deficiency syndrome
ANA	American Nurses' Association
AMA	against medical advice; or American Medical Association
BP	blood pressure
bpm	beats per minute
cal	calorie
CBC	complete blood count
CDC	Centers for Disease Control and Prevention
CHO	carbohydrate
CO_2	carbon dioxide
CPR	cardiopulmonary resuscitation
CT	computed tomography (also CAT)
CVC	central venous catheter
dl	deciliter (100 mL)
ECG	electrocardiogram (also EKG)
EEG	electroencephalogram
EMG	electromyography
EOMS	extraocular movements
g	gram
GI	gastrointestinal
HIV	human immunodeficiency virus
JCAHO	Joint Commission on Accreditation of Health-care Organizations

I & O	intake and output
ICN	International Council of Nurses
IM	intramuscular
IV	intravenous
IVP	IV push
IVPB	IV piggyback
kcal	kilocalorie
kg	kilogram (1000 g)
L	liter
LPN	licensed practical nurse (also LVN, licensed vocational nurse)
MAR	medication administration record
mEq	milliequivalent
mg	milligram (one thousandth g)
mL	milliliter (one thousandth L)
mm Hg	millimeters of mercury
mph	miles per hour
MRI	magnetic resonance imaging
NANDA	North American Nursing Diagnosis Association
NAPNES	National Association for Practical Nurse Education and Service
NCLEX-PN	National Council Licensure Examination for Practical Nurses
NCLEX-RN	National Council Licensure Examination for Registered Nurses
NEX	nose, earlobe, xiphoid process
NKA	no known allergies
NLN	National League for Nursing
NPO	*nil per os*, nothing by mouth
NREM	nonrapid eye movement (sleep phase)
NSS	normal saline solution
NWB	nonweight bearing
O_2	oxygen
OTC	over the counter (eg, nonprescription)
QA	quality assurance
PACU	postanesthesia care unit

Timby BK: *Fundamental Skills and Concepts in Patient Care, Sixth Edition* © 1996 Lippincott-Raven Publishers

PaCO$_2$	partial pressure of carbon dioxide; that which is dissolved in plasma	RBC	red blood cell
PaO$_2$	partial pressure of oxygen; that which is dissolved in plasma	REM	rapid eye movement (sleep phase)
		RN	registered nurse
PCA	patient-controlled analgesia	R/O	rule out; either confirm or eliminate
PEG	percutaneous endoscopic gastrostomy	ROM	range of motion
PEJ	percutaneous endoscopic jejunostomy	SAD	seasonal affective disorder
PERRLA	pupils equally round and respond to light and accommodation	SaO$_2$	oxygen saturation; percent of hemoglobin molecules saturated with oxygen
PET	positron emission tomography	SNF	skilled nursing facility
pH	degree of acidity or alkalinity	SSE	soap suds enema
PICC	peripherally inserted central catheter	TPN	total parenteral nutrition
PPN	peripheral parenteral nutrition	TPR	temperature, pulse, and respirations
PWB	partial weight bearing	WBC	white blood cell
		WHO	World Health Organization

North American Nursing Diagnosis Association (NANDA) Accepted Nursing Diagnoses

✓Activity Intolerance
Activity Intolerance, Risk for†
Adjustment, Impaired
Airway Clearance, Ineffective
Anxiety
Aspiration, Risk for†
Body Image Disturbance
Body Temperature, Risk for Altered†
Breastfeeding, Effective
Breastfeeding, Ineffective
Breastfeeding, Interrupted
Breathing Pattern, Ineffective
Cardiac Output, Decreased
Caregiver Role Strain
Caregiver Role Strain, Risk for†
Communication, Impaired Verbal
Confusion, Acute*
Confusion, Chronic*
Constipation
Constipation, Colonic
Constipation, Perceived
Coping, Defensive
Coping, Ineffective Community*
Coping, Ineffective Individual
Decisional Conflict (Specify)
Decreased Adaptive Capacity: Intracranial*
Denial, Ineffective
Diarrhea
Disuse Syndrome, Risk for†
Diversional Activity Deficit
Dysreflexia
Energy Field Disturbance*
Enhanced Community Coping, Potential for*
Environmental Interpretation Syndrome, Impaired*
Family Coping: Compromised, Ineffective
Family Coping: Disabling, Ineffective

Family Coping: Potential for Growth
Family Processes, Altered
Family Processes, Altered: Alcoholism*
Fatigue
Fear
Fluid Volume Deficit
Fluid Volume Deficit, Risk for†
Fluid Volume Excess
Gas Exchange, Impaired
Grieving, Anticipatory
Grieving, Dysfunctional
Growth and Development, Altered
Health Maintenance, Altered
Health-Seeking Behaviors (Specify)
Home Maintenance Management, Impaired
Hopelessness
Hyperthermia
Hypothermia
Incontinence, Bowel
Incontinence, Functional
Incontinence, Reflex
Incontinence, Stress
Incontinence, Total
Incontinence, Urge
Infant Behavior, Disorganized*
Infant Behavior, Risk for Disorganized*
Infant Behavior, Potential for Enhanced Organized*
Infant Feeding Pattern, Ineffective
Infection, Risk for†
Infection Transmission, Risk for†
Injury, Risk for†
Injury, Risk for Perioperative Positioning*
Knowledge Deficit (Specify)
Loneliness, Risk for*
Memory, Impaired*
Noncompliance (Specify)

Timby BK: *Fundamental Skills and Concepts in Patient Care, Sixth Edition* © 1996 Lippincott-Raven Publishers

Nutrition, Altered: Less Than Body Requirements
Nutrition, Altered: More than Body Requirements
Nutrition, Altered: Potential for More Than Body Requirements
Oral Mucous Membrane, Altered
Pain, Acute
Pain, Chronic
Parent–Infant Attachment, Risk for Altered*
Parental Role Conflict
Parenting, Altered
Parenting, Risk for Altered†
Peripheral Neurovascular Dysfunction, Risk for†
Personal Identity Disturbance
Physical Mobility, Impaired
Poisoning, Risk for†
Post-Trauma Response
Powerlessness
Protection, Altered
Rape Trauma Syndrome
Rape Trauma Syndrome: Compound Reaction
Rape Trauma Syndrome: Silent Reaction
Relocation Stress Syndrome
Role Performance, Altered
Self-Care Deficit
    Bathing/Hygiene
    Feeding
    Dressing/Grooming
    Toileting
Self-Esteem, Chronic Low
Self-Esteem, Situational Low
Self-Esteem Disturbance

Self-Mutilation, Risk for†
Sensory/Perceptual Alterations (Specify) (visual, auditory, kinesthetic, gustatory, tactile, olfactory)
Sexual Dysfunction
Sexuality Patterns, Altered
Skin Integrity, Risk for Impaired†
Skin Integrity, Impaired
Sleep Pattern Disturbance
Social Interactions, Impaired
Social Isolation
Spiritual Distress
Spiritual Well-Being, Potential for Enhanced*
Suffocation, Risk for†
Swallowing, Impaired
Therapeutic Regimen, Effective Management of: Individual*
Therapeutic Regimen, Ineffective Management of
Therapeutic Regimen, Ineffective Management of: Community*
Therapeutic Regimen, Ineffective Management of: Family*
Thermoregulation, Ineffective
Thought Processes, Altered
Tissue Integrity, Impaired
Tissue Perfusion, Altered (Specify Type) (renal, cerebral, cardiopulmonary, gastrointestinal, peripheral)
Trauma, Risk for†
Unilateral Neglect
Urinary Elimination, Altered
Urinary Retention
Ventilation, Inability to Sustain Spontaneous
Ventilatory Weaning Response, Dysfunctional
Violence, Risk for: Self-Directed or Directed at Others†

* New diagnoses added in 1994.
† These diagnoses have changed terminology from "High Risk for" to "Risk for."

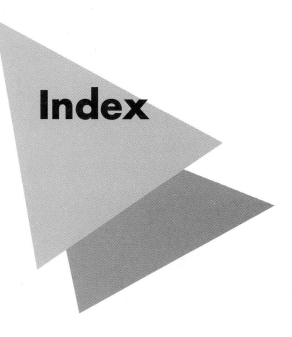

Index

Page numbers in *italics* indicate figures; those followed by *t* indicate tables; those followed by *d* indicate displays; and those followed by *s* indicate skills. Nursing diagnoses are capitalized.

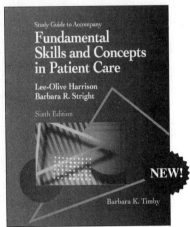
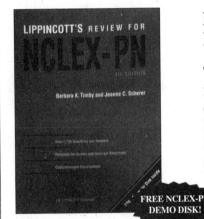
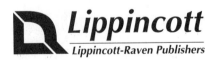